SALEM HEALTH

Adolescent
Health & Wellness

SALEM HEALTH
Adolescent Health & Wellness

First Edition

Volume 1
Advice from Teens – Grief and Loss

Editor

Paul Moglia, PhD
South Nassau Communities Hospital
Oceanside, NY

SALEM PRESS
A Division of EBSCO Information Services, Inc.
IPSWICH, MASSACHUSETTS

GREY HOUSE PUBLISHING

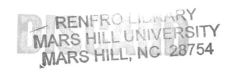
Publisher's Cataloging-In-Publication Data
(Prepared by The Donohue Group, Inc.)

Adolescent health & wellness / editor, Paul Moglia, PhD, South Nassau
 Communities Hospital, Oceanside, NY. -- First edition.

 3 volumes : illustrations ; cm. -- (Salem health)

 Includes bibliographical references and index.
 Contents: Volume 1. Advice from Teens-Grief and Loss -- volume 2. Health and Illness: Diseases and Conditions-Relationships: Friends, Family, and Dating -- volume 3. School and Jobs: Skills for Success-Your Emotional and Mental Health.
  ISBN: 978-1-61925-545-6 (3-volume set)
  ISBN: 978-1-61925-807-5 (vol. 1)
  ISBN: 978-1-61925-808-2 (vol. 2)
  ISBN: 978-1-61925-809-9 (vol. 3)

 1. Teenagers--Health and hygiene--Encyclopedias. 2. Health behavior in adolescence--Encyclopedias. 3. Teenagers--Mental health--Encyclopedias. 4. Teenagers--Drug use--Encyclopedias. 5. Teenagers—Sexual behavior--Encyclopedias. 6. Teenagers--Life skills guides--Encyclopedias. I. Moglia, Paul. II. Title: Adolescent health and wellness III. Series: Salem health (Pasadena, Calif.)

RA777 .A36 2015
613.0433

FIRST PRINTING
PRINTED IN THE UNITED STATES OF AMERICA

PUBLISHER'S NOTE

Adolescent Health & Wellness is a new title in the Salem Health series. It is designed to address three major areas that typically affect adolescents: physical and emotional issues; non-health topics with tremendous potential impact, like safe sex, paying for college, bullying, and leadership; and socially relevant issues, like shopping locally and recycling.

Other titles in the Salem Health series include *Psychology & Behavioral Health; Magill's Medical Guide; Addictions & Substance Abuse; Complementary & Alternative Medicine; Infectious Diseases & Conditions; Genetics;* and *Cancer,* a new edition of which is due out Spring 2016. *Adolescent Health & Wellness* broadens the scope of those who will benefit from the current and informative material that Salem Health is known for.

This new first edition comprises three volumes, 483 articles, and 19 major categories. In addition to material updated from other Salem Health titles, *Adolescent Health & Wellness* includes over 130 brand new articles, notably on current topics of vital interest to 13 to 21 year-olds, their parents, guardians, and caregivers. They include *Biracial Heritage, Tanorexia, ADHD Medications, Smokeless Tobacco, Cyberbullying, Asthma, Teenage Suicide, Insomnia, Personal Hygiene, Sexual Harassment, Body Image,* and *Changing Passwords.*

ORGANIZATION AND FORMAT
Articles in *Adolescent Health & Wellness* range from one to eight pages in length. Each begins with an italicized summary of the topic, and the text continues in clear, concise language, thoughtfully punctuated with helpful subheads. All articles include a list of Further Reading,

annotated for additional insight, and See Alsos to guide the reader to supplemental material throughout the work. *Adolescent Health & Wellness* also includes three appendixes and a general index.

RESOURCES AND INDEXES
A complete Table of Contents appears at the beginning of each volume. Appendixes and Index appear at the end of volume three.

APPENDIXES:
- Four Glossaries – Psychological Terms, Green Terms, Healthy Eating Terms, and Prescription Drug Terms
- Web Sites and Organizations – more than 150 annotated web site listings and organizations relevant to adolescents, young adults, and their young adult network
- Mediagraphy – more than 50 films and books with adolescent themes and characters, all with detailed descriptions
- Subject Index – alphabetically lists all the significant people, places and concepts covered in this set

ACKNOWLEDGMENTS
Salem Press gratefully acknowledges Editor Paul Moglia, Ph.D., whose introduction to the work follows this Publisher's Note. Salem Press also thanks the many contributors whose names and affiliations follow Dr. Moglia's introduction.

EDITOR'S INTRODUCTION

Adolescent Health & Wellness (AHW) is an overview of and guide through the exciting and exacerbating, confident and confusing, and triumphant and despairing years from puberty through young adulthood. This stage of development houses the greatest potential for growth as well as the greatest potential of risk throughout the lifecycle. Stationed between the ridges of autonomy, individual identity, and uniqueness, and the cliffs of family membership, societal role identification, and the panicky need of peer acceptance, adolescence is a biopsychosocial tug-of-war.

I want to stand out, be extraordinary, appreciated, and valued that I am my own person. My adulthood will bring me more things, and yet, I am afraid that those whose attentions I crave will not accept me. Will the hand I raise to be called upon be ignored? Will the hand I move to touch pull away? I need to be different, and I need to be the same, to be one standing alone, and one peer standing with many.

Marked by extremes and contrasts, adolescence is where the importance of being a part of a family is seemingly eclipsed by being apart from that same family. Energy, enthusiasms, and drives outpace introspection, listening, and prudence. Words that connate the convection currents of adolescent winds include strength, virility, stamina, heartache, individuation, higher order intellectual development, self-sacrifice, service to others, and even heroism. Wisdom, perspective, and insight are usually not among these. Their absence reflects the challenges adolescents face and, more so, the risks. Each year in the United States, 6,000 adolescents leave home and never return.

The challenges adolescents face are paralleled by the challenges of their adult caregivers: when to let life's lessons do the instruction; when to hold to zero tolerance; when to call for another lap. Adult parenting, teaching, and coaching fluid adolescents requires discretion and boldness, being friend and foe, letting go while holding on, and above all, the emotional intelligence to know when to make which call.

Adolescent Health & Wellness is both a review of most adolescent topics and a guide over those fogged waters. We have divided topics loosely into a range of categories. In **Schools and Jobs,** we discuss adolescent economics,

education, and finances. In **Critical Skills**, we present articles on writing, networking, interviewing, and public speaking, among others. You'll read about savings plans for college, career and self-identity, studying abroad, internships, managing time, and the balancing act student athletes perform. In **Staying Safe,** we warn about piercings and infection, advise how to cope with bullying, and address the potentially deadly issue of texting while driving. **Diversity** discusses religion and spirituality, stereotyping, LGBT youth and their parents' and peers' acceptance.

Change is the only constant and change brings loss. For youth, it is hard to reconcile that profound pain can be natural and that learning to grieve well is healthy, even healing. In spite of the objective health of this population, most adolescents will have to cope with some profound loss. In **Grief and Loss,** *AHW* offers advice to help friends cope, how to manage romantic loss, and how to grieve the death of a parent or guardian.

We live in a digital age. Unlike those born only half a generation earlier, virtually all adolescents use the Internet daily and automatically. The Internet, like adolescence, is full of promise, possibility, and unforeseen risk. In **Going Online**, we present articles on scams and spam, cyberbullying, and having a relationship online.

As part of Salem's Health series, this edition includes a significant number of health topics in two related sections, **Disabilities and Disorders** and **Health and Illness: Diseases and Conditions.** Here you will find articles on asthma, common infections like tonsillitis, developmental disorders like fetal alcohol and fragile X syndromes, congenital heart disease, and PKU. Other topics include the autoimmune disorder lupus, the common and contagious pink eye, and a condition almost universally faced at some point in adolescence—insomnia.

AHW is also a guide about wellness. In **Going Green** and **Nutrition and Staying Fit,** we discuss fracking, buying local, managing weight, staying fit, the freshman fifteen, playing sports, stretching, and sports drinks. Indeed, as sex is the singular demarcation between childhood and adulthood, we also present articles on sexuality, sexual health, and sexual practice in **Sexuality and Sexual Health**. Our writers review, in adolescent vernacular, sexually transmitted infections, birth control, having safe, pleasurable sex, and virginity.

Wellness suggests happiness and a life of emotional health; such are possible only as life challenges are faced, managed, and overcome. A number of articles address the issue of attachment, a primary developmental task in adolescence: connecting to maintain identity and history, yet disconnecting to form a maturing identity and future. You will read about immature behavior fulfilling the immature needs of the attention-seeker, ways to sustaining wellness, how to ask for psychological help, and how to approach those who provide it. We also include an academically grounded, yet lay-friendly review of the different theoretical approaches these professionals take. In **Drugs, Alcohol, and Addictions,** we speak to steroid abuse, tanorexia, and living below the threshold of bulimia, a condition far more widespread than most adults suspect. Also touched upon is the hub of adolescent identity and its social psychology, including the painful sting of being outside of a clique, being a victim in an abusive relationship, and understanding the psychodynamics of female friendships.

Perhaps, *AHW*'s most innovative section is **Advice from Teens,** including topics teens have identified as important to their phase of life. Written by adolescents, this section includes peer advisement on volunteering and giving back to community, finding that first job, joining the military and, indicative of pubic health trends, being gluten-free. And **Health Myths** explains why cell phones do not cause brain cancer.

In all, we offer nearly 500 topics in a something-for-everyone marketplace. No one work can be comprehensive on this topic. The concerns, needs, and interests of the 13-year-old are often forgotten by the 20-year-old preoccupied with different things. We present a menu of interests, however, that provides scientifically based, culturally aware, and pragmatically conceived overviews of a remarkably broad-range of topics, each with information on how to easily learn more. All of us involved in readying these three volumes have a shared intent: helping adolescents and helping those who help them. We hope we have met your need.

It has been my privilege to edit this new, first edition Salem Press Health title. I love this stage of the human life cycle with its over-developed sense of justice and its underdeveloped sense of balance. I connect with adolescent energy and enthusiasm and believe direction and intervention here pay handsome benefits in adult prevention and productivity. My role as editor involved adding to the philosophical discussions of what the nature of this work should be, to its organization, to editing all new material. My work was informed from my own adolescence, which saw the emergence of adulthood later in me than in many, to my years teaching high school, and my subsequent 30 years of clinical practice treating adolescents.

But even these layers of experience would not enable me to rise to the task of editing this work. For that, I whole-heartedly thank these wonderful people: Alexandra Sabrina Blanchard, recent honors graduate of Pace University in New York City for her sharp eye, due diligence, and timely completion of every task and request. Grey House's friendly and increasingly fearless editorial assistant, Melissa Rose. No one's time was more occupied, day-to-day, for these many months in seeing this work grow from competing embryonic ideas to the birth of triplet volumes. Only she knows how often she tugged at my shirtsleeve to point out something I had missed or forgotten. The matchless Laura Mars, Vice President, Editorial, at Grey House once again, encouraged my work and refined my judgment as only an expert in this industry can. She was the other oar in the boat that saved me from what happens when only one oar enters the water. Jean Busi Moglia, my wife for these many, where-did-the-time-go, years. She manages to balance, better than I ever could, supporting my work while worrying that I'm doing too much of it. Our three children: Jenna, Michael, and Briana Frances who are, how fortuitous for *AHW*, just crossing over the cusp of adulthood coming from adolescence. They provided invaluable perspective, advice, and insight. They actively contributed to the work from beginning to end. Without their support from heart and head, whatever value I've added to *AHW* would surely be less.

Paul Moglia, PhD
Glen Cove, New York

CONTRIBUTORS

Christopher M. Aanstoos
University of West Georgia

Maria Adams

Richard Adler
University of Michigan Dearborn

Rick Alan
Medical writer and editor

Debra A. Appello
Brick, NJ

Tammi Arford

Bryan C. Auday
Gordon College

Catherine Avelar
Cornell University of Veterinary Medicine

Buffie Longmire Avital
*National Development and Research Institutes, Inc.,
Public Health Solutions*

Mihaela Avramut
*Verlan Medical Communications, American Medical
Writers Association*

Pamela J. Baker
Bates College

Thomas E. Baker
Professor Emeritus, University of Scranton

Jane Piland-Baker
Former Instructor and Counselor, Marywood University

Anita Baker-Blocker
Ann Arbor, Michigan

Veronica N. Baptista
Stanford Medical Group

Christina Barrett
St. Joseph Hill Academy, Staten Island, New York

Erica Bass

Lawrence W. Bassett
*University of California, Los Angeles, School of
Medicine*

Robert J. Baumann
University of Kentucky

Stephen R. H. Beach
University of Georgia

Susan E. Beers
Sweet Briar College

Lauren Behrman
White Plains, New York

Tanja Bekhuis
TCB Research

Michael S. Bendele
Indiana University-Purdue University, Fort Wayne

Robert A. Bendele
Ivy Tech Fort Wayne

Raymond D. Benge, Jr.
Tarrant County College

Janet Ober Berman
Temple University School of Medicine

Matthew Berria

Jacquelyn Berry
State University of New York at New Paltz

Krishna Bhaskarabhatla
*Saint Joseph's Regional Medical Center, Mount Sinai
School of Medicine*

Jennifer Birkhauser
University of California, Irvine

Virginiae Blackmon
Fort Hays, Texas

Paul R. Boehlke
Wisconsin Lutheran College

Wanda Bradshaw
Duke University School of Nursing

Barbara Brennessel
Wheaton College

Courtney Brogle
St. Joseph Hill Academy, Staten Island, New York

Mitzie L. Bryant
St. Louis Board of Education

Faith Hickman Brynie
Bigfork, Montana

Fred Buchstein
John Carrol University

Amy Webb Bull
Tennessee State University School of Nursing

Michael A. Buratovich
Spring Arbor University

John T. Burns
Bethany College

Jamie Stockslager Buss

Rosslynn S. Byous
University of Southern California, Keck School of Medicine

Byron D. Cannon
University of Utah

Lauren M. Cagen
University of Tennessee, Memphis

Mary Calvagna

James J. Campanella
Montclair State University

H. Richard P. Capriccioso
University of Phoenix

Christine M. Carroll
American Medical Writers Association

Rosalyn Carson-DeWitt

Brittany Casey

Mariel Cataldi

Layla Cavitt

Anne Lynn S. Chang
Stanford University

Emmanuel L. Chandler
Cincinnati Children's Hospital Medical Center

Karen Chapman-Novakofski
University of Illinois

Paul J. Chara, Jr.
Northwestern College

Archana Chatterjee
University of South Dakota, Sanford School of Medicine

Richard W. Cheney, Jr.
Christopher Newport University

Philip Cheng
Sleep Disorders Center, Henry Ford Health System

Kausalya Chennapragada
Saint Joseph's Regional Medical Center, Mount Sinai School of Medicine

Andrea Chisolm

Marcin Chwistek

Maryalice Citera
State University of New York at New Paltz

Rose Ciulla-Bohling
Lansdale, PA

Lisa M. Cockrell

Maria Conte

Sarah Crawford
Southern Connecticut State University

Julia D'Alessio
Saint Joseph Hill Academy, Staten Island, New York

Tish Davidson
Fremont, California

Elizabeth Davies
University of St. Francis

Rhianon Davies

Harrison Davis

LeAnna DeAngelo
Arizona State University

Everett J. Delahanty, Jr.
Manhattanville College

Patricia J. Deldin
University of Michigan

Shawkat Dhanani
Veterans Administration, Greater Los Angeles Healthcare System

M. Casey Diana
Arizona State University

Sandra Ripley Distelhorst
Vashon, Washington

Duane L. Dobbert
Florida Gulf Coast University
Kimberly Duris

Stephanie Eckenrode
New York, New York

Russell Eisenmann
McNeese State University

Dina Elnaggar
South Nassau Communities Hospital Family Medicine Residency Program, Oceanside, New York

Merill Evans
Tucson, Arizona

C. Richard Falcon
Roberts and Raymond Associates, Philadelphia, Pennsylvania

L. Fleming Fallon, Jr.
Bowling Green State University

Sharea Farmer
Rutgers University & Orleans Technical College

Reza Fazeli

K. Thomas Finley
State University of New York, Brockport

Robert M. Flatley
Kutztown University

Dale L. Flesher
University of Mississippi

Felicity Flesher
Carleton College

Barbara Flor
Mechanicsville, Pennsylvania

Tracy O. Franklin
University of Kansas

Katherine B. Frederich
Eastern Nazarene College

Paul J. Frisch
Nanuet, New York

Christi N. Gandham
Oceanside, New York

Bianca Garcia
South Nassau Communities Hospital

Lenela Glass-Godwin
Texas A&M University

Kimberly Glazier
Yeshiva University

Christian V. Glotfelty

James S. Godde
Monmouth College

Virginia L. Goetsch
West Virginia University

Jennifer R. Goldschmied
University of Michigan

Diane C. Gooding
University of Wisconsin-Madison

Rick Gorvett

Hans G. Graetzer
South Dakota State University

Meredith M. Griffin

Sara M. Grossi
Florida International University, Herbert Wertheim College of Medicine

Wendy C. Hamblet

Stephen Hampe
Walden University

Angela Harmon

Jasper L. Harris

Peter M. Hartmann
York Hospital, Pennsylvania

H. Bradford Hawley
Boonshoft School of Medicine, Wright State University

Daniel Heimowitz
National Psychological Association for Psychoanalysis

Carol A. Heintzelman
Millersville University of Pennsylvania

Jennifer Hellwig

Diane Andrews Henningfeld
Adrian College

Julie Henry

Stephen Henry
South Nassau Communities Hospital

Martha M. Henze
Boulder Community Hospital, Colorado

Margaret L. Herzog
Adelphi University

Jennifer M. Hickin

Jane F. Hill
Bethesda, Maryland

Carl W. Hoagstrom
Ohio Northern University

Robert A. Hock
Xavier University

David Wason Hollar, Jr.
Rockingham Community College

Christine G. Holzmueller
Glen Rock, Pennsylvania

David L. Horn

Howard L. Hosick
Washington State University

Mary Hurd
East Tennessee State University
Glenn Hutchinson

Loring J. Ingraham
George Washington University

Tracy Irons-Georges
Glendale, California

Vicki J. Isola
Hope College

Shelley A. Jackson
Texas A&M University, Corpus Christi

Louis B. Jacques
Wayne State University School of Medicine

Bruce E. Johansen
University of Nebraska at Omaha

Christen Johnson
Wright State University Boonshoft School of Medicine

Cheryl Pokalo Jones
Townsend, Delaware

Claire B. Joseph
*South Nassau Communities Hospital, Oceanside,
New York*

Karen E. Kalumuck
The Exploratorium, San Francisco

Clair Kaplan
Yale University School of Nursing

Susan J. Karcher
Purdue University

Armand M. Karow
Xytex Corporation

Oriaku A. Kas-Osoka
Cincinnati Children's Hospital Medical Center

John C. Keel

Patricia Griffin Kellicket

Ing-Wei Khor
Discovery Institute of Medical Education

Michael R. King
University of Rochester

Hillar Klandorf
West Virginia University

Robert T. Klose
University College of Bangor

Terry J. Knapp
University of Nevada, Las Vegas

Jeffrey A. Knight
Mount Holyoke College

Marylane Wade Koch
University of Memphis

Ernest Kohlmetz

Diana Kohnle

Padma Komerath

Felícitas Kort
New York, New York

Robin M. Kowalski
Clemson University

Steven A. Kuhl
V and R Consulting

Jeanne L. Kuhler
Auburn University, Montgomery

Stephania Lairet
*Florida International University, Herbert Wertheim
College of Medicine*

Amanda Backer Lappin
The University of Kansas

Kevin T. Larkin
West Virginia University

David M. Lawrence
J. Sargeant Reynolds Community College

Katharine Lawrence
Florida International University, Herbert Wertheim College of Medicine

Amanda Lefkowitz

Stefan Leonte
Chicago, Illinois

Leon Lewis
Appalachian State University

Scott O. Lilienfeld
Emory College

Stan Liu
University of California, Los Angeles, School of Medicine

Chad T. Lower

Elizabeth T. Lynn
South Nassau Communities Hospital, Oceanside, New York

Nancy E. Macdonald
University of South Carolina at Sumter

Paul D. Mageli
Kenmore, New York

Christina Maher
St. Joseph Hill Academy, Staten Island, New York

Daus Mahnke

Janet Mahoney
Monmouth University

Thomas E. Malloy

Mary E. Markland
Argosy University

Sergei A. Markov
Austin Peay State University

Theresa Mastronardi
South Nassau Communities Hospital, Oceanside, New York

Grace D. Matzen
Molloy College

Richard D. McAnulty
University of North Carolina at Charlotte

Krisha McCoy

David S. McDougal
Plymouth State College of the University System of New Hampshire

Christine Degnon McFarlin
Florida International University, Herbert Wertheim College of Medicine

Wayne R. McKinny
University of Hawaii School of Medicine

Richard L. McWhorter
Prairie View A&M University

Ralph R. Meyer
University of Cincinnati

Robert D. Meyer
Chestnut Hill College

Mira Mikhael
New York, New York

Elva B. Miller
Harrisonburg, Virginia

Roman J. Miller
Eastern Mennonite College

Randall L. Milstein
Oregon State University

Eli C. Minkoff
Bates College

Beatriz Manzor Mitrzyk

Eugenia F. Moglia
Glen Cove, New York

Paul Moglia
South Nassau Communities Hospital, Oceanside, New York

Robin Kamienny Montvilo
Rhode Island College

Rodney C. Mowbray
University of Wisconsin, LaCrosse

Martin Mrazik
University of Alberta

Virginia C. Muckle

Beverly Nancy

Kimberly A. Napoli

Donald J. Nash
Colorado State University

Alexander R. Nelson

Elizabeth Marie McGhee Nelson
Christian Brothers University

Elizabeth M. Nielson
John Jay College of Criminal Justice

Jane C. Norman
Tennessee State University

Annette O'Connor
La Salle University

Ayn Embar-Seddon O'Reilly
Capella University

Cherie Oertel
University of Kansas

David A. Olle
Eastshire Communications

Dawn Ortiz
Milan, New York

Randall E. Osborne
Phillips University

Oliver Oyama
Duke/Fayetteville Area Health Education Center

Maria Pacheco
Buffalo State College

Beverly B. Palmer
California State University, Dominguez Hills

Robert J. Paradowski
Rochester Institute of Technology

Allan D. Pass
National Behavioral Science Consultants

Elyssa Pearlstein
University of Michigan

Joseph G. Pelliccia
Bates College

E. E. Anderson Penno

Gabrielle Perk
St. Joseph Hill Academy, Staten Island, New York

Susan H. Peterman

Christina Hamme Peterson
Rider University

Elizabeth Peterson

Carol Moore Pfaffly
Fort Collins Family Medicine Center

Vicky Phares
University of South Florida

Nancy A. Piotrowski
Capella University and University of California, Berkeley

Luzanna Plancarte
*South Nassau Communities Hospital, Oceanside,
New York*

Darleen Powars
Los Angeles County-USC Medical Center

Marie President
Sequoia Medical Associates

Debra S. Preston
University of North Carolina at Pembroke

Victoria Price
Lamar University

Judith Primavera
Fairfield University

John Pritchard

Ganson Purcell, Jr.
Hartford, Connecticut

Lydia R. Qualls
Kennedy Center at Vanderbilt University

R. Christopher Qualls
Emory and Henry College

Lillian M. Range
Our Lady of Holy Cross College

Virginia Reece

Wendy E. S. Repovich
Eastern Washington University

Peter D. Reuman
University of Florida

Alex K. Rich

Alice C. Richer
Norwood, Massachusetts

Cheryl A. Rickabaugh
University of Redlands

Mary Beth Ridenhour

Benjamin Riley
Nyack College

Bernadette Riley
*South Nassau Communities Hospital, Oceanside,
New York*

Gina Riley
City University of New York, Hunter College

Dianne Scheinberg Rishikof

Connie Rizzo
Columbia University

Gina Robertiello
Felician College

James L. Robinson
University of Illinois, Urbana-Champaign

Eugene J. Rogers
Chicago Medical School

Carol A. Rolf
Rivier College

Laurie B. Rosenblum

John Alan Ross
Eastern Washington University

Kaitlin Ross
*West Kendall Baptist Hospital
Florida International University*

Jacquelyn Rudis

Claudia Datleader Ruland

Lauren Ruvo
Harvard Graduate School of Education

Diane Safer

Frank A. Salamone
Iona College

Tulsi B. Saral
University of Houston, Clear Lake

David K. Saunders
Emporia State University

Elizabeth D. Schafer
Loachapoka, Alabama

Rosemary Scheirer
Chestnut Hill College

Miriam E. Schwartz
UCLA Geffen School of Medicine

Rebecca Lovell Scott
College of Health Sciences

Sibani Sengupta
American Medical Writers Association

Felicisima C. Serafica
Ohio State University

Gregory B. Seymann
University of California, San Diego School of Medicine

Uzma Shahzad
*South Nassau Communities Hospital, Oceanside,
New York*

Diane W. Shannon

Michael Shaughnessy
Eastern New Mexico University

June Shepherd
Eastern New Mexico University

Martha A. Sherwood
University of Oregon

R. Baird Shuman
University of Illinois, Urbana-Champaign

Sanford S. Singer
University of Dayton

Virginia Slaughter
University of Queensland, Australia

Jane A. Slezak
Fulton Montgomery Community College

Genevieve Slomski
New Britain, Connecticut

Dwight G. Smith
Southern Connecticut State University

Jane Marie Smith
Butler County Community College

Laura B. Smith

Roger Smith
Portland, Oregon

Janet A. Sniezek
University of Illinois at Urbana- Champaign

Lisa Levin Sobczak
Santa Barbara, California

Ballaro Sprague

Mark Stanton
Azusa Pacific University

Sharon W. Stark
Monmouth University

William D. Stark
Monrovia, California

Lloyd K. Stires
Indiana University of Pennsylvania

Wendy L. Stuhldreher
Slippery Rock University

Laura Tahir
New York, New York

Rebekah Tanner
Onondaga Community College

Sue Tarjan
Santa Cruz, California

Alyssa Tedder-King
University of Kansas

Janice Tedford
Gordon College

Bethany Thivierge
Technicality Resources

Venkat Raghavan Tirumala
Western Kentucky University

Leslie V. Tischauser
Prairie State College

James T. Trent
Middle Tennessee State University

John V. Urbas
Kennesaw State College

Maxine M. Urton
Xavier University

Leonardo Fonseca Valadares

Nicole M. Van Hoey
Arlington, Virginia

Charles L. Vigue
University of New Haven

Joseph C. Viola

Jessica Vitale
St. Joseph Hill Academy, Staten Island, New York

Linda Volonino
Canisius College

Scott R. Vrana
Purdue University

John F. Wakefield
University of North Alabama

Elaine F. Walker
Emory University

Catherine J. Walsh
Mote Marine Laboratory

Melissa Walsh

Andrew Walter
Allyson Washburn
Institute on Aging/Jewish Home

Marcia Watson-Whitmyre
University of Delaware

Ann L. Weber
University of North Carolina at Asheville

Marcia J. Weiss
Point Park College

S. M. Willis

Bradley R. A. Wilson
University of Cincinnati

Stephen L. Wolfe
University of California, Davis

Bonnie L. Wolff

Karen Wolford
SUNY Oswego

Debra Wood
Orlando, FL

Michael Woods

Robin L. Wulffson
American Medical Writers Association

Susan J. Wurtzburg
University of Utah

Frederic Wynn
County College of Morris

Danielle Wysokowski
St. Joseph Hill Academy, Staten Island, New York

W. Michael Zawada
University of Colorado Health Sciences Center

Debra Zehner
Wilkes University

Ross Zeltser

Ming Y. Zheng
Gordon College

Ling-Yi Zhou
University of St. Francis

Thomas G. Zimmerman
*South Nassau Communities Hospital, Oceanside,
New York*

Therese Zink
Wright State University, Boonshoft School of Medicine

COMPLETE LIST OF CONTENTS

VOLUME 1

VOLUME 2

Health and Illness:
Diseases and Conditions

Health Myths

Infections

Nutrition and Staying Fit

Relationships: Friends, Family, and Dating

VOLUME 3

School and Jobs: Skills for Success

Sexuality and Sexual Health

Staying Safe

Vaccines and Vaccinations

Your Body

Your Emotional and Mental Health

Appendixes

Advice from Teens

Being gluten-free

There are different reasons why someone may decide to eat a gluten free diet. Some have celiac disease, which is an autoimmune disorder. When a person with celiac disease eats gluten, the body mounts an attack on the small intestine, which over time results in intestinal damage and can compromise nutrient absorption. The only known treatment for celiac disease is to eat a strictly gluten free diet. Some people have what is known as gluten intolerance or gluten sensitivity, which has very similar symptoms as celiac disease. However, gluten intolerance is not an autoimmune disorder, and as a result, individuals with gluten intolerance sometimes have a less severe onset of symptoms and don't experience any intestinal damage.

INTRODUCTION

In order to understand why some people live a gluten free lifestyle, we need to know what gluten actually is. Gluten is a protein that is found in wheat. More specifically, gluten is the protein in wheat that holds food together and keeps it from coming apart. In other words, gluten is the "glue" that holds everything together. Make no mistake: gluten is not wheat. It is a protein found in wheat. People who cannot eat gluten usually cannot eat wheat because gluten is one of the proteins that is contained in wheat. However, having a wheat allergy is different than having celiac disease or a gluten intolerance or sensitivity. People who choose to life a gluten free lifestyle generally do so for one of three reasons. Some have an autoimmune disorder known as celiac disease, in which eating foods containing gluten triggers an immune response that attacks the small intestine, which decreases the body's ability to absorb nutrients through food. Symptoms of celiac are different from person to person and range from frequent stomach aches to chronic diarrhea to rashes and joint pain. Some have a condition known as gluten intolerance, which is sometimes referred to as "gluten sensitivity" or "non celiac gluten sensitivity". In this article, the terms "gluten intolerance" and "gluten sensitivity" will be used celiac disease. However, unlike celiac disease, for those who have gluten intolerance or gluten sensitivity, gluten does not cause an autoimmune reaction. As a result, people who suffer from gluten intolerance usually do not experience intestinal damage. Individuals who have gluten intolerance also tend to sometimes experience a less severe onset of symptoms than those who have celiac disease. Some

people, despite having no symptoms relating to celiac or gluten intolerance also choose to avoid foods containing gluten as a lifestyle choice.

CELIAC DISEASE

As stated in the introduction, celiac disease is an autoimmune disorder. When an individual with celiac disease eats gluten, the body is triggered to attack the small intestine, which compromises the body's ability to absorb and retain nutrients from food. Symptoms vary widely, which makes celiac disease difficult to detect and diagnose. There are over 300 different symptoms of celiac disease and it is actually possible to have celiac disease without experiencing any symptoms at all. This is somewhat rare and is known in the medical field as asymptomatic celiac disease. People can be affected by celiac disease regardless of age, race, or gender. However, it is a proven fact that there is a genetic component to the likelihood of getting celiac disease. According to Celiac Central, 5-22 percent of people who have celiac disease have a first degree relative that has celiac disease.

DIAGNOSIS

Because of the wide range of symptoms that celiac disease can cause, celiac disease is often difficult to diagnose. According to Celiac Central, 83% of Americans who have celiac disease are not diagnosed or misdiagnosed, with the average case of celiac disease taking 6-10 years to be correctly diagnosed. Celiac is typically tested for by a blood test for gluten antibodies and a small bowel biopsy to assess damage to the gut. To be diagnosed, a person must still be eating a non gluten free diet at the time of being tested. Because the person has to continue eating gluten in order to be officially diagnosed, some people will instead go on an elimination diet to determine whether choosing a gluten free lifestyle will get rid of their symptoms. If you choose to do this, it is important to note that it is nearly impossible to know for certain whether you have celiac disease or gluten intolerance unless you have been tested, as they both cause very similar symptoms. Both celiac disease or gluten intolerance require eating a strictly gluten free diet if you get diagnosed or find out through an elimination diet.

TREATMENT

The only proven treatment for celiac disease is to strictly avoid eating all foods that either contain gluten or that have been cross contaminated with foods that contain gluten. Cross contamination is when foods that do not contain gluten are prepared on the same surfaces and equipment as foods that do contain gluten. For example, French fries are naturally gluten free. However, restaurants often fry French fries using the same equipment that they use to fry gluten containing foods such as onion rings and chicken fingers. As a result, if you have celiac disease, you can't eat foods that are cross contaminated with foods that contain gluten. Cross contamination is difficult to avoid in restaurants, but if you are a good self advocate and inform your server that you have celiac disease and explain what that entails, you have a better chance at avoiding cross contamination.

GLUTEN INTOLERANCE OR SENSITIVITY

Gluten intolerance, which is also known as gluten sensitivity or non celiac gluten sensitivity causes symptoms that are nearly identical to celiac disease. The difference between celiac disease and gluten intolerance is that celiac disease is an autoimmune disorder and gluten intolerance is not. Individuals who have gluten intolerance typically experience a less severe onset of symptoms in response to eating gluten than those who have celiac disease experience. Also, people who have gluten intolerance usually do not suffer any intestinal damage, which is not the case with celiac disease. Gluten intolerance has only recently been accepted as a legitimate medical condition by the medical field. For many years, the majority of doctors and people working in the medical profession dismissed gluten intolerance as an illegitimate condition, but at the present time doctors are becoming more aware of the validity of gluten intolerance.

DIAGNOSIS

There is currently no widely accepted test for gluten sensitivity. Tests for celiac disease often come up negative in those who have gluten intolerance. Often, people determine that they have gluten intolerance by going on an elimination diet, in which the patient will eliminate different potential allergens from their diet to determine which food group(s) are causing symptoms. If symptoms significantly improve after the patient eliminates gluten from their diet, than the patient may have gluten intolerance. The elimination diet can be self-administered or done under the guidance of a physician and/or nutritionist.

TREATMENT

As is the case with celiac disease, the only way to effectively treat gluten intolerance or gluten sensitivity is to eat a completely gluten free diet.

GOING GLUTEN FREE AS A LIFESTYLE CHOICE

In the last couple of years, more and more people have been choosing to live a gluten free lifestyle. Recently there has been much more awareness of celiac disease and gluten sensitivity and as a result, more and more people are choosing to eat a gluten free diet. This awareness has resulted in a huge increase in availability and sales of gluten free pastas, breads, cakes, and other gluten free versions of foods that normally contain gluten. Some people choose to live a gluten free diet because they claim that it is healthier, helps with weight loss, and boosts energy among many other reasons. A gluten free lifestyle has also been recommended by some to decrease symptoms of autism. In this section we will explore the validity of two of the most common reasons that people live a gluten free lifestyle even if they do not technically have to for medical reasons.

GOING GLUTEN FREE TO LOSE WEIGHT

Going gluten free to lose weight has been one of the most popular reasons for trying to live a gluten free lifestyle in the past couple of years. Does a gluten free diet actually help people to lose weight? Strictly adhering to a gluten free diet does make fast food less accessible, and whole, less processed foods such as fruits, vegetables, and some meat more accessible, which can lead to living a healthier diet and as a result, possibly losing weight. Also, strictly adhering to a gluten free diet requires more awareness of what you are eating, which may lead to making healthier food choices, which can contribute to weight loss. However, eating a gluten free diet is not automatically healthier than eating a normal diet, and there is no proven link between eating a gluten free diet and losing weight. In fact, many people who choose to go on a gluten free diet to lose weight actually gain weight after going gluten free, especially those that eat a lot of gluten free prepared foods such as gluten free breads, pastas, cookies, and cakes. The bottom line is that eating a healthy diet is statistically proven to help maintain a healthy weight. Going gluten free is not a proven weight loss diet.

GOING GLUTEN FREE TO INCREASE ENERGY

Some people claim that they experience a boost of energy from adhering to a gluten free diet. As is the case for going gluten free to lose weight, going on a gluten free diet causes you to become more aware of what you are eating, which can result in the person consuming more fruits, vegetables, and less processed foods. If the person has no symptoms directly relating to celiac disease or gluten sensitivity, this increase in energy probably stems from eating a healthier, more balanced diet, as people who eat a balanced diet generally claim to have more energy whether they are eating a gluten free diet or not. It is not statistically proven that eating a gluten free diet boosts energy levels.

CONCLUSION

As a teen, it is important to realize the impact nutrition has on your life. If you feel that you may have symptoms relating to celiac disease or gluten intolerance, you can either get tested or first choose to go on an elimination diet to see if you have an allergy or sensitivity to a certain food group. Your physician or nutritionist can assist you in planning out an elimination diet. Remember, if you get tested for celiac disease and tests come back negative, you can still have gluten intolerance. This is why it can be helpful to go on an elimination diet before getting tested for celiac disease. If you are considering choosing a gluten free diet in order to lose weight or boost energy, it is important to note that there is no proven link between going gluten free and losing weight and/or boosting energy levels. It is statistically proven that people who eat a healthy and balanced diet that includes lots of fruits and vegetables tend to maintain a healthy weight and have higher energy levels as a result of eating a healthy diet.

FURTHER READING

Ahern, S. J. (2009). *Gluten free girl: How I found the food that loves me back…And how you can too.* Hoboken, NJ: John Wiley & Sons. This book is a first-hand account of how Shauna Ahern (founder of the website Gluten Free Girl and The Chef) found out that she could not eat gluten. The book discusses how to eat a healthy and delicious diet while staying strictly gluten free, and focuses on the importance of finding out what foods you can eat instead of what you can't eat. Ahearn's positive attitude shines through throughout the book, and it is a great read for anyone who is considering a gluten free lifestyle.

Gluten Free Girl and The Chef. (n.d.). New to gluten free? Retrieved from http://glutenfreegirl.com/new-to-gluten-free/. This article is a comprehensive guide to starting to live a gluten free lifestyle. The article is written by Shauna James Ahern, who has celiac disease and has a very successful blog (glutenfreegirl.com) This blog contains advice for living a gluten free lifestyle, gluten free recipes, and posts about her various life experiences living gluten free.

National Foundation for Celiac Awareness. (2014). Retrieved from http://www.celiaccentral.org/. The National Foundation for Celiac Awareness website features lots of accurate and in depth information about celiac disease. Contains information about symptoms, risk factors, essential facts, being diagnosed, related conditions, and much more. The website also has some handy resources, many gluten free recipes, and an events page which features various celiac disease related events.

WebMD. (n.d.). Celiac disease health center. Retrieved from http://www.webmd.com/digestive-disorders/celiac-disease/celiac-disease-topic-overview. This article from WebMC.com gives an explanation of what celiac disease is and goes over common symptoms, diagnosis, and treatment. The article also instructs the reader as to what an individual with celiac disease can and cannot eat, and what to watch out for when reading food labels. It also briefly goes over some disorders that can be mistaken for celiac disease.

Benjamin Riley

SEE ALSO: Celiac Disease; Gastrointestinal System, The; Nutrition; Staying in a Healthy Weight Range; Vegetarian Diet

Dealing with peer pressure

Peer pressure is a universal phenomenon that causes people—namely teenagers—to give into the wants of their peers rather than their original beliefs or intentions. Unfortunately, this can have an adverse effect on individuals and lead them to comply in potentially harmful situations. By looking at the consequences of certain scenarios and at ways to resist them, a person facing peer pressure can cope and also realize that he or she is not alone in facing these issues.

INTRODUCTION

"Peer pressure" is a term both widely-known and widely-feared. Children, adolescents, teenagers, and even adults are often faced with it: the conflict of having to choose between their wants and the wants of others. According to psychology professor Philip Zimbardo, famed for his studies on conformity, the desire to conform is driven by a need to be accepted and liked by a group of people (Zimbardo, 1971). This need drives individuals to comply in situations they wouldn't normally consider.

While the archetypical peer pressure scenario usually consists of drugs and/or alcohol, peer pressure may also be experienced in different ways. For example, an individual may feel compelled to become more intimate in a relationship than he or she would like to be. Another person may be pressured to join in on bullying, or someone else could feel the need to conform in a less harmful situation, such as in the way he or she dresses. It may be very difficult to get through many of these situations. However, regardless of the scenario, there are definitive ways to deal with the challenges posed by peer pressure, no matter how difficult it may seem.

DANGEROUS SUBSTANCES

Alcohol is one of the most commonly abused substances and is normally distributed to teens at parties, concerts, or at a friend's house when there is no parental supervision. Other drugs, such as marijuana ("pot"), "molly," heroin, and cocaine, are slightly more difficult to obtain but still pose a major issue. Aside from addiction, abuse of these drugs (or even one time use for certain substances) can lead to other serious long-term effects such as permanent brain damage, nerve damage, damage to the cardiovascular system, kidney failure, and liver failure, just to name a few (*Long Term Drug Addiction*, n.d.). While these effects seem far-away and implausible, they have, do, and will happen.

When being offered a dangerous substance, it is important for one to keep those effects in mind. There are other consequences involved, too, such as getting caught by a parent or making poor decisions due to clouded judgment. It could also be a violation of one's own beliefs. It's vital that the person remember all the consequences in order to say "no" with firm conviction. If one is confident and adamant, most people will take "no" for an answer. However, if the person offering continues to persist, the best solution would be to ignore that individual and to walk away. Leaving (either the conversation or the party entirely) is the best way to escape an uncomfortable and

potentially dangerous situation. People not wanting to take drugs should distance themselves from friends who try to pressure them into doing so.

In the case of teenagers, this usually isn't the favorite way to go. Walking away removes one from the pack, causing him or her to feel isolated, to fear being excluded from future events, and to worry about no longer being liked by that group of people. A good solution to this would be for the person to find like-minded individuals to spend time with during those events or to hang out with in lieu of going to a place where drugs are going to be offered. That way, one will always have friends that he or she can count on for acceptance and understanding. It is irrational to believe that everyone abuses substances. If one individual is uncomfortable with a situation, there are always at least several others who feel similarly.

PRESSURE IN RELATIONSHIPS

While this topic normally applies to girls being pressured by their boyfriends, it is possible for *either* gender to feel sexually pressured in a relationship. This is a very difficult and sensitive issue, as the person being pressured usually cares for the other individual and does not want to risk losing him (or her). In order to keep the other person happy, she may give in, contrary to her personal values and risk health consequences such as teen pregnancy or sexually transmitted infections. Other pressures may stem from outside of the relationship, such as television shows that make regular sexual activity appear normal. A girl may go further sexually in order to impress her friends or to make herself seem more appealing to other boys. A person who feels that she may eventually give into sexual pressure should talk to someone close to her about the issue. This will help her to see a new perspective on things and to reexamine her priorities.

To avoid such a situation, it is important to have a conversation early in the relationship discussing one's personal stance on sexual actions. That way, the partner may be less likely to suggest anything further down the road. One could also have that conversation as soon as the pressure begins. As with alcohol or drugs, the best solution is to just say no and to leave if it continues.

If the other person threatens to end the relationship if his sexual advances aren't met, then it is in the girl's best interest to end the relationship herself. This will bolster her confidence and allow her some closure after being pressured and threatened. While it may not be easy, it has to be done in order to maintain one's self respect and to end the pressure entirely. A conditional relationship has no real foundation and is thus not a relationship at all.

BULLYING

Giving into negative peer pressure not only harms oneself, but also poses a danger to others, especially in the case of bullying. When a person is targeted by bullies, it is difficult for that individual to find a peer to defend him or her. The majority of neutral parties partake in what is known as the diffusion of responsibility, in which no one goes to the person's aid because they assume that someone else will. In addition, because no one is moving to help the bullying victim, others are less likely to stand out and be the first to say something in the individual's defense. This also stems from fear: the neutral parties fear being the next victim. In this light, the bully is pressuring the other kids into either staying out of the situation entirely or joining in on the attack.

When dealing with bullying, regardless if it's in middle school or high school, it's vital that an adult is notified. It's hard for peers of the bully or of the target to stop it on their own, but an authority figure such as a parent or a teacher can handle the situation. While no one wants to be labeled a "snitch" or become the next target, notifying an adult can easily be done quietly, such as via email or text message, so that he or she remains anonymous to the bullies. It is very important for one to keep in mind that there is a possibility that if he doesn't say something, no one else will.

If facing pressure to join in on the bullying, the person must stick to what he or she knows is right. As in the case of the individual avoiding dangerous substances, a person being pressured to bully should find people who are also against bullying to both befriend and to act as a support system.

In any instance of peer pressure, one must remember to stay true to his or her own beliefs, no matter how difficult it may seem.

FURTHER READING

Lickerman, A. (n.d.). The diffusion of responsibility. Retrieved from: https://www.psychologytoday.com/blog/happiness-in-world/201006/the-diffusion-responsibility. The author further explains the phenomenon of the diffusion of responsibility while providing a real-life example of the danger it poses.

Long term drugaAddiction effects. (n.d.). Retrieved from http://www.drugabuse.net/drug-addiction/long-term-drug-addiction-effects/. This article lists the short and long term damages of drug addiction, useful for anyone considering experimenting with drugs or trying to talk someone else out of doing so.

Teens for life -- Join the revolution. (2009) Retrieved from http://www.teensforlife.com/hot-topics/peer-pressure/. This provides an in-depth and relatable discussion on the importance of sticking to one's morals and avoiding negative peer pressure.

Your life counts. (n.d.). Retrieved from: http://www.your-lifecounts.org/blog/20-ways-avoid-peer-pressure. This article helps strengthen resolve against peer pressure while also educating readers on dealing with it.

Zimbardo, P. (2006). *The Lucifer Effect*. Retrieved from: http://www.lucifereffect.com/index.html A very informative and interesting site chronicling and discussing professor Philip Zimbardo's famous Stanford Prison Experiment on conformity.

Maria Conte

SEE ALSO: Abstinence; Binge Drinking; Bullying; Dealing with Bullying; Marijuana; Sexual Harassment; Teen Pregnancy

Ending an unhealthy friendship

Making friends is a rewarding part of life. However, there are times when this relationship changes from being fulfilling to toxic. Even in the instances when the friendship is not necessarily toxic, it is common for friends to drift apart and to no longer have as much in common as they once did. Ending a friendship can be very emotional, stressful, and taxing for a person. Young people may feel there are social repercussions for ending particular friendships; however, not ending a friendship when it is no longer fulfilling is more detrimental than any other social repercussion.

INTRODUCTION

Friendships are a very rewarding part of a person's life. We often rely on our friends for support as well as enjoy the social pleasures they bring to our lives. Having friends makes people feel less lonely, which is why people place such an importance on not only making friends, but also keeping them. It is not uncommon for people to drift apart and for friendships to change. Oftentimes when friendships change, we feel at a crossroads about whether or not we should end the friendship or if we should continue putting forth the time and effort that is required of any kind of relationship. The decision to end a friendship is a difficult one and it often comes with much sadness and even feelings of guilt; however, there are many times when despite these feelings this is the best possible decision for all parties. Ending a friendship is not an easy decision to make; however, when it is well thought out and done right, it will not be long until it feels like the right decision.

ENDING A FRIENDSHIP

Friendships bring a lot of happiness; however, when a friendship starts to deteriorate the time spent with that friend will begin to feel like it is doing more harm than good. It can often be difficult to recognize and acknowledge that the relationship is no longer as good as it once was, especially when the person has been a part of your life for a long period of time; however, if you have ever made a resolution to make your life happier and more complete, ending a friendship is sometimes necessary. While all relationships are different, the main source of conflict arises when a person does not feel honored or respected. When a person does not feel respected or honored, emotions ranging from feeling a little hurt to extreme sadness occur, which makes it difficult to be around the person who makes us feel this way. While sometimes friends say or do things that upset us, the feeling of needing to end a friendship usually happens after consistently feeling devalued.

The need to end a friendship is not something that can be decided overnight. Rather, it is a process of evaluating the benefits of staying in the relationship (the person makes you feel good, you have fun when you are together) versus the costs (the person always makes fun of you, you are unable to be yourself when you are with that person). If the costs outweigh the benefits of staying with your friend, then it is likely time to consider ending the friendship.

WAYS TO END A FRIENDSHIP

There are two approaches to ending a friendship that depend on the circumstances. The first approach is a "formal break up." During the "formal break up" the friends will sit down together and have a conversation around why the friendship is no longer working. There will likely be feelings of anger or sadness and the person who is getting "broken up with" might feel defensive. Feelings of rejection are also likely. While this approach might seem daunting, by letting your friend know why the friendship cannot continue, you are letting him or her know upfront

about your feelings, which gives them the chance to try to fix their behavior that has led you to feel this way. Formally "breaking up" with a friend is best when the friend has been a part of your life for awhile or your friend has done something so horrible that it is imperative that you confront them.

The second approach is to just allow the friendship to fade away. In this approach you slowly phase the person out of your life. It involves telling the person that you are busy whenever they invite you to do something or when you are in a small group you act polite but do not go out of your way to spend time with them. This approach is most appropriate when you have not known the person for very long or they are a part of your social circle. By using the "fade away" approach there is no formal rejection, which can make it easier for the other person to justify why the two of you are not longer spending as much time together as you once did.

TOXIC FRIENDSHIPS

Friendships, like any relationship, are about giving and taking. However, when one person in the relationship is giving more than he or she is receiving from his or her friend, it may be a sign that the friendship is toxic. When a friend constantly needs you for absolutely everything, it can be tiring especially when that friend does not return the support. Along with feeling like the other person is constantly taking up all of your time and energy, another sign that a friendship is toxic is when you dread seeing the person. Since friendships are voluntary relationships, it is probably time to end the friendship if there are feelings of dread every time the person is calls or tries to hang out with you.

Another sign of a toxic friendship is when the friendship is never consistently fun. The relationship jumps from being great to awful rather quickly, which can lead to emotional exhaustion. The unpredictable nature of this relationship can lead to emotional distress such as feeling anxious, nervous, or in some instances depressed. Again, friendships are voluntary relationships, which is why it is imperative that this relationship benefits both parties. When friends are in constant turmoil or can't seem to agree on much of anything, it can lead to feelings of extreme uncertainty as well as all of aforementioned emotional impacts.

ENDING A FRIENDSHIP VERSUS A ROMANTIC RELATIONSHIP

The media constantly sensationalizes the breaking off of romantic relationships. It is not uncommon to see a group of girl friends in a movie eating out of pints of ice cream while they cry over their ex-boyfriends. However, ending a friendship can be just as taxing as a traditional break up. People often go into romantic relationships calculating the potential risks and benefits, whereas not as many people do that with friendships. Rather, it is common to go into a friendship thinking there is not nearly as much risk as a romantic relationship, since it is unlikely that it will end with as much pain. However, this is not always true. When a romantic relationship ends, it is common for people to offer some kind of explanation about why the relationship did not work, whereas when a friendship ends it is harder to justify the need to cut that person out of your life. While it might be more difficult to explain to people why the friendship had to end, it does not make ending a friendship any less painful.

Another reason that ending a friendship can be as, if not more, difficult than ending a romantic relationship is that we often rely on our close friends to be a constant part of our lives. The close friendship that is nurtured and developed over the course of many years, leads to a certain level of reliance on the friend. It is expected that that person will be able to support you regardless of what is going on, which is why when that source of support changes or ends completely, it is emotionally difficult to overcome.

Ending a close friendship can be extremely daunting because unlike romantic relationships, there are no dating sites for friends. It appears much more difficult to find friends; especially close ones, than it does to find a new romantic interest. At the time the friendship ends, it might seem nearly impossible to go out and make new friends; however, it does not have to be this way. Getting involved with different activities in your community, school, or church will help ease the pain that is felt when a friendship ends. By getting integrated in different activities, exposure to new people will be maximized and it will reassure you that making friends outside of your previous friendship is possible.

EMBRACE THE ENDING

It might seem counterintuitive to embrace the ending of a friendship, since the relationship with someone close to you has ended. However, if a friendship has ended it is often because the relationship was no longer benefit-ting both parties. While it might seem daunting to no longer be able to call that person a "friend," it is important to not be afraid of the unknown. When a friendship ends, feelings of uncertainty as well as questions such as "whom will I hang out with?" and "who will be my friend?" are likely to surface. It is important to remember that this friendship did not end because it was a great friendship; rather it ended because it was no longer a good match for either of you.

Similar to the ending of a romantic relationship, there will be a period of missing the friendship you had as well as reminiscing about the good times that the two of you had together. Remembering the good times is important, but it is also necessary to take responsibility for the ending of the friendship and remember why the friendship ceased in the first place. This is a time for self-reflection regarding what you value and want out of a friendship as well as what you do not want. By doing this, you will be able to better embrace the ending of the friendship as well as realize your self worth.

FURTHER READING

Firger, J. (2015, January 2). "How to recognize (and end) a toxic friendship". Retrieved May 22, 2015, from http://www.cbsnews.com/news/how-to-spot-and-end-a-toxic-friendship/. An article on how to recognize toxic friendship as well as how to end the relationship.

Lickerman, A. (2013, August 25). How to end a friendship. Retrieved May 22, 2015, from https://www.psychologytoday.com/blog/happiness-in-world/201308/how-end-friendship. An article on how to end a friendship that begins with a personal anecdote, which helps to explain how to end a friendship when you are younger.

Wilding, M. (2014, January 9). Surviving a friendship break up. Retrieved May 22, 2015, from http://psychcentral.com/blog/archives/2014/01/09/surviving-a-friendship-break-up/. This article discusses the ways to get over a friendship break up. It offers good advice that is easy to understand and apply to daily life.

Lauren Ruvo

SEE ALSO: Decision Making; Helping Friends Cope; Interpersonal Skills; Self-Esteem; Separation Anxiety

Ending unhealthy relationships

Identifying, understanding, and ending an unhealthy relationship is a difficult process no-matter the age of the individuals involved, and often produces complicated and conflicting emotions. Being able to recognize unhealthy relationship behaviors and understand the detrimental consequences are important, but often overlooked relationship skills, especially in adolescence and young adulthood, when romantic relationships are a more novel experience. Teens and young adults turn to peers, parents, and other trusted adults when they face relationship difficulties, but they and their supporters are often unaware of where to seek additional information and help, and have fears about doing so.

INTRODUCTION

Adolescent dating violence (ADV) has received a plethora of research attention over the past decade, even though adult and young adult intimate partner violence has long been a major public health concern. Increasing awareness of the high prevalence of emotional and physical abuse that can take place in adolescent relationships has spurred organizations around the United States to take action and begin funding programs to increase preventative efforts and survivor supports. Nearly one fourth of adolescents have experienced unhealthy dating relationships. ADV is not exclusive to gender, sexual orientation, or age and is defined by the Centers for Disease Control as "physical, sexual, or psychological/ emotional violence within a dating relationship, including stalking." (CDC, 2014)

It comes as a surprise to many young people that physical and/or sexual violence aren't the only markers of dating violence and unhealthy relationships. Psychological and/ or emotional abuse or violence is an even more common expression of an unhealthy relationship than physical violence. This can look like manipulation, stalking, isolation, name-calling, insults, and any other form of degradation of a romantic partner. This repeated behavior can lead to depression, anxiety, difficulties with body image and self-esteem, suicidal ideation, substance use, and the dissolution of healthy relationships on the part of the individual receiving such damaging messages. Despite all the grief caused by a relationship that exhibits these qualities with or without a physical abuse component, ending a relationship with someone who is deeply cared for can be emotional, difficult, and scary. Knowing how

to ask for needed support and planning for safety is instrumental in such situations.

WARNING SIGNS

If you suspect that you or someone you care about is in an unhealthy relationship there are often warning signs that may confirm your suspicions, however, it's important to remember that just because you can't see the signs does not mean that a relationship is healthy behind closed doors. Changes in mood, behavior, and appearance are three hallmarks of a person who is in an unhealthy relationship. The person may be dressing differently because that is a way in which their partner is controlling them, or in order to hide signs of physical violence. They may become noticeably depressed, irritable, or nervous and as a result of physical or emotional violence, or at the partner's urging may begin to engage in risky behaviors including risky sexual behavior, substance abuse, or other risk-taking. A decline in participation in group activities previously enjoyed is also another frequent behavior change in those who are in an unhealthy relationship. Defensiveness, loss of confidence, and apathy about school or work are also common characteristics that may indicate an unhealthy relationship. Being aware of these signs and willing to talk about them openly when you have concerns can be crucial for your safety or the safety of someone you care about.

TALKING TO OTHERS ABOUT AN UNHEALTHY RELATIONSHIP

Individuals in an unhealthy relationship often experience a great deal of difficulty talking to others about their relationship. This can be due to fear, shame, denial, or a whole host of emotions, however, talking to peers and adults is incredibly important to ensuring your safety if you think you are in an unhealthy relationship. Teens and young adults often turn to their peers first because of the perception, and sometimes reality, that their peers will be more understanding than parents or other adults in the person's life. Peers can be a positive source of support, but research has shown that peers are often hesitant to tell friends when they believe a relationship might be unhealthy. Generally, this is because they want to be seen as supportive and have a greater reluctance to confront their friends in a situation that may cause discord.

In addition, individuals experiencing an unhealthy relationship are often reluctant to share the degree to which psychological and/or physical abuse is happening. This may be because of a desire to protect the reputation of their partner; it may be due to denial of the extent to which the unhealthy behaviors are happening, or a combination of both. Another possible explanation is that the individual on the receiving end of abusive behavior is unsure whether the behaviors are unhealthy or not. Peers can help by openly listening, and expressing the full degree of their concern to a friend in an unhealthy relationship, as well as being aware of what behaviors are unhealthy and sharing their observations with a friend they feel might be in an unhealthy relationship.

Parents, although not many young individuals' first choice, are frequently the first non-peer adult whose advice and support is sought. Many males in unhealthy relationships might go to parents first, as their concerns may be minimized by peers, or seen as "unmanly." Often young people expect their parents to overreact or demand that they end the unhealthy relationship against their will, or before they are ready to do so. While parents are less reluctant than peers to express the extent of their concern about an unhealthy relationship and will often openly share their opinions about ending the relationship, it is important that the individual in the relationship feel supported and heard, and is helped to make a decision of their own accord.

Parents may also have the ability to share and teach relationship skills, such as conflict resolution, which may be helpful in ending the relationship, or giving the young person a new strategy to try if they aren't yet ready to end the relationship. Parents can help by being a safe place to bring relationship concerns, fully listening to their child's concerns before interrupting with opinions or demands. Parents can also help their adolescent and young adult children learn to make healthy relationship choices by helping evaluate concerns and options without making demands or punishing the individual in some way (grounding the individual, taking away their keys or cell phone, etc.). Self-efficacy and self-esteem are built by handing difficult situations and doing so on one's own terms.

Teens and young adults may also turn to other adult individuals that they determine to be safe and supportive. Often times, this may be a coach, teacher, youth pastor, a friend's parent, or someone else they have regular contact with. They can provide support in the same way that both a peer and a parent might. It is important for peers, parents, and other adults working with young people to be able to identify and talk about unhealthy relationship behaviors, including psychological and emotional violence. An important part of listening and supporting someone who is in an unhealthy relationship is to try and speak as neutrally as possible about the partner committing the unhealthy acts. This means part of creating a safe space requires discussing the unhealthy behavior without name-calling, verbally attacking, or generalizing the behavior to the partner's character because doing so often makes it more difficult for the person wanting help and support, and they may stop discussing their concerns, or feel shamed in some way.

It's also important to be aware of local agencies that may be able to help with safety planning when needed and provide additional support. These agencies include domestic violence centers, counseling agencies, law enforcement, and other social service agencies. Finally, ending a relationship, even an unhealthy one, is difficult. It is important to allow the individual ending a relationship to feel the full gamut of emotions and not to dismiss or ignore them. If there is concern about anxiety or depression, or any other mental health concerns, discussing them with a counselor may be helpful.

PLANNING FOR A SAFE EXIT

If a relationship has been tumultuous and dating violence has occurred, regardless of whether it was physical, psychological, or both, a safe plan for leaving the relationship is an important precaution, and there are several factors to consider. These include: what does the individual in the relationship want? If they want the abuse to stop, but don't want to leave the relationship, then efforts to create a safety plan and help may be perceived as unsupportive. This is an important question to answer first. Second, have they tried to end the relationship before? What was the result? It is important to be as prepared as possible for the partner's reaction. Will they threaten harm to themselves or others? Will they respond manipulatively? Third, what resources are available to the individual, and which should they tap into to ensure their safety and support? Safety planning can be an empowering experience for the individual and will help them feel supported. Resources that can be helpful include, but are not limited to school counselor's, law enforcement, local domestic violence centers (which often have adolescent specific resources and/or support groups), and friends' parents.

FURTHER READING

Centers for Disease Control and Prevention. (2014). *Understanding teen dating violence.* Retrieved June 10,

2015 from http://www.cdc.gov/violenceprevention/pdf/teen-dating-violence-factsheet-a.pdf

Kulze, L. (2011, July 27). Teaching teens to have healthy breakups. *Newsweek Web Exclusives.* Retrieved from: http://www.thedailybeast.com/articles/2011/07/27/teen-breakups-start-strong-programs-aims-to-make-them-safer.html. This article reviews the importance of prevention efforts and helping teens engage in both healthy relationships and healthy break-ups. The article also discusses a fatal ADV incident following a break-up that made national headlines in 2011. Finally, several experiences teens have had with both physical and emotional violence are shared.

www.loveisrespect.org. This national campaign's website hosts a plethora of tools, tips, and articles on healthy relationships, safety planning, and ending unhealthy relationships. Resources are available for young people and those supporting them including a healthy relationship quiz, warning signs, and advice on how to get help for yourself or someone else.

www.breakthecycle.org. Another empowering national campaign to end relationship violence, this website provides information on recent research on ADV, legal services, and has links to LGBT domestic violence information and survivor services, which are often overlooked. Break the Cycle's blog, programs, and policy advocacy are helpful resources for parents, peers, and those in unhealthy relationships.

http://www.loveisrespect.org/is-this-abuse/power-and-control-wheel/. The interactive power and control wheel reproduced by loveisresepct.org is an excellent resource for anyone questioning whether a behavior is a healthy or unhealthy relationship behavior and encompasses the expression of physical, emotional, and sexual abuse.

Tracy O. Franklin

SEE ALSO: Abusive Relationships; Date Rape Drugs; Dealing with Peer Pressure; Helping Friends Cope; Resiliency; Romantic Breakups; Sexual Consent; Teenage Suicide

Finding your first job

Finding a job as a teenager is hard, especially when you aren't sure what you are doing. This article provides advice on how to find a job as well as how to apply for one. It can be tricky, but being informed beforehand will be a big benefit. Hopefully this article helps you understand what is needed to find your first job.

INTRODUCTION

Teenagers don't realize how much money they spend every week. No matter if it's on stuff for school, food, or clothing, they are spending more money now than ever before. Since teens need more money, and only few still have an allowance, it is time for them to start looking for a job. Having a job teaches teens responsibility and trains them for a future career. Finding your first job can be difficult if you don't know what to do. Here are some helpful steps that can be used to increase the chances of you getting the job.

Simply explained, the steps include creating your résumé, getting working papers, finding places you feel comfortable working, and preparing and handling an interview. Just because you apply for a job doesn't mean you will always get it. If you don't get the first job you apply to, don't be discouraged, there are plenty of jobs that are available.

PUTTING TOGETHER YOUR RÉSUMÉ

The first thing to do when looking for your first job is to make sure you have a résumé. Résumés are organized lists of your education history, accomplishments, work experience, and interests. A résumé begins with your personal information, like your name, address, phone number, and social security number. After your personal information, list your educational history and accomplishments

Résumés help employers get to know who you are without formally meeting you yet. They help highlight what you can offer a prospective employer. Résumés help employers ask you questions during an interview that focus on your strengths and abilities. A résumé is your first impression in the job world. There are great résumé builder websites that will help you organize your information in an appealing way.

GETTING YOUR WORKING PAPERS

After creating your résumé, the next important step is obtaining working papers. If you are under 18 years old, you need papers explaining that you are a minor enrolled in school. This ensures that you are able to work part-time while attending school. To get your working papers, all you have to do is go to your school and ask a faculty member, like a secretary or academic dean, for working papers. They will be happy to make them for you. Make sure to make copies of these papers and bring them to every job interview you attend.

LOOKING NEAR AND FAR

The hardest part about finding a job is actually finding places that are hiring. An easy way of finding places is checking for flyers in your school or in local neighborhood spots. Be on the lookout for job opportunities like shoveling or babysitting. These are easy ways to get into the working world. Most schools will have flyers up for summer job opportunities as well. If you look in the windows of stores in your community, you have a good shot at finding a few places with a "Help Wanted" sign in the window. Also if you live in a close neighborhood, it's more likely for you to get a job since they already know who you are.

When these two ways don't work, and you still can't find a place that is hiring, next look in the newspaper or online. There is always a page in the newspaper with job opportunities. The only problem with searching in the newspaper is you don't know if it will be a stable job or a one-time thing. Searching for a job online can get your job search by opening you up to jobs outside your community. You provide these sites with some personal information and résumé and you are then added to a pool of potential workers. Employers can then find you. The issue with these sites is you aren't guaranteed a job right away, or ever. This doesn't mean don't try. The biggest point of the job search is making sure you feel comfortable in the work you are doing.

BECOMING KNOWN

After you have found a few places you would like to work you should let them know you want the job. Most places will give you an application to fill out. Since you probably won't meet with the manager or owner at this early stage your application will let them know you are interested. Not all places accept applications, but if they do, make sure to bring it back in a timely fashion. This shows you really want the job. When given the application, the easiest thing to do is bring it home and use your résumé to help you fill it out. After returning the application, wait for a call, email, or letter inviting you to an interview. If you never receive anything, don't feel hopeless. It probably means they had a lot of applications to go through, or they found someone for the job before you handed in your application. It doesn't mean you aren't able to work somewhere else, which is why it is important to send in

applications at a few different places to increase your chances of employment.

THE INTERVIEW

The interview is possibly the most important part of the job finding process. This is the make it or break it point for the job. It's ok to be nervous, the interviewer understands. To lessen your nervousness, make sure you are fully prepared. Interviews can be in a group, individually, or on the phone. Group interviews are less scary because it consists of about eight people all in the same position as you. It's less stressful and more laid back than an individual interview. Individual interviews mean being one on one with the person who will possibly be hiring you. The questions they ask will not be hard questions. Most will be about yourself, why you want the job, and what you can offer to make the business better. Make sure to bring your résumé and working papers to the interview as well. The interviewer might not take them, but it's better to be safe than sorry. Interviews over the phone can happen as well. Make sure you are placed somewhere that you won't lose the connection during the call. Also, since you aren't face to face, have your résumé ready. You can use it like a cheat sheet in case you get nervous and blank out.

During any type of interview, remember to be polite. If you are meeting your interviewer make sure to dress appropriately. Don't be afraid to ask questions; interviewers would love to answer your questions. It shows you are truly interested in the job. More than one interview may be conducted, meaning they are looking at you for the position. As long as you continue to show interest and keep a positive outlook, getting the job will be a breeze.

FURTHER READING

Care.com: Find child care, senior care and pet care and more. (n.d.). Retrieved from: http://www.care.com/ .If you are looking for a job involving taking care of others, this website takes your information and puts you into the system. People can then see who you are and can ask you directly to work for them.

How to land your first job. (n.d.). Retrieved from: http://www.snagajob.com/teen-jobs/first-job/. This site gives more information on finding your first job. It also discusses different kinds of jobs suitable for teenagers. It gives tips on résumés and the importance of maintaining a family friendly social media life.

Resume builder | Free resume builder | LiveCareer. (n.d.). Retrieved from: http://www.livecareer.com/

resume-builder. This website is great for helping you build your résumé. It takes your information and organizes it to look professional.

The smart teenager's guide to getting a job in high school. (2013, November 1). Retrieved from: http://www.theprospect.net/the-smart-teenagers-guide-to-getting-a-job-in-high-school-8749. This website focuses on the interview and relates the personal accounts of job seekers.

Danielle Wysokowski

SEE ALSO: Carrer Testing; Cover Letter and Résumé Writing; Interviewing

Joining the military

The United States Military consists of the brave that ensure the land of the free. Today, enlistment is voluntary and the decision to join the armed forces cannot be taken lightly. There are many factors to consider and many sacrifices to be made. Service can be rewarding in numerous ways, but the risks are high and plenty.

INTRODUCTION

The United States Army can be traced back to the Second Continental Congress in 1775. Over the course of almost 250 years, the United States Military has evolved into a dynamic and elite force in the world. Since the draft era is over, joining the military is voluntary. Enlisted members and officers play different roles in the U.S. Military. Enlisted members can be seen as the muscle of the military, while officers can be seen as the brain. Joining the Military is a big decision and recruits should make this decision well informed. Serving in the military is an honorable sacrifice. The idiom "freedom isn't free" proves to be true because military men and women give their lives to protect personal freedoms. Members forego time with their loved ones and regular daily life. Things that civilians take for granted, such as eating dinner with family or friends, sleeping in the comfort of one's own bed, or just the normalcy of everyday life, are traded for service. Potential recruits should educate themselves as much as possible on the enlistment process and military experience in order to make the right decisions. No matter what branch a soldier occupies or rank a soldier earns, every individual contributes to protecting the United States. The military is unified in

that all members are working toward the common goal of securing freedom.

ENLISTED MEMBERS VS. OFFICERS

To enter as an enlisted member, a GED (General Education Development certificate) is usually required. Even though it is not required, many enlisted members have their bachelor's degree. Enlisted members carry out the hands-on duties in the military. While combat is the conventional way to serve one's country, approximately 91 percent of enlisted military jobs are non-combat. Any job that can be found in a major city can almost always be found in the United States Military.

To become a manager in the military, or a commissioned officer (CO), one must get a college degree or move up the ranks. Officers that receive their seniority by moving up the ranks are called mustangs and are greatly respected. During war, personnel showing exceptionally strong leadership skills can be given battlefield commissions and promotion to CO. Officer programs are competitive. Congress must approve flag officers. Flag officers rank higher than captain. Commissioned Officers usually have at least a bachelor's degree, but a good number of officers have their master's or higher degrees. Their job is to carry out leadership and administrative operations. CO's have authority over all enlisted personnel plus other officers under their command. Along with greater managerial responsibilities, commissioned officers also enjoy a higher pay and ranking as well as more privileges. Some officers function as doctors and lawyers.

Enlisted members can become non-commissioned officers (NCO) by advancing through the ranks and then completing officer training. Non-commissioned officers are also referred to as a "non-com" or "sub-officer." Sergeant, Corporal, and Petty Officer are non-commissioned officers. They receive orders from officers and make sure those orders are followed through by lower-ranked military personnel. The major difference between a CO and an NCO is that CO's have a higher level of authority.

REQUIREMENTS

Each branch of the military has different requirements; however, they all share the same basic qualifications. The minimum qualifications to serve in any branch of the United States Armed Forces are that one must be a U.S. citizen or permanent resident alien, be at least 17 years of age, have a high school diploma, and pass a medical exam. Each branch of service also has its own height and weight requirements. The Armed Services Vocational Aptitude Battery (ASVAB) is a test that determines what a recruit will do in the military. The higher a recruit scores, the more options he/she will have when beginning his/her military career. The ASVAB aids recruits in deciding what military job would be best for them. ASVAB preparation and practice tests are available at military.com. Practice tests are also available at a local recruiting office. However, special preparation is not required. ASVAB tests math, English, and science skills, coding speed, auto and shop information, mechanical comprehension, assembling objects, and electronics information. ASVAB scores are commonly referred to as the Armed Force Qualification Test (AFQT) score. The AFQT determines if a recruit can enlist in the U.S. Army or not. Military Entrance Processing Station (MEPS) is where applicants complete the enlistment process. MEPS determines if a recruit can serve in the United States Armed Forces under military regulations, policies, and federal law. MEPS includes a medical evaluation. After the physical requirements and ASVAB standard of the desired branch of service are met, a service liaison counselor explains job opportunities and recruits take the oath of enlistment.

The Air Force protects domestic and foreign interests of the United States with a concentration on air power. To join the Air Force, one must be between 17-27 years old, have no more than two dependents, and score at least a 50 on the ASVAB. The Air Force can assign jobs to recruits while at MEPS, but will usually ask recruits to make a list of desired vocations and then put recruits on a waiting list.

The Army, the oldest branch, guards the safety of America along with its resources. To join the Army, one must be between 17-34 years old, have no more than two dependents, and receive at least a 31 on the ASVAB.

The Coast Guard exists within the Department of Homeland Security and is responsible for protecting the general public, the environment, and the American economic and security concerns that persist in any maritime area, including U.S. coasts, ports, inland waterways, and international waters. To join the Coast Guard, one must be between 17-39 years old, have no more than two dependents, pass the ASVAB with a score of at least 45, and be willing to serve on or around the water. During wartime, the Coast Guard becomes part of the Navy.

The Navy preserves the right to trade and travel liberally across the oceans. It by and large safeguards

overseas national interests. To join the Navy, one must be between 17-34 years old and score at least a 50 on the ASVAB. The Navy gives recruits a job while at MEPS.

The Marine Corps works closely with the Navy and is often first to fight in combat situations. To join the Marines one must be between 17-29 years old, meet exact physical, metal, and moral standards, and pass the ASVAB with a score no less than 32.

All age limits may vary based on active-duty, prior service, or reserve. Applicants 17 years of age require parental consent. Women have contributed to the military since the American Revolution in 1775, where they served as nurses and caretakers. However, it wasn't until 2013 that women were permitted to fight in combat roles. Women are eligible to enlist in all occupational fields in the military with a few exceptions. In the Marines, they cannot enlist in the combat arms specialties in infantry, tank, and amphibian tractor crew. Women also cannot serve in the Navy Seals or on submarines.

TRAINING

Once a recruit has decided to enlist, they must begin to train for their career. Basic Training is usually referred to as "boot camp." Basic Training is seven to twelve weeks, depending on the service branch, of rigorous physical exercise. On top of building physical strength, Basic Training builds mental strength. Recruits learn about military history and tactics. About 90 percent of recruits complete Basic Training despite the challenging nature of the program. Preparing for boot camp can help make training easier. Learning military jargon, exercising regularly, and practicing basic speed training routines can help recruits make good impressions on their drill instructors as well as lessen the labor of this high-stress environment.

Advanced Individual Training (AIT) is the next step of training. AIT prepares recruits for specific career fields. Learning takes place in classrooms at skill-training school and in field exercises. At AIT, recruits learn their Military Occupational Specialty (MOS). AIT can last anywhere from two to twelve months. The training takes places at various military sites across the country.

THINGS TO CONSIDER

Taking orders without question is heavily emphasized in the military. Questioning orders can put lives at risk. Non-conformists may have trouble giving up their basic liberties at certain times. Sedition is punished with dishonorable discharge. G.I. stands for "Government

Issue," meaning enlisted members are property of the government. Once officially enlisted, there is no turning back. A majority of first-term enlistments entail an obligation to four active years and two inactive years. Contracts are not easy to get out of. The only time a recruit can reconsider joining the reserve is after his or her service term. Moving also plays a large role in the military life.

LONG-TERM EFFECTS

Joining the service is a life-altering experience. Service members grow and develop as individuals while they contribute to their country. Joining the military whips people into shape. Recruits leave in peak physical condition. Discipline is a major concept taught to service members. Appropriate conduct is stressed. People that have served are not viewed as lazy in a business setting; in fact, many people respect veterans in a professional setting. As self-confidence and decisiveness are heavily emphasized in the military, these two traits become part of a recruit's strengths. Members learn to work as part of a group or to assume leadership roles. The military provides college tuition support for service members during and after serving. Service members are provided with free medical care for themselves, and are eligible to get health insurance for the rest of their family at a low deductible cost. In addition, service members are offered life insurance and retirement plans from the military. The military gives 30 paid vacation days per year to each service member. At no cost, service members can travel on available military aircraft and stay at bases overseas.

Members join at their own risk. Sometimes soldiers return home wounded or don't return at all. Veterans can suffer from an array of psychological disorders such as post-traumatic stress disorder (PTSD), anxiety, and depression. As a coping mechanism, some turn to alcohol or drugs and develop a substance addiction.

READY TO MAKE THE COMMITMENT?

If you are seriously interested in pursuing a career in the military, contact a recruiter. A recruiter can answer any questions you may have about serving in the military and help you with the enlistment process.

FURTHER READING

Becoming a military officer. (n.d.). Retrieved from: http://todaysmilitary.com/joining/becoming-a-military-officer. This article reviews the benefits of being an officer and the necessary steps to become one. It explores options for recruits, such as academics and ROTC.

O'Brien, Marco. (n.d.). What you should ask the recruiter. Retrieved from: http://www.military.com/join-armed-forces/questions-when-joining-the-military.html?comp=7000023451786&rank=1. This article discusses important questions that recruits should ask their recruiter. It also lists items needed to start the enlistment process. Furthermore, the author explains that recruiters need full knowledge of a recruit's medical and legal record.

Substance Abuse and Mental Health Services Administration. (2014, September 29) Veterans and Military Families. Retrieved from: http://www.samhsa.gov/veterans-military-families. This article gives the facts and figures regarding how many veterans are affected by mental disorders. It also discusses how the mental health of military families can be affected.

Jessica Vitale

SEE ALSO: Military Families; Leadership Skills

Living with allergies

Allergies are caused by an overreaction of the immune system to an allergen, which can be many substances that are foreign to the body. Allergens are usually not toxic and only pose a threat when a person is prone to these immune system overreactions. Due to the immune system being a large factor in a person's allergies, there is research that connects allergies to a person's stress level. The treatment used by a healthcare practitioner will vary depending on the type, duration and severity of the allergies. Symptoms of these allergies may be constant or vary depending on the concentration of the allergen they come in contact with and some allergies will have different symptoms than others. Anaphylaxis, the most severe form of allergic reaction, can be fatal if not treated immediately.

INTRODUCTION

The topic of allergies is relatable to close to 40% of the population worldwide who suffer from some kind of hypersensitivity or symptoms of allergies from a certain allergen. The most common kinds of allergens are common substances such as pollen, pet dander, or certain kinds of foods. The first studies of allergies were conducted relatively recently, the conceptual idea of an allergy only first being thought of in 1906 by Clemens von Pirquet. The hypersensitivity that was observed after overexposure to an allergen such as pollen or foods was known as an "allergy." In the last century, different kinds of testing (skin and blood testing for example) have become available in order to prevent any kind of life threatening or otherwise dangerous allergic reactions and treatment options have not only become available, but have become extremely popular as daily medications. Without medications, different parts of the body can be affected by the allergens. The nose can undergo swelling and sneezing, often with an allergy to pollen or pet dander. During these reactions, the eyes may experience itching, redness and watering. Skin may experience rashes, hives or itching. The most dangerous symptoms are related to the airways. Coughing and wheezing may be signs of constriction of the airways, which are common signs of anaphylaxis. Treatment of allergies can vary but the most obvious form of treatment is complete avoidance of the allergen. In the cases of unavoidable contact with the allergen, an antihistamine or emergency measures such as epinephrine may be administered.

CLINICAL IMPLICATIONS OF STRESS'S EFFECT ON ALLERGIES

Stress is the body's response to external stimuli that may be threatening or overwhelming to a person. Research has shown that if a person is stressed, they may be affected physically as well as emotionally and mentally. Physical problems that result from stress may be caused by a decrease in immune system function. This phenomenon happens as a result of the "fight or flight" reaction. The body focuses on the problem at hand and some other internal processes are neglected. Hormones are released by the sympathetic nervous system such as adrenaline, which can provide strength in times of acute stress and emergency situations. Although this is a useful adaptation, in times of constant stress, it may have negative effects.

Cortisol's purpose in the body is to suppress inflammation and is the regulator of the response of the body to stress. The body can become accustomed to levels of cortisol in the body, however, causing cortisol to lose its effectiveness. During times of chronic stress, the body's response to stress is skewed and the body is more susceptible to experiencing hypersensitivity to certain allergens and showing symptoms of allergies. For example, a child whose parents are going through a divorce and are experiencing an extremely stressful home life may be more

likely to suffer from allergies. Conversely, when a person is experiencing positive emotions, their body responds more positively to allergens.

MANAGING SYMPTOMS AND LIVING WITH ALLERGIES

Histamines are chemicals made by the immune system, which allow the body to protect itself against foreign bodies that may be harmful. The overreaction of the body causing the allergy occurs when these histamines overreact to an allergen. Airborne allergens such as pollen, pet dander or dust come in contact with the body through the airways and eyes. Because of this, common symptoms may include itching, watering and redness in the eyes. A person can experience sneezing or runny nose, coughing, wheezing or tightening of the airways among many other possible symptoms. Antihistamines are usually used to treat these kinds of allergies. Prescription medications as well as "over the counter" medications can be used to treat these allergies. Antihistamines are used to block histamines and therefore block the ongoing allergic reaction. Antihistamines can also be used as a preventative measure to stop seasonal allergies that are pervasive. Regularly taking an antihistamine-based medication has been shown to improve seasonal allergies overall. Food allergies are present in only 5% of children and 4% of adults. Food allergies take place when there is an "overreaction" of the immune system to a certain kind of food. When this happens, the body fights off the food as if it is a dangerous substance when in reality, it isn't. The symptoms caused by this allergic reaction can be far ranging. Mild food allergies may consist of rashes or itching but more severe allergies may lead to anaphylaxis, which hinders breathing, leads to a change in heart rate and blood pressure, may include gastrointestinal distress and may cause death. Injecting epinephrine from an EpiPen can delay the reaction and allow a person to be treated for the allergy immediately. Those with severe allergies are always urged to carry an EpiPen at all times.

Skin reactions are extremely common in allergies and represent the majority of allergic reactions. Kinds of rashes, itching, swelling, redness, inflammation or a bumpy texture are common signs of allergic skin reactions. One usual form of skin allergy is the condition eczema. Skin may dry out, becoming itchy and irritated and inflamed. If the area becomes infected, fluid-filled sections of skin may begin appearing. Urticaria, otherwise known as hives, is a condition involving large and often itchy bumps on the skin that may last from hours to weeks. Urticaria may take place as a result of any kind of allergen, including a rare reaction resulting from a sensitivity to hot and cold.

FUTURE DIRECTIONS

In dealing with allergies, consulting a doctor or allergist is recommended, but not always necessary. By involving a professional in the care of allergies, an appropriate treatment plan and the full extent of options can be provided. Treatment for allergies can completely rectify potentially life-threatening symptoms. Being fully educated about allergies may also help a person understand their own individual health needs regarding their allergies.

FURTHER READING

Allergy Statistics | AAAAI. (n.d.). Retrieved May 22, 2015. Retrieved from: http://www.aaaai.org/about-the-aaaai/newsroom/allergy-statistics.aspx. This article discusses statistical facts about allergies in America. The author goes into depth and talks about each type of allergy, allergic reaction, and its statistics in America.

Montoro, J., Mullol, J., Jáuregui, I., Dávila, I., Ferrer, M., Bartra, J., ... & Valero, A. (2009). Stress and allergy. *J Investig Allergol Clin Immunol*, 19(Suppl 1), 40-47. This article discusses the biomedical and psychological aspects of allergies. This article discusses the relationship between mental and emotional stress and the physical aspects of allergic reactions.

The fight or flight response: Our body's response to stress. (n.d.). Retrieved May 28, 2015, from: http://www.youngdiggers.com.au/fight-or-flight. This article speaks about the human fight or flight reaction. The article discusses stress and how the body handles emergency situations. Understanding how the body processes outside dangers is important to understanding the body's ability to deal with allergens.

What are allergies? (n.d.). Retrieved May 25, 2015, from: http://www.medicalnewstoday.com/articles/264419.php. This article includes in-depth information about what an allergy really entails and why they occur. This article also talks about the common symptoms of different kinds of allergies.

Christina Barrett

SEE ALSO: Allergies; Rashes; Stress

On becoming a mother

Pregnancy is always a time of transition, but becoming pregnant as a teenager may come with extra challenges. One of those challenges involves overcoming existing stereotypes people seem to have regarding teen motherhood. Although raising a child is a huge responsibility, many teens and young adults have raised healthy and happy children through positive parenting. During pregnancy and beyond, familial support is essential. Continuing one's education is also important. Although economic support may be needed initially, by getting a college or graduate degree, young parents can create an economically stable environment for their growing child.

INTRODUCTION

Becoming a mother at any age is a transition, but becoming a mother as a teenager comes with some unique challenges. These challenges are not roadblocks. However, knowledge of the challenges is important so that they can be faced realistically.

One of the biggest challenges is overcoming the stigma that comes with being a teen mother, as many individuals seem to feel as if teens are physically, economically, academically, and emotionally unprepared for the responsibilities that come with being a good parent. Many people also get their information about teen parenting from the mainstream media or from reality television shows, both of which have agendas of their own. Thankfully, the stigma of being a young mother has decreased in recent years, as individuals have generally become more accepting of diverse mothering experiences. The "perfect mother" is no longer the middle class, well-educated mother who is married and has a home with a large backyard. You will soon find out that there are many ways to be a good mother, and that no mother or situation is ever perfect.

The day that you find out you are become a mother may paradoxically be one of the most exciting and scariest days of your life. Exciting because a baby will be born, and you will be the one responsible for it; scary for that exact same reason. Know and make peace with the fact that your own childhood has ended at that moment. Life is not about you anymore... instead, it is about the child that will soon be placed in your arms. This does not mean you will not be able to achieve all the many goals and dreams that you have for yourself. It just means that there will be another person to consider when thinking about those dreams and goals.

FIND YOUR SUPPORT PEOPLE

These people may initially include your partner, your parents, your friends, and the OB/GYN or midwife that you choose. Make sure that their support is unconditional and focused on the health and safety of you and your baby. Support received from your family is important, even if the news of the pregnancy wasn't initially taken well.

If you have a partner, make sure that your partner is on board with the decisions you make for your child. If your partner is not on board, for whatever reason, be prepared to make decisions (and parent), on your own. You can indeed do anything you set your mind to, with a partner or alone. Your child will become your biggest motivation, as you will want to create the best life possible for him or her.

Later on, support may be found in those you meet through your experience in being a mother. Your child's pediatrician can be a great support to you, so choose him or her well. Find a pediatrician that you respect, and who is non judgmental and open minded about your role as a young mother. Share any questions or concerns you may have about your baby with this doctor. If you choose to breastfeed, your local chapter of La Leche League can be a wonderful place to meet other moms and find support and acceptance.

TAKE CARE OF YOURSELF

It is so important that you take care of yourself during the pregnancy, because by taking care of yourself you are also caring for the baby growing inside you. Make prenatal care a priority, and attend all your scheduled doctor or midwife's appointments. Pay attention to your diet, making sure you are eating healthfully and regularly. Make sure you hydrate properly, and take any prenatal vitamins or supplements prescribed to you by your obstetrician or midwife. Sign up for and attend any labor/delivery or birth preparation classes that are available to you. Attend new mother/new parent classes as well. Take time to learn about what is happening to you at each stage of your pregnancy. Books like *What to Expect When You Are Expecting* are really helpful here. There are also apps you can download that take you through what is happening during each week of your pregnancy, focusing on the baby's growth in utero as well as the physical changes you should be expecting as the pregnancy progresses.

CONTINUE YOUR EDUCATION

Make plans to continue your education while pregnant and as a new mother. If you are in high school, continue attending classes as far into your pregnancy as possible. After that, make plans to make up work during the time you may be at home after the baby is born. Homeschooling or online schooling is also an option, and may allow you to spend time with your baby after he or she is born even as you take classes and work through high school.

If you are of college age, do not let having a baby affect your decision to continue your education. In fact, continuing your education may be the best decision you ever make for both you and your child. Many colleges and universities have child care centers on campus, where trained child care workers or early childhood education majors will watch your baby while you take classes. Most colleges also offer online classes, so you can continue your education while being home with your child. If finances are an issue, contact your schools' Financial Aid Office. Federal financial aid is always available in the form of loans, grants, and scholarships.

MONEY DOES MATTER, BUT LESS THAN YOU THINK

One of the biggest concerns of any parent centers on how they will "pay" for their child. The truth is, babies are not that expensive. If you choose to breastfeed your baby, you will not only be providing him/her with superior nutrition, but you will also save money by not having to buy formula or bottles. Diapers do cost money, but many diaper companies will send coupons and special deals if you call and explain your financial situation. Many second hand stores sell baby clothing, towels, and crib sheets very inexpensively. Baby nurseries can be created on a budget, and secondhand cribs and changing tables are easy to find.

The one thing that is suggested you do purchase new is a car seat. Almost all health insurance companies, including Medicaid, will offer car seats for free for pregnant or new mothers. State police and fire departments may also offer car seats free to low income mothers, so do call them as well.

Your local WIC (Women, Infant, and Children) office may also be able to provide some financial support. WIC is a federally funded supplemental nutrition program that can offer supplemental food, health care referrals and nutrition assistance to pregnant, nursing, or non nursing mothers with children up to the age of five years old.

MAKE A PLAN TO RAISE YOUR SOCIOECONOMIC STATUS

Although raising a baby itself can be done on a budget, costs do increase as your child gets older. Make a plan to get your family into as positive a financial situation as possible during the years your child is young. An easy way to do this is to continue your education, as a college or graduate degree can lead to a higher income, and more career prestige and freedom later on. While you are continuing your education, take on a small part time job, do freelance work, or babysit other children for extra money. Remember, mothering a young child never closes off opportunities. Instead, mothering motivates you to become a strong, successful, independent woman so you can be a good role model for your child.

OTHER TIPS

Challenge other people's assumptions about what teen pregnancy looks like by constructing pregnancy and young motherhood as a positive experience. Devote this period in your life to becoming the best mother you can possibly be. Read and play with your child often, as quality time spent with your child increases a child's cognitive, linguistic, and social intelligence. When you practice positive, loving, attentive parenting, you end up with a positive, loving, attentive child.

Before you know it, your child will be a young adult, and your time spent actively mothering will decrease. Take time to enjoy these precious days.

FURTHER READING

La Leche League International. (2014). Retrieved from http://www.llli.org/.. La Leche League's mission is to provide information, guidance, and support for the pregnant and breastfeeding mother. LLL's website is full of information regarding breastfeeding and parenting, and local La Leche League meetings are a great way to meet new and pregnant mothers in your area. La Leche League leaders are also available via phone 24 hours per day to answer questions and concerns regarding breastfeeding.

Murkoff, H. & Mazel, S. (2008). What to expect when you are expecting. New York: Workman Publishing. A must have for pregnant women. Explains week by week fetal development, as well as the physical and emotional changes that happen during pregnancy. Addresses almost all pertinent questions about pregnancy and childbirth, including issues surrounding nutrition, sexuality, and lifestyle trends.

Vianna, N. (2014, May 30). Natasha Vianna: Changing the meaning of teenage motherhood. [Video File]. Retrieved from https://www.youtube.com/watch?v=MJUS4r_41fY..This TED talk by Natasha Vianna centers on her experiences as a teen mom. Within the talk, she discusses gender expectations with regards to sexuality, her experience being pregnant in high school, and the overall stigma that still surrounds teenage mothers. She concludes the talk by asking society for more open mindedness and acceptance of young mothers.

Gina Riley

SEE ALSO: Pregnancy Health Myths; Teen Pregnancy

Owning a credit card

This article is a brief overview of the world of credit cards. Several different topics will be addressed including: (1) what is a credit card (2) the advantages of a credit card (3) the disadvantages of a credit card (4) how to choose the right credit card and (5) what to do once you have the credit card. When finished with this article, a list of further resources will be provided in order to enable you to do your own research in addition to this article.

INTRODUCTION

The goal of this article is to educate you, the reader, on the world of credit cards and how to live safely in this world. Everyone has heard the horror stories of someone winding up with thousands in credit card debt and losing everything or of being taken advantage of by the credit card companies. The way to avoid this is to educate yourself on credit cards and the dangers they can bring about. Although there are dangers to having a credit card, do not be discouraged from applying for a credit card, they can do as much good as they can do bad. The important part is to be educated on the topic and to be smart about your finances. Hopefully this article will lead you on the path of good credit score and a secure financial future

WHAT IS A CREDIT CARD?

What is credit? According to *Economics for Everybody* (1976), credit is "buying it now and paying for it later", essentially it is a form of borrowing. When using a credit to buy items you are receiving merchandise that you agree to pay for later while in the meantime the credit card company gives you the means to initially afford this merchandise. Basically you are using the money of the credit card company to buy something that you don't have the money for. One of the most common forms of credit is the credit card. Credit cards, also known as "plastic money" can be used at many different venues including airlines, restaurants, and stores.

ADVANTAGES OF OWNING A CREDIT CARD

Credit cards allow a purchaser to buy what they want when they don't have the funds. This can include items like cars, food, electronics, or vacations. This can make purchases a lot easier for the consumer, giving them the opportunity to buy something they may want or even need when they do not have the money. Depending on how responsibly you deal with your payments, your credit card can establish your financial character and credibility. This means that if you have a good credit history, like keeping up with payments, companies like banks and car dealerships are more willing to give you a loan on a car knowing that you are dependable enough to make the payments. A credit card holder is also ready for emergencies. For example, if you were to have engine trouble while driving on the highway and need to be towed but have no cash. Having the credit card allows you to be able to put the charge on the credit card and pay for the purchase later. With the use of credit cards, you don't have to carry a lot of cash or any cash at all, therefore lowering your chances of having your money stolen. Credit cards are highly convenient, taking out a card and swiping it in one easy motion versus taking out cash, counting it, and making sure you get the right change back. The process is a lot faster with a credit card.

DISADVANTAGES OF OWNING A CREDIT CARD

Credit cards often encourage a person to spend beyond their means. Due to the fact that all you have to do is swipe a card and you get these items, a person will often think that they have a lot more money to spend then they actually have. It is very easy to keep swiping the card without realizing how much you are spending, it isn't until the bill comes that you realize how much you have actually spent. Along with that, a person can easily neglect to pay credit card bills until eventually the payments pile up put you find yourself in debt. Sometimes the bills add up to be much more than the person can pay off. When carrying a credit card, you run the risk of identity theft.

Technology has become very advanced, making it easy for someone to get your credit card information and use that info to make purchases under your identity. When this happens a person has basically stolen your identity and is most likely accumulating thousands of dollars in debt that you will potentially be stuck with if it can't be proven that it wasn't you making the purchases.

HOW TO CHOOSE THE RIGHT CREDIT CARD

There are several different types of credit card, which one is best depends on your current financial situation. Each type of credit card offers different terms, payment plans and fees. The law requires that credit card companies must provide their like Annual Percentage Rate (APR) which is the annual interest rate you will be charged on the balance on the credit card. Most credit card companies charge more than one APR depending on the type of credit card it is and the transaction that it will be used for. It is important to pay attention to the types of fees and charges that each credit card carries. Essentially the type of credit card you choose depends on your financial situation and what you plan to use the credit card for. The best plan is to research the companies you are thinking of applying to, make sure to read all of the terms and conditions and then use that information to determine which is best for someone in your financial situation. Although it is important to choose a credit card that will suit you best, once you choose it doesn't mean you're stuck with that card forever. There is always the possibility of switching to another credit card if the one you're using isn't working for you. For example if the interest rates become too high on a certain credit card, it may be beneficial to switch to another credit card with lower interest rates. While this can sometimes be a complicated process, it is important to remember that you have the means to switch to another card if it will suit you better. Be cautious about "interest free" or "no payment period" if you don't pay off the full balance before the end of the grace period all interest is compounded on that day.

WHAT TO DO ONCE YOU HAVE A CREDIT CARD

Never pay only the minimum payment; the smallest possible amount you are allowed to pay on the bill. Many companies will allow you to pay the minimum balance of the balance you owe the company. The problem is that there are interest charges on the remaining balance. Although you may think you're buying a lot and only paying a minimum charge for it, you will in fact wind up paying much more than what the original item cost due to the interest you are paying on the existing balance. For example you buy a TV on credit and start paying the minimum payments every month, in addition to those payments you will also be paying interest on the rest of the bill that you still haven't paid off. The bigger the balance, the more interest. It will take a longer amount of time to pay the bill like this and with the addition of interest payments you will wind up paying a considerably larger sum than what the TV actually cost. If you were to pay off the bill in payments larger than the minimum amount it would take a smaller amount of time and the less interest to pay off the bill.

Always keep yourself updated on the status of your account. Most credit card companies have an app or online portal where you can go online and keep track of your charges. It is very easy to buy a lot of items on credit and then lose track of how much you are actually spending. Don't let this balance get too high; the higher it is, the more interest you pay. It is also important to keep track of your credit card balance in order to ensure that no unexpected charges are accruing on your card.

Join a credit monitoring company. These companies are designed to monitor your credit card transactions in order to prevent rogue charges and identity theft. Some well-known and dependable companies include Equifax and Transunion. Both are easily accessible online and will provide information on how to utilize their services.

Keep track of your credit score. Your credit score is a three digit number that keeps track of how well you handle your credit and debt. The higher the credit score, the better. A good credit score is usually 720 or above and will enable you to be a better candidate for things like loans. There are many credible websites that will give you your credit score for free. If your credit score is not good, then it is vital that you work to improve your credit score by paying your bills on time, keep your balances low, and avoid opening new credit accounts unless absolutely necessary.

Be aware of any fees that your credit card company is charging. This includes fees like late charges and interest charges. Companies can change their policy at any time and start charging you with the new policy terms that may include charges you weren't aware of. It is important to look over your credit card bill and be aware of any unexpected charges.

FURTHER READING

Antell, G., Harris, W., & Gómez, C. (1976). Chapter 12: Using consumer credit wisely. In *Economics for everybody* (3rd ed). New York: Amsco School Publications. *Economics for Everybody* provides a simple explanation as to what credit is. It provides clear and concise explanations of what credit is and how to use it. The pages selected specifically go into detail about credit cards and their uses as well as their advantages and disadvantages.

Geffner, M. (2011, January 3). 6 facts about credit card APR. *Bankrate*. Retrieved from: http://www.bankrate.com/finance/credit-cards/6-facts-about-credit-card-apr-1.aspx   This website explains what APR is and the different types of APR a credit card holder may encounter. It explains the difference between APR and fees, how and if an APR rate may decrease, and how to pay an APR off.

Micieli, J. (2015, April 28). How to review your credit report. *Credit Karma*. Retrieved from: https://www.creditkarma.com/article/how-to-review-your-credit-report This article explains what a credit report is, how reports may differ, and how to avoid negative reports. The author gives several solutions to avoid varying credit reports and how to fix those reports should they be misconstrued.

Sherrier, J. (n.d.). Credit card glossary terms to know for first-time card users. *CreditCards.com*. Retrieved from: http://www.creditcards.com/credit-card-news/credit-card-glossary-terms-first-credit-card.php. This website provides a list of terms for first time card users. It is a good resource to help understand the world of credit cards and the specific language involved in order to be better prepared for owning a credit card.

Julia D'Alessio

SEE ALSO: Budgeting; Identity Theft; Money; Spam and Scams

Paying for college

As tuition continues to increase, it becomes more arduous to amass the funds necessary to finance a college education. More students enroll in higher education each year to expand their horizons. The various forms of financial aid can serve to abate economic struggles based on the information provided in a Free Application for Federal Aid. Grants and scholarships do not need to be repaid while student loans must be paid with interest. The most effective form of financial aid is being prepared to cover college expenses.

INTRODUCTION

Financing a college education is one of the most common problems facing most American families. For some it is seen as merely turning over hard-earned dollars to already well-endowed universities. It is not uncommon for financially unstable families with members in college to resort to scrimping on food and sacrificing necessities. Highly intellectual, qualified students from underprivileged backgrounds sometimes cede prestigious educations at renowned colleges and universities, such as Ivy Leagues, because of the inadequacy of some financial aid programs or because of the notoriety of extracting student loans.

According to Sandy Baum, a senior fellow at the Urban Institute in Washington, D.C., who specializes in college tuition trends, family income has remained generally static in recent years as tuition continues to become a larger percentage of family annual expenses. Almost a century ago, most Americans believed that a college education was exclusive to the wealthy aristocracy. The Servicemen's Readjustment Act of 1944, also known as the G.I. Bill, served to amend this belief and increase enrollment into higher education. The doctrine provided World War II veterans with funds for college education, increasing university enrollment by roughly 2.5 million students nationwide. The unexpected success of the bill galvanized the federal government's decision to institute the National Defense Education Act (NDEA) in 1958, which provided opportunities for scholarships and loans, further expanding college enrollment. In the 1970s, pervasive inflation deteriorated public and federal investment in higher education. The immediate struggle for colleges to recoup their dissolved funding has been the most influential circumstance in increased college tuition over the years, proving that costly tuition is simply in the interest of the institution.

It has become increasingly paramount that students and families take conscientious steps in financing college education. The continuous evolution of education has created more respective college expenses, such as on-campus living, daily expenses for food and clothing, and involvement in extracurricular activities. Recognizing the dangers of debt can be a fundamental step in managing the college financial process.

WHY PEOPLE AGREE TO PAY FOR COLLEGE

College is undeniably a major financial investment. However, with ever-changing cultural and societal values, Americans have learned to esteem intellect more than opulence. New data from the United States Department of Labor has revealed a gradual increase in college enrollment rates since the correlational study began in 1959. An increased demand for higher education is likely reflective of the unsteady job market. A Bachelor's Degree is a corporeal job guarantee. Very few jobs provide self-sustaining incomes on a high-school diploma. The American attitude has become "spend money now, make money later."

Beyond these practical vindications to consider a college education lie more personal and self-actualizing reasons. Higher education is an opportunity for personal as well as intellectual growth as the student expands his or her horizons. Taking college-level courses in a campus setting contributes to expanded knowledge of the community as well as one's own interests. The student receives a unique opportunity to cogitate his or her life goals and to utilize the resources provided by the institution to achieve said goals.

FINANCIAL AID AND FAFSA

According to the New York State Financial Aid Administrators Association, financial aid is a sum of money offered by a number of various sources to help a student cover his or her college expenditures. Financial aid is available to all students and can cover tuition, additional fees, books, supplies, room and board, and transportation. The primary determinants of financial aid are the federal government, state governments, colleges and universities, and private institutions. Need-based financial aid programs are based on the respective college's tuition and the family's financial status. To be eligible for financial aid in most colleges and universities, a student must be a U.S. citizen with a valid Social Security Number or an eligible non-citizen, have a high school diploma or GED certificate, be associated with a suitable major, and maintain good academic status.

Each family is expected to contribute a percentage to a student's college tuition. How much a family commits depends upon its financial status and is known as the Expected Family Contribution (EFC). A student's EFC is determined by the Board of Education when the Free Application for Federal Student Aid (FAFSA) is proffered. The financial information provided by the FAFSA is analyzed by a federal processor and results are sent to the financial aid offices of the colleges and universities chosen by the student. A completed FAFSA that is submitted by the requisitioned deadline is the first step to being considered for federal financial aid. Generally, the FAFSA may be filed with the Department of Education beginning January of each year. Missing deadlines can harm financial aid opportunities and result in higher education expenses.

GRANTS

Grants are a form of financial aid most often determined by financial status and administered on federal, state, or college levels. Grants do not have to be repaid unless the student leaves the school before a certain enrollment period ends. Some federal grants and most state grants have less strict income criteria and are more concerned with the student's major, yet financial background is significant. FAFSA is a sufficient source of information for some federal grant programs, while others require distinct applications.

A Federal Pell Grant is given to undergraduate students from low-income families. According to the Federal Student Aid Office, the maximum Federal Pell Grant award will be $5,775 for the 2015 - 2016 school year. This grant can be given for a maximum of twelve semesters through deduction of school costs or direct payment. Students who have received a Federal Pell Grant and are experiencing serious financial adversity will receive a college-based Federal Supplemental Educational Opportunity Grant (FSEOG), providing between $100 and $4,000 per year in aid. Administration of FSEOGs are on a first-come, first-serve basis as each college receives limited funding for this form of aid.

SCHOLARSHIPS

A scholarship is a form of financial aid that may be awarded by a college, business, association, institution, or private industry based on need, academic merit, or proficiency in certain interests. Scholarships do not have to be repaid and are crucial to bridging the gap between college tuition and EFC. Because a wide variety of scholarships are available, all students are encouraged to search for scholarship eligibility in all areas, primarily by filing the FAFSA. Even students from high-income backgrounds who do not think they are eligible for financial aid should file the FAFSA annually in order to maintain academic scholarships.

STUDENT LOANS

Extracting a student loan involves borrowing money that must eventually be repaid with interest. According to the College Board, interest is the additional fee for borrowing money that is charged usually once a month and is equal to a percentage of the amount borrowed. The more money borrowed, the higher the interest rate and the more the student must repay after graduation. Excessively borrowing money can lead to debt, so it is important for loans to be withdrawn only when imperative. The two main options for student loans are federal student loans and private loans.

For most, federal student loans are the primary option as they are usually less expensive and are easier to repay. Federal loans allow for a six-month grace period after the student graduates or leaves school. Most federal loans have fixed interest rates and flexible repayment terms. The loan is paid in monthly installments that are fairly adaptable based on income and financial adversity. According to the Consumer Financial Protection Bureau, interest rates are reliable and range from 3.86% to 6.41% of the amount borrowed. Federal Perkins Loans have a 5% interest rate and are endowed by colleges predominantly to students of very low income backgrounds. Federal Direct Subsidized Loans, also based on financial need, have interest that is paid by the government while the student is in college and a borrowing limit that increases for each year of schooling the student completes. Federal Direct Unsubsidized Loans, for which all students are qualified, add interest to the amount borrowed and do not have to be paid until after graduation. Federal Parent or Graduate PLUS Loans allow parents or graduates to borrow total college tuition minus financial aid or scholarships received by the student. Almost all students are applicable to receive federal loans, yet those with greater financial adversity will receive lower interest rates. The amount of money borrowed is limited to the cost of each respective college, yet more specific limits vary based on financial status and the type of loan. A portion of wages and tax refunds may be assumed by the government if payment responsibilities are neglected. On average, an undergraduate student can expect $5,500 to $12,000 per year of student loans, while a graduate can expect $8,000 to $25,000 per year. Options for federal student loans should be taken advantage of foremost. Special regard should be given to Federal Perkins Loans and Federal Direct Subsidized Loans.

Private loans, most commonly offered by banks, are generally more expensive than federal loans and offer payment terms with very limited flexibility. Private loans allow the student to borrow more money with lower interest rates based on the ability to repay. Grace period, interest rates, and loan limits vary and are often subject to change during the student's years in college. Banks and similar financial institutions charge the highest interest rates as they are based on credit. Some private organizations and colleges offer lower interest rates, sometimes less than those of federal loans. Interest is always charged while the student is in school. Private loans may charge other fees in addition to interest. Eligibility for private loans is based upon the type of loan. State Agency Loans are endowed by the state to students attending a college in that state. Traditional Bank Loans, endowed by commercial banks, are the most common and require a co-signer, who is legally obligated to pay the loan in the case that the student is unable. School loans are specific to each college and have fixed interest rates. It is recommended that the student explores all other possible options, such as scholarships or a low-cost school, before extracting a private loan.

PREPAREDNESS

A national study of college students and parents conducted by Sallie Mae found that fewer than two in five families had a proposition for paying their child's college tuition before he or she enrolled. Students from families who planned ahead were more likely to pursue a Bachelor's Degree and less likely to narrow school choice based on tuition. Planning to pay for college provides an opportunity to utilize a variety of resources, such as college cost calculators or scholarship programs. Saving money now will make financing a college education less arduous.

FURTHER READING

Federal Student Aid: An Office of the U.S. Department of Education. (n.d.). Retrieved May 26, 2015, from: https://studentaid.ed.gov/sa/. This website provides information about the types of financial aid and determines eligibility. It offers help in completing the FAFSA, repaying loans, and preparing for college.

How America pays for college. (2014). Retrieved May 29, 2015, from: http://news.salliemae.com/files/doc_library/file/HowAmericaPaysforCollege2014FNL.pdf This document provides an in-depth analysis of how American families invest in undergraduate education. The study was conducted by Sallie Mae, a financial services company specializing in education.

Paying for college. Consumer Financial Protection Bureau. (n.d.). Retrieved May 29, 2015, from: http://www.consumerfinance.gov/paying-for-college/. This is the official website of the Consumer Financial Protection Bureau. It provides information regarding student loans and banking and allows you to compare financial aid offers or repay student debt.

Student Financial Aid Services Inc. (n.d.). Retrieved May 26, 2015, from: https://www.fafsa.com/home. This is the official FAFSA website, which provides FAFSA services and a thorough explanation of student financial aid. A list of FAFSA deadlines is included.

What is financial aid? | NYSFAAA. (2015). Retrieved May 28, 2015, from: http://www.nysfaaa.org/docs/student_family/what_is_finaid.html. This website explains the significance of financial aid and lists all types of grants, scholarships, and loans.

Mira Mikhael

SEE ALSO: Finding the Right College; First Generation College Students; Money

Staying fit freshman year

Balancing weight throughout different stages of life is difficult to do. Individuals can go through many different times in their lives that can greatly affect the way they take care of themselves. Often times when people become concerned about their weight, they will start to weigh themselves. When stepping onto a scale it can be intimidating, but it increases awareness of how to manage weight. Once the problem is known, then a solution can be brought about. For most people, working towards a goal to lose weight is found to be hard. The key to reaching that goal is motivation and consistency.

INTRODUCTION

Occasionally, when transitioning into different stages of life the activities or sports that one once participated in are no longer important. The things that were once important could have been a big factor in staying fit. A transition is needed to adapt to different ways of staying fit and living a healthy life. Staying fit helps boost self-esteem and endurance. By making healthy choices a person begins to look better and the body begins to feel better. Eating healthy can also put someone into a better mood. For example, people who are sad tend to eat fatty

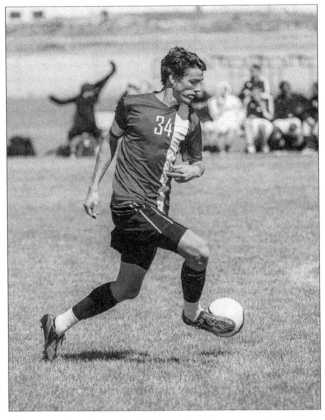

Photo: iStock

foods. Participating in exercise provides health benefits such as: lowering blood pressure, cholesterol levels, and preventing obesity. Adapting to a healthy lifestyle can be challenging at times, but it is worth it. When an individual's body begins to change for the better, it gives that individual the motivation to keep pushing forward.

TIPS ON HOW TO STAY HEALTHY THROUGHOUT LIFE

Joining a gym can be a wonderful and effective experience. Signing up for weekly classes with friends can be a cheap and useful way to stay fit while also having fun. Classes are also very motivational because it involves a group of people who are all working hard together doing the same thing. At gyms fitness instructors lead a variety of classes. One type of class is zumba. Zumba is a fun and enjoyable way to exercise through dance routines, and it helps to burn many calories. Other classes such as yoga, kickboxing, Pilates, boot camp conditioning, spinning, and aqua fit are also great classes one can take advantage of at a gym. These classes are common ways

to get an effective exercise in during a person's busy day and a start on the road to staying fit.

Playing a sport consists of hard work, dedication, sportsmanship, and responsibility. Sports will increase stamina and help to balance weight. They also help prevent most athletes from using alcohol and drugs. A large number of athletes are dedicated and will refrain from doing anything that harms their health. Teammates count on each other and expect each teammate to take on the responsibility that was given to each individual. Playing a sport also helps academically because students have to be on a time schedule. After a long day of practice, most athletes have a set agenda when it comes to finishing homework. When having a time schedule, most students who are athletes feel that there is no time to fool around. Immediately after practice is finished it is most likely straight to homework, dinner, and sleep.

Sleep affects the body and causes health consequences when cut short. People with a lack of sleep have been seen to have health conditions or obesity. One study reports, "People who slept less than six hours per night on a regular basis were much more likely to have excess body weight, while people who slept for eight hours per night had the lowest relative body fat of the study group." Sleeping benefits are extensive and help the human body repair tissues that were used in earlier activity which will increase health benefits.

FAST FOOD AND ITS EFFECTS

Fast food is a cheap and quick way to stop for something to eat, but is it worth it? Consuming fast food daily is harmful to the human body. Fast food is processed food that contains added sugar, carbohydrates, harmful fats, and a lot of sodium. Fast food is usually low in protein and does not give the body the energy that it needs to survive throughout the day.

Fast food contributes to high cholesterol and high blood pressure. These factors make an individual's heart pump harder eventually leading to heart disease. Fast food also leads to a shortness of breath including asthma and sleep apnea. These breathing problems can lead to serious effects such as: diabetes, stroke, headaches, and heart attacks.

Just because fast food may be reasonably priced, does not mean you should consume it. The human body pays a greater price when consuming food with little or no nutritional value. Fast food may lead to various illnesses and also cause acne and weight gain.

WHAT TO SUBSTITUTE UNHEALTHY FOODS WITH

There are many ways to substitute unhealthy foods when it comes to those cravings that you just cannot get rid of. One craving that many people face is the craving for chocolate. When chocolate is swallowed it results into a good feeling, mainly from dopamine being released. Chocolate contains magnesium which can also be obtained from nuts, seeds, vegetables, and fruit.

Sugary food contains chromium, carbon, phosphorus, sulfur, and tryptophan. Most meats, berries, vegetables, sweet potatoes, and dairy products can be substituted for sugary foods and sweets.

WHY READING FOOD LABELS IS IMPORTANT

The nutritional information found on a food labels can a help in reaching weight goals. Food labels can help to limit the amount of fat, sodium, sugar, and cholesterol that is consumed. Food labels help one monitor how many calories they are consuming. It is important to realize that calories mentioned on labels are for one serving.

Reading the food labels makes it easy to compare one brand to another. If two types of brands with different nutritional information are compared, it is easier to choose the healthier one.

DON'T BE INTIMIDATED BY THE NUMBER ON A SCALE

Stepping onto a scale can be intimidating, but it increases awareness of how to manage weight. People should not weigh themselves daily, it is important to weigh themselves ideally in the morning on a weekly basis. This technique gives an individual a chance to see the differences in their body. Body weight change is not a steady process, and it can often fluctuate. Balancing weight is a learning process and only improves with time.

The number on the scale is not important. Rather than going by a number, go by the way you feel and how you think you look in the mirror. You must take into consideration that muscle weighs more than fat.

SLOW AND STEADY WINS THE RACE

Do not be overwhelmed by the amount of things you think you need to do in order to reach your weight goals. If you focus on one thing at a time you will eventually see improvement. Once improvement is noticed it is most likely that you will have the motivation to keep moving forward. If you stay motivated and work hard consistently, then you should have no problem. When noticing a positive change in your body, make sure to be happy even

if it is something as small as losing a pound. Keep in mind that small changes lead to big goals being achieved.

FURTHER READING

Isagenix Products - Weight Loss Solutions - Isagenix. com. (n.d.). Retrieved from: http://www.isagenix.com/ en-US/products. Isagenix offers dietary supplements and other nutritional cleansing products. This 30-day cleansing method helps lose weight, give energy boosts, reduce cravings for unhealthy food, improve muscle tone, and balance digestion.

Weight Watchers - Success starts here. (n.d.). Retrieved from: https://welcome.weightwatchers.com. The Weight Watchers program revolves around a point system. Portions of food are assigned to points. If a food is low in fat it is worth fewer points, therefore, you are able to eat more food throughout the day without using up all your points.

Jenny Craig. (n.d.). Retrieved from: http://www.jennycraig.com. Jenny Craig is a weight loss and weight management corporation. Jenny Craig sells its own pre-made meals to teach weightwatchers about how to eat healthy.

Gabrielle Perk

SEE ALSO: Food Labels; Maintaining Wellness; Nutrition; Staying in a Healthy Weight Range

Teen parenting: Putting your baby up for adoption

Current popular media including the movie Juno, *and the reality documentary TV series "16 and Pregnant" detail the challenges and struggles of pregnant teens who choose to parent their babies, often with little or no support from the biological father. Pregnant teens who are faced with a pregnancy they are not prepared for, are faced with difficult decisions, including the option of making an adoption plan for their unborn babies.*

INTRODUCTION

Becoming pregnant during adolescence presents serious and major challenges. For many young women there are difficult choices to be made to either parent the baby, terminate the pregnancy or make an adoption plan. Each of these choices comes with life-altering consequences. Many young women are in denial, or don't recognize the symptoms of pregnancy and find that it is too late for them to terminate the pregnancy. For others, strong religious beliefs take the option of abortion off the table. For those teens who are opposed to abortion, and recognize that they are not ready for parenting and don't have the financial resources or family support to raise their babies, an adoption plan can be a viable alternative. While studies show that adoption is often recommended to pregnant teens by their physicians, this is a very difficult option to consider.

COMMON MISPERCEPTIONS ABOUT ADOPTION FOR BIRTHPARENTS

In a national survey published in 2007 by the US Department of Health, evidence was provided that illustrates common fears and misconceptions about adoption. Some of the most common fears for birthparents are the question of whether adoptive parents will love their adopted children as much as a biological child, whether the child will hate their birthparents for having made an adoption plan, and whether they will ever see their child again. The survey data reveals that adopted children receive as much or more parental attention as biological offspring. Adoptive parents cherish the time they have with their children, reading to them and singing to them more frequently as compared to biological children, having frequent family dinners, reporting close relationships, and indicating that they would make the decision to adopt again.

Birth mothers often fear that their children will hate them for having made an adoption plan. The statistics did not support this fear, either, as they show that 90 percent of adopted children over age 5 have positive feelings about their adoption. Birth mothers also are afraid that they might never see their child again. The data show that most adoptions are at least semi-open with an exchange of pictures and letters, and that 100% of all birth mothers can choose the amount of openness in the adoptive relationship, and can select a family that would agree to their request. According to this study 67% of private adoptions have pre-adoption agreements that allow for some degree of openness in the adoption, and the remaining adoptions that don't have these agreements, are at the request of the birth mother. Many birth mothers also fear that their child won't be told of their adoption, though statistics show that 99% of adopted children 5 and older know of their adoption, and have been told their own unique adoption story.

When compared to unwed teenage mothers who choose single parenthood, those who choose adoption were found to be more likely to "have higher educational aspirations and finish school. Those same mothers who choose adoption were less likely to live in poverty and receive public assistance than mothers who keep their children. They delay marriage longer, are more likely to marry eventually, and are less likely to divorce. They are more likely to be employed 12 months after the birth and less likely to repeat out-of-wedlock pregnancy. They are no more likely to suffer negative psychological consequences, such as depression, than are mothers who rear children as single parents." (Henney et al, 2007)

REACHING THE DECISION TO MAKE AN ADOPTION PLAN

Following the discovery of pregnancy, there can be a great deal of emotional distress while considering your options. For some, friends and the biological father are the only ones to speak to, for those afraid to tell their parents, there may be a trusted relative, pastor, teacher, coach, counselor, or doctor. Many teens, though, hide their pregnancies from parents and community due to feelings of shame and wishing to avoid negative consequences.

When the decision is reached to proceed with an adoption plan, there are two choices to be made-- whether to work through an adoption agency, or to go the route of private adoption. Working with an agency, may require relocating to the state where the agency is located. The agency itself may provide assistance with housing, legal matters, medical care and counseling, along with support in choosing an adoptive family for the baby, and support through the process of labor and delivery. The agency will also screen adoptive families and act as a liaison between the adoptive family and the birth mother.

Going through a private adoption can begin by responding to an adoption ad that is online or in a local or national newspaper. A typical adoption ad may look something like this: ADOPT: Musical, adventurous married couple and 4 y.o. daughter from MI looking to adopt again. Stay-at-home mom & professional dad. Expenses paid. www.LindaBobAdopt.com 888-123-5555. By calling this number and speaking with the prospective parents a birth mother will get a sense of who the potential adoptive parents are and what their life is like. It can help to have a list of questions prepared. If it appears that there is a potential match between the adoptive family and the birth mother's wishes, the next step would be to have contact with the adoption attorney of the prospective parents. Sometimes connections are not made through an ad, but through people who know of a couple looking to adopt, or other forms of networking. The process is the same, however once a potential match is identified. Once the connection is made with the adoption attorney, information is exchanged. The prospective birth mother will fill out forms about herself and her family. For prospective adoptive parents, there is a process they must go through to be qualified to adopt, which includes fingerprinting, and a 'homestudy' in which a licensed social worker interviews each of them and visits their home and prepares a report. The application of the prospective adoptive couple is shared, including the home study, and a story with photos about their life. If the birth mother and prospective parents agree to work together, more medical information is disclosed.

The US Department of Health & Human Services (childwelfare.gov) provides a great deal of information on their website regarding federal laws related to adoption, and how the laws vary state to state. It explains emotional, practical and legal issues, and offers a variety of resources for helping you if you are thinking about make an adoption plan.

When interviewing potential families, focus on the most important elements. Look for stable marriages, financial stability and family support. Look for a family whose values are consistent with what you wish for your child. Be mindful of the way it feels to interact with each of the family members. Hobbies or interests that match those of your family members can also increase the match or fit. For example, if there is musical talent or athletic ability in the birth parent's family, looking for a family that engages in those activities can increase the chances that these will be part of the child's life.

MEETING THE PROSPECTIVE ADOPTIVE PARENTS
It may be possible to meet the prospective adoptive family prior to the birth. Depending on each person's comfort level, there is a wide range of ways the adoptive family can participate in the pregnancy and birth. In some cases, the prospective adoptive mother may accompany the birth mother to doctor's appointments and/or be in the delivery room. In other cases, the birth mother or adoptive parent may prefer not to meet at all, or only meet after the termination of parental rights papers have been signed. This is all determined on a case by case basis, and worked out between the individuals involved.

LEGAL ASPECTS
Every state has a unique set of laws governing adoption. Proceeding with an adoption requires formally terminating the parental rights of both birth parents. This is done before a judge. If the adoptive parents live in a different state, and are travelling with the baby, they must have filed for and received permission to travel. This is called the "Interstate Compact". Following the placement, there is a process where the family is seen by a social worker who does a post-placement visit and files a report. Ultimately, the adoption is finalized by a judge.

EMOTIONAL ISSUES AROUND THE ADOPTION
Many birth parents choose adoption as a way of giving their unborn children a better life than they feel they would be able to give them. Other reasons include allowing themselves to focus on their own lives, their socioeconomic position, and to avoid the stigma of single parenthood in the family and community. While each birth mother's experience is unique, there are some common themes that emerge in the literature having to do with grief, guilt, and healing from the loss.

GRIEVING THE LOSS
Making an adoption plan, and anticipating the loss of a child can be quite traumatic for many birth parents. This is often a grueling decision that birth mothers struggle with for months. Frequently they may be quite ambivalent. Following the birth of the baby and the actual surrendering of the baby, birth mothers can experience the same kind of grief that follows a death. (Romanchik, 1999) The loss of a baby to adoption is an ambiguous loss, or the loss of someone who is still alive. Society does not have set rituals for dealing with this kind of loss, and many birth mothers will feel that they are expected to 'get over it', or not deserve sympathy or empathy because they have 'chosen' this outcome. This makes it more difficult for the loss to be acknowledged and the normal process of grief to proceed. In some situations, where the pregnancy was hidden, the birth mothers are closed off from the support they need in the community to help them grieve.

Many birth parents may mourn the loss of their child for their lifetime, and think frequently about the child they placed for adoption. There is a continuing need for support and self acceptance for young women who have made such a difficult and mature decision at an early time in their lives.

MOVING ON WITH LIFE

In order to reach resolution, it is necessary for a birth mother to resolve her grief, make peace with her decision, incorporate being a birth parent into her identity, and overcome the effect of the experience on other relationships in her life. There are a number of strategies to help oneself move forward. One can develop rituals or traditions that commemorate the child and the decision. For some adoptive and birth parents creating an 'entrustment ceremony' that allows the birth parent to say goodbye to their child and to entrust the care of the child to the adoptive family. Other ongoing rituals can be created to commemorate the child's birthday or other special milestone day for the child.

Educating oneself about adoption and the experience of other birth parents can help decrease the feeling of being alone in this loss. Journaling or writing serves as an outlet where one can create a record of feelings and observations. It can be an emotional outlet, and help in recalling details and gaining perspective over the years. Professional counseling can help birth parents replace unrealistic fantasies with reality and improve self-esteem. Post adoption support groups and mentoring for birth parents can help birth mothers heal and look forward in their lives.

This poem honors the importance of both birth mothers and adoptive mothers in the life of a child.

Legacy of an Adopted Child

Once there were two women who never knew each other.
One you do not remember, the other you call mother.
Two different lives, shaped to make your one...
One became your guiding star, the other became your sun.
The first gave you life and the second taught you to live it.
The first gave you a need for love, and the second was there to give it.
One gave you a nationality, the other gave you a name.
One gave you a seed of talent, the other gave you an aim.
One gave you emotions, the other calmed your fears.
One saw your first sweet smile, the other dried your tears.
One gave you up ... that's all she could do.
The other prayed for a child and God led her straight to you.
And now you ask me, through your fears,
the age old question unanswered throughout the years...

Heredity or environment, which are you the product of?
Neither, my darling ... neither.
Just two different kinds of love.

~ Author Unknown ~

FURTHER READING

Henney, S. M., Ayers-Lopez, S., McRoy, R. G., & Grotevant, H. D. (2007). "Evolution and resolution: Birthmothers' experience of grief and loss at different levels of openness". *Journal of Social and Personal Relationships*, 24, 875–889. This article presents a longitudinal study that looked at birthmothers experiences when adoptions were at different levels of openness.

McLaughlin, SD, Manninen DL, Winges LD. (1998) "Do adolescents who relinquish their children fare better or worse than those who raise them?" *Family Planning Perspectives*, 20:1, 25-32. This article presents the findings of research studies that show that birthmothers who place their babies for adoption are likely to fare better economically, educationally and have more successful marriages when they eventually marry. These authors also found that adopted children are also likely to fare well.

Silber, K, and Dorner, PM. (1991) *Dear Birthmother, Thank-you For Our Baby*. San Antonio, TX: Corona Publishing Co. This book presents the experience of open adoption through the use of actual letters between birthfamilies and adoptive families.

Romanchik, B. R. (1999). *Birthparent Grief*. Royal Oak, MI:R-squared Press. Guidebook for understanding the stages and realities of grief that are unique to the birthparent placing a child for adoption.

Lauren Behrman

SEE ALSO: Abortion; Adopted Teens, Your Identity, and Searching for Your Birth Parents; Peer Pressure; Separation anxiety; Teen Pregnancy

Time management

The key to time management lies within the understanding of how the brain perceives the construct of time. Several theories abound, trying to explain the science to managing time and to increasing awareness of how to effectively accomplish tasks within an allotted time frame.

Understanding both the science of time management and its antonym, procrastination, have proven to be very effective in using time appropriately and effectively with physical and mental benefits.

INTRODUCTION

Scientists have trouble finding an exact definition for the term "time management," but the most widely agreed upon understanding of it is the planning and execution of activities. It is therefore a twofold concept-- it involves both the preparation and the actual doing of the idea. Though it may appear counterintuitive, it is vital to dedicate some time to the organization of ideas and seeing to the completion of the tasks. And oddly enough, it is that time spent planning that is so essential to proper time management; without it, a person would be blindly acting out assignments. A plethora of literary sources agree that with proper time assessment a person can feel more in control of their time, more content with academic or professional careers, and most of all less stressed. Additionally, individuals who exercise time management report high productivity and numerous benefits from extra free time. Many researchers and theorists have explored what happens to a person psychologically and biologically when planning a course of action. Moreover, for many to fully comprehend time organization, it is easier to compare it with its complete opposite-- procrastination, the act of delaying tasks and "putting off" assignments to very last-minute.

THE SCIENCE TO MANAGING TIME

Many see the perception of time as the key to understanding time management. One major theory in this field of study is the Planning Fallacy. Pioneered by researchers Roger Buehler, Dale Griffin, and Michael Ross, it is the concept that a person underestimates how long a task will require of them, particularly if he or she spends a large amount of planning time foreseeing a pleasant outcome without accounting for possible obstacles. Professor Douglas Hofstadter's law states that no matter

how much planning goes into an activity, every task takes longer than anticipated. Alternatively, other studies turn to past experiences with similar circumstances rather than looking to at the future; they find that previous experience provides both a realistic result as well as a fairly accurate gauge for how long the activity will take. The University of Belgium conducted a study in which they found that the more details imagined on a future project, the more imminent and critical it feels.

Perhaps the reason time management may be so difficult to achieve for some is because of the nature of the brain. According to Dr. Timothy A. Pychyl, the limbic system (the portion of the brain primarily concerned with instinct and emotion) uses its reflexes to avoid activities that cause distress. In other words, it is an unconscious coping mechanism to evade tasks considered unpleasant. In the same study, Pychyl found that the prefrontal cortex may be both a newer and weaker portion of the brain. Because this portion of the brain is where the response to problems originates, it requires active thought and energy to generate a solution. However, particularly if the problem at hand is unpleasant, the limbic system reacts

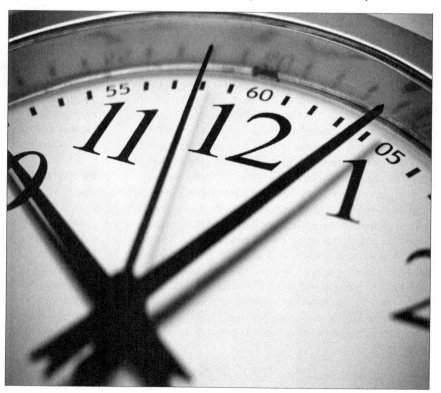

Photo: iStock

and creates a drive to ignore the task. But when an individual carves out the proper time to plan before acting, a surge of dopamine is released in the brain, producing a euphoric feeling of accomplishment.

UNDERSTANDING TIME MANAGEMENT IN COMPARISON TO PROCRASTINATION

Perhaps the key to understanding how to properly manage time is to understand what happens when time is improperly managed through procrastination. A coping mechanism for avoiding displeasing tasks, it leads to higher stress levels than if the task was completed sooner. Again, the limbic system's response to unpleasant situations tends to push people to not accomplish the assignment, leaving less time to accomplish it as well as a variety of physical symptoms associated with heightened anxiety-- nausea, headache, weakness of limbs, etc. The two main types of procrastination are linked to behavior and decisions respectively. In one form of procrastination, a person self-sabotages to avoid action; in the other, a person avoids conflict and decisions. Both involve a multitude of psychological factors, including negative self-image, anxiety, high stress, and more.

A study from Carleton University found that nearly half of procrastinators found that their habit has been detrimental to their happiness. Joseph Ferrari from DePaul University in Chicago found that procrastination could be an unconscious method of rebellion, particularly for those with very strict parents. Clary Lay from York State, Toronto published the General Procrastination Scale, which takes into consideration dreams and obligations. He also found that chronic procrastinators have a genetic makeup so that they are actually neurologically disorganized thinkers, and they cannot help but procrastinate.

Having proper time management does just the opposite—it boosts productivity, reduces stress, and the release of neurotransmitters such as dopamine creates a happy feeling that further boosts productivity. The process of collecting oneself and allotting time to finish a job is surprisingly more effective than going into a plan without the proper planning it requires, even leading to successes both short-term (such as good test grades or commendation on work presentations) and long-term (such as graduating with honors or receiving a promotion).

STRATEGIES TO ACCOMPLISH PROPER TIME MANAGEMENT

Mastering effective time management skills may seem daunting, but with a few basic skills, it can prove to be quite easy. Maintain a routine using a planner or daily "to-do" list. Use of one of these makes managing time easier, helping to establish continued, long-term success. Specifically making a habit of organizing time and factoring in distractions and the Planning Fallacy help a person prioritize his or her time and learn to value it. In this modern age of technology, it helps to ignore and even turn off electronic devices, apps, and social media to direct all focus to the task at hand.

Another one of the most important time management skills is sleeping. An exhausted brain cannot think as quickly or with as much clarity as a well-rested brain can. Proper rest is also physiologically important; with sleep being such a vital life process disrupting it could lead to health complications as well. Shorter breaks should be used to refocus energy on the matter at hand, and longer weekend breaks and vacations should be used to retain long-term productivity. Proper nourishment is just as important for keeping the mind alert and attentive.

CLINICAL IMPLICATIONS

Having knowledge and insight into the concept of time management through the concepts of time itself and procrastination have proven to be quite beneficial. With an understanding of the various theories associated with the construct of time as well as comprehension of its polar opposite procrastination, one can take this knowledge and go forth with strategies to succeed.

FURTHER READING

Booth, F. (2014, August 28). "30 Time Management Tips for a Work-Life Balance". *Forbes*. Retrieved from: http://www.forbes.com/sites/francesbooth/2014/08/28/30-time-management-tips/. This article provides helpful tips to live a life with effective time management skills.

Herbet L. (2013, June 13). "How Your Brain Perceives Time (and How To Use It To Your Advantage)". *Lifehacker*. Retrieved from:http://lifehacker.com/how-your-brain-perceives-time-and-how-to-use-it-to-you-511184192. This article evaluates the theories many researchers hold on the perception people have of time and how they manage their time.

Letham, S. (n.d.). "The Procrastination Problem". *Success Consciousness*. Retrieved from: http://www.successconsciousness.com/guest_articles/

procrastination.htm. This article examines the study of procrastination. Using scientific studies, it attempts to fully explain different concepts associated with procrastination and poor time management.

Spencer, A. (n.d.). "The Science Behind Procrastination". *Real Simple*. Retrieved from: http://www.realsimple. com/work-life/life-strategies/time-management/procrastination. This article delves further into the ideas of Dr. Pychyl and the effect of the brain's structure on time management.

Courtney Brogle

SEE ALSO: Decision making; Managing Time: The Adult Perspective

Volunteering and community service

The following article deals with the topic of volunteering and community service for teenagers. With the use of published studies, statistics, and quotes by famous leaders and activists, the positive effects of volunteering on teenagers are outlined. These include physical, mental, social, and vocational benefits attributed to volunteer work. Ways of becoming involved in local organizations or independent service work are also outlined with a link to a particular organization, Do Something, which provides a multitude of ideas and opportunities. The article concludes with helpful tips for teenagers interested in volunteering to ensure a positive and successful experience.

INTRODUCTION

The Merriam-Webster Dictionary defines volunteering as, "offering to do something without being forced to or without getting paid to do it." This action acts in combination with the act of community service, which is defined by Google as "voluntary work intended to help people in a particular area." Since the time of colonization, Americans have been initiating, working towards, and establishing nonprofit and community service geared organizations. It is proven that participation in community service projects and volunteering both locally and abroad as a teenager can have lifelong positive benefits on both mental and physical health. Enforcing positive action and habits starting from a young age can lead to a healthy, happy, and productive life in the future. The seeds of a life-long dedication to service, expansion of viewpoints, and collaboration among others are instilled

within teen volunteers through their work. There are many resources and possibilities for involvement both within local programs and beyond. National non-profit organizations, local service groups, or independently established movements are all potential outlets for teenage volunteering. Many individuals throughout history have advocated for the positive aspects of reaching out and assisting others including Audrey Hepburn. In a famous quotation she stated, "As you grow older, you will discover that you have two hands, one for helping yourself and the other for helping others." By instilling volunteer habits in a teenager, this understanding and call to take action to enact change will come even sooner. There has been a documented increase in the amount of teen volunteers over the years. The following outlines the key reasons to volunteer and its positive benefits. Assistance on getting involved and helpful volunteering tips are also located below.

BENEFITS OF VOLUNTEERING

The benefits of volunteering are endless especially for teenagers. Getting involved within their community, learning life skills, and understanding their role and capacity to enact change can all positively enrich a teen's life. Volunteering and committing to an organization, event, or activity will teach time management, productivity, and responsibility. A study at the University of Pennsylvania by a Wharton professor, Cassie Mogliner, for the *Harvard Business Review* found that those who volunteer their time feel a balance and find they have more time. Skills that promote organization, dedication, work ethic, and perseverance are all attributed to the work of volunteers and prove very beneficial to the character development of a teenager. There is a particular development of social responsibility linked to a broadened global perspective and understanding of the value of education and everyday resources. A new sense of humility and gratitude can be forged in the service of others. Multiculturalism and understanding of the shared identity and needs of all people around the world can be directly grasped through hands-on volunteering. College applications and résumés can be enforced with the skills, connections, and abilities developed through involvement with a community service organization. A study conducted in 2012 at the University of Michigan for the publication, Monitoring the Future, found that 40 percent of high school seniors who planned to finish college were already active volunteers.

Volunteering allows a teen to develop new skills and pursue areas of potential interest. By honing in on skills and attributes beginning as a young adult, a teen can be prepared to enter future academic and vocational endeavors. Interests exemplified through work done as a teen can lead to a life-long calling and discovery of a particular passion. Winston Churchill stated, "We make a living by what we get, we make a life by what we give." By establishing new connections and bonds with like-minded individuals, a great support system is created for a teen. Sharing in a common cause and contributing towards its success directly enforces critical thinking skills. Social skills are developed through shared activity and striving for a common goal. Volunteering allows an active participation and application of academic knowledge and skills towards everyday problems and their solutions. While students are given factual information and written knowledge in a classroom setting, community service allows this knowledge to be applied and strengthened. Participation in volunteer work has shown a decrease in a teenager's likelihood of participating in illegal and harmful activities.

Volunteering promotes overall well being, both mentally and physically. A report published by the Corporation for National and Community Service found that "those who volunteer have lower mortality rates, greater functional ability and lower rates of depression" going forward in life. Active movement and interaction with peers and mentors develops a teen into a well-rounded and high-functioning adult. Interaction and hands-on volunteer work grants teens a global perspective and better understanding of society and the world around them. Volunteering promotes self-confidence, fulfillment, and happiness. There is a great reward and sense of satisfaction derived from helping others. As a teen, finding a personal role in society can sometimes be challenging. By directly doing something to benefit someone or something else, a teen will gain a sense of pride, value, and identity. No matter how young, all people have the ability to make a positive difference in the world. Studies have proven an actual "happiness effect" linked to volunteer and community service work. In a report published by Harvard Health Publications, the London School of Economics found that there was a direct positive correlation in the relationship between the frequency of volunteering and an inclination to be happy. There was a 16% rise in happiness levels for those who volunteered weekly.

VOLUNTEER IDEAS AND OPPORTUNITIES

There are many outlets for volunteer work spanning a variety of interests. Whether dealing with the environment, hunger and poverty relief, animal welfare, community development and infrastructure, human rights, or politics, there are both local and national organizations in need of teen volunteers. Teens can volunteer in both large and small-scale settings. As Mother Teresa stated, "Do small things with great love." Any contribution that can be made proves influential no matter how big or small. Assisting with everyday tasks at home is an easy way to perform an act of community service. Visiting and talking to elderly family members or mentoring and tutoring young relatives are each positive contributions made without the sole intention of personal gain. Within a hometown or community, local soup kitchens and community centers can provide positions assisting with outreach programs and volunteer events. Nationally, nonprofit organizations, such as, The American Cancer Society, Special Olympics, and Habitat for Humanity provide youth leadership and volunteer programs within their campaigns, events, and advocacy. High school clubs provide a platform for student-led and hands-on work. Many organizations provide the ability to form local chapters and branches making it easy for teens to form their own movement. For those interested in even more service-based immersion, community

Christina Maher took this image on a summer 2014 service trip to Costa Rica. It shows the distribution of school supplies collected to donate to a local impoverished school.

service programs exist abroad allowing students to travel and assist others around the world. The organization, Do Something, outlines a variety of ways in which teenagers can get involved in a variety of volunteer ideas and opportunities. By keeping one's perspective and options open, an array of resources and chances for worthwhile service can be found.

TIPS FOR OPTIMIZING THE VOLUNTEER EXPERIENCE

There are a few tips to ensure that volunteer work as a teenager is worthwhile. The first is to remember safety and always follow sanitation, health codes, and protective measures. Being open to new experiences, people, and activities can broaden a teen's perspective and lead to a life-long path. By incorporating passions, interests, and hobbies the best match in a community service program can be discovered. It is important to ask questions and fully understand your role, commitment, and participation. Knowing what to expect by asking questions and doing research prior to serving will allow the most comfort and transitional ease. As a teen, it is easy to become discouraged or feel insignificant. It is key to remember that anyone has the ability to change the world with the right work ethic and dedication. Setting a personal goal and timeline will allow a sense of achievement and fulfillment while eliminating the daunting and overwhelming stresses of taking on a large task all at once. Finally, it is vital to the entire experience to approach volunteering as a positive and fun activity. In participating in new experiences, helping others, meeting new people, and finding one's identity and passions, a teen can have a truly enjoyable and rewarding experience in volunteering and community service!

FURTHER READING

Child Trends Databank. (2014). Volunteering. Available at: http://www.childtrends.org/?indicators=volunteering - See more at: http://www.childtrends.org/?indicators =volunteering#sthash.BaxYKMHw.dpuf. This article outlines specific positive trends related to student's academic and vocational plans in relation to service work. Through the presentation of graphics and statistics the correlation found through study is clearly outlined.

DoSomething.org/ America's largest organization for youth volunteering opportunities. (n.d.). Retrieved from: https://www.dosomething.org. This organization provides an online resource for teenagers looking for effective and feasible volunteer and community service opportunities. There are many resources spanning a variety of opportunities and subject matters allowing students to have easy access to community service and inspiration to enact change.

Mogilner, C. (2012, September 1). You'll Feel Less Rushed If You Give Time Away. Retrieved from: *Harvard Business Review*. This article discusses the positive benefits of volunteering. In this study, the positive correlation between committing time to service work and personal freedom, organization, and enjoyment is proven.

Simple Changes, Big Rewards: A practical, easy guide for healthy, happy living- Harvard Health. (n.d.). Retrieved from: http://www.health.harvard.edu/ special-health-reports/simple-changes-big-rewards-a-practical-easy-guide-for-healthy-happy-living. In this article, researchers for Harvard Health identified actual positive physical and mental benefits and an inclination towards happiness associated with volunteering and community service.

Christina Maher

SEE ALSO: Self-Esteem; Time Management

Critical Skills

Cover letter and résumé writing

Cover letter and résumé writing are critical skills that are sometimes neglected in formal curriculum. As a result, these documents are often misconceived as documents of "objective accomplishments", not unlike a transcript. In this articler, cover letter and résumé writing is presented as much more effective when approached as a crafted argument of fit as determined by the employer, and that each application should be tailored to the specifications of the job description.

INTRODUCTION

Despite being required for almost all employment, résumé and cover letter writing is seldom taught in standard curriculum. Often résumé and cover letters are born out of necessity, cobbled together in response to an application deadline and subsequently recycled for all future applications. As someone who has served on multiple admissions and hiring committees, I frequently lament the applications that land in the reject pile due to issues on the résumé or cover letter that would have been easy fixes.

The most common misconception of résumé and cover letter writing is that these are objective documents of your accomplishments, not unlike a transcript. However, what counts as an "accomplishment" is often based on what the applicant is proud of, or what his/her peers have deemed remarkable. This would all work splendidly if not for the problem that accomplishments valued by the applicant may not be similarly valued by an employer. For example, while winning the regional science fair in physics may be a source of pride for an applicant, it may be less valuable for a job that relies heavily on people skills.

In truth, a résumé and cover letter is more like a persuasive argument than a transcript. These documents should convince the employer that you are the best fit for the position by presenting a collection of supporting evidence. Consider this analogy: If you were buying a birthday cake for someone you want to impress, the smart strategy would be to figure out what flavors and texture they like, and use that information to pick the best cake. Since people have widely varying tastes, the optimal cake will differ based on the individual's preferences. This philosophy runs throughout this article, which will focus more on the artful crafting of an argument in résumé and cover letter form, rather than the basic mechanics of building a résumé or cover letter.

FIRST RULE OF WRITING: KNOW YOUR AUDIENCE

As with all good writing, the first step is to understand who your audience is, and how they will be reading your writing. In this case, the audience is usually an employer looking to hire someone to do something specific. Note that the two variables of interest here are 1) the person, and 2) the requisite skills to for the job. The specific attributes of the two variables can vary widely between jobs. For example, customer service jobs may require someone who can behave extrovertly for sustained periods of time, whereas blogging for an organization may require someone who can function independently. Similarly, the requisite skills for an information technology specialist (e.g., familiarity with programming languages) can be very different from that of a wedding planner (e.g., familiarity with the latest trends in the wedding industry). Therefore, it behooves you to first understand 1) what kind of a person the employer is looking for, and 2) what skill sets are valuable to the employer.

So how do you secure this information? The easiest place to look is in the job description. A well-written posting should contain most of the information necessary for a targeted résumé and cover letter. To illustrate this, let us go through an example of a job posting for a retail associate:

Figure 1. Example job description for a retail associate.

A careful reading of this job description should yield an understanding that this employer is likely looking for someone who:

- **Behaves extrovertly**
  "providing excellent customer service to patrons"
- **Clearly organized**
  "ensuring that all products are organized by the approved 'store map'"
- **Meets strict deadlines and works well under pressure**
  "complete the freight process within the designated time"
- **Aware of and attuned to their environment and is adaptable**
  see "attend to in-store customers…when other sales associates are unavailable"
- **Leads and manages well**
  "proactively engaging in investigation and correction of any potential issues or discrepancies"

RETAIL AND MERCHANDISE ASSOCIATE

Responsibilities for the Retail and Merchandise Associate (RMA) includes efficient processing an inventory of products, and providing excellent customer service to patrons in-store as needed.

The RMA must complete the freight process within the designated time, and must do so by following the standardized sorting and stocking guidelines. RMAs are responsible for ensuring that all products are organized by the approved "store map", including proactively engaging in investigation and correction of any potential issues or discrepancies.

The RMA should attend to in-store customers who require assistance when other sales associates are unavailable.

Additional Information:
- Previous sales/customer service experience is desirable, but not required
- Strong interpersonal and communication skills needed
- Must be able to read, write, and count for accurate documentation
- Familiar with technology in order to utilize traning tools and process inventory
- Candidates should enjoy interacting with people

Figure 1.

In the case that the job description is more ambiguous, there are a few other ways in which this information may be obtained. Firstly, most companies have mission statements describing their values and goals, from which specific attributes and skills should naturally follow. For example, Google's states:

"Google's mission is to organize the world's information and make it universally accessible and useful."

Even from this one-sentence statement, a careful reading should yield useful information. On first read, you likely noticed that words "organize", "universally", and "useful". This should immediately communicate that Google is likely interested in applicants who 1) have strong organizational skills, 2) can think BIG, and 3) are simultaneously pragmatists. If you read even more carefully, you may notice that they tasked themselves with the grandiose goal of "organizing the world's information". This indicates that resourcefulness and creativity are likely valuable attributes/skills, as they are probably necessary in order to tackle the seemingly impossible task of organizing all of the information in the entire world. The mission statement also ends with the word "useful", which qualifies that big-thinking must not remain a fantasy, and that the most competitive applicants will likely be someone who can translate lofty abstract ideas into real-world outcomes. Finally, the words "universally accessible" may also connote a value of social justice and equal opportunity.

In the case that neither the job description nor the mission statement is helpful, you can always be proactive and contact human resources or the hiring associate to obtain this information. This can be achieved with simple questions like, *"I am extremely interested in the _____ position at your company, and I wanted to know what kind of employee you are looking for, and what skill sets will be valuable to you?"* When executed appropriately, this may simultaneously be informative and communicate enthusiasm as well as thoughtfulness.

BE SELECTIVE ABOUT CONTENT

Once you have identified the attributes and skills that are the best fit for the position, the rest should follow logically. Each piece of information on your résumé and cover letter should be strategically selected based on the relevant attributes and skills. The simplest method is to showcase experiences that demonstrate the specific skills or attributes desired by the employer. For example, you may write about your experiences on student council to showcase leadership skills, or volunteering at an animal shelter to illustrate compassion. Keep in mind that life experiences are rarely unidimensional, which means that different aspects of the same experience can be highlighted to demonstrate various skills and attributes. For instance, you may focus on your successful campaign for student council to illustrate interpersonal skills in connecting with a larger student body, or instead focus on your responsibilities as treasurer on student council to demonstrate accounting and money management skills.

PUTTING IT TOGETHER: RÉSUMÉ

Armed with the strategic collection of evidence, the final step is to amass them into a document with precision and impact. In returning to the first lesson, decisions in writing (including wording, organization, and formatting) should be guided by who your audience is and how they will be reading your writing. In most cases, your audience will be the employers. Obtaining employment is also a competitive process, so employers are likely sifting through large amounts of applications with limited time and energy. As a result, employers rarely spend more than 30 seconds per résumé, with some research indicating an average as short as 6-seconds per résumé!

With limited time, the challenge is to present yourself as an ideal fit for the position in as few words as possible. The document must be easy to read (i.e., clean font, clear sections), and present compelling evidence about your fit for the position. Here are some general guidelines specific for résumés:

Be concise. For example, "I helped with writing the script and directing the annual school musical" can be shortened to "Assisted in creative writing and direction of musical".

BULLET POINTS ARE YOUR FRIEND
One page constraint often aids with conciseness

Use action verbs. These are verbs that succinctly communicate skills and attributes. For example, instead of "Served on Yearbook Committee", you may write "Collaborated with peers to publish and distribute a 200 page yearbook" to illustrate interpersonal skills, and organizational skills in managing large tasks.

Do an internet search of "action verbs" for a full database of action verbs

Follow the general structure. Most résumés follow a standard format, and employers will likely expect to see specific information in specific places. Not following the standard format can be risky because it may disrupt the flow of information and require additional effort to re-orient to your résumé.

Most résumés begin with your name, followed by contact information, an objectives section, your education, selected honors/awards, your (strategically selected) experiences, and any other relevant skills

Do an internet search of "résumé structure" to see examples

Visual presentation matters. Just like how your attire in an interview communicates specific attributes, visual presentation on a résumé can be leveraged to your advantage.

Efficient use of space can demonstrate organizational skills

Creative formatting may communicate innovation, though this should be carefully considered (see guideline 3)

PUTTING IT TOGETHER: COVER LETTER
A common error of cover letter writing is duplication of the résumé, except in prose form. The cover letter is your opportunity to communicate the larger context in which the evidence on your résumé fits. For example, your cover letter may state that your ability for critical thinking under pressure will be an asset to the employer, as exemplified by successful performances in competitive circumstances. This is then followed by a résumé that might include leadership roles in team sports, volunteering in disaster relief efforts, and/or medals won in chess competitions. The cover letter not only explicitly communicates why you should be hired, but also allows you to guide the reader through the contents on your résumé. Finally, your cover letter should also be concise and easy to read, as the same time pressure applies to both the cover letter and the résumé.

FURTHER READING
Brizee, A., Jarrett, N., Schmaling, K. (2010, April 2). What is an action verb? *Owl Purdue*. Retrieved from: https://owl.english.purdue.edu/owl/resource/543/01/. This article reviews what an "action verb" is and how it should be used. A link is also included for a list of action verbs categorized by skill sets.

Brizee, A., Olson, A. (2011, December 14). What is a cover letter? *Owl Purdue*. Retrieved from: https://owl.english.purdue.edu/owl/resource/549/01/. This article reviews what an cover letter is, and contains further links such as video instructions and sample documents.

Giang, V., & Stanger, M. (2012, November 29). How to write the perfect résumé. *Business Insider*. Retrieved from: http://www.businessinsider.com/how-to-write-the-perfect-resume-2012-11?op=1. This article reviews the general principles of writing an effective résumé, and also provides mechanical details regarding the formatting of a résumé (e.g., where to put your name, how to make use of space, etc.)

Philip Cheng

SEE ALSO: Finding Your First Job; Interpersonal Communication

Interpersonal communication

Interpersonal communication is the process of sending and receiving messages. Interpersonal communication is effective when the message is received as the sender intended. This process can involve written communication, nonverbal communication, or face-to-face communication.

INTRODUCTION

Perhaps the most important critical skill to master is effective communication because it helps others to understand you, increases your understanding of others, increases others' positive feelings toward you, and decreases conflict.

Communication is the process of sending and receiving messages. Communication is effective when the message is received as the sender intended. This process can involve written communication, nonverbal communication, or interpersonal communication.

WRITTEN COMMUNICATION

Letters, papers, books, magazines, scripts, notes, texting, and social media all use written communication to convey a message. To be effective, written communication requires more than just jotting down a few words. It requires constructing the message to appeal to a particular audience and proofreading to catch any phrases that might cause a misunderstanding as well as grammatical errors.

NONVERBAL COMMUNICATION

"It's not what you say, it's how you say it" describes the importance of nonverbal communication. According to Albert Mehrabian, only 7% of a message is conveyed through words. Thirty-eight percent is conveyed through vocal paralanguage (intonation, pitch, regional accent, hesitations). This paralanguage reveals our gender, age, geographic background, level of education, emotional state, attitudes, and our relationship with the person spoken to. Other nonverbal elements such as facial expression, gestures, physical appearance, posture, and proxemic behavior, comprise 55% of the message conveyed. Judgments are made based on these physical nonverbal elements and some of them are cultural or out of one's conscious control. Misunderstanding can then arise. Suspending judgment, not assuming anything based on a person's cultural group membership, and ask-ing the other person their interpretation of their nonverbal communication helps dispel misunderstandings.

An important message that is sent through nonverbal behavior is whether you are paying full attention to the other person. If you sit facing that person with an open posture, slightly leaning forward, and making good eye contact, that person will know you are interested in what they are saying. Attending to the other person with these nonverbal cues also will cause the other person to like you more since everyone wants to feel listened to. Besides showing you are paying attention to the other person, smile. A smile goes a long way in establishing a good relationship. And, when one smiles, the other person usually smiles back, making you feel less nervous. As the saying goes, "smile and the whole world smiles with you."

FACE-TO-FACE COMMUNICATION

Face-to-face communication involves at least two people in a meaningful exchange. The sender intends to affect the response of a particular person or persons. The message may be received in the way it was intended or it may get distorted. So the sender needs to monitor how the message is sent and then how it was received by asking for feedback. In this way, any confusion or misunderstanding can be reduced.

SENDING MESSAGES EFFECTIVELY

Although saying what is on one's mind seems effortless, it really takes a great deal of skill to send a message so that the receiver does not become defensive and then distort the sender's message. For example, people who are straightforward with the messages they send, avoid the distortions that can occur when a person just hints at what they have in mind or they tell a third person, hoping the message will get to the intended recipient indirectly.

Owning one's messages by using "I" instead of "you" reduces the receiver's defensiveness. Notice the difference when you hear "I am concerned that you are spending too much time with her" instead of "You are spending too much time with her". Another skill involved in sending effective messages is being complete and specific as well as separating fact from opinion. A specific and complete statement is, "When you look away from me, I feel you are being insincere" as opposed to the vague and opinionated statement, "Nobody likes people who don't look at people."

One way of diminishing the natural tendency of the receiver to engage in mindreading, that is reading more into the message than what was sent, is for the sender to ask for feedback. The sender can ask, "Can you let me know your understanding of what we just talked about?" Or, "What is your reaction to what I just said?"

ROADBLOCKS TO INTERPERSONAL COMMUNICATION

Often, the sender does not stop to think how the message is going to be received before sending it. You, as the sender, may be in a rush to say what is on your mind. Or you may be thinking about what you want to say rather than closely paying attention to what the other person is saying before formulating a response. As Stephen R. Covey said, "Most people do not listen with the intent to understand; they listen with the intent to reply. They are either speaking or preparing to speak. We all want to be heard--that is why we speak. But most of the time we are so busy speaking that we don't listen. We don't listen to the other person. We don't even listen to ourselves."

For effective communication to occur, you must monitor yourself for at least the following three roadblocks that intensify interpersonal problems rather than alleviate them.

The first roadblock is judging, as in "You're just jealous" or "That's really wrong." The second roadblock is avoiding the other's concerns, as in "That happened to me too and it was awful" or "Don't worry, things will work out fine". The third roadblock is sending solutions, as in "You ought to do this …", or "Go make friends with someone else", or "If you do that, you'll be sorry."

You can prevent these roadblocks from occurring by pausing instead of giving a quick reaction to what the other person said. Before giving a reply or even initiating a conversation, it is important to listen to yourself. Notice any thoughts you are having or any strong emotional response that is arising. Instead of just impulsively expressing these thoughts, stop and ask yourself, "Am I saying this for my benefit rather than for having a good relationship with the other person?"

Listening closely and actively to what the other person is saying affects interpersonal communication even more than how a message is sent. When employers were asked to describe the communication skill they considered most important, listening was the number one response. Yet the average worker listens at only a 25 percent efficiency level.

Research also shows that immediately after a ten-minute presentation, a normal listener can recall only 50 percent of the information presented. After 48 hours, the recall level drops to 25 percent. This dismal state extends to students listening to a lecture. A researcher activated an alarm at sporadic intervals and asked the students to write down their thoughts and moods at that moment. About 20 percent of the students, men and women, were pursuing erotic thoughts. Another 20 percent were reminiscing about something. Only 20 percent were actually paying attention to the lecture; with 12 percent actively listening.

Poor listening not only causes a decrease in academic performance, but it can lead to interpersonal conflict as well as frustration and a breakdown in communication. Yet, most people do not develop the ability to listen actively.

One of the reasons people do not make the effort to develop listening skills is they think they have more to gain by speaking than by listening. One big advantage of speaking is that it seems to give the speaker a chance to control others' thoughts and actions. Telling the other person what they should do is easier than first listening to what they want to do.

Another apparent advantage of speaking is the chance it provides to gain the admiration, respect, or liking of others. Tell jokes, and everyone will think, "there's a fun person". Offer advice, and they'll be grateful for the help. Make them impressed with your wisdom by pontificating. As you can quickly imagine, none of these strategies really work. Thus, there is a false assumption that the way to win friends and influence people is to talk rather than listen.

Finally, talking gives a person the chance to release energy in a way that listening can't. When you are frustrated, the chance to talk about your problems can often help you feel better. In the same way, you can often lessen your anger by letting it out verbally. And, sharing your excitement with others by talking about it helps when you feel as if you will burst if you keep it inside.

Although it's true that talking does have some advantages, it's important to realize that listening can pay dividends, too. Being a good listener is one good way to help others with their problems—and what better way is there to gain their appreciation? As for controlling others, it may be true that it's hard to be persuasive while you are listening, but your willingness to hear others out will often encourage them to think about your ideas in return. Like defensiveness, listening is often reciprocal: People get what they give.

Sometimes, even if a person wants to listen well, they're hampered by a lack of skill. A common but mistaken belief is that listening is like breathing, an activity that people do well naturally. "After all," the common belief goes, "I've been listening since I was a child. I don't need to study the subject in high school or college." The truth is that listening is a skill much like speaking: Virtually everybody does it, though few people do it well.

In today's rushed society, there are several reasons people don't listen well. The first reason is message overload. The amount of communications received through verbal and digital forms every day makes carefully attending to everything impossible. Almost half the time people are awake they are listening to verbal messages from teachers, co-workers, friends, family, salespeople, and total strangers, not to mention radio, television, and digital media. Research has shown people spend an average of five hours or more a day listening to people talk, 4 hours 28 minutes watching television and 5 hours 46 minutes with digital media. It looks like there is very little time spent in silence.

Another reason people don't always listen carefully is that they're often wrapped up in personal concerns that are of more immediate importance to them than the messages others are sending. It's hard to pay attention to someone else when you are anticipating an upcoming test or thinking about the wonderful time you had last night with good friends.

RECEIVING MESSAGES EFFECTIVELY

All of us are guilty of forming snap judgments, evaluating others before hearing them out. We also often listen to only what we want to hear. This tendency is greatest when the speaker's ideas conflict with our own. To really listen to another person is to set aside all of your distractions, expectations, judgments, anxieties, and self-concerns. Take a slow deep breath and open your ears, eyes, and heart to give center stage to the other person.

By focusing on the other person, you are putting him/her at ease and creating an atmosphere of trust. You may think it is important to talk about yourself to create a good impression, but just the opposite is true. Everyone wants to be listened to, so by attending to the other person instead of nervously talking about yourself, you are creating the best impression. To be listened to and acknowledged as heard is the greatest gift we can give or receive.

HOW TO SHOW YOU ARE LISTENING

As was mentioned in the section on nonverbal communication, show you are paying attention to the other person by adopting an open posture, leaning forward, and making eye contact. Then listen so closely to the other person that you can state back, in your own words, the essence of what you heard that person say. This is called paraphrasing. Paraphrasing is not a parroting of the other person's words. Paraphrasing involves listening to the other person's key ideas and then stating that person's ideas in your own words. Basically, you are listening for the primary content of what the person is saying and repeating the essence of that back. You might say something like, "It sounds like you are saying...." Then, after you have stated the essence of what you heard, you can assess the effectiveness of your paraphrase by listening to and observing the person's response. If your paraphrase is accurate, the person will, in some way, verbally or nonverbally, confirm its accuracy and usefulness.

Effective paraphrasing is not a trick. Rather, it is an attitude, an attitude that expresses, "I really want to know what you mean." The paraphrase response is a way of activating that attitude. We can't fake attitudes. If we believe that: (a) we know it all, (b) the speaker will say what we would say, and so we know what he is going to say before he says it, or (c) we should listen to words, not people... then we will never be able to, or want to, check out what the other person means. We will be psychologically deaf, and will never "hear" anything new. If, however, we do want to benefit from other person's perspective and we assume that we don't know it all, then the paraphrase can be a powerful expression of the attitude: "I'd like to hear clearly what you're trying to say," "Is this what you are saying?" This attitude of genuine interest is essential to all human relations.

Suppose a classmate tells you, "It's just a rough time for me—trying to work and keep up with school assignments. I keep telling myself it will slow down someday." You first ask yourself, "What has this person told me?" (That it's hard to keep up with everything he has to do.) Next you ask yourself, "What is the content of this message—what person, object, idea, or situation is the person discussing?" (Trying to keep up with work and school.) Finally you give a response, in your own words, such as, "It sounds like you're having a tough time balancing all your commitments" or "There are a lot of demands on your time right now."

When we paraphrase the listener relinquishes the leadership role, and "follows" the other person through the conversation. Sometimes, too, paraphrasing feels artificial when we first practice it. But, with added practice, paraphrasing sounds more natural.

An effect of paraphrasing is that the conversation slows down (which has the added benefit of giving us a chance to think). When someone puts you on the spot, your best defense is to just listen and paraphrase. This buys you time to think about your response and helps the other person hear what/he she really said when you feed it back to him/her via a paraphrase. Also, paraphrasing invites the other person to talk more. It leaves you less time to make your own points, but it helps you figure out what the other person really wants to hear. It also helps the other person focus on what they are saying. Often people do not listen to what they are saying. Paraphrasing helps them hear the essence of the message they are sending so they can come to their own conclusions. Finally, paraphrasing leads to understanding and generates feelings of being understood. It creates warmth and trust in the relationship.

To show you are listening at an even deeper level, use empathy. Empathy is the ability to identify with another person's experience. Empathy literally means "to feel in"--to stand in another's shoes, to get inside his/her feelings. It is listening so closely to another person that you can feel what he/she is feeling. And then it is the communication of this empathic understanding that creates trust, closeness, safety, and growth in relationships.

Empathy has been demonstrated to be one of the most important qualities for healthy relationships and for an individual's psychological health. Since the 1950s, empathy has been theorized to be essential for an individual's healthy development and has been identified as one of the most important skills parents need to develop psychologically healthy children. Empathy is essential for successfully resolving conflicts between individuals, between opposing groups of people, and even between nations.

It is important to use empathy in all your relationships but especially when:

- The other person is defensive. Empathy breaks down defenses faster and better than any other technique. Even if the other person comes back with another defensive remark, just keep using empathy. Say nothing else but a reflection of the other person's feelings, experiences, and behaviors. Don't let yourself get triggered into arguing or becoming defensive yourself. Just keep replying with empathic reflections of what you hear the other person saying.
- You want to create a deeper relationship. Empathic responses help the other person feel safe enough to tell you what is really bothering them. They encourage the other person to express their deeper feelings, not just their surface thoughts. Empathy begets empathy. So the more empathy you show, the more empathy you receive. People like people who show empathy, feel closer to them, and want to be with them.

- An empathic response identifies the central feeling and the central meaning, experience, or behavior in the other person's message. The basic formula for communicating empathy is "You're feeling…because…." Suppose a friend tells you, "My mother never lets me do anything on my own. She's looking over my back on everything, and when she's not doing that she's going through my things in my room." You could reply with, "You're saying that your mother both goes through your belongings and is always doing things for you," which is a paraphrase. Or you could reply with, "You're angry at your mother because you would like to be more independent from her and she is holding on," which is an empathic response.

GIVING FEEDBACK

Feedback gives clients an understanding of how others may view them. It is a reflective mirror, like empathy is, but it concentrates on the performance or behavior of the client whereas empathy deals with the statements the client makes.

Written and oral feedback is used in performance evaluations in families, education, sports, and business. The intent is to create behavior change and effective learning. Yet, in all of these settings, feedback is often given in a way that damages the relationship or the receiver. Damage occurs when the feedback concentrates on traits rather than behavior. Some of the common traits focused on are: adaptable, quick-tempered, cooperative, honest, bossy, loyal, pessimistic, impulsive, and sincere. Whether the traits are positive or negative ones, they describe characteristics of the person that are difficult to change. Instead, feedback that is based on specific, observable behaviors leads to increased learning, fewer opportunities for misunderstandings, and gives clear criteria for what is and is not acceptable performance. Feedback does not give conclusions about the "goodness" or "badness" of behavior; it simply describes the behavior that is observed. When giving feedback based on behavior, think, "Who did what, when, and how?"

Feedback is effective when it is given:

- After asking the receiver's permission
- As promptly as possible after the observed behavior
- In a nonjudgmental way. For example, say, "When you look away from me, I feel you are being insincere," as opposed to "Nobody likes people who don't look at people." Or, say, "I saw you relax and heard your joy as you went through that exercise," as opposed to, "You did that exercise very well."
- About the individual's specific and observable behavior, as opposed to his character or intention. It is concrete, not vague, and only deals with behavior. For example, "You aren't able to get along with the group" is not as helpful as "You had two arguments with Ginny that upset both of you, and now you are disagreeing strongly with Lois."
- About the individual's strengths as well as his or her weaknesses.
- By being checked-out with the receiver to see how your feedback was received. Ask, "How do you react to that?" to begin a discussion between the two of you that doesn't end until both of you feel the feedback was accurately received and determine how useful it was.

HANDLING CONFRONTATION

Confrontation can occur when you are trying to make a request or refuse a request. Some situations in which you might want to refuse a request are (a) resisting sales pressure, (b) refusing an unfair demand. Some situations in which you might want to initiate a request are (a) asking a favor of someone, (b) asking a person who is annoying you to stop. Some people often avoid making reasonable requests of others. And, when they do make them, they appear apologetic or do not expect the request to be accepted. Some people have trouble saying no and, instead, give excuses for not complying when they really just don't want to. Other people sound demanding, coercive, and hostile in requesting, and resentful and hostile in refusing.

Assertive responding is an important way of getting your point across without increasing the other person's anxiety and creating a defensive reaction. The first step is to learn to make "I" statements instead of "you" statements. Here are some typical "you" statements that show aggression or passivity instead of appropriate assertion.

"Don't ever do that again."

"You're such a slob. You are always leaving everything all over the place."
"Can't you see I'm already overburdened?"

Stop blaming the other person and, instead, tell the other person what you want. To change these statements into "I" statements use the following formula to tell the person how you feel and what you want.
"I feel…when you…and I want…."

The "I feel" part of the statement stops the other person from becoming defensive because it focuses on you rather than the other person. So the other person is able to hear you better. The "when you" part of the statement is a pure description of what is bothering you about the other person's behavior.

Remember, to just describe the behavior and leave out all evaluation. A good way to notice whether you are putting in any evaluation is to look at any adverbs or adjectives you might have in the statement. Take the adverbs and adjectives out and you will be closer to a pure description. It is the adjectives and adverbs that give the evaluative tone that puts the other person on the defensive.

For example: "You're such a slob. You are always leaving everything all over the place." This statement contains an adjective, "slob," and an adverb, "always." If you take out the adjective and the adverb, you have a pure description. "You're leaving everything all over the place."

The third part of the statement is a request for a change in the other's behavior. You may not get that change because you can never change the other person; you can only change yourself. But, changing yourself to at least request what you want honestly with an assertive statement makes you feel better and at least gives the other person a choice.

Before you make an assertive statement, though, you must make an empathic statement. When you are asserting your position you want the other person to accurately hear what you have to say. The other person won't hear you accurately if he/she is anxious and defensive. So, to prevent the other person from getting defensive or to disarm an already defensive person, make an empathic reflection. Then, state your assertion.

For example, if your friend criticizes you with, "You're not a good listener. Every time I try to talk with you, you act like you are just waiting for me to shut up so you can talk." You would first make an empathic reflection such as, "You feel I don't really listen to what you have to say…

that I'm just waiting for you to finish so I can say what I want to say."

Then you can make an assertive statement about your own feelings such as, "Sometimes I have a difficult time trying to figure out what the main point is when you are giving me a long story about something. I would like you to be a little less wordy."

Confrontations can often lead to disagreements. What do you do when you get into a disagreement with someone? Do you try to convince the other person that you are right? If that is your strategy, you may win the argument but lose a friend. Or you may lose both. What you really want is a way to find solutions to a disagreement or conflict where everyone, including yourself, wins.

Most people think about disagreements in terms of conflicting solutions. We prematurely define the problem in terms of "either-or" solutions. For example, your parent says, "I'm angry that so often when I ask you to complete your household chores you say you can't because you have to do your homework" and you reply with "But I have to do my homework and isn't it the most important thing?" Because each of you defined the problem of what is important in terms of solutions you are now having a disagreement.

The first step in resolving this disagreement is to accurately paraphrase or use an empathic response such as "You're upset because you think I use homework as an excuse for not doing my household chores." You do not have to agree with your parent's statement; you just have to let him/her know you understand what is being communicated. Or your parent might give you an empathic reflection such as, "Homework is important to you." It really only takes one person making an empathic response to break the impasse and to move the conversation to the next level, which is to change the solutions into a mutual goal. A mutual goal might be, "In the limited amount of time we have after school there are two things that need to be done; household chores and homework." Now the two of you can brainstorm possible ways to reach this goal. For example, you might agree that you both participate in household chores for one-half hour immediately after you come home from school and then you have uninterrupted time before and after dinner to finish your homework. You have handled this confrontation in a way that both of you feel respected and having your needs met.

Interpersonal communication is a set of skills that require practice but, once these skills become your usual way of communicating, you will find your relationships to be more successful and satisfying.

FURTHER READING

Bolton, R. (1986). *People Skills: How To Assert Yourself, Listen To Others, and Resolve Conflicts.* New York: Simon and Schuster. This paperback book was published a while ago but it is still available and it contains additional information and specific examples of the skills mentioned in this article.

Wood, J. F. (2016). *Interpersonal Communication: Everyday Encounters.* Independence, KY: Cengage Publishing, 2016. This book can be obtained online and it expands the information in this article by including ways to deal with many of the communication issues of today's relationships.

Beverly B. Palmer

Interpersonal skills and technology

In today's world, interpersonal skills do not just relate to in-person interactions. Strong interpersonal skills now also relate to an individual's ability to effectively communicate with people through technology-based settings such as emails, texts and social media sites. While there are some similarities regarding how interpersonal skills present within face-to-face versus remote settings there are also important differences. Building one's interpersonal skills within the technology-medium is essential in today's era, which embraces technology-based methods for communication.

INTRODUCTION

The meaning of interpersonal skills has greatly expanded over the past couple of decades. Prior to the emergence of the Internet and cellular phones, interpersonal skills were basically limited to in-person interactions. However, the abilities, advancement, and pervasiveness of today's technology have changed the way society as a whole interacts and communicates. While face-to-face communication remains an integral part of life, technology-based communication such as texting, emailing and social networking (e.g., Facebook, Twitter, Instagram) has become a standard part of day-to-day communication. Due to the high prevalence of email, text and social media forums as a standard way of communication, the aim of this article is to highlight both how interpersonal skills present within technology-based communication mediums and why having strong interpersonal skills related to one's email, texting and social media use are so important.

EMAILING AND TEXTING

The emergence of email began in the 1970's, with 1972 widely accepted as the invention point of email as we know it today. However, it was not until the 1990's that email became mainstream in our society. Since its inception, the use of emailing as a form of communication has exponentially increased. Reports from 2012 show that 144.8 billion emails are sent worldwide every day and the email rates are projected to increase to 206.6 billion emails per day in 2017. Email is the most widely used facility of the Internet.

Similarly, texting is also a relatively recent medium tracing its entry into popular usage in the 1990's. The popularity of texting grew on the back of the massive technology boom in the personal mobile phone industry. The convenience and appeal of communicating by text was, and continues to be, immense; people can send messages instantly from anywhere. The convenience of text is so strong that it is the preferred form of communication for many people, particularly amongst younger individuals.

Since emailing and texting are common avenues for both professional and social interactions, the importance of having strong interpersonal skills in these areas is essential. However, when communicating via email or text valuable interpersonal information that is inherent to in-person communication is absent; the missing components relate to eye contact, body language, and rate of speech. Therefore, the remaining key interpersonal skills associated with email and text are the following: 1) Tone of voice intended by the writer, 2) Tone of voice interpreted by the receiver, 3) Intended meaning of the words typed, and 4) Interpretation of the meaning of the words typed.

TONE OF VOICE

Tone of voice relates to the emotion or attitude of how one's words are being conveyed. Some descriptors for tones of voice include but are not limited to: happy, angry, optimistic, negative, rude, empathic, frustrated or sarcastic. The tone of voice adds significant meaning to the words being stated, but if misunderstood can be highly problematic since misunderstanding the tone of a message creates an entirely new meaning. Further-

more, interpreting the tone of voice from written words compared to an in-person verbal exchange increases the likelihood of the tone of voice being misjudged. When speaking directly with someone their body language and facial expressions add helpful information to help guide the listener to interpret the speaker's tone in the correct, intended manner. Additionally, their rate of speech and volume can also serve to guide listeners to correctly decipher their intended tone. However, emails and texts do not allow one the privilege of assessing the speaker's nonverbal behaviors for cues on how to read their tone of voice.

As recipients of an email or text all we have to go by are the words and punctuation contained in the written message. For example, a person emails or texts a friend about going to the movies and the friend responds, "No, I can't today." The friend reading the reply could take the message in many different ways, based on the perceived tone of voice they attribute to the text when reading the message. Some possible interpretations could include, feeling their friend was abrupt or disinterested or upset, which may in turn lead the person to feel sad or annoyed with their friend. Or perhaps the person thinks their friend is busy and therefore feels appreciative that their friend wrote back, even though it was a short message. Ultimately, the person can only guess at what their friend really meant by their reply; clearly not ideal communication!

Another example is a manager giving feedback to a team member on a completed task in a work setting, "Changes need to be made. Let's discuss." The manager sending the email may have been very impressed by the piece of work, however, did not have a lot of time to compose a longer message; they wanted to let the employee know they have looked at the piece of work. The employee would have no way of knowing the manager's intention, and the fact they liked the work. The employee only has the words of the email to go by – they are left to imply the tone. From their perspective they might interpret a whole range of things from the email; the work they prepared was not of good quality – "changes need to be made", which in their mind translates to the manager not being happy – the email was short and direct. There is a big disconnect between what the employee takes from the email, and what the manager actually feels. This is all due to the incorrect tone coming through, which a receiver can only construct from a very limited amount of information available in the written message.

Without being able to *hear* the actual tone it is challenging to properly identify how the person sending the message intended it to come across. This highlights why it is so important for the person writing the email or text to relay their tone clearly. The tools available to control tone include punctuation, sentence length, and word choice. The extra time you spend ensuring that your punctuation reflects your intended tone and that you have carefully chosen the words to convey your message properly, the stronger your interpersonal skills will become.

MEANING OF WORDS

Word choice serves two functions in written communication; firstly, it directly provides the meaning understood by recipients, secondly, it indirectly contributes to the tone of the message. When we write an email or text to somebody we are seeking to communicate a message to the individual; our ultimate goal is for the individual to understand the message. It is crucial to remember that when interacting with people this way, particular attention needs to be given to the words used. The words people read directly impact their understanding of and reaction to the message.

Using the example above of the movie invitation, the response "No, I can't today," is pretty clear in meaning to the recipient. However, is this the meaning intended by the sender? Additionally, could there be a different choice of words used to reply to the initial invitation, so as to achieve better communication? From the recipient's perspective the words of the message indicate their friend is unable to go to the movies today. Can they go tomorrow? How about next week? Or do they not want to go at all? Based solely on the message that was sent there is no way of knowing. However, were the friend to have chosen their words better, their message would have been much more effective. A better response could have been, "No, I can't today. I'd like to go though. How about next week?" or "I don't want to see that movie but thanks for the offer!" By including more detail in the message through a different choice of words the friend is able to communicate their position much more clearly. Choosing your words carefully as the sender of a message reduces the onus of the reader to try and decipher what you mean based on the limited cues inherent in written communication.

SOCIAL MEDIA

The advent of social media has heralded unparalleled interaction and connection between individuals. Its reach across the globe and sharing based platform allows for communication to occur between people who have never even met before. While there are many benefits and significant positives to social media, users need to be aware of how they use social media so as to avoid the pitfalls presented by the numerous platforms.

Similar to emails and texts, social media is primarily a written based medium, whether that is text only or also pictures. As such it is subject to the same limitations; eye contact, body language, and rate of speech is removed. Users of social media therefore need to be vigilant to ensure they create their messages carefully to be understood as intended. However, unlike email and texts, the sharing nature of social media presents some unique areas to take into consideration around interpersonal skills. The two biggest areas to be aware of are; people sharing posts, and information residing on the internet permanently.

SHARING POSTS

The ability for information to be disseminated through social media so quickly is built on the function of it being able to be shared by users. A post can be shared between many, many people who spread it extremely quickly, in the extreme making it viral. It is very difficult for the original poster to have any control over their post in this circumstance. The inability to control such rapid dissemination demands that users be vigilant about their posts, particularly as it exposes individuals to miscommunication that can lead to unfavorable outcomes. In some cases this can be harmless, however, it can have real life consequences.

An additional feature of the sharing aspect that is important to understand revolves around the fact that people are able to post and share anything they want. That includes information about you! This creates a fusion between events in the real world and the cyber world; think of social media as a giant scrapbook where everybody has control over what is included in the scrapbook. The demands placed on interpersonal skills are huge!

INFORMATION RESIDING PERMANENTLY ON THE INTERNET

If you say something you regret in-person more often than not the situation is short lived. For example, you may be temporarily embarrassed, or you may have angered somebody but you are usually able to smooth it out shortly afterwards. However, information that finds itself into social media has a much more permanent nature. Even for posts that you originate, you only have very limited control. The availability of this information presents a unique interpersonal frontier: people formulate opinions, pass judgment, and make decisions based on something online. It is not uncommon for both prospective and current employers trawling through social media accounts to get information about individuals. Due to the very real consequences related to social media activity it is important to keep in mind the same key concepts when expressing yourself via Facebook as you do when writing an email or text.

TAKEAWAY MESSAGE

The ability to communicate with people without actually being in their presence is amazing and has many positive implications. It is important however to realize how speaking to someone face-to-face versus via technology requires a different interpersonal skill set. Without being able to see the other person, read their body language, or hear their tone of voice the words used to convey a message whether by email, text or a social media page are extremely important. Understanding the basic principles that are the foundation for effective technology-based communication and then actively building these interpersonal skills has immense value in today's technology dominant society.

FURTHER READING

Barclay, J. (2013). Text messaging: Does it destroy relationships? *Snowdrift*. Retrieved from: http://www.snowcollegenews.com/text-messaging-does-it-destroy-relationships/. This article discusses that while texting has benefits, the ease and frequency in which people's texts are misinterpreted can lead to significant negative outcomes. The author focuses on how texts have lead to many break-ups, specifically among college students.

Demangone, A. (2014). That's not what I meant! – Technology and miscommunication. *National Association of Federal Credit Unions*. Retrieved from: http://www.cuinsight.com/thats-not-what-i-meant-technology-and-miscommunication.html. This article focuses on how easily technology-based communication can be misinterpreted. It highlights the importance that the person writing the message take time when composing the email to increase the likelihood that the intended and received message are the same.

Ferrazzi, K. (2013). How to avoid virtual miscommunication. *Harvard Business Review*. Retrieved from: https://hbr.org/2013/04/how-to-avoid-virtual-miscommun/. This article discusses how simple things can be misinterpreted when communication occurs remotely versus in-person. The author outlines six techniques to help increase the accuracy and effectiveness of technology-based communication.

Winerman, L. (2006). E-mails and egos. *American Psychological Association*. Retrieved from: http://www.apa.org/monitor/feb06/egos.aspx. This article discusses how the message intended in an email is often quite different than the actual message received. The inability to accurately convey one's tone of voice when writing an email is a key component that causes the discrepancy between the intended and received message. The authors discuss how people need to learn to see how others may perceive their message.

Stefan Leonte and Kimberly Glazier

SEE ALSO: Interpersonal Communication

Interviewing

Interviewing is one of the most popularly adopted methods to select and recruit productive employees. Interviewee competences are critical to obtaining attractive job offers, the first step to success in the workplace. Adolescents face a developmental task to construe their identity, a part of which is career identity. One meaningful path is to get working experience through employment. In modern society, adolescence is probably the first time in life for a youngster to go through a formal interviewing process to be hired for a job.

INTRODUCTION

This article focuses on interviewee skills , and not interviewer skills, because realistically, the majority of the adolescents will be interviewees.

According to the late psychologist Erik Erikson, adolescents' developmental task is to construe identity ("who you are"). In this process, career becomes a salient part to adolescence and many start to participate in the labor force. If work is balanced well with school, employment can be beneficial to adolescent development. The longitudinal data from the Youth Development Study of high school students showed benefits of employment to the "steady workers" (< 20 hours per week most of the

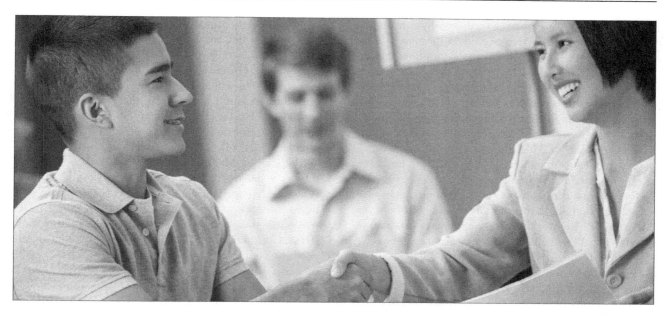

Photo: iStock

time) and "occasional workers" (< 20 hours per week in a few months only), giving them a sense of accomplishment. Supported by work experience they were strong at achieving educational goals, accumulating savings and bettering their time management skills. Another group, identified as "the most invested workers" (> 20 hours per week most of the time), also benefited. Employment gave them an opportunity to practice agency and helped them move faster into their self-selected career path to achieve a full-employee identity. In addition, obtaining job-related training, receiving mentoring, and enjoying advancements in the workplace were positively associated with the adolescents' self-efficacy. Negative effects like work stress tended to be short-lived, and more noticeably, might actually have fostered psychological resilience and expanded stress management skills.

INTERVIEWING BASICS

Only employment interviewing is discussed here but the information is applicable to other types of interviewing for different purposes, e.g., for admission to colleges/ graduate programs or for scholarships.

For the sake of reliability (consistency) and validity (job-related qualifications), employment interviews are most likely to be structured, i.e., a pre-determined set of designed interview questions will be asked to all of the job candidates in the same way by all interviewers and there is a standardized scoring key to evaluate each

candidate's performance, although the level of structure may vary.

Adolescents should be prepared for all three phases in an employment interview: the pre-interview phase, the actual interviewing phase, and the post-interview phase. A face-to-face interview may have only one interviewer or a panel of interviewers. Interviews may be conducted in an alternative medium: a phone interview or a video interview.

TYPICAL INTERVIEW QUESTIONS

Interview questions are designed to assess the candidate's personality, knowledge and skills, quality of thinking, ability to handle difficult situations, values and ethics, motivation, career goals, etc. Michael G. Aamodt, an American industrial and organizational psychology professor at Radford University, has listed six types of interview questions:

Clarifier questions – to clarify information in the application files. Work-history questions belong to this group. Be prepared to answer questions such as "Why are you applying for this job?" "Why do you want to leave your current job?" or "Why do you seek jobs sporadically?" Your answers should highlight your career interest, motivation for career development, and realistic necessities such as location and school commitment. You should avoid mistakes like criticizing former employers/coworkers, complaining about previous jobs, or emphasizing benefits.

Disqualifier questions – to disqualify a candidate if he/she cannot satisfy the specific requirements of the job. For example, if the job requires the employee to work on night shifts, a candidate who answers "no" to "Are you able to work on night shifts?" is disqualified for this job.

Skill-level determiners – to tap the applicant's job-relevant skills. Applicants for a receptionist position may be asked questions about computer skills and using software to schedule and file. Brainteasers may be included in an interview for competitive jobs that require logical reasoning and creative thinking.

Past-focused questions (behavioral questions) – to get information about the candidate's previous behavior. For example, "Share with me an example of how you reacted to negative feedback from your teacher or boss."

Future-focused questions (situational questions) – to get information about the candidate's probable behavior in the future. For example, "Imagine that you are a waiter/waitress in a restaurant and a customer becomes impatient with the long waiting. How would you handle this situation?"

Organization fit questions – to find out if the candidate will fit into the culture of the company/work unit. For example, the candidate may be asked to tell the interviewer about his/her preference for team-based work or independent work.

THE PRE-INTERVIEW PHASE

Caldwell and Burger have reported the power of social preparation and background preparation in predicting interview success (getting subsequent interviews or job offers). Social preparation is to utilize social resources (teachers, school counselors, parents, friends, someone in the company, and people in similar jobs) for advice and information about the company and the position. Background preparation is to research the company to learn as much as possible about it and the job. Study the company's website. Find brochures, news and business reports in the career center, public libraries, and business publications. Read the information carefully. Get educated about the company's location, history, mission and values, objectives and plans, current status, brand products, recent changes, management and people, etc.

Preparation is not just for gathering information to answer the interviewer's questions but also is for you to prepare questions for the interviewer. You may ask questions about the specific job (e.g., responsibilities, authority), growth opportunities (e.g., training, promotion), or peers and management (e.g., culture of the work

unit, immediate supervisor). Prioritize your questions. Caution: Do not ask any question about the information already given to you, e.g., in the ad/brochures or on the website. Otherwise, you are telling the interviewer that you have not done your homework. Remember, your questions are not just questions; they are part of the interviewing because they tell something about you – your conscientiousness, intelligence, personality, and career interests and goals.

Preparation should include practice. Practice your role as a job interviewee. Get feedback and improve. Role play again. Familiarity helps reduce anxiety and nervousness. Practice improves speech fluency. Pay attention to your articulation, volume, tone, rhythm, and stress. Get rid of "um," "like," "and," or "you know." Keep good eye contact with "the interviewer." Emphasize with proper gestures without excessive hand movements. Body should be relaxed but alert.

Get familiar with the interview location and how to get there. On the interview day, give yourself plenty of time to arrive at the interview site 10-15 minutes earlier than the scheduled interview time. Never be late for an interview. Dress appropriately. Look clean. Smile. Be professional and friendly to all the people you meet once you set your feet on the site of the company (you never know who that person is and what role that person plays in hiring). If possible, decline coffee (you may spill it and look clumsy and messy). Keep mentally alert and focused. Organize all of the materials you will need during the interview neatly and get into the interview room with confidence.

If it is a phone/video interview, find a quiet location without any distraction or interference. Check the device, volume, clarity of the visual images, and all of the connections. Have a back-up plan in case technology fails. Familiarize yourself with how to operate the machine(s).

THE INTERVIEWING PHASE

The interviewer will start interviewing with a brief welcoming introduction. Give a warm greeting with a firm handshake. Respond to "small talk" naturally. Take your seat with a comfortable position without casualness. The interviewer then proceeds to give you some information about the position and the company, and/or explain the interviewing process. Listen attentively. Make some mental notes as the information may be usable later when you answer or ask questions. After this information giving phase comes the time for you to answer the interviewer's questions. Listen carefully to get an accurate understanding of each question. If you are not sure about what is being asked, politely ask for clarification. Provide focused answers in specific and personalized language that goes straight to the point (demonstrating your clear way of thinking). Speak up and speak clearly with good eye contact. Do not ramble or use vague/general expressions (indicator of a cloudy mind or lack of knowledge). Cite specific examples to vividly illustrate the key points. Avoid reciting a memorized answer. Interact with the interviewer and monitor your approach. When it is your turn to ask questions, select a couple of job/company-related questions that can show your independent thoughts, values, and goals. You may also develop questions based upon what the interviewer has been saying on the spot. When the interview approaches conclusion, you may inquire about the timeline for the decision making and also, encourage the interviewer to contact your references. Leave a good impression that you are interested and enthusiastic. Remember to thank the interviewer.

If this is a phone interview without visual imaging, be aware that you are deprived of non-verbal and paralinguistic cues (e.g., facial expressions, eye contact). Your articulation and speech features become even more important here than in a face-to-face interview. It is advisable to dress up so that you won't get too relaxed and lose your alertness.

Here is a last note specific to adolescents. While it is important to effectively deliver your job-relevant qualifications, it is equally, if not more, important to convince the interviewer that you have great potential. Show your career interest and goals, motivation and enthusiasm, modesty and willingness to learn and improve, and courage to welcome challenges.

THE POST-INTERVIEW PHASE

Remember to do follow-up work after an interview in a timely manner. Send a thank-you note right after the interview. Be patient and wait. After a week or two, you may send a letter or make a call to the contact person reinforcing your continued interest, and provide new supportive documents, if any. But do not be a stalker. After two such inquiries without a reply, it is a sign for you to move on.

Reflect critically upon your interview experience. Find strengths to keep and weaknesses to improve. You may even contact the interviewer for constructive feedback. There may be other opportunities.

CONCLUSION

Being mindful of the developmental process in an all-rounded way and garner successful experiences in various activities (e.g., schoolwork, sports, volunteering)to contribute to building the many elements for successful interview performance, including self-efficacy, healthy attribution style and locus of control, emotional intelligence, cognitive competencies/skills, oral/written communication skills, social competencies/skills, and critical self-reflection skills. All-rounded adolescents are highly likely to get interview opportunities. They will be able to do conscientious preparation and perform well in the actual interviews.

Adolescents should also be mindful of cultivating adaptive flexibility in thinking and behavior. Exploration, commitment, and insightful self-reflection will enable adolescents to gradually achieve flexibility in its mature form. In the context of interviewing, the ability to monitor, regulate and adapt one's response to the specific interview situation appropriately is essential. While "under" is not desired, "over" destroys appropriateness. Over-confidence is arrogant and reveals narrow-mindedness. Being over-zealous may convey a sense of fakeness or sound flattery.

FUTURE DIRECTION

Programs and workshops for training interviewee skills tend to focus on interview preparation (gathering job/company information, practicing answers to likely questions, generating questions to ask). Social skills training typically include impression management (e.g., dress, handshake) and responding to questions (e.g., verbal delivery, non-verbal behavior, eye contact). However, the effectiveness of such training is not clear as findings from evaluative studies are inconsistent.

Effectiveness of training is typically measured by the ratings from mock/potential recruiters and the success rates of getting subsequent interviews or job offers. But a challenging question here is whether what is delivered in the interview is in fact what is perceived and picked up by the interviewer. The answer is uncertain because any interview is a dynamic interviewer-interviewee interaction with many factors coming into play. Huffcutt and his colleagues' theoretical model is recommended here for future research considerations and theory building. In their model, six clusters of influencing factors are identified: 1. The interviewer-interviewee dynamics (interviewee social effectiveness, interviewer personality); 2. Interviewee state influences (self-efficacy, interview motivation and anxiety); 3. Supplemental preparation (interview training, interview experiences); 4. Interview designs (level of structure, interview mediums, pre-interview information); 5. Demographic/personal characteristics (cultural background, attractiveness, race and gender); and 6. Interviewer information processing effects (memory limitations, simplifying heuristics [mental shortcuts], biases and errors). We have little empirical knowledge about their dynamic relationships; let alone causal links. Systematic research is needed to equip us with evidence-based knowledge in this regard. That knowledge will help improve interviewee training; how to deliver job-specific qualifications in an adaptively flexible way with interviewer variables taken into consideration. This will certainly benefit adolescent interviewees tremendously when they are at the beginning of their career.

FURTHER READING

Aamodt, M. G. (2016). *Industrial/Organizational Psychology: An Applied Approach* (8th ed.). Boston, MA: Cengage Learning. A segment of Chapter 4 describes types of employment interviews and interview questions, as well as how to conduct interviews.

Caldwell, D. F., & Burger, J. M. (1998). "Personality characteristics of job applicants and success in screening interviews". *Personnel Psychology* 51, 119-136. The paper reports the mediating functions of personality traits of conscientiousness, extraversion, and openness to experience in the associations of social preparation and background preparation to interview success.

Huffcutt, A. I., Van Iddekinge, C. H., & Roth, P. L. (2011). "Understanding applicant behavior in employment interviews: A theoretical model of interviewee performance". *Human Resource Management Review*, 21, 353-367. doi:10.1016/j.hrmr.2011.05.003. The authors present a theoretical model composed of multiple factors in interviewer-interviewee dynamics and ideas for future research.

Mortimer, J. T. (2011). *The Benefits and Risks of Adolescent Employment* (PMCID: PMC2936460). Retrieved from http://www.ncbi.nlm.nih.bov/PMC2936460/. This document reviewed the longitudinal Youth Development Study and identified four types of high school students who participated in employment.

Ling-Yi Zhou

SEE ALSO: Finding Your First Job; Friendship Between Parents and Adult Children; Time Management

Leadership

What makes a great leader? Leadership is comprised of basic human traits that any individual can embrace and develop. Understanding the basic components of leadership and then implementing the areas in your own unique and individualized manner is an essential aspect of being a great leader. Everyone is different and therefore leadership traits work in ways that reflect a person's uniqueness and individuality.

INTRODUCTION

The traditional concept of leadership evokes images of individuals in positions of authority; an established hierarchy with defined roles and responsibilities. However, is there more to leadership than a title and position? Surely 'leadership' does not simply happen once you reach a particular position. What is the real substance that lies behind leadership that allows an individual to be looked upon as a leader? This article explores the characteristics and actions instrumental to the act of leading.

A commonly accepted definition of leadership is "the action of leading a group of people." What does this actually mean though? If you were told to go and "lead a group of people," what would that actually mean? There are countless ways people could interpret the aforementioned task. Instead of attempting to create one standard definition of leadership we instead focus in detail on the individual aspects that feature in good leadership. The features have been grouped into four overarching categories: Moral Traits, People Oriented Traits, Task Oriented Traits, and Improvement Focused Traits. It is important to understand that while key leadership characteristics can be individually identified, in practice they frequently intertwine with one another.

MORAL TRAITS

An important aspect for leadership relates to the person's overall integrity. Some people have a talent for speaking in a persuasive and enticing manner but their end objectives are not well intentioned. While they may appear to be leaders due to their charisma and ability to get others to listen to them, these types of individuals are not honest and therefore lack an essential aspect of genuine leadership: being trustworthy. Real leaders do not hide their motives nor do they operate under false pretences.

The question then arises, how do leaders gain other's trust? Trust grows over time as a leader's words and actions translate into reality. Therefore, it is highly important for leaders to be open and honest in what they say and what they actually do. While strong leaders genuinely do have other's best interests in mind it is equally important for leaders to not make promises that cannot be kept, even if the promises are well-intentioned. In essence, real leaders while they strive to create high quality outcomes also genuinely care about those working for them and treat people with respect.

PEOPLE FOCUSED TRAITS

Similar to the moral focused traits, this area shares the underlying principle of caring about others. However, it also highlights the need for leaders to understand how each individual's personality and abilities impact their work. Being aware of peoples' work styles along with the areas they excel and struggle in, is a first important step. Great leaders take it a step farther and tailor their leadership approach based on the individual characteristics of the person. For example, if one person thrives when working independently and creatively while another person performs best when given specific guidelines and deadlines, a strong leader knows how to tailor tasks to match each individual's preferred working style.

Additionally, great leaders have a positive energy that motivates people and also builds others' self-confidence. While some people use the fear tactic to get results, real leaders do not resort to scaring others. They lead by cultivating a supportive environment that focuses on utilizing people's strengths, building upon their areas of weakness, and igniting their motivation and passions.

TASK ORIENTED TRAITS

The ability to have a vision and break that end goal down into smaller, objective, and more manageable steps is an important quality for leadership. Often people have grand plans but fail to make their target goal because the road needed to reach the end result is too ambiguous or difficult. A strong leader is able to see the larger and the smaller picture at the same time and successfully implement a strategic plan to reach both goals. Good leaders commit to their plans without being inflexible and rigid and are always open to ways to enhance the process. Often times the wide range of options can overwhelm an individual; strong leaders are knowledgeable about the pros/cons of the different routes but are able to make a decisive decision and be accountable for their choice. Sometimes when a "leader" makes a decision the person does everything in their power to make that option

work. The ability to see when a plan is not working and admit to the fact is not a sign of weakness but rather one of great strength. Strong leaders maintain composure in difficult situations and modify plans in a rational versus panic-like state; the emphasis is placed on how to reach the goal and what steps need to be taken in order to get closer to the desired outcome.

IMPROVEMENT FOCUSED TRAITS

Another essential component of leadership is one's ability to both give and receive feedback. Knowing how to provide helpful feedback is highly important. Some people are hesitant to give constructive feedback and only focus on peoples' strengths, while other individuals tend to focus on the negatives. Leaders understand the importance of equally focusing on both the positive attributes of others while also highlighting their areas for improvement. At the same time, true leaders also ask others for feedback on their own performance (e.g., the leader's strengths and areas to improve), and moreover actually make modifications based on the suggestions received. Strong self-reflection and self-awareness skills coupled with a genuine openness to feedback from others makes people respect, trust and want to listen to the leader's instructions or advice.

In addition to inviting and embracing feedback from individuals that work for the leader, another important aspect related to strong leadership rests in the leader's proactive approach to seeking counsel and advice from people both within and outside the group/agency. Soliciting suggestions from others generates additional ideas; having a wide range of options allows the leader to consider more techniques and strategies to implement. Another key factor within this Improvement Focused Traits domain is the leader's ability to communicate clearly and effectively. When instructions are not clearly outlined it increases the likelihood of mistakes being made. Confusion regarding the task at hand not only causes the workers to feel frustrated but it also reduces the efficiency of the overall work. Therefore, it is important that leaders are able to provide clear instructions when allocating tasks to individuals and provide people with both positive and constructive feedback.

ANYONE CAN BE A LEADER

The aforementioned are characteristics that can be championed by anybody. The characteristics are not reserved for only certain people, or people in certain positions. By displaying the above qualities every individual can be deemed a leader in some capacity. True leadership is the recognition that people bestow upon you; simply telling people what to do does not make one a leader. A position of power does not make one a leader. Unless individuals truly view and relate to the 'leader' as their leader, there is no leadership, simply a person with a title. Every company has a CEO, not every company has a leader. All teams have a captain, not every team has a leader.

Everybody has his or her own style. People tend to associate the concept of a leader with someone who is extroverted and exudes self-confidence. Leaders can be, but by no means "have" to be confident, charismatic individuals. The range of personality types of well-known and admired leaders ranges greatly. The real key to being a true leader is to embody the positive leadership elements that are attainable to people across all personality types.

FURTHER READING

Ashkenas, R. (2015). "Seven Mistakes Leaders Make In Setting Goals". *Forbes*. Retrieved from: http://www. forbes.com/sites/ronashkenas/2012/07/09/seven-mistakes-leaders-make-in-setting-goals/. This article focuses on the importance of goal setting but also describes common ways in which the goal setting process, if done incorrectly, can have counterproductive side effects. It outlines seven common pitfalls.

Folkman, J. (2013). "The Best Gift Leaders Can Give: Honest Feedback". *Forbes*. Retrieved from: http://www.forbes.com/sites/joefolkman/2013/12/19/the-best-gift-leaders-can-give-honest-feedback/. This article highlights how strong leaders are both able to give constructive feedback and receive constructive feedback. It talks about how leaders who give constructive feedback are viewed more positively than leaders who do not.

Horsager, D. (2012). "You Can't Be a Great Leader Without Trust. Here's How To Build It". *Forbes*. Retrieved from: http://www.forbes.com/sites/forbes-leadershipforum/2012/10/24/you-cant-be-a-great-leader-without-trust-heres-how-you-build-it/. The article emphasizes how to be a true leader you must be trustworthy. Being in a position of authority does not automatically make people trust you. The article outlines eight key components for helping to build your trustworthiness.

Silverstein, R. (2010). "Good People Make Good Leaders". *Entrepreneur*. Retrieved from: http://www.

entrepreneur.com/article/206832. This article discusses the importance of leaders treating other people with respect and honouring their accomplishments both professional and personal.

Stefan Leonte and Kimberly Glazier

Networking

In today's competitive climate, networking is a valuable tool for young adults to develop. Networking opportunities can arise through social media, extracurricular activities, hobbies, and interests. The first step in networking is being aware of the opportunities that exist, so that they can help you with your future wants. Whether you are networking for a career goal, social interest, or college, this article will provide guidelines to help you navigate the process of using networking to attain your goals.

INTRODUCTION

Networking is a skill that many leaders learned early on. It can be practiced and learned in a variety of settings. The first thing to do to encourage networking is to pick a field, college, profession or interest that you would like to learn more about and find like-minded sites or individuals who can help you succeed in these fields. Networking is an important social skill, as it can help you meet individuals that can help you attain your professional and personal goals. Social connections can help you get access to resources or people that can help you get a job, get into the college of your dreams, or master a hobby. Seeking out networking opportunities can help you improve your résumé or find a mentor in your field of interest. It can also help you develop social and communication skills.

There are many social media sites that contain blogs or chat rooms where you can communicate with people who share the same interests as you. If it is a specific college you want to go to, social networking can be a good way to start. A recent study has shown that 92% of teenagers go online daily (Lenhart, 2015), and in this decade, social media has become a requirement for succeeding at networking. Some online sites where young adults connect include Facebook, Tumblr, Instagram, Twitter, Vine and Pheed. It is very important to maintain a professional environment with everything you post. Realize that your words, photos, and videos will be scrutinized carefully and that future job employers and college admission counselors will be viewing your postings. What you post and write can be used against you, so be very cautious with what you chose to put on social media. With that precaution in mind, online sites have proven to be a successful part of the networking process. In this day and age if you do not have access to social media, you are at a great disadvantage, and may be seen by some to be behind in technology.

Networking can help you create a career portfolio, and can give you access to leaders in your field of interest. One way to increase your chances of in-person networking is to attend career or college days. These usually occur at high schools, colleges, or at specific locations that are usually posted online. While you are at one of these events, ask about the possibility of shadowing a student, employee, or member of the faculty. This is a great way to further enhance your networking skills and gain valuable work experience.

In-person networking opportunities can teach you a lot about yourself and the way you handle the networking process. During the process you can evaluate yourself on how you associate with others. Body language is an important non verbal communication skill that should be considered and developed. Remember to smile, focus, and maintain an open demeanor. Sit up straight, and try not to cross your hands in front of your chest or hunch. These nonverbal clues can all be learned or unlearned to help navigate the networking process. Wearing a name tag can also help at networking events, and can serve as a reminder to the person you are talking with. While you network in a social setting, remember to ask open-ended questions, as this allows the person you are talking with to share more about themselves. Listen carefully and with interest to what the person in front of you is saying.

Expressing yourself verbally, with clarity, is also a key part of the networking process. Many young adults have found something in common with the person they speak with, and this commonality can provide one with a serious connection that may be able to help in the future. At networking events, save business cards or pamphlets, and write follow up thank you notes if you spend a significant amount of time with a key individual. If it is a college event, try to schedule an interview with an alumni member before you leave. Remember that networking can provide you with an opportunity to meet a mentor who can help you with your goals. Networking opportunities can also arise through friends and family,

so remember to let people know you are interested in a certain goal or college, and ask if they have any connections they might introduce to you.

Being a successful networker does mean you have to be present at events, and show up at meetings. These events provide you an excellent opportunity to meet people who have attained the goals you would like to. While at the events, walk around the room, and see if you know someone or see a familiar face. If not, go up to someone friendly, shake his or her hand, and introduce yourself and your grade level. If you recognize that this person is someone that is key in your field, be sure to express that you have read their article, social media post, or something that tells them you are aware of their importance and reputation. People love to talk about themselves and their accomplishments, and this will put you both at ease. Realize that networking opportunities are available all over. At airports, cafes, or even your local coffee shop, you can run into a person who will help you advance your profession, or who knows something about the admission process of the college of your choice. It is important to see networking as a valuable opportunity to help you attain your goals.

Always dress the part for a networking event. Wearing professional clothing is important. Depending on personal preferences and events, you can decide if you want to cover up identifying features such as tattoos or extra piercings. Some people are judgmental, and at an interview or networking event you are being judged and evaluated by the person in front of you. Remember to always act professionally at a networking event or interview. Show up on time and do not use questionable language, slang, or street terminology when communicating with the person you are interviewing or networking with, no matter how laid back you perceive them to be.

The hope is that after your networking opportunity or interview, you receive the job, volunteer opportunity, or college acceptance letter! Congratulations! At an appropriate time, you can then ask your network connection to write you a letter of recommendation for future employment or academic opportunities. This letter can prove your value and your connection with your networking contact. Ask for both a paper and electronic copy of the letter of recommendation, and be sure to save your electronic letters on your computer, and your print letters in a paper-based portfolio.

FURTHER READING

Christian, C. & Bolles, R. (2010). *What Color is Your Parachute for Teens: Discovering Yourself, Defining your Future* (2nd ed.). Berkley, CA: Ten Speed Press. A book about finding your strengths and interests at an early age, so that you can decide what type of schooling, job, or career is right for you. This book includes profiles of individuals who have leveraged their strengths to find their dream job.

Cohen, S., Dwane, A., deOliveira, P., & Muska, M. (2011). *Getting In! The Zinch Guide to College Admissions and Financial Aid in the Digital Age.* New York: Cliff Notes. A short, well-researched, current guide for mastering the college admissions process. Includes information on college admissions offices, application guidelines, choosing the right college, athletic recruiting, and scholarship/financial aid opportunities. This book also contains helpful sections on college essay assistance and waiting for an answer after the application process.

Kouzes, J.M. & Posner, B.Z. (2012). *The Leadership Challenge: How to Make Extraordinary Things Happen in Organizations.* San Francisco: Jossey Bass. A book about how individuals can create positive change within their organization by engaging in practices of modeling, shared vision, challenge, action, and heart based encouragement. Provides information on forward moving leadership, integrating tenets of intrinsic motivation and desires in planning and doing within corporations, companies, and non-profit organizations.

Lenhart, A. (2015, April). Teens, Social Media & Technology Overview – 2015. *Pew Research Center.* Retrieved from http://www.pewinternet. org/2015/04/09/teens-social-media-technology-2015/. A review of social media and technology use in teenagers. Trends include increased use of smartphones and mobile devices, as well as continuing use of social media platforms like Facebook and Twitter. Use of Instagram, Snapchat, Tumblr, and Google+ is also discussed.

Rath, T. (2007). *Strengths Finder 2.0.* Washington, D.C.: Gallup Publishing. This is a classic book about finding and leveraging your strengths in the classroom, at work, during interviews, and at home. Purchase of this book in electronic or print format comes with a code that allows you to take an online assessment that highlights your five signature strengths.

Bernadette Riley and Gina Riley

SEE ALSO: Interpersonal Communication; Leadership; Social Media and Etiquette

Public speaking

Public speaking permeates almost all aspects of our lives. However, despite its significance, the fear it stirs in people leads many to try and avoid it; for some, at all costs! Through their avoidance people ultimately serve to only short change themselves. By choosing to confront the fear elicited from the mere thought of public speaking, over time it can be overcome. Exposure work is a strong ally in conquering the fear associated with public speaking.

INTRODUCTION

The thought of giving a speech or presentation in front of an audience makes most people want to run and hide. The comedian Jerry Seinfeld uses humor to emphasize how strongly people fear speaking in front of others, "According to most studies, people's number one fear is public speaking. Number two is death. Death is number two. Does that sound right? This means to the average person, if you go to a funeral, you're better off in the casket than doing the eulogy." While most people try to avoid public speaking at all costs, the reality is it is nearly impossible to completely avoid. The more that public speaking is avoided, the more anxious people feel when "forced" to make a presentation or speech. This chronic avoidance leads to missed opportunities and prevents personal growth. The aim of this article is to highlight the prevalence and benefits of public speaking and to describe specific steps to transform public speaking from an anxiety provoking to enjoyable experience.

PUBLIC SPEAKING: MORE THAN GIVING SPEECHES

Public speaking includes but is broader than simply giving a speech to an audience; it refers to any time when a speaker orally communicates with an audience. The following are all examples of public speaking: giving a class or work presentation, sharing a story to a group of people, reading aloud to others, speaking up during a team meeting to express your ideas, giving a toast, and auditioning for a show. The range of activities that involve a public speaking component are numerous and span social, academic and professional settings. Over the past couple of decades the importance that employers place on applicants' public speaking abilities has increased substantially. However, unfortunately, people's fear of public speaking has remained elevated.

OVERCOMING THE FEAR OF PUBLIC SPEAKING

There is an extensive body of literature that suggests the most effective way to overcome one's anxieties is to face the fear head on in a gradual and systematic fashion. This process is formally referred to as exposure work. For individuals who fear public speaking (which according to research is the majority of people) exposure work directly targets this fear. Since the main focus is to confront one's fear, at the beginning of the exposure people feel an increase in anxiety; this is an expected and necessary part of exposure work. However, the anxiety does decrease with repeated exposures, and the initial fear of public speaking lessens. As the anxiety lowers, one's self-confidence in their public speaking abilities typically increases.

While exposures are highly effective there are three key components that are important in order to truly benefit from them. The first two essential factors are the *frequency* and *consistency* of the exposure work, which determines both how quickly results are felt and how long the results last. Frequency refers to how often the exposures are conducted. Doing one presentation or answering a question in class once a month, or even once a week, will likely not lead to a significant reduction in one's anxiety of giving presentations or speaking up in class. When first starting out with exposure work, doing multiple exposures per day is important. The second aspect, consistency, refers to continuing to do the exposures on a regular basis. Doing five exposures on Monday but then waiting until the following Monday to do another five exposures has good frequency (5 exposures per day vs. 1 exposure per day) but lacks the consistency (once a week vs. once a day). The reason that frequency and consistency are important is because the fear of public speaking has become so ingrained within

the individual that in order to change one's perception of public speaking the person needs to create a new association of public speaking. This new perception is obtained through experience; the more often and more consistent the experiences occur the more quickly the new mindset becomes the natural way of thinking and believing.

DETERMINING WHERE TO START

The third key component for exposures relates to the systematic and gradual nature of the exposure work. For example, if an individual has a fear of public speaking then giving a presentation in front of an audience of 100 people would likely be far too overwhelming. Starting with this exposure would likely be too difficult to accomplish, and if attempted initially may lead to even more anxiety of public speaking. Depending on the individual's anxiety the presentation can start as basic as the following: presenting aloud to just oneself; looking at oneself in the mirror while presenting; presenting to one other person you feel comfortable with; presenting to a couple

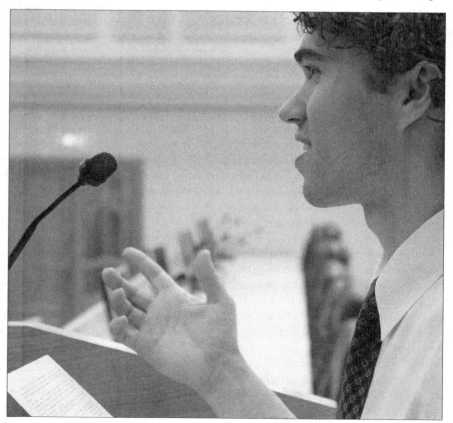

Photo: iStock

of people you feel comfortable with; presenting to someone you feel less comfortable with; presenting to a small group of people. If needed, the exposure presentations to others could start with having the audience member(s) initially not looking at the speaker during the presentation and then working up to having the audience face the presenter. Eventually the process could include having the audience member ask a question(s) after the presentation. For more difficult exposures, the questions can be more challenging or even express disagreement with an aspect of the presentation. The possible variations with creating the exposure hierarchy are countless and the key is for each person to develop their own hierarchy that has a range of exposures, including some that are anxiety provoking but manageable and others that initially would be extremely challenging or "impossible" for the person to complete. Starting with the more manageable items allows the person to gain a sense of mastery and accomplishment and eventually makes the initial "impossible" tasks seem less scary and more doable.

WHEN TO USE IMAGINAL EXPOSURES

Sometimes it may be impossible for the individual to make one or more presentations a day (or even a week) to audiences. Similarly auditioning for a play on a daily basis for most people is not feasible. In these situations, imaginal exposures can be used. For imaginal exposures the presenter should imagine they are standing in front of an audience. The key is for the person to truly immerse themselves in the situation by visually seeing and mentally and/or verbally describing all the details of the event. All five senses (sight, smell, hearing, taste and touch) should be incorporated when visualizing and describing the situation; this is important as it helps increase how real the exposure feels.

Another time to use imaginal exposures is when the situation itself may be too overwhelming at first. For example, if the person has a fear of public speaking related to having conversations with a group of people, imaginal exposures would be a good place to start. The same rules apply here; the imaginal exposure should involve the person visualizing and describing the situation in as much detail as possible (which includes using the five senses). During the exposure the person should engage in an imaginal conversation in which the individual is an active contributor to the conversation.

REAL LIFE IMPORTANCE

Public speaking is a skill. It is something that is learned and mastered. Ralph Waldo Emerson acknowledges how public speaking abilities are not inherent within an individual; he believed "All great speakers were bad speakers at first." Often times the biggest barrier to mastering the art of public speaking relates to individuals' fear of speaking in front of others and their resulting desire to minimize or avoid public speaking opportunities. It is very difficult to enjoy an activity whether it be socializing at a party, making a toast, or giving a speech or presentation when one is feeling high levels of anxiety. The good news is that by frequently confronting the fear in a systematic and consistent manner the anxiety related to public speaking scenarios decreases. By reducing the fear associated with these situations space opens up for the once present anxiety to be replaced with feelings of confidence, mastery, excitement and happiness.

FURTHER READING

Adams, M. (2015). Public speaking 101 – Become a great storyteller. *EDGE*. Retrieved from: http://www.worldchampionsedgenet.com/resources/articles/becoming-a-great-storyteller/. This article emphasizes how learning to master the art of storytelling is integrally intertwined with becoming an exceptional public speaker. Specific strategies to increase one's storytelling abilities are outlined.

Branson, R. (2013, February 4). Richard Branson on the art of public speaking. *Entrepreneur*. Retrieved from: http://www.entrepreneur.com/article/225627. This article discusses the author's fear of public speaking. It also describes how he learned to overcome his fear, and how his ability to do so directly led to the elevated and international success of his company.

Writing Commons. (n.d.) Why is public speaking important? Retrieved May 4, 2015, from: http://writingcommons.org/open-text/genres/public-speaking/844-why-is-public-speaking-important. This article describes the following three common types of public speaking: informative, persuasive, and entertaining. It also outlines the significant role that public speaking plays in all individuals' lives and highlights how building one's public speaking abilities simultaneously improves one's critical thinking abilities.

Zeoli, R. (2014, April 16). Seven principles of effective public speaking. *American Management Association*. Retrieved from: http://www.amanet.org/training/articles/Seven-Principles-of-Effective-Public-Speaking.

aspx. This article talks about how public speaking is a skill that is learned. It proceeds to outline seven key principles that help teach individuals how to improve their public speaking abilities.

Kimberly Glazier and Stefan Leonte

SEE ALSO: Anxiety; Interpersonal Communication; Interpersonal Skills and Technology; Leadership Skills

Writing

Writing is one of the most essential skills that anyone should develop not only as an employment skill, but as part of a rewarding, educated life. Today we live in a world that is rich in access to information. As always, command of basic skills (such as spelling and grammar) remains important, but in addition, writers must learn how to explore vast amounts of information, then choose and organize what is relevant to a specified task.

INTRODUCTION

The ability to organize one's thoughts in written form is an essential skill in most professional employment, including sometimes surprising places. The desk sergeant in a police precinct house, for example, appreciates a police officer who can spell, compose cogent sentences, and communicate relevant information in an accurate and comprehensive manner. Police officers fill out a large number of reports that require narrative description.

Today's informational landscape, with its constant barrage of information, contains its own dangers, and requires a degree of focus and purpose. In any given profession, the same basic skills may be applied, but adapted to different traditional formats. For example, while police compile incident reports, news reporters write stories, social workers must keep case notes, and lawyers file briefs.

WRITING IN A WORLD OF TMI (TOO MUCH INFORMATION)

To begin, define a subject as precisely as possible. This allows a writer to navigate oceans of information by fashioning precise search terms, so he or she will emerge with a cogent body of notes that will save time when composition begins. Create a computer file into which you will place all information relevant to the subject. Enter your sources (complete with the URL if you are

working on the internet) when you first encounter them. Working "backwards" – retrieving sources long after first consulting them – can be very difficult in a world that is drowning in information. As you compile source material, do not forget the scope and size of an assignment, as well as your deadline.

Once you have assembled an array of notes and sources, you begin to make this body of work your own by paraphrasing and, where appropriate, using direct quotation to tell the reader how a given source is thinking and feeling. In some contexts, direct quotation can be very useful and, with credit, it is not plagiarism. Be aware, however, that too much quotation from a single source may exceed "fair use" as defined by copyright law, and require written permission. Even short excerpts (usually more than two lines) of song lyrics and poetry may exceed fair use. Limits on prose are looser. The United States Copyright Law does not define "fair use" precisely. Direct quotation using internet sources is very easy (copy and paste), so do not be tempted to use it when your own words are more appropriate. Professional journalists have been fired for lifting other peoples' work via the internet without credit. This is very easy to do, and just as easy to find (with a simple web search).

As you work your way through a body of notes, you will begin not only to paraphrase sources (or quote directly), but also to organize your work. Move each piece of information up if you have an idea of where it may fit, or down if you do not. Delete if information is not useful, if it repeats what you already have done, or if you do not have the word allowance to include so much detail. You do not need to be perfect at this stage, so don't agonize. You'll get another chance.

WRITERS' WORKING CONDITIONS

As a writer, you are what you read. Reading does more than supply information for writing projects. It teaches you subconsciously how to write. Reading, a writer is absorbing spelling, sentence structure, and other basics. Make time each day for pleasure reading.

Writing is work and, as such, requires time independent of other activities, including social media. In a world where everyone is expected to be "plugged in" all the time, carving out time for writing can be very difficult, but it is essential. Serious writers must spend a few hours each day alone with their keyboards. In our world of information overload, this can be a challenge.

A writer must learn to self-edit, and to act as a critic of his or her own work before submitting to editors or other authority figures. With that in mind, many professional editors discourage "sloppy copies," the practice of handing rough work off so that someone else can correct errors. While such practice may fill a pedagogical purpose in elementary school, its use in a professional context is an indication that a writer may be ignorant of the basics of spelling and sentence composition.

Along the same line, be very wary of "auto-correct" in word-processing software. Machines cannot judge context, and results can be very humorous. In one instance, for example, a reference to Martin Luther's 95 theses (tacked to a church door in Wittenberg, Germany during 1517), came up "feces." Only a machine would make such an error. Only a human being could catch it.

YOUR SUBCONSCIOUS CAN WORK WITH YOU

Everyone who writes has been faced with a deadline, facing a blank screen, staring at a clock, worried that the creative "sap" no longer runs. The deadline, the blank screen, and the ticking clock (symbolic of the deadline, and impending failure) forms a negative feedback loop, otherwise known as "writer's block."

At this point, a writer can try to force the creative process, but this usually fails. The mind is an unruly partner, and trying to whip it into action does little but reinforce the block. It's time to work with the subconscious – take a walk, or a shower. Wash the dishes. Lay on the couch and close your eyes, and put yourself in a mode in which the subconscious will work on your problems. After that, go back to work.

Never be without a piece of scrap paper and a pen. Your subconscious may feed you an idea when you are required to be doing something else. Jot down a few key words that will stimulate memory when you can sit down at the keyboard. In this way, stray thoughts can be collected and elaborated later. These are the building blocks of effective composition.

FURTHER READING

LaRocque, P. (2013). *The Book on Writing: The Ultimate Guide to Writing Well*. Berlin, DE: Grey and Guvnor Press. LaRoque, a master writer, shares advice on the art and craft of composition.

Provost, G. (1985). *100 Ways To Improve Your Writing*. New York: New American Library. Provost provides quick, breezy, instruction on writing; in a decades-old title that has not gone out of print, or out of style.

Strunk, W., Jr. and White, E.B. (Eds.). (1999). *The Elements of Style*. 4th ed. New York: Longman. A classic, erudite practical guide to style and the basics of English composition.

Writing Skills: Success in 20 Minutes A Day. (2012). LearningExpress. 5th ed. This workbook contains basic advice on how to develop writing skills in an academic context.

Zinsser, W. (2006) *On Writing Well: The Classic Guide To Writing Nonfiction*. 30th anniversary ed., 7th ed., revised and updated. New York:HarperCollins. New York: Harper Perennial. This title (like Strunk and White) is a classic guide that focuses on writing quality.

Bruce E. Johansen

SEE ALSO: Cover letter and Résumé Writing; Study Skills

Disabilities and Disorders

Anorexia nervosa and bulimia nervosa

Anorexia and bulimia nervosa are disorders characterized by a distorted body image, an intense fear of becoming obese, and a desperate attempt to lose weight. These disorders most frequently occur in female adolescents, and they present serious health risks.

INTRODUCTION

Anorexia nervosa and bulimia nervosa are two types of eating disorders. They are illnesses with a biological basis modified by emotional and cultural factors. Anorexia literally means a severe loss of appetite, while nervosa means nervousness. Actually, the word anorexia is somewhat of a misnomer, given that most people with anorexia nervosa have not lost their appetites.

HISTORY OF THE DISORDERS

Anorexia is a disorder that can be traced as far back as the twelfth century, when it was associated with religion—saints refused food to get closer to God. The disorder was specifically named as a diagnosis in 1874, when Sir William Gull published an article giving the disorder its present name.

The binge/purge behavior of bulimia has been around for centuries, and bulimia nervosa was identified as a disorder in the 1930s but was thought to be a form of anorexia. Bulimia nervosa was not named as a disorder separate from anorexia until the late 1970s, when both disorders began receiving media attention with stories of girls and women refusing to eat and dying from the behavior. Probably the most famous case at that time was that of Karen Carpenter, a singer who died at age thirty-two of heart failure caused by anorexia. There is evidence to suggest that the incidence of both disorders in the United States has increased since the 1970s. The increased emphasis on thinness within American society is a likely explanation for the increase in eating disorders.

SYMPTOMS

The disorder of anorexia nervosa consists of three prominent symptoms, according to the fifth edition of the American Psychiatric Association's *Diagnostic and Statistical Manual of Mental Disorders* (DSM-5). The first symptom is an abnormally low weight for one's age, height, and physical condition due to significant restriction of energy intake. Because many people with anorexia nervosa (known as anorectics or anorexics) are secretive about their eating behaviors and cover their weight loss with clothing, they are not diagnosed until they have already lost significant amounts of weight. The second symptom of anorexia nervosa can take the form either of an intense fear of gaining weight or being fat or of behavior that prevents weight gain. This second symptom has been labeled weight phobia by some researchers because of the anorectic's anxiety toward food and the desperate attempts the person makes to avoid food. The third major symptom of the syndrome is distorted body image. Distorted body image, which sometimes takes the form of body dysmorphic disorder, involves the anorectic seeing herself or himself as obese when in reality she or he is extremely underweight. Because of this, during treatment, anorectics are not allowed to know their weight. Premenopausal women with anorexia nervosa also often experience the absence of at least three menstrual cycles in a condition known as amenorrhea, which is caused by being severely undernourished. The lack of nutrients affects the hypothalamic, pituitary, gonadal axis, causing the lack of hormones that result in amenorrhea.

Bulimia nervosa refers to the recurring cycle of binge eating, a short period of excessive overeating, followed by purging or other compensatory behaviors as drastic efforts to lose the weight gained by binge eating. For the bulimic, binging has two components: eating large amounts in a limited amount of time and feeling a lack of control while eating. Purging may be accomplished through several means, including vomiting (done either by gagging oneself or through the consumption of certain drugs) and the use of laxatives, diuretics, or enemas; other inappropriate compensatory behaviors include fasting or strict dieting and excessive exercising.

To be diagnosed with bulimia, according to the DSM-5, a person must engage in the cycle of binge eating and compensatory behaviors at least once per week, on average, for three months. It is likely that the number of bulimics reported would be higher without this strict criterion. However, bulimia should not be confused with binge eating disorder, which, according to the DSM-5, is characterized by binge eating that is not followed by inappropriate compensatory behaviors such as purging.

HEALTH PROBLEMS

Numerous health problems may occur as a result of anorexia or bulimia. The health problems of anorectics include an abnormally low heart rate and low blood pressure as well as irregular heart functioning, often resulting in heart failure. Fatigue is common, and bone thinning (osteopenia) may lead to osteoporotic fractures if left untreated. Dehydration can lead to kidney failure, and lack of body fat combined with the change in hormones makes it difficult to regulate body temperature. Anorectics may develop lanugo hair over their bodies, including the face, to help with temperature regulation. The death rate for anorexia nervosa is one of the highest for any mental health condition, and generally, the longer the condition lasts, the higher the death rate.

Most of the health complications of bulimia are related to the purging behaviors. Electrolyte imbalances, particularly potassium reduction, can occur from all purging behaviors and can lead to irregular heartbeats and possibly heart failure and death. Vomiting leads to the erosion of tooth enamel and a variety of disorders affecting digestive organs. A significantly lower number of people are thought to die from bulimia as compared with anorexia. Those with binge eating disorder exhibit the same health consequences as anyone with obesity, so heart disease and type 2 diabetes are common.

When compared with obesity, which in some cases can be the result of an eating disorder, anorexia and bulimia are rare. According to a 2012 report by the Centers for Disease Control and Prevention, approximately 35.7 percent of American adults and 16.9 percent of American children are obese. In contrast, an estimated 0.6 percent of American adults will have anorexia during their life, according to 2007 statistics compiled by the National Institute of Mental Health. The incidence of anorexia among adolescents, especially female adolescents, however, is significantly higher than in the general population. Bulimia is likewise estimated to occur in 0.6 percent of American adults, and again, the incidence of bulimia among adolescents is estimated to be significantly higher. A subpopulation in which the incidence of eating disorders is higher is athletes. The type of eating disorder seems to correlate with the sport. In individual sports, in which lower weight is an advantage or looks are a factor, anorexia is more common, and in team sports, bulimia is more common. Male and female athletes show similar rates of eating disorders because the disorders are related to the sport and athletic performance.

CAUSES AND EXPLANATIONS

The proposed causes of anorexia and bulimia can be grouped into four categories: biological, sociocultural, familial, and psychological. The notion of biological causes of anorexia and bulimia involves the idea that anorectics and bulimics have specific brain or biochemical disturbances that lead to their inability to maintain a normal weight or eating pattern. One biological explanation researched for the occurrence of anorexia and bulimia is the existence of an abnormal amount of certain brain neurotransmitters, especially norepinephrine and serotonin. Neurotransmitters are chemical messengers within the brain that transmit nerve impulses between nerve cells.

In contrast to biological explanations, sociocultural causes are factors that are thought to exist within a society that lead certain individuals to develop anorexia or bulimia. Joan Brumberg, a historian of anorexia, has outlined the sociocultural forces of the late nineteenth and twentieth centuries that many believe promoted the increased incidence of eating disorders among women. These societal forces included an emphasis on weight reduction and aesthetic self-control and the treatment of women as sexual objects. The most prominent of these suggested cultural factors is the heightened importance placed on being thin.

Some researchers believe that particular family types cause certain of their members to develop anorexia and bulimia. For example, family investigators believe that a family whose members are emotionally too close to one another may lead one or more family members to strive for independence by refusing to eat, according to Salvador Minuchin, Bernice Rosman, and Lester Baker. Other researchers believe that families whose members are controlling and express an excessive amount of hostility toward one another promote the occurrence of bulimia. Some research also shows genetic tendencies; that is, if a parent had an eating disorder, it is more likely that one or more of his or her children will also be diagnosed with one, even if the parent is no longer exhibiting symptoms.

The most prominent of the suggested psychological causes for anorexia and bulimia are those expressed by researchers who take psychoanalytic or cognitive behavioral perspectives. For example, cognitive behavioral theorists emphasize the role of distorted beliefs in the development and continuation of anorexia and bulimia. These distorted beliefs include that the person is attractive only if she or he weighs a certain number of pounds, usually a number well below normal weight, or that consuming certain types of foods (such as carbohydrate-rich foods) will automatically make a person fat.

TREATMENTS

Numerous treatments have been used for individuals who have anorexia or bulimia, but they can be broadly grouped into the categories of medical and psychological therapies. If symptoms are life threatening, these disorders are treated in a hospital, and if they are more manageable, these disorders can be treated on an outpatient basis.

Before the 1960s, medical therapies for anorexia included such radical approaches as lobotomies and electroconvulsive therapy (ECT). The first goal for the treatment of anorexia is to ensure the person's physical health, which involves restoring the person to a healthy weight. Reaching this goal may require hospitalization. Although a controversial treatment, various types of tube feeding continue to be used when a patient's malnutrition from anorexia poses an imminent risk of death. Tube feeding can be accomplished either intravenously or by inserting a tube via a patient's nasal cavity into the patient's stomach.

Once a person's physical condition is stable, treatment usually involves individual psychotherapy and family therapy, during which parents help their children learn to eat again and maintain healthful eating habits on their own. Behavioral therapy also has been effective for helping anorectics return to healthful eating habits. Supportive group therapy may follow, and self-help groups within communities may provide ongoing support. There are a number of in-patient treatment facilities that specialize in anorexia throughout the United States. The most effective treatment no matter the location is team treatment addressing all three areas of concern. A physician treats the medical conditions and potentially the mental aspects if drugs are required, a counselor manages the behavioral aspect, and a dietician manages the dietary component.

When treating bulimia, unless malnutrition is severe, any substance abuse problems that may be present at the time the eating disorder is diagnosed are usually treated first. The next goal of treatment is to reduce or eliminate the person's binge eating and purging behavior. Behavioral therapy has proven effective in achieving this goal. Psychotherapy has proven effective in helping prevent the eating disorder from recurring and in addressing issues that led to the disorder. Studies have also found that fluoxetine (Prozac), an antidepressant, may help people who do not respond to psychotherapy. Some bulimics also exhibit obsessive-compulsive disorder (OCD), and drugs appropriate for OCD also help reduce the bulimic behaviors. As with anorexia, family therapy is also recommended.

The family treatment of anorectics involves the therapist seeking to change the interactions among family members that serve to maintain the self-starvation of the patient. In attempting to change family interactions, the family therapist might address the parents' overprotectiveness or the way family members manipulate one another's behavior. For bulimics, the family therapist would seek to lower the amount of family conflict or to redirect conflict between the parents away from the bulimic.

Another frequently employed method of treatment for bulimia is group therapy. Group treatment initially involves educating bulimics about their disorder, including its negative health consequences. The group experience provides members with the opportunity to share with fellow bulimics regarding their eating problems and to find support from one another in overcoming bulimia. In addition, the therapist or therapists initiate discussions regarding healthful eating and exercise habits as well as specific ways to end the cycle.

A final issue involved in surveying the different interventions for anorexia and bulimia is the effectiveness of these treatments. A meta-analysis of one hundred studies of anorectics in 1988 found only small differences between the various types of treatment in the amount of weight gained during therapy, although behavioral treatments appeared to work faster. A negative impact of changes in health insurance coverage for anorectics has been shorter treatment times and poorer outcomes. Definitive research shows that the closer anorectics are to their ideal weight on discharge, the less likely they are to be readmitted, even if that requires a longer treatment initially. Managed care generally allows a certain amount of time or certain number of treatment sessions rather than basing coverage on return to normal weight.

Less research has been conducted investigating the effectiveness of different therapies for bulimia. No single therapy for bulimia, however, whether medical or psychological, has shown clear superiority in its effectiveness as compared with other interventions. More important was when treatment began. Patients with bulimia nervosa demonstrated a better recovery rate if they received treatment early in their illness.

PREVENTION AND REMAINING QUESTIONS

Research has begun to focus on the prevention of eating disorders. Catherine Shisslak and colleagues have suggested that preventive efforts should be targeted at female adolescents, given that they are at increased risk for developing an eating disorder. One of the most important ideas that has come out of research on eating disorders is that outcomes are much better when treatment begins early. Research also suggests that if the disordered eating behaviors are caught when they begin and before they have reached diagnostic criteria, development of the eating disorder may be prevented. These preventive efforts should focus on issues such as the physical, emotional, and social changes that occur in maturation. Also, information regarding diet and exercise should be provided, and the connection between emotions and eating should be discussed, as should ways to resist the pressure to conform to peers' and societal expectations regarding appearance.

With evidence of the increasing prevalence of anorexia and bulimia and binge eating disorder, it is important to learn more regarding the causes and effective treatment methods of these disorders. Some of the questions that remain to be definitively answered are why certain groups have a greater likelihood of developing anorexia and bulimia (notably, white female adolescents), whether the underlying causes of anorexia are different from those of bulimia, and whether a more effective treatment can be developed for those with anorexia or bulimia.

FURTHER READING

American College of Sports Medicine. "The Female Athlete Triad." *Medicine &; Science in Sports &; Exercise* 39.10 (2007): 1867–82. Print.

Arnold, Carrie. *Decoding Anorexia: How Breakthroughs in Science Offer Hope for Eating Disorders.* New York: Routledge, 2013. Print.

Bruch, Hilde. *The Golden Cage: The Enigma of Anorexia Nervosa.* Cambridge: Harvard UP, 2001. Print.

Brumberg, Joan J. *Fasting Girls: The History of Anorexia Nervosa.* Rev. ed. New York: Vintage, 2000. Print.

Centers for Disease Control and Prevention. "Overweight and Obesity." *Centers for Disease Control and Prevention.* CDC, 16 Aug. 2013. Web. 17 Feb. 2014.

Chambers, Natalie, ed. *Binge Eating: Psychological Factors, Symptoms, and Treatment.* New York: Nova Science, 2009. Print.

Dawson, Dee. *Anorexia and Bulimia: A Parent's Guide to Recognising Eating Disorders and Taking Control.* New York: Random, 2012. Print.

Fairburn, Chrisopher G., and Kelly D. Brownell. *Eating Disorders and Obesity: A Comprehensive Handbook.* New York: Guilford, 2005. Print.

Gordon, Richard. *Eating Disorders: Anatomy of a Social Epidemic.* 2nd ed. New York: Blackwell, 2000. Print.

Minuchin, Salvador, Bernice L. Rosman, and Lester Baker. *Psychosomatic Families: Anorexia Nervosa in Context.* Cambridge: Harvard UP, 1978. Print.

National Eating Disorders Association. http://www.nationaleatingdisorders.org/.

Natl. Inst. of Mental Health. "Statistics: Eating Disorders." Natl. Inst. of Mental Health. *US Dept. of Health and Human Services,* 2007. Web. 17 Feb. 2014.

Ogden, Jane. *The Psychology of Eating: From Healthy to Disordered Behavior.* Malden: Wiley, 2010. Print.

Sacker, Ira M., and Marc A. Zimmerman. *Dying to Be Thin: Understanding and Defeating Anorexia Nervosa and Bulimia.* New York: Warner, 2001. Print.

Walsh, Timothy B. "Fluoxetine for Bulimia Nervosa Following Poor Response to Psychotherapy." *American Journal of Psychiatry* 157 (2000): 1332–34. Print.

R. Christopher Qualls;
updated by Wendy E. S. Repovich

SEE ALSO: Eating Disorders

Asperger syndrome

Asperger syndrome is a mild form of autistic spectrum disorder characterized by deficiencies in social and communication skills. It is differentiated from other autism spectrum disorders by normal early development and the absence of a language delay. Individuals with Asperger syndrome have obsessive interests in narrow subjects to the exclusion of everything else. This makes people with Asperger syndrome relationally awkward and emotionally stunted, but their ability to intensely focus on one thing makes them adept at certain tasks that others would find tedious and uninteresting.

INTRODUCTION

Asperger syndrome (AS) is an autistic spectrum disorder (ASD) characterized by deficits in social interaction and communication, fixated interests, and repetitive, stereotypical behaviors. AS differs from other ASDs in that language skills and cognitive development tend to be relatively normal. AS is one of the five pervasive developmental disorders (PDDs) recognized by mental health professionals; the other four are childhood disintegrative disorder, Rett syndrome, pervasive developmental disorder (not otherwise specified), and autism.

The incidence and prevalence of AS vary substantially from one study to another, ranging from 0.03 to 4.84 per 1,000 people. Males are 1.6 to 4 times more likely to have AS than females.

The lack of standardization of diagnostic instruments for AS causes the majority of AS cases to be identified later in life when a patient experiences relational problems that result from the extremely literal and logical thought processes symptomatic of AS. Diagnosing AS and understanding these features can help close family members and friends adequately deal with them, and adult interventions that consist of training the AS individual in the right ways to communicate and deal with other people can enrich the lives of the AS patients and all those who interact with them. Without a proper diagnosis and intervention, AS individuals go from one failed relationship to another which can cause deep disappointment, depression, social withdrawal and isolation, and increased suicide risk.

Because of the tendency for AS individuals to have almost obsessive interests and their ability to focus on problems or subjects for long periods of time, AS has been dubbed the "geek syndrome" on the Internet. This characteristic of AS individuals makes them ably suited for tasks that most people would find impossible. This can make AS individuals some of the most creative and productive members of society, as illustrated by several famous people with AS that include Nobel Prize-winning economist Vernon Smith, electropop rocker Gary Numan, and Satoshi Tajiri, creator of Pokémon.

HISTORY

Eva Sucharewa, a Russian neuroscientist, was the first person to formally describe the symptoms of AS in a 1926 paper. In 1944, the Austrian pediatrician Hans Asperger published similar clinical descriptions of the condition that would later bear his name. Asperger based his diagnosis on detailed observations of four boys from his medical practice in Vienna. All four boys began to speak at approximately the same time as other children, but they had difficulty using pronouns correctly, and the content of their speech was abnormal and pedantic and consisted of lengthy discussions on their favorite subjects. They often repeated a word or phrase over and over again in a stereotypical fashion. Asperger also noted that these boys displayed impaired two-way social interaction, a complete disregard for the demands of their environ-

ment, repetitive and stereotyped play, and isolated areas of interests. At school, the boys routinely talked back to and sassed their teachers, hit and verbally abused other children, and lashed out and knocked objects over. They seemed to have no regard for the feelings of others or the consequences of their actions. Asperger called their condition "autistic psychopathy." Furthermore, those with this condition were capable of creative and original innovation in their chosen fields and showed excellent, logical abstract thinking. Because of their ability to talk at length and in great detail about their favorite subject, Asperger referred to these boys as "little professors." Unfortunately, because Asperger published in German and during wartime, his work was not widely read.

The German psychiatrist Gerhard Bosch first used the term "Asperger's syndrome" in a 1962 monograph. The British physician Lorna Wing popularized this term in the English-speaking medical community in her influential and widely-read 1981 publication of a series of case studies of children who showed similar symptoms. Wing considered AS part of the "autistic continuum" and thought that AS could be a mild variant of autism in intelligent children. The third edition and revised third edition of the *Diagnostic and Statistical Manual of Mental Disorders* (DSM-III) adopted Wing's views of AS but did not provide any specific definition or diagnostic criteria for it. The first systematic studies of AS appeared in the late 1980s and the diagnostic criteria for Asperger's syndrome were outlined 1989. At this time, Asperger's original work became more widely available in English when Uta Frith, an early autism researcher, translated his original paper in 1991. AS became a distinct diagnosis in 1992, when it was included in the 10th edition of the World Health Organization's diagnostic manual, *International Classification of Diseases* (ICD-10), and in 1994, when it was added to the fourth edition of the DSM.

In May 2013, the publication of the fifth edition of the DSM subsumed AS into the overarching category of ASD and designated AS as a mild form of ASD. This reclassification was based on work from several psychiatric research groups that failed to find significant differences between AS and high-functioning autism (HFA). However, more recent analyses of AS and HFA have demarcated distinct clinical and neurological features between these two conditions, and some mental health professionals think that future DSM editions will distinguish AS from HFA.

SIGNS AND SYMPTOMS

AS is a "wide spectrum" disorder which means that the characteristics of those diagnosed with AS vary substantially from person to person. There are, however, particular features commonly observed in the majority of AS patients.

Obsessive interests. Many children with AS become experts on a single object or topic, often to the exclusion of other topics. These compulsive interests can range from household objects such as vacuum cleaners and lawn mowers to model cars, trains, or computers, and they will usually collect, list, and number their objects of interest. The acquisition of large amounts of information on their topic of interest motivates AS children to incessantly talk about it, but their conversations with other people will consist of a collection of facts without any useful synthesis of those facts. Their desire to speak only of their singular interest makes conversation with them difficult.

Distinctive speech patterns. AS individuals often speak in a monotone voice, devoid of rhythm and with a limited range of intonation. Children with AS often lack the capacity to properly modulate the volume of their voices and must be routinely reminded to speak softly. AS children can possess large vocabularies for their age, and the pedantic content and sometimes formal nature of their speech can cause them to sound much older than they actually are.

Routines. People with AS tend to rigidly adhere to various rules, rituals, and methodical routines, and disruptions of these routines can generate anxiety or even anger. An AS child, for example, might take the same route to school every day and wear particular outfits for specific days of the week. They also may engage in repetitive behaviors including finger flapping or twisting or whole body movements and can occasionally include self-injury. Echolalia, the routine repetition of a word or phrase, is sometimes observed. AS children also show obsessions with objects and how they are arranged (e.g., they may spend hours lining up toy cars or trains).

Diminished social and communication skills. AS individuals have trouble reading social cues and tend to give inappropriate social and emotional responses. They have difficulty interpreting gestures, vocal inflections and changes in tone, and facial expressions. AS individuals also show alexithymia which is difficulty describing or even identifying emotions. They lack social skills that most people take for granted. For example, AS individuals often fail to detect when the listener has lost interest in their monologues. They also do not easily understand irony, jokes, or sarcasm, and they tend to not understand the figurative use of language. AS individuals may not understand basic rules of social engagement such as the appropriate topics for conversation or the proper distance to stand next to someone. Because of their inability to master the rules of social interaction, AS individuals may come off across as insensitive or uncaring. Additionally, because of their tendency to talk about their singular interest, AS individuals often spend a good deal of time alone. Social isolation can cause them to become withdrawn and inured to any desire for companionship or depressed and anxious.

Motor and sensory difficulties. Though not a required sign of AS, many AS children display poor physical coordination, and they typically show delayed mastery of physical skills such as riding a bicycle or tying their shoes. Their gait is sometimes bouncy and odd. They may also have poor handwriting. AS children are often sensitive to loud noises and unfamiliar textures. Particular foods are often eschewed because of the way they feel in their mouths.

CAUSE

The precise cause of AS is presently unknown. Inheritance studies have firmly established that AS and ASD run in families. Several twin studies in which the AS rates of identical twins who were separated at birth and adopted by different families were compared with nonidentical twins subjected to the same conditions have confirmed a significant genetic contribution to the development of AS. However, the precise genes responsible for the onset of AS have not been definitively identified, and it is likely that AS is due to more than one gene. The candidate genes that have been identified encode enzymes that help synthesize neurotransmitters and neurotransmitter receptors, nerve cell adhesion molecules and migration factors, proteins involved in gene expression (transcription factors), cell signaling molecules, and several others. Nevertheless, the role these genes play in the development of AS remains unclear.

In a few cases, exposure of the fetus to particular chemicals during the first eight weeks after conception has been linked to AS. Other environmental factors might also contribute to the cause of AS. Brain scans of AS patients, while revealing abnormalities in particular AS patients, have not established that such structural defects are common to most AS patients.

DIAGNOSIS

No standardized diagnostic tests exist for AS. There are several screening instruments in use such as the Autism Diagnostic Interview-Revised which consists of a semi-structured parent interview and the Autism Diagnostic Observation Schedule which includes a conversation and play-based interview with the child. Unfortunately, the absence of standardization of AS screening instruments may cause children to receive disparate diagnoses from different physicians.

Typically, the child first receives an initial diagnosis during his or her routine check-up by the family doctor. This is followed by a more extensive series of tests by a medical team that consists of psychologists, neurologists, psychiatrists, speech therapists, and others who specialize in diagnosing AS children. The team usually assesses the child's verbal and non-verbal communication skills, speech patterns, ability to carry on a conversation and the content of their conversations, motor coordination, and cognitive abilities. Interviews with the parents to determine the developmental history of the child are also used to confirm the diagnosis.

THERAPIES

There is no cure for AS, but several available interventions can help AS children and adults manage their condition and live more fulfilling lives. Applied behavior analysis teaches AS children social skills to help them more successfully interact with other people. Cognitive behavior therapy gives AS children the skills they need to manage stress and temper tantrumsand mediate their obsessive interests and repetitive routines to live more balanced lives. Occupational therapy can help AS children overcome their clumsiness and improve their coordination. Social communication intervention is a speech therapy program designed for AS children to help them learn how to master the back-and-forth nature of normal conversation.

In some cases medications can ameliorate the symptoms of AS. Such medications include the anti-psychotic medicine risperidone (Risperdal) which can reduce irritability, aggression, repetitive behavior, and depression in AS children. Likewise stimulants such as methylphenidate (Ritalin, Concerta, Metadate) and clonidine (Catapres) can reduce the hyperactivity that afflicts high-functioning AS children. Another group of drugs called the selective serotonin reuptake inhibitors (SSRIs) can effectively reduce the repetitive interests

and behaviors in adults with AS but is not indicated for children or adolescents.

AS CULTURE

Because of the Internet, AS individuals have formed their own communities and refer to themselves as "aspies." Internet sites such as the Wrong Planet site provide ways for AS individuals to connect with each other.

AS individuals have lobbied to change the perception of AS from a neurological disease that needs to be treated or cured to a difference that has its advantages. Some have even argued that AS should be removed from the DSM. However, it is the judgment of most mental health professionals that even though AS individuals can make positive contributions to society, their emotional difficulties that result from lack of empathy makes it useful to include AS in the DSM.

FURTHER READING

Attwood, T. (2008). *The complete guide of Asperger's syndrome.* London, UK: Jessica Kingsley. A very readable and useful compendium of case studies, research summaries, and personal anecdotes by a clinical psychologist who specializes in AS.

Cook O'Toole, J. (2012). *The Asperkid's (secret) book of social rules: The handbook of not-so-obvious social guidelines for tweens and teens with Asperger syndrome.* London, UK: Jessica Kingsley. A self-help book for young people with AS by a mother with AS.

Emlet, M. R. (2011). *Asperger syndrome.* Greensboro, NC: New Growth Press. An informative, sensitive book on AS by a Christian counselor who is also a physician and writes for pastors and lay workers who want to know more about AS children and adults.

Smith Myles, B., & Southwick, J. (2005). *Asperger syndrome and difficult moments: Practical solutions for tantrums, rage and meltdowns.* Shawnee Mission, KS: Autism Asperger Publishing Company. Practical advice for parents of AS children by a recognized AS expert.Welton, J. (2003).

Can I tell you about Asperger syndrome?: A guide for friends and family. London, UK: Jessica Kingsley. For children between ages 7-15 on how to successfully deal with family members or friends who have AS.

Michael A. Buratovich

SEE ALSO: Autism Spectrum Disorder

Attention-deficit hyperactivity disorder (ADHD)

Attention-deficit hyperactivity disorder is one of the most common disorders of childhood and adolescence, and it can also be one of the most disturbing and debilitating disorders that a child or adolescent can experience. Research into this disorder has identified its primary causes; however, it remains a difficult disorder to treat effectively.

INTRODUCTION

Attention-deficit hyperactivity disorder (ADHD) is one of the most extensively studied behavior disorders that begin in childhood. Thousands of journal articles, chapters, and books have been published on the disorder. There are a number of reasons this disorder is of such interest to researchers and clinicians. The two primary reasons are that ADHD is a relatively common disorder of childhood (it is regarded as a childhood disorder although it can persist into adulthood) and that there are numerous problems associated with ADHD, including lower levels of intellectual and academic performance and higher levels of aggressive and defiant behavior.

In national and international studies of childhood emotional and behavioral disorders, ADHD has been found to be relatively common among children. Although prevalence estimates range from 1 to 20 percent, most researchers agree that between 3 and 7 percent of children could be diagnosed as having ADHD. The fifth edition of the *Diagnostic and Statistical Manual of Mental Disorders: DSM-5*, published by the American Psychiatric Association in 2013, describes the diagnostic criteria for ADHD. To receive the diagnosis of ADHD according to DSM-5, a child must show abnormally high levels of inattention, hyperactivity-impulsivity, or both when compared with peers of the same age. The DSM-5 lists two sets of behavioral symptoms characteristic of ADHD. The first list contains nine symptoms of inattention such as "often has difficulty sustaining attention in tasks or play activities," while the second list contains nine symptoms of hyperactivity-impulsivity such as "often talks excessively" and "often has difficulty awaiting turn." To be diagnosed with ADHD, a child must exhibit at least six symptoms from at least one of the lists. Although many of these behaviors are quite common for most children at some point in their lives, the important point to consider in the diagnosis of ADHD is that these behaviors must be in excess of the levels of behaviors most frequently exhibited for children of that age and that the behaviors must cause functional impairment in at least two settings (for instance, at home and at school). Additionally, it is expected that "several inattentive or hyperactive-impulsive symptoms were present prior to age twelve."

Boys tend to outnumber girls in the diagnosis of ADHD, with the male-to-female ratio estimated at 2:1 to 9:1, depending on the source. ADHD boys tend to be more aggressive and antisocial than ADHD girls, while girls are more likely to display inattentive symptoms.

ASSOCIATED PROBLEMS

There are a number of additional problems associated with ADHD, including the greater likelihood of ADHD boys exhibiting aggressive and antisocial behavior. Although some ADHD children do not show any associated problems, many ADHD children show deficits in both intellectual and behavioral functioning. For example, a number of studies have found that ADHD children score an average of seven to fifteen points below normal children on standardized intelligence tests. It may be, however, that this poorer performance reflects poor test-taking skills or inattention during the test rather than actual impairment in intellectual functioning. Additionally, ADHD children tend to have difficulty with academic performance and scholastic achievement. It is assumed that this poor academic performance is a result of inattention and impulsiveness in the classroom. When ADHD children are given medication to control their inattention and impulsiveness, their academic productivity has been shown to improve.

ADHD children have also been shown to have a high number of associated emotional and behavioral difficulties. As mentioned before, ADHD boys tend to show higher levels of aggressive and antisocial behavior than ADHD girls and normal children. Additionally, it is estimated that up to 50 percent of ADHD children have at least one other disorder, and the DSM-5 now allows ADHD to be included in a comorbid diagnosis with autism spectrum disorder. Many of these problems are related to depression and anxiety. Many ADHD children also have severe problems with temper tantrums, stubbornness, and defiant behavior. It is also estimated that up to 50 percent of ADHD children have impaired social relations; that is, they do not get along with other children. In general, there are many problems associated with ADHD, and this may be part of the reason that researchers have been so intrigued by this disorder.

Researchers must understand a disorder before they can attempt to treat it. There are a variety of theories on the etiology of ADHD, but most researchers have come to believe that there are multiple factors that influence its development. It appears that many children may have a biological predisposition toward ADHD; in other words, they may have a greater likelihood of developing ADHD as a result of genetic factors. This predisposition is exacerbated by a variety of factors, such as complications during pregnancy, neurological disease, exposure to toxins, family adversity, and inconsistent parental discipline. Although a very popular belief is that food additives or sugar can cause ADHD, there has been almost no scientific support for these claims. Because so many factors have been found to be associated with the development of ADHD, it is not surprising that numerous treatments have been developed for the amelioration of ADHD symptoms. Although numerous treatment methods have been developed and studied, ADHD remains a difficult disorder to treat effectively.

DRUG THERAPIES

Treatments of ADHD can be broken down into roughly two categories: medication and behavior or cognitive behavior therapy with the individual ADHD child, parents, or teachers. It should be noted that traditional psychotherapy and play therapy have not been found to be effective in the treatment of ADHD. Stimulant medications have been used in the treatment of ADHD since 1937. The most commonly prescribed stimulant medications are methylphenidate (Ritalin and Concerta), pemoline (Cylert), and dextroamphetamine (Dexedrine). As of 2014, the Federal Drug Administration (FDA) had approved three nonstimulant medications to treat ADHD. Strattera was the first nonstimulant drug approved and is prescribed to both children and adults. Intuniv and Kapvay are approved for children ages six through seventeen. Behavioral improvements caused by medications include better impulse control and improved attending behavior. Overall, approximately 75 percent of ADHD children on stimulant and nonstimulant medication show behavioral improvement, and 25 percent show either no improvement or decreased behavioral functioning. The findings related to academic performance are mixed. It appears that these medications can help the ADHD child with school productivity and accuracy but not with overall academic achievement. In addition, although ADHD children tend to show improvement while they are on a stimulant or a nonstimulant medication, there are rarely

any long-term benefits to their use and can, in general, can be seen as only a short-term management tool.

Antidepressant medications such as imipramine and fluoxetine (Prozac) have also been used with ADHD children. These medications are sometimes used when stimulant medication is not appropriate (for example, if the child has motor or vocal tics). Antidepressant medications, however, like stimulant and nonstimulant medications, appear to provide only short-term improvement in ADHD symptoms. Overall, the use or nonuse of medications in the treatment of ADHD should be carefully evaluated by a qualified physician (such as a psychiatrist). If the child is started on medication for ADHD, the safety and appropriateness of the medication must be monitored continually throughout its use.

BEHAVIOR THERAPIES

Behavioral and cognitive behavior therapy has been used with ADHD children, their parents, and their teachers. Most of these techniques attempt to provide the child with a consistent environment in which on-task behavior is rewarded (for example, the teacher praises the child for raising his or her hand and not shouting out an answer) and in which off-task behavior is either ignored or punished (for example, the parent has the child sit alone in a chair near an empty wall, a "time-out chair," after the child impulsively throws a book across the room). In addition, cognitive behavior therapies try to teach ADHD children to internalize their own self-control by learning to "stop and think" before they act.

One example of a cognitive behavior therapy, which was developed by Philip Kendall and Lauren Braswell, is intended to teach the child to learn five "steps" that can be applied to academic tasks as well as social interactions. The five problem-solving steps that children are to repeat to themselves each time they encounter a new situation are the following: Ask "What am I supposed to do?" and then ask, "What are my choices?" Concentrate and focus in; make a choice and ask, "How did I do?" (If I did well, I can congratulate myself, and if I did poorly, I can try to go more slowly the next time.) In each therapy session, the child is given twenty plastic chips at the beginning of the session. The child loses a chip each time he or she does not use one of the steps, goes too fast, or gives an incorrect answer. At the end of the session, the child can use the chips to purchase a small prize; chips can also be stored in a "bank" to purchase an even larger prize in the following sessions. This treatment approach combines the use of cognitive strategies (the child learns self-instructional steps) and behavioral techniques (the child loses a desired object, a chip, for impulsive behavior).

Overall, behavioral and cognitive behavior therapies have been found to be relatively effective in the settings in which they are used and at the time they are being instituted. Like the effects of medication, however, the effects of behavioral and cognitive behavior therapies tend not to be long lasting. There is some evidence to suggest that the combination of medication and behavior therapy can increase the effectiveness of treatment. In the long run, however, no treatment of ADHD has been found to be truly effective, and in a majority of cases, the disorder persists into adulthood.

HISTORY AND CHANGING DIAGNOSTIC CRITERIA
Children who might be diagnosed as having ADHD have been written about and discussed in scientific publications since the mid-1800s. A focus on ADHD began in the United States after an encephalitis epidemic in 1917. Because the damage to the central nervous system caused by the disease led to poor attention, impulsivity, and overactivity in children who survived, researchers began to look for signs of brain injury in other children who had similar behavioral profiles. By the 1950s, researchers began to refer to this disorder as "minimal brain damage," which was then changed to "minimal brain dysfunction" (MBD). By the 1960s, however, the use of the term MBD was severely criticized because of its overinclusiveness and nonspecificity. Researchers began to use terms that more specifically characterized children's problems, such as "hyperkinesis" and "hyperactivity."

The *Diagnostic and Statistical Manual of Mental Disorders* (DSM), first published by the American Psychiatric Association in 1952, is the primary diagnostic manual used in the United States. In 1968, the second edition, called DSM-II, presented the diagnosis of "hyperkinetic reaction of childhood" to characterize children who were overactive and restless. By 1980, when the third edition (DSM-III) was published, researchers had begun to focus on the deficits of attention in these children, so two diagnostic categories were established: "attention-deficit disorder with hyperactivity (ADD with H)" and "attention-deficit disorder without hyperactivity (ADD without H)." After the publication of DSM-III, many researchers argued that there were no empirical data to support the existence of the ADD without H diagnosis. In other words, it was difficult to find any children

who were inattentive and impulsive but who were not hyperactive. For this reason, in 1987, when the revised DSM-III-R was published, the only diagnostic category for these children was "attention-deficit hyperactivity disorder (ADHD)."

With the publication of the fourth version of the manual, the DSM-IV, in 1994, three distinct diagnostic categories for ADHD were identified: ADHD predominantly hyperactive-impulsive type, ADHD predominantly inattentive type, and ADHD combined type. The type of ADHD diagnosed depends on the number and types of behavioral symptoms a child exhibits. Six of nine symptoms from the hyperactivity-impulsivity list but fewer than six symptoms from the inattention list lead to a diagnosis of ADHD predominantly hyperactive-impulsive type. Six of nine symptoms the inattention list but fewer than six symptoms from the hyperactivity-impulsivity list lead to a diagnosis of ADHD predominantly inattentive type. A child who exhibits six of nine behavioral symptoms simultaneously from both lists receives a diagnosis of ADHD combined type.

The eighteen criteria used in the DSM-IV to diagnose ADHD were carried over to the DSM-5, which was published and released in 2013. The wording criterion for onset of ADHD has been changed, however, from "some" of the inattentive or hyperactive "symptoms that caused impairment were present before age seven years" in the DSM-IV to "several" inattentive or hyperactive "symptoms were present prior to age twelve" in the DSM-5. The DSM-5 also added a reduced symptom threshold for adults with a minimum of five symptoms (as opposed to the six required for children) for both the inattention and the hyperactivity/impulsivity aspects of the disorder.

Although the diagnostic definition and specific terminology of ADHD will undoubtedly continue to change throughout the years, the interest in and commitment to this disorder will most likely persist. Children and adults with ADHD, as well as the people around them, have difficult lives to lead. The research community is committed to finding better explanations of the etiology and treatment of this common disorder.

FURTHER READING
Alexander-Roberts, Colleen. *The ADHD Parenting Handbook: Practical Advice for Parents from Parents.* Dallas: Taylor Trade, 1994. Print.

Barkley, Russell A. *Attention-Deficit Hyperactivity Disorder: A Handbook for Diagnosis and Treatment.* 3d ed. New York: Guilford Press, 2005. Print.

Goldstein, Sam, and Joy Jansen. "The Neuropsychology of ADHD." *In The Neuropsychology Handbook,* edited by Arthur MacNeill Horton, Jr., and Danny Wedding. 3d ed. New York: Springer, 2007. Print.

Hallowell, Edward M., and John J. Ratey. *Driven to Distraction: Recognizing and Coping with Attention Deficit Disorder.* New York: Random House, 2011. Print.

Kendall, Philip C., and Lauren Braswell. *Cognitive-Behavioral Therapy for Impulsive Children.* 2d ed. New York: Guilford Press, 1993. Print.

Parker, Charles E. *New ADHD Medication Rules: Brain Science and Common Sense.* 2nd ed. New York: Köehler Books, 2013. Print.

Ramsay, Russell J. *Cognitive-Behavioral Therapy for Adult ADHD: An Integrative Psychosocial and Medical Approach.* 2nd ed. New York: Routledge, 2015. Print.

Wender, Paul H. *ADHD: Attention-Deficit Hyperactivity Disorder in Children and Adults.* New York: Oxford University Press, 2000. Print.

Vicky Phares; updated by Virginia Slaughter

SEE ALSO: ADHD Medications

Autism spectrum disorder

Autism, a poorly understood, nonschizophrenic psychosocial problem, includes great social unresponsiveness, speech and language impairment, ritualistic play activity, and resistance to change. Research on the causes of autism suggests multiple risk factors. A wide variety of treatments are available, and they can be tailored to suit the needs of individual children and their families.

INTRODUCTION

The modern term "autism" was originated by Leo Kanner in the 1940's. In "Autistic Disturbances of Affective Contact" (1943), he described a group of autistic children; he viewed them as much more similar to one another than to schizophrenics, with whom they generally had been associated. Until that time, the classical definition for autism (still seen in some dictionaries) was "a form of childhood schizophrenia characterized by acting out and withdrawal from reality." Kanner believed that these children represented an entirely different clinical psychiatric disorder. He noted four main symptoms associated with the disorder: social withdrawal or "ex-treme autistic aloneness"; either muteness or failure to use spoken language "to convey meaning to others"; an "obsessive desire for maintenance of sameness"; and preoccupation with highly repetitive play habits, producing "severe limitation of spontaneous activity." Kanner also noted that autism, unlike other types of childhood psychoses, began in or near infancy and had both cognitive and affective components.

Over the years, several attempts have been made to establish precise diagnostic criteria for autism. The criteria that are given in the current edition of the American Psychiatric Association's *Diagnostic and Statistical Manual of Mental Disorders: DSM-IV-TR* (rev. 4th ed., 2000), are onset prior to thirty-six months of age; pervasive lack of responsiveness to other people; gross deficits in language development and, if speech is present, peculiar patterns (such as delayed echolalia and pronoun reversals); bizarre reaction to environmental aspects (resistance to change); and the absence of any symptoms of schizophrenia. These criteria are largely a restatement of Kanner's viewpoint.

In the first decade of the twenty-first century, the prevalence of autism has been estimated at around 1 in 150 children. Study of the sex distribution shows that it is approximately three to four times as common in male as in female children. The causes of autism have not been conclusively determined, although the possibilities are wide-ranging and said to be rooted in both biology and environment. One of the most controversial proposals in the 1990's was that the mumps, measles, and rubella (MMR) vaccination that is given at approximately eighteen months of age caused at least some forms of autism because the timing of the vaccine often corresponds with the earliest detected symptoms of autism. However, researchers in the United States and Europe have determined that this vaccine does not cause autism. This is based on the fact that vaccination rates held steady throughout the 1990's at almost 97 percent of children, yet the rate of autism diagnosis increased sevenfold during the same time period.

Research on physiological causes of autism indicate a genetic component: Siblings of autistic children are fifty times more likely to be diagnosed with autism than children who do not have an autistic brother or sister. Other potential physiological causes include abnormal neurochemistry, low birth weight, and brain abnormalities such as reduction of tissue in the cerebellum and enlarged ventricles in the cerebrum.

DSM-IV-TR CRITERIA FOR AUTISM

AUTISTIC DISORDER (DSM CODE 299.00)
Six or more criteria from three lists

1) Qualitative impairment in social interaction, manifested by at least two of the following:
- marked impairment in use of multiple nonverbal behaviors (eye-to-eye gaze, facial expression, body postures, gestures)
- failure to develop peer relationships appropriate to developmental level
- lack of spontaneous seeking to share enjoyment, interests, or achievements with others
- lack of social or emotional reciprocity

2) Qualitative impairments in communication, manifested by at least one of the following:
- delay in, or total lack of, development of spoken language, not accompanied by attempts to compensate through alternative modes of communication such as gesture or mime
- in individuals with adequate speech, marked impairment in ability to initiate or sustain conversation
- stereotyped and repetitive use of language or idiosyncratic language

- lack of varied, spontaneous make-believe play or social imitative play appropriate to developmental level

3) Restricted, repetitive, and stereotyped patterns of behavior, interests, and activities, manifested by at least one of the following:
- preoccupation with one or more stereotyped and restricted patterns of interest abnormal in either intensity or focus
- apparently inflexible adherence to specific, nonfunctional routines or rituals
- stereotyped and repetitive motor mannerisms (hand or finger flapping, complex whole-body movements)
- persistent preoccupation with parts of objects

Delays or abnormal functioning in at least one of the following areas, with onset prior to age three:
- social interaction
- language as used in social communication
- symbolic or imaginative play

Symptoms not better explained by Rett Disorder or Childhood Disintegrative Disorder

Largely because of Kanner's original sample (now known to have been atypical), many people believe that autistic children come from relatively wealthy, professional families. Subsequent studies have indicated that this is not so. Rather, autistic children come from families within a wide socioeconomic range, and more than 75 percent of them score in the moderately intellectually disabled range on intelligence tests before, or in the absence of, effective treatment.

The behavior that characterizes autism strongly suggests that the disorder is related to other types of neurologic dysfunction. Identified neurological correlations include soft neurologic signs (such as poor coordination), seizure disorders, abnormal electroencephalograms, and unusual sleep patterns. This emphasis on neurologic (or organic) explanations for autism is relatively new; autism was previously thought to be an entirely emotional disorder.

The difficulties that autistic children show in social relationships are exhibited in many ways. Most apparent is a child's failure to form social bonds. Autistic children are typically less "cuddly" and affectionate than children without autism, though they do show attachment toward their parents and prefer them to strangers. In their peer groups, however, children with autism rarely initiate interactions with other children, preferring to play alone and often showing avoidance or aggression when other children try to join in. Autistic children tend to avoid direct eye contact and often look through or past other people. Unlike nonautistic children, older autistic children rarely indulge in any cooperative play activities or strike up close friendships with peers.

Another characteristic is disordered communication. Early nonverbal communication such as gaze following and pointing to share information is delayed or fails to emerge. Sometimes speech does not develop at all. When speech development does occur, it is very slow and may even disappear again. A prominent speech pathology in autism is either immediate or delayed repetition of something heard (such as a television commercial) not in a meaningful way but as a simple parroting back; these phenomena are called immediate and delayed echolalia, respectively. Another characteristic is lack of true language comprehension, shown by the fact that an autistic child's ability to follow instructions often depends on situational cues. For example, such a child may understand the request to come and eat dinner only when a parent is eating or sitting at the dinner table.

Behavior denoting resistance to change is often best exemplified by rigid and repetitive play patterns, the interruption of which results in tantrums and even self-injury. Some autistic children also develop very ritualistic preoccupations with an object or a schedule. For example, they may become extremely distressed with events as minor as the rearrangement of furniture in a particular room at home.

TREATMENT

Autistic children can be very frustrating to both parents and siblings, disrupting their lives greatly. Often, having a child diagnosed with autism causes grief and guilt feelings in parents. According to Mary Van Bourgondien, Gary Mesibov, and Geraldine Dawson, this can be ameliorated by psychodynamic, biological, or behavioral techniques. These authors point out that all psychodynamic therapy views autism as an emotional problem, recommending extensive psychotherapy for the individual with autism and the rest of the family. In contrast, biological methodology applies psychoactive drugs and vitamins. Finally, behavioral therapy uses the axioms of experimental psychology, along with special education techniques that teach and reinforce appropriate behavior.

Psychodynamic approaches are based on the formation of interpersonal relationships between the child and others. One example is holding therapy, which involves the mother holding the child for long periods of time so that a supposedly damaged bond between the two can be mended. The intervention technique called Floortime, in which the therapist or parent joins the child in his or her activities and follows the child's lead in play, is a more active method of establishing a bond with a child.

Biological methods of treatment attempt to influence how the brain receives and processes information. Sensory integration is favored by occupational therapists who take the perspective that the nervous system of the autistic child is attempting to regain homeostasis, causing him or her to behave oddly. The approach involves trying to meet the child's sensory needs through a "sensory diet" of activities throughout the day, such as close physical contact, balance exercises, and moving to music. Drug therapies include antiseizure medications, tranquilizers, stimulants, antidepressants, and antianxiety medications that have varying results. One of the most controversial drug therapies is the injection of the hormone secretin, which reportedly causes remarkable improvements in the symptoms of some children but no change in others. Dietary interventions include megadoses of vitamins and minerals that could have very harmful side effects and are not reliably beneficial. Some parents cut out food additives or coloring, or follow a gluten-free and casein-free regimen that eliminates all milk and wheat products from their autistic child's diet. Only anecdotal evidence exists of the effectiveness of these and other special diets.

The last category of therapies is behavioral or skill-based techniques. The Treatment and Education of Autistic and Related Communication Handicapped Children (TEACCH) Treatment and Education of Autistic and Related Communication Handicapped Children program emphasizes modifying the environment to improve the adaptive functioning of individuals given their unique characteristics and teaching others to accommodate autistic children at their particular level of functioning. In contrast, applied behavior analysis programs, such as those advocated by Norwegian psychologist Ivar Lovaas, involve manipulating the environment only for the initial purpose of shaping an individual's skills toward more normal functioning, with the eventual goal of mainstreaming the child with his or her typically developing peers in the regular education setting, an outcome that is estimated to be more likely for children whose treatment begins by two or three years of age.

All these varying therapeutic techniques have their supporters, but no single intervention is recognized to work for all children with autism. In general, the most effective treatment involves a mixed program tailored to the individual child.

CHANGING PERCEPTIONS

As defined by Kanner in the 1940's, autistic children were at first perceived to be victims of an affective disorder brought on by their emotionally cold, very intellectual, and compulsive parents (so-called refrigerator mothers). The personality traits of these parents, it was theorized, encouraged such children to withdraw from social contact with them and then with all other people.

In the years that have followed, additional data, as well as conceptual changes in medicine and psychology, have led to the belief that autism, which may actually be a constellation of disorders that exhibit similar symptoms, has a biological basis that may reside in subtle brain and hormone abnormalities. Increasingly since the beginning of the twenty-first century, scientists and practitioners have begun to refer to autism spectrum disorders (ASD) to capture the fact that children as well as adults with autism vary widely in terms of the severity of their symptoms, their strengths and weaknesses, and their responses to different treatments.

FURTHER READING

Baron-Cohen, Simon. *Autism and Asperger Syndrome (The Facts)*. New York: Oxford University Press, 2008. This volume by one of the world's experts on autism and related disorders provides a broad overview of the indicators and diagnosis of autism, its biological bases, and various treatments.

Frith, Uta. *Autism: A Very Short Introduction*. New York: Oxford University Press, 2008. This brief volume outlines the research on the brain bases of autism and integrates the results with modern theories of the disorder.

Grandin, Temple. *Thinking in Pictures: My Life with Autism*. London: Vintage Press, 2006. A firsthand account of what it is like to be a high-functioning person with autism. Grandin overcame early difficulties with communication and social relationships to become a successful animal scientist, professor, and expert on her own disorder, autism.

Greenspan, Stanley I., and Serena Wieder. *Engaging Autism: Using the Floortime Approach to Help Children Relate, Communicate, and Think*. Cambridge, Mass.: Da Capo Lifelong Books, 2006. This book first describes autism, highlighting the positive as well as the negative elements of autistic behavior, then describes the Floortime approach to intervention and therapy and reviews the research on its effectiveness.

Maurice, Catherine, Gina Green, and Stephen C. Luce, eds. *Behavioral Intervention for Young Children with Autism: A Manual for Parents and Professionals*. Austin, Tex.: Pro-Ed, 1996. With the mother of two children who were diagnosed with autism and successfully treated with behavior therapy among its editors, the book provides clear guidance for parents embarking on

a search for effective treatment methods for their children. Included is information on the effectiveness of various treatments, funding behavior therapy, working with educators and other professionals, and what is involved in behavior therapy.

Sanford S. Singer; updated by Virginia Slaughter

SEE ALSO: Asperger Syndrome; Siblings With Autism

Bipolar disorder

Bipolar disorder is a serious mental illness that is characterized by depressive and manic episodes. Advanced neurobiological research and assessment techniques have shown this disorder to have biochemical origins and a genetic element. Research indicates that stress may play a role in the precipitating recurrence of episodes. The main treatment interventions include lithium, mood-stabilizing anticonvulsants, antipsychotics, and psychotherapy.

INTRODUCTION

Although mood fluctuations are a normal part of life, individuals with bipolar disorder experience extreme mood changes. Bipolar disorder, or bipolar affective disorder (also called manic-depressive disorder), has been identified as a major psychiatric disorder characterized by dramatic mood and behavior changes. These changes, ranging from episodes of high euphoric moods to deep depression, with accompanying behavioral and personality changes, are devastating to those with the disorder and perplexing to the loved ones of those affected. The National Institute for Mental Health (NIMH) reported that approximately 2.5 percent of the US population over the age of eighteen suffers from bipolar disorder. The disorder is divided fairly equally between men and women.

Clinical psychiatry has been effective in providing biochemical intervention in the form of mood stabilizers such as lithium carbonate or valproate, which both stimulate the release of the neurotransmitter glutamate in order to stabilize or modulate the ups and downs of this illness. Lithium treatment is most effective when treating individuals with pure mania, which is characterized by periods of euphoria and depression. Mood-stabilizing anticonvulsant medications, such as oxcarbazepine (Trileptal), carbamazepine (Tegretol), and lamotrigine (Lamictal) are often used to treat bipolar.

Atypical antipsychotic medications, antidepressants, electrocovulsive therapy (ECT), and nonmedical therapies such as sleep management and psychotherapy are increasingly utilized to treat individuals with bipolar disorder. Psychotherapy is seen by most practitioners as a necessary adjunct to medication.

SYMPTOMS

In the manic phase of a bipolar episode, individuals may experience inappropriately good moods, or "highs," or may become extremely irritable. During a manic phase, they may overcommit to work projects and meetings, social activities, and family responsibilities in the belief that they can accomplish anything; this is known as manic grandiosity. At times, psychotic symptoms such as delusions, severe paranoia, and hallucinations may accompany a manic episode. These symptoms may lead to a misdiagnosis of other psychotic disorders such as schizophrenia. Although it may be difficult to arrive at a differential diagnosis between schizophrenia and bipolar disorder when a person is acutely psychotic, a long-term view of the individual's overall symptoms and functioning can distinguish between the two disorders.

The initial episode of bipolar disorder is typically one of mania or elation, although in some people, a depressive episode may signal the beginning of the disorder. Episodes of bipolar disorder can recur rapidly—within hours or days—or may have a much slower recurrence rate, even of years. The duration of each episode, whether it is depression or mania, varies among individuals but normally remains fairly consistent for each individual.

TYPES

According to the fifth edition of the *Diagnostic and Statistical Manual of Mental Disorders* (DSM-5, 2013), which is the diagnostic manual of the American Psychiatric Association, there are several types of bipolar disorder. Bipolar disorder specifiers are categorized according to the extent of severity; the types of the symptoms; the changes in activity, energy, and mood; and the duration of the symptoms.

Bipolar I disorder is characterized by alternating periods of mania and depression. At times, severe bipolar disorder may be accompanied by psychotic symptoms such as delusions and hallucinations. For this reason, bipolar I disorder is also considered a psychotic disorder. The prevalence of bipolar I disorder is divided fairly equally between men and women. However, women report more episodes of depression than men and are more likely to be diagnosed with bipolar II disorder.

Bipolar II disorder is characterized by alternating episodes of a milder form of mania (known as hypomania) and depression. In bipolar II disorder, although there is an observable change in mood and functioning, the hypomanic episode causes less severe impairment than that seen in mania. It is very rare for an individual's diagnosis to change from bipolar II disorder to bipolar I disorder.

CYCLOTHYMIA

Cyclothymic disorder is a form of bipolar disorder in which hypomania alternates with a low-level, chronic depressive state. Seasonal affective disorder (SAD) is characterized by alternating mood episodes that vary according to seasonal patterns; the mood changes are thought to be related to changes in the amount of sunlight and accompanying effects on an individual's circadian rhythm and levels of the hormone melatonin.

In the northern hemisphere, the typical pattern is associated with manic symptoms in the spring and summer and depression in the fall and winter. Manic episodes often have a shorter duration than the depressive episodes. Bipolar disorder must be differentiated from depressive disorders, which include major depression (unipolar depression) and dysthymia, a milder but chronic form of depression.

COMORBIDITY

Clinical comorbidity is the existence of two or more disorders in the same individual. in In 2011, the Archives of General Psychiatry (now JAMA Psychiatry) reported on a World Mental Health survey conducted by researchers from Harvard University. The survey found that 75 percent of participants with bipolar spectrum disorder also met the criteria for at least one other psychiatric disorder, with anxiety disorder as the most prevalent co-occurring condition. Less than half of those with bipolar disorder reported receiving mental health treatment for the condition. Other frequently occurring comorbid disorders are attention-deficit hyperactivity disorder (ADHD), personality disorders, and substance use disorder.

CAUSES

The causes of bipolar disorder are not fully understood. However, family, twin, and adoption studies indicate that genetic factors play a major role. The Depression and Bipolar Support Alliance reports that approximately two-thirds of individuals with bipolar have at least one close relative with the disorder. In fact, it is not uncommon to see families in which several generations are affected by bipolar disorder. Serotonin, norepinephrine, and dopamine, brain chemicals known as neurotransmitters that regulate mood, arousal, and energy, respectively, are thought to be altered in bipolar disorder.

One theory is that bipolar disorder is associated with dysregulation in brain regions that are implicated in emotion such as the amygdala and basal ganglia. This theory is supported by functional brain imaging studies that indicate that during cognitive or emotional tasks, people with bipolar I disorder show different patterns of activity in the amygdala. In terms of structural brain imaging, people with bipolar disorder also display differences in the volume of activity in certain regions such as the amygdala and basal ganglia.

A diathesis-stress model has been proposed for some psychosomatic disorders such as hypertension. This model has also been applied to bipolar disorder. In a diathesis-stress model, there is a susceptibility (the diathesis) for the disorder. An individual who has a diathesis is at risk for the disorder but may not show signs of the disorder unless there is sufficient stress. In this model, a genetic, structural, or biochemical predisposition toward the disorder (the bipolar diathesis) may lie dormant until stress triggers the emergence of the illness. The stress may be psychosocial, biological, neurochemical, or a combination of these factors.

A diathesis-stress model can also account for some of the recurrent episodes of mania in bipolar disorder. Investigators suggest that positive life events, such as the birth of a baby or a job promotion, as well as negative life events, such as divorce or the loss of a job, may trigger the onset of episodes in individuals with bipolar disorder. Stressful life events and the social rhythm disruptions that they cause can have adverse effects on a person's circadian rhythms. Circadian rhythms are normal biologic rhythms that govern such functions as sleeping and waking, body temperature, and oxygen consumption. Circadian rhythms affect hormonal levels and have significant effects on both emotional and physical well-being. For those reasons, many clinicians encourage individuals with bipolar disorder to work toward maintaining consistency in their social rhythms.

Investigators have compared the course of bipolar disorder to kindling, a process in which epileptic seizures increase the likelihood of further seizures. According to the kindling hypothesis, triggered mood episodes may leave the individual's brain in a sustained sensitized state that makes the person more vulnerable to further episodes. After a while, external factors are less necessary for a mood episode to be triggered. Episode sensitization may also account for rapid-cycling states, in which the individual shifts from depression to mania over the course of a few hours or days. Some individuals are diagnosed with a subtype of bipolar disorder known as rapid cycling bipolar disorder, which is defined as four or more episodes per year. Rapid cycling is characterized by poorer outcome.

IMPACT

The burden of bipolar disorder is considerable. In addition to experiencing functional impairment during illness episodes, many people with bipolar disorder experience ongoing functional impairment between episodes. In 2002, the World Health Organization (WHO) reported that bipolar disorder was responsible for more adjusted life-years than any form of cancer or such major neurologic diseases as Alzheimer's and epilepsy. It was estimated that bipolar disorder was the sixth leading cause of disability worldwide among adults between the ages of fifteen and forty-four. Bipolar disorder is associated with the highest rate of suicide out of all of the psychiatric disorders. According to Kay Redfield Jamison, one of the foremost experts on bipolar disorder, approximately 50 percent of people with bipolar disorder attempt suicide at least once during their lives. In one large-scale study, when asked to rate their perception of their well-being in terms of their culture, values, and how they live in relation to their goals, standards, and expectations (that is, their quality of life), individuals with bipolar disorder rated their quality of life lower than members of the general population did. Indeed, study findings suggest that quality-of-life ratings are poorer in bipolar disorder than they are in anxiety disorders and in depression but are better than compared with quality-of-life ratings in schizophrenia.

Organizations such as the National Alliance on Mental Illness (NAMI) and support groups such as the Depressive and Bipolar Support Alliance (DBSA) have provided a way for people with bipolar disorder to share their pain as well as to triumph over the illness. Many people have found comfort in knowing that others have suffered from the mood shifts, and they can draw strength from one another. Family members and friends can be the strongest supporters and advocates for those who have bipolar disorder or other psychiatric illnesses. Many patients have credited their families' constant, uncritical support in addition to competent effective treatment including medications and psychotherapy, with helping them cope with the devastating effects of the illness. As many as 15 percent of those with bipolar disorder commit suicide; this reality makes early intervention, relapse prevention, and treatment of the disorder necessary to prevent such a tragic outcome.

TREATMENT APPROACHES

Medications have been developed to aid in correcting the biochemical imbalances thought to be part of bipolar disorder. Lithium carbonate is effective for the majority of individuals who take it. Many brilliant and successful people have reportedly suffered from bipolar disorder and have been able to function successfully with competent and responsible treatment. Some people who have taken lithium for bipolar disorder, however, have complained that it robs them of their energy and creativity. They say that they actually miss the energy associated with manic phases of the illness. This perceived loss, some of it realistic, can be a factor in relapse associated with lithium noncompliance.

Other medications have been developed to help those individuals who are considered lithium nonresponders or who find the side effects of lithium intolerable. Anticonvulsant medications, such as divalproex sodium (Depakote), carbamazepine (Tegretol), and lamotrigine (Lamictal), which have been found to have mood-stabilizing effects, are often prescribed to individuals with bipolar disorder. During the depressive phase of the disorder, electroconvulsive therapy (ECT) and lamotrigine (Lamictal) have also been administered to help restore the individual's mood to a normal level. Phototherapy is particularly useful for individuals who have Seasonal Affective Disorder (SAD). Atypical antipsychotic medications such as risperidone (Risperdal), olanzapine (Zyprexa), and quetiapine (Seroquel) have also been prescribed to individuals with bipolar I disorder for the treatment of mania.

Cognitive behavior therapy is a form of therapy that addresses an individual's beliefs, assumptions, and behaviors to improve that person's emotional responses and health. Interpersonal social rhythms therapy encourages individuals to achieve and maintain stable routines, emphasizing the link between regular routines and moods, whereas the interpersonal component of the therapy focuses on the interpersonal issues that arise in individuals' lives. Psychotherapy, especially cognitive behavior therapy or interpersonal social rhythm therapy, is viewed by most practitioners as a necessary adjunct to medication. Indeed, psychotherapy has been found to assist individuals with bipolar disorder in maintaining medication compliance.

Local mental health associations are able to recommend psychiatric treatment by board-certified psychiatrists and licensed psychologists who specialize in the treatment of mood disorders. Often, temporary hospitalization is necessary for complete diagnostic assessment, initial mood stabilization and intensive treatment, medication adjustment, or monitoring of an individual who feels suicidal.

FURTHER READING

Correa, R., et al. "Is Unrecognized Bipolar Disorder a Frequent Contributor to Apparent Treatment Resistant Depression?" *Journal of Affective Disorders* 127 (2012): 10–18. Print.

Deckersbach, Thilo, et al. *Mindfulness-Based Cognitive Therapy for Bipolar Disorder.* New York: Guilford, 2014. Print.

Goodwin, Frederick K., and Kay R. Jamison. *Manic Depressive Illness.* 2d ed. New York: Oxford University Press, 2007. Print.

Jamison, Kay R. *An Unquiet Mind.* New York: Knopf, 1995. Print.

Miklowitz, David J. *The Bipolar Disorder Survival Guide: What You and Your Family Need to Know.* New York, N.Y.: Guilford, 2002. Print.

Miklowitz, David J., and Sheri E. Johnson. "The Psychopathology and Treatment of Bipolar Disorder." *Annual Review of Clinical Psychology* 2 (2006): 199–235. Print.

Merikangas, Kathleen, et al. "Prevalence and Correlates of Bipolar Spectrum Disorder in the World Mental Health Survey Initiative." *Archives of General Psychiatry* 68.3 (2011): 241–51. Print.

Post, RM, and P. Kalivas. "Bipolar Disorder and Substance Misuse: Pathological and Therapeutic Implications of their Comorbidity and Cross-Sensitisation." *British Journal of Psychiatry* 202 (2013): 172–76. Print.

Yatham, Lakshmi N., and Vivek Kusumakar, eds. 2nd ed. New York: Brunner-Routledge, 2009. Print.

Diane C. Gooding and Karen Wolford; updated by Diane C. Gooding

See Also: Depression; Stress

Body dysmorphic disorder

A perceptual and cognitive disturbance in which people are preoccupied with one or more imagined bodily defects. Preoccupation occurs even though bodily appearance is objectively well within the range of normal. People with body dysmorphic disorder (BDD) find some aspect of their physical appearance loathsome. They commonly complain about minor flaws such as facial wrinkles, freckles, facial hair, baldness, or some other feature that is repugnant: shape of the chin, nose, eyebrow, for example. Treatment usually involves combinatory therapy: use of a selective serotonin reuptake inhibitor (SSRI) and cognitive behavioral therapy (CBT).

INTRODUCTION

Amusement park goers often enjoy viewing themselves in "carnival mirrors" which distort their bodies to make them seem hideously deformed: stretched tall and thin, squashed short and thick, or bulging in the midsection. Fans of this entertainment enjoy the images because they know them to be optical illusions. Though not as extreme, people who suffer from BDD perceive some aspect of their physical selves as grossly deformed and become preoccupied in attempting to improve, remove, or hide it. Believing the misperception is their reality promotes self-hatred, depression, social embarrassment and isolation. They are often confused that others are not repulsed.

Though the psychiatric and psychological communities did not formally recognize BDD until 1987, Italian psychiatrist, Enrico Morselli described it in some of his patients more than a century earlier. Patients reported feeling ugly or complained of having horrific physical defects even though others never noticed them. Morselli noted that these patients were depressed and miserable, often tormented by obsessions over the imagined deformity, and named this disorder dysmorphophobia. Today, body dysmorphic disorder (BDD) is understood as an involuntary preoccupation with an imagined, or actual but slight, defect in appearance. The anxiety and rumination about the defect causes enough psychological distress that it impairs social, educational, and occupational functioning even to the point of social isolation.

POSSIBLE CAUSES

While the causes of BDD are not entirely known, experts feel a combination of triggers is responsible. Like many mental disorders, brain chemicals responsible for how brain cells communicate with each other, neurotransmitters, seem to play a major role. Serotonin, a chemical linked to mood, is one that is of particular interest in developing BDD and treating it.

Additional evidence suggests one or more genetic factors may be at work, especially in persons with a family history of BDD. The specific genetic action remains unknown, however. The presence of BDD among family members though also supports the idea that family environmental factors, like the expectation of flawless appearance in a family of models, actors, athletes, the socially prominent, or public figures, may play a role though research suggests genetics is the more important player.

Environmental and cultural reinforcement may also play a large role. Over the years, society has become obsessed with achieving perfect physical appearance, and the obsession fuels a huge economy. Advertisements for makeup, hair products, cosmetic surgery, tanning salons, diet pills and plans all attest to the obsession with improved, and for some the obsession with perfect, appearance. The media constantly presents perfectly-sculpted superstars whom millions aspire to emulate but who cannot possibly duplicate stars' flawless physical appearance.

DIAGNOSING BDD

The American Psychiatric Association's *Diagnostic and Statistical Manual of Mental Disorders* (DSM-III-R) officially recognized BDD in 1987 as a variant of obsessive-compulsive disorder. In 1999, it refined its view, designating BDD as a discrete disorder in the DSM-IV-R. The primary symptom is an involuntary obsessive focus on a particular body part or feature that is normal or near-normal in appearance. Often, people with BDD are most concerned with some part of their face. Common flaws like acne, blemishes, scars, or wrinkles can be intensely scrutinized for hours. Frequent symptoms of BDD are incessant mirror-gazing or comparing one's features to others. People with BDD may also be obsessed with grooming such as plucking eyebrows, skin-picking, or shaving. Often, these activities cause significant skin damage which stresses afflicted persons even more, resulting in exhaustive efforts to camouflage the defect with makeup, clothes, or frequently plastic surgery. BDD should be suspected when behaviors of inspecting, treating, and/or camouflaging consume enough time and energy to interfere patients' work, school, finances or social life, or when grooming becomes ritualistic. People with BDD often appear generally anxious or worried.

BDD differs from other body image disorders such as what occurs in anorexia nervosa. People with BDD are obsessed over a defect (slight or imagined) in a specific part of the body. People with anorexia nervosa have the perceptual distortion that their bodies are as a whole overweight; they misperceive skin plasticity as fat tissue.

BDD results from a complex combination of biological, psychological and environmental factors though their precise interactions are not fully understood. BDD does have striking similarities to obsessive compulsive disorder, and these similarities may help to explain why many of the same treatments for OCD are also effective for it. Because its symptoms are easily mistaken for OCD and other disorders like major depression, BDD is often misdiagnosed. Some studies suggest 1-2% of the world's population meet all diagnostic criteria for BDD, but others put this percentage much higher.

WHO SUFFERS

BDD occurs in men and women equally, typically developing when appearance begins to matter a lot: adolescence or early adulthood with average onset between 16 and 17. Older adults can develop obsessive concerns about the physical effects of normal aging and develop BDD. People with BDD seek cosmetic surgery and dermatological procedures much more often than other groups seeking elective surgical interventions. Because BDD symptoms overlap with OCD symptoms, and because people with BDD are often too ashamed of their "defective" feature, they often do not seek help and their BDD remains undiagnosed and untreated.

TREATMENT OPTIONS

The first-line treatment of BDD involves taking an SSRI and starting CBT counseling in conjunction. SSRI's are generally effective in treating other conditions whose symptoms are similar to those in BDD, like major depressive disorder and OCD, both conditions in which serotonin levels are low and both of which get better as serotonin levels increase—at least to a point. It would be dangerous to assume that the more serotonin one has, the happier and more care free he or she would be.

BDD often requires higher doses than those prescribed for depression and more similar to those prescribed for OCD. The SSRI's used typically include fluoxetine (80mg/day), sertraline (200 mg/day), paroxetine (40-60 mg/day), and citalopram (40-60 mg/day). Patients are typically treated at the maximum effective and tolerated dose for 12-16 weeks before any symptoms might

improve. If successful, use of the medication should continue indefinitely as relapse after discontinuation is high though this is a decision that should only be reached between the provider and the patient. Sometimes, when the patient has tried a second or third SSRI without success, the psychiatrist might recommend a medicine from the group known as the "anti-psychotics" which like the antidepressants are effective for many other conditions than the category they are in, psychosis. Common antipsychotics used for BDD are olanzapine or risperidone.

The cognitive part of CBT involves identifying and rethinking patient's self-loathing and disparaging thoughts. Then, through repetitive exposure, systematic desensitization, and step-wise implementation of adaptive behavioral strategies, CBT attempts to systematically remove the harmful and maladaptive behaviors associated with patients' coping with BDD on their own. Though widely practiced, not all psychologists or other mental health providers are specifically trained in CBT. People with BDD should seek out from among those with training and experience, the providers they believe they will develop effective therapeutic rapport: professionals who will challenge patients to work hard and support them in non-judgmental ways as they strive to meet the challenge of defeating this emotionally painful and socially limiting condition.

FURTHER READING

Claiborn, James and Cherry Pedrick, *The BDD Workbook: Overcoming Body Dysmorphic Disorder and End Body Image Obsessions.* Oakland, CA: New Harbinger, 2004. Solid, useful introduction to this widely under-recognized condition. Exercises are practical and while not requiring supervision, do not constitute professional clinical treatment on their own.

Mayo Clinic Staff, *Body dysmorphic disorder.* Clear, second-person and plain spoken overview of the condition, how it develops, how it can be diagnosed and effectively treated. Available on-line or in print. Rochester, MN: The Mayo Foundation for Medical Education and Research, 2009. www.mayoclinic.com/health/body-dysmorphic-disorder/DS00559.

Phillips, Katharine A. *The Broken Mirror: Understanding and Treating Body Dysmorphic Disorder.* New York, NY: Oxford, 1998. Perhaps the classic work on BDD written for the lay audience. This is a hopeful, helpful, and well-informed approach to understanding BDD's various manifestations and their treatment. Clinical vignettes are particularly illustrative and illuminating.

Wilhelm, Sabine. *Feeling Good about the Way You Look: A Program for Overcoming Body Image Problems.* New York, NY: Guildford, 2006. Directly focused on the person suffering with BDD, this is a cognitive behavioral approach for starting self-treatment and includes the author's thoughts about medication and focused psychotherapy. Is also helpful for those who have concerns that a friend or family member might have BDD.

Paul Moglia and Thomas G. Zimmerman

SEE ALSO: Body Image and Girls; Body image and Guys

Cerebral palsy

A motor disability evident early in life (often by one year of age and certainly by age two) that is caused by a brain abnormality present by the end of the newborn period (one month of age) and unchanged after that time.

CAUSES AND SYMPTOMS

Cerebral palsy is not a single disorder. Rather, it is a group of disorders that affect the brain at some time before a child is one month old, resulting in a lack of normal control of movements. While problems with making normal movements may be apparent at birth, this symptom is often not noticeable until the child is nine or ten months of age; on occasion, it may not be apparent before eighteen or twenty-four months of age because the areas of the brain that control movement are immature and not very effective early in life. Until the child reaches an age at which these areas are functional, a lack of function may go unrecognized. For example, problems using the legs may not be evident until the child is old enough to try to walk. Sometimes, a child is so severely affected that the motor problems-noticeable as either decreased or increased motor tone, or tension on the tendons-may be apparent in the first days or months of life.

Abnormal motor function can have both negative and positive symptoms. Negative symptoms can include the inability to do normal motor activities such as reach for a toy, pick up a raisin with the fingers, or walk. Positive symptoms can consist of abnormal movements such as the involuntary flexion of the foot when trying to walk, resulting in toe walking, or the persistence of primitive reflexes (such as the Moro reflex), which impede voluntary movements. These positive manifestations can result in unusual arm or leg postures that make some of these children easily recognizable. On the other hand, many children with cerebral palsy do not have these symptoms and are normal in appearance. Others have motor problems so mild that they are never diagnosed but are simply considered clumsy or maladroit.

By definition, any brain abnormality that causes cerebral palsy is not progressive, which means that the brain does not deteriorate. Actually, most children with cerebral palsy show improved motor coordination as they become older. A child with mild cerebral palsy at one year of age may be able to move normally by the second grade. Children correctly diagnosed with cerebral palsy early in life may no longer suffer from the disorder later in life. Therefore, the number of children with cerebral palsy decreases with age. The rate in developed countries is approximately two per one thousand school-age children. The vast majority of children with cerebral palsy reach adulthood, with most having a full life span. As a group, those who are never able to walk are more likely to die younger.

There is no single cause of cerebral palsy. Any abnormality of the brain that can develop either in utero or before the infant is one month old can cause cerebral palsy. Cerebral palsy is more common among children born prematurely; they account for approximately one-third of all children with cerebral palsy. One theory holds that these children develop a brain abnormality while in the womb which causes the child both to be born prematurely and to have cerebral palsy. Alternatively, especially among very low birth weight infants, their difficult first weeks of life may cause intraventricular hemorrhage and brain injury, most commonly of the white matter adjacent to the lateral ventricles. The pattern referred to as diplegia, in which the legs are more severely affected than the arms, is characteristic in premature infants with cerebral palsy.

Approximately 78 percent of term infants who develop cerebral palsy are healthy at birth. Only later, when they reach the appropriate developmental stage, does their condition become apparent. It is widely believed that these children have a brain abnormality that occurred while the brain was developing in the womb. The underlying cause of such abnormalities is unclear. About 22 percent of term infants with cerebral palsy are unwell at birth. These children have had various physiological insults-including stroke, infection, or lack of oxygen-either in the womb or at the time of birth. Children who suffer a lack of oxygen or hypotension (low blood pressure) during the birth process account for about 10 percent of infants who develop cerebral palsy. Sometimes, maternal hemorrhage or placental abnormalities deprive the infant of oxygen. Errors committed by the delivering doctor or midwife are an uncommon cause of cerebral palsy. Enhanced fetal monitoring during labor and delivery using electronic devices and delivery by cesarean section have not lowered the rate of cerebral palsy.

Since cerebral palsy is a motor disorder, it is classified by motor patterns. Children with cerebral palsy are generally divided into two major groups: those with increased tone (also called spasticity) and those with decreased tone. This is a somewhat artificial distinction since some children have decreased tone in infancy and increased tone later in life, while others may have decreased tone when lying down but increased tone when sitting or standing. A major advantage of this division is the recognition that persistent and severe decrease in motor tone makes walking more difficult, while increased tone makes the development of contractures (shortened tendons) more likely. In addition, children are classified by pattern of limb involvement. The common pattern in children born prematurely is diplegia, in which the legs are more severely affected than the arms. About 50 percent of children affected with diplegia are able to walk. Another common pattern is hemiplegia, in which the arm and leg on one side are affected and the other side is normal. The arm is more severely involved than the leg, and the prognosis for walking is good, with almost all these children able to walk if they do not have any other motor problem. When all four limbs are involved, the condition is called quadriplegia (or double hemiparesis or tetraplegia). These youngsters have the least likelihood of being able to walk and are most likely to have associated problems such as mental retardation. The pattern wherein the limbs produce markedly abnormal movements whenever the child attempts voluntary movements is uncommon. These abnormal movements can be sharp and sudden in nature (called chorea) or slower and more writhing (called athetosis), although often the movements are a combination of the two patterns and thus not easily classified. In the past, this motor pattern was caused by severe hyperbilirubinemia (a very high accumulation of bilirubin) shortly after birth. Today, modern therapies such as exchange transfusion and light therapy usually prevent the bilirubin level from rising to dangerous levels.

The motor impairment can affect more than the child's limbs. Speech, chewing, drinking, and swallowing can be abnormal when the motor disability affects the

---

INFORMATION ON CEREBRAL PALSY

Causes: Unknown; likely a brain abnormality that develops in utero
Symptoms: Lack of normal control of movements, unusual arm or leg postures, weak muscle tone, facial distortion, labored speech
Duration: Chronic
Treatments: None

---

face, tongue, and lips. This is most commonly seen in children with quadriplegia. It is widely noted that many of these children have weak face muscles and tend to keep their mouths open and to drool. When speech is affected, the patient often speaks slowly, has a nasal quality to the voice, and has poor enunciation. When

this disability is severe, patients may find it impossible to speak any intelligible words even when their understanding of speech is not affected. Children with this type of motor problem may have difficulty with the fine lip and tongue movements necessary for chewing and may be able to eat only soft foods. Some of these children also have difficulty handling liquids such as water and may choke on clear liquids; they may prefer thickened soft foods. The motor disability can be severe enough that the swallowing movements of the esophagus and stomach are disturbed. Normally, there is a well-organized progression of such movements that propel food down the esophagus and through the stomach into the intestines. When this normal motor progression does not occur, children may regurgitate their food, since the food is inadvertently propelled up and out instead of down and into the intestines. This is referred to as reflux. When present to a minor degree, reflux can be merely a cosmetic problem, and the child may need to wear a bib much of the day. When present to a more severe degree, reflux can interfere with normal nutrition. Having food returning into the mouth in a child who has difficulty coordinating swallowing can lead to aspiration, the inadvertent passage of food down the windpipe and into the lungs, which can cause frequent bouts of pneumonia.

The brain abnormalities that cause cerebral palsy can produce other brain-related disabilities. In a survey of children with cerebral palsy in Atlanta, 75 percent had another disability, 65 percent had mental retardation, 46 percent had epilepsy, and 15 percent had sensory loss. Many of the children had more than one additional disability. Children with quadriplegia are the most likely to have other disabilities.

TREATMENT AND THERAPY

Only in unusual circumstances is there any direct treatment available for the brain abnormality that causes the motor disability of cerebral palsy. On the other hand, a variety of resources are available for helping the child cope with motor problems. Physical aids such as wheelchairs, walkers, and crutches have long been available. Modern ones are extremely adjustable and made of lightweight and durable materials. Lightweight plastic can be custom molded and fitted to supplement or replace the more traditional leg braces. Physical therapy helps interfere with involuntary and primitive reflex patterns that hinder voluntary movements. Therapy can also facilitate normal patterns of arm and leg use. Occupational therapy focuses on developing fine motor skills and improving the ability to dress, eat, write, and perform other daily activities. To be successful, all these therapies must be done every day.As a practical matter, this means performing the activities at home with parental assistance under the periodic supervision of a therapist. Orthopedic surgery, when used judiciously, can improve muscle aalance, release contractures, and correct scoliosis. The surgeon must consider carefully how the child's growth in height and weight in the years following the surgery might affect the outcome either favorably or adversely.

Abnormal tone is difficult to alter. No medicines exist that can increase tone, while several medications such as diazepam, dantrolene, and baclofen can sometimes decrease tone for children who have spasticity. Side effects such as sleepiness greatly limit the use of such medications. In addition, many children have both weakness and increased tone. The tone often helps them do activities such as standing, since the tone stiffens their legs. The loss of tone can actually make the child less able to stand. Asurgical procedure called posterior rhizotomy can decrease the tone for children with diplegia who have mild gait abnormalities. These youngsters can walk with minimal assistance, usually walking up on their toes, and they have no problem with truncal balance. In this surgical procedure performed on the lower back, some of the sensory (posterior) innervating nerves to the leg muscles are severed. The procedure can produce some postoperative sensory loss, which usually disappears. Long-term adverse effects include weakness and scoliosis. It is generally believed that to be effective,

the procedure should be accompanied by an aggressive program of physical therapy.

School programs have become increasingly sophisticated in assisting pupils with motor disabilities. Techniques include the use of computers for written work as well as computers with voice simulators for youngsters who cannot speak adequately to participate in the classroom. All schools in the United States are required to be physically accessible to motor-disabled students and to structure gym and recess programs so that all students can participate.

Medications are available that can help control muscle spasms and seizures. Spasticity may be treated with botulinum toxin, baclofen, diazepam, or tizanidine. Glycopyrrolate can be prescribed to help ease drooling. Pamidronate can be given to help treat related osteoporosis.

PERSPECTIVE AND PROSPECTS

The Centers for Disease Control and Prevention reported in September 2012 that cerebral palsy is the most common motor disability to occur during childhood, with an estimated global incident rate of 1.5 to more than four cases per thousand live births or children in a defined age group. The brightest hope lies in research to understand better the abnormalities of fetal development that lead to cerebral palsy, in the expectation of finding preventive measures. In addition, since premature infants are disproportionately represented among those with cerebral palsy, the prevention of prematurity and improvements in the management of children born prematurely also provide hope for decreasing the occurrence of the disorder. Newer medicines such as gabapentin that hold the potential for decreasing the adverse effects of increased tone with fewer side effects are also appearing. Finally, the potential of computers and computer-assisted physical devices to help motor-impaired persons is being actively explored.

FURTHER READING

Centers for Disease Control and Prevention. "Facts about Cerebral Palsy." *CDC*, May 18, 2012.

Centers for Disease Control and Prevent. "Data & Statistics for Cerebral Palsy." *CDC*, Sept. 7, 2012.

Geralis, Elaine, ed. *Children with Cerebral Palsy: A Parent's Guide.* 2d ed. Bethesda, Md.: Woodbine House, 1998.

Grether, Judith K., and Karin B. Nelson. "Maternal Infection and Cerebral Palsy in Infants of Normal

BirthWeight." *Journal of the American Medical Association* 278, no. 3 (July 16, 1997): 207-11.

Hutton, J. L., T. Cooke, and P. O. Pharoah. "Life Expectancy in Children with Cerebral Palsy." *British Medical Journal* 309, no. 6952 (August 13, 1994): 431-35.

Kramer, Laura Shapiro. *Uncommon Voyage: Parenting a Special Needs Child.* 2d ed. Berkeley, Calif.: North Atlantic, 2001.

MedlinePlus. "Cerbral Palsy." *MedlinePlus*, Mar. 25, 2013.

Pimm, Paul. *Living with Cerebral Palsy.* Austin, Tex.: Raintree, 1999.

Stanton, Marion. *The Cerebral Palsy Handbook.* London: Vermilion, 2002.

Swaiman, Kenneth F., Stephen Ashwal, and Donna M. Ferriero, eds. *Pediatric Neurology: Principles and Practice.* 4th ed. Philadelphia: Mosby, 2006.

United Cerebral Palsy. *UCP*, 2013.

Wood, Debra. "Cerebral Palsy." *Health Library*, Feb. 1, 2013.

Robert J. Baumann

SEE ALSO: Brain, The; Muscular Dystrophy

Dyslexia

Dyslexia is often defined as severe reading disability in children of otherwise average or above-average intelligence; it is thought to be caused by neuropsychological problems. Dyslexia frustrates afflicted children, damages their self-image, produces grave maladjustment in many cases, and decreases their adult contributions to society.

INTRODUCTION

The ability to read quickly and well is essential for success in modern industrialized societies. Several researchers, including Robert E. Valett, have pointed out that an individual must acquire considerable basic cognitive and perceptual-linguistic skills to learn to read. First, it is necessary to learn to focus one's attention, to concentrate, to follow directions, and to understand the language spoken in daily life. Next, it is essential to develop auditory and visual memory with sequencing ability, word-decoding skills, a facility for structural-contextual language analysis, the ability to interpret the written language, a useful vocabulary that expands as needed, and

speed in scanning and interpreting written language. Valett has noted that these skills are taught in all good developmental reading programs.

Dyslexia may make it difficult to distinguish letters and words that are mirror images of each other. Yet 20 to 25 percent of the population of the United States and many other industrialized societies, people who otherwise possess at least average intelligence, cannot develop good reading skills. Many such people are viewed as suffering from a neurological disorder called dyslexia, a term that was first introduced by a German ophthalmologist, Rudolph Berlin, in the nineteenth century. Berlin meant it to designate all those individuals who possessed an average or above-average performance intelligence quotient (IQ) but who could not read adequately because of an inability to process language symbols. Others reported children who could see perfectly well but who acted as though they were blind to the written language. For example, they could see a bird flying but were unable to identify the word "bird" written in a sentence.

Although the problem has been redefined many times over the ensuing years, the modern definition of dyslexia is still fairly close to Berlin's definition. The American Psychiatric Association's *Diagnostic and Statistical Manual of Mental Disorders: DSM-IV-TR* (rev. 4th ed., 2000) labels this condition "reading disorder" and defines it as reading achievement substantially below that expected given chronological age, measured intelligence, and age-appropriate education that interferes significantly with academic achievement or activities of daily living requiring reading skills.

BRAIN DEVELOPMENT

Two basic explanations have evolved for dyslexia. Many physicians propose that it is caused by either brain damage or brain dysfunction. Evolution of the problem is attributed to accident, to disease, or to faults in body chemistry. Diagnosis is made by the use of electroencephalograms (EEGs), computed tomography (CT) scans, and other related technology. After such evaluation, medication is often used to diminish hyperactivity and nervousness, and physical training procedures called patterning are used as tools to counter the neurological defects.

In contrast, many special educators and other related researchers believe that the problem is one of dormant, immature, or undeveloped learning centers in the brain. The proponents of this concept encourage the correction of dyslexic problems by emphasized teaching of specific reading skills to appropriate individuals. Although such experts also agree that the use of appropriate medication can be of value, they lend most of their efforts to curing the problem by a process called imprinting,Imprinting which essentially trains the dyslexic patient through use of often-repeated, exaggerated language drills.

Another interesting point of view is the idea that dyslexia may be at least partly the fault of the written languages of the Western world. Rudolph F. Wagner has pointed out that children in Japan exhibit an incidence of dyslexia that is less than 1 percent. One explanation for this, say Wagner and others, is that the languages of the Western world require reading from left to right. This characteristic is absent in Japanese—possibly, they suggest, making it easier to learn.

Several experts, among them Dale R. Jordan, recognize three types of dyslexia. The most common type—and the one most often identified as dyslexia—is visual dyslexia: the lack of ability to translate observed written or printed language into meaningful terms. The major difficulty here is that afflicted people see certain letters backward or upside down. The result is that, to them, a written sentence is a jumble of letters whose accurate translation may require five times as much time as would be needed by an unafflicted person.

AUDITORY DYSLEXIA AND DYSGRAPHIA

The other two problems viewed as dyslexia are auditory dyslexia and dysgraphia. Auditory dyslexia is the inability to perceive individual sounds of spoken language. Despite having normal hearing, auditory dyslexics are deaf to the differences between certain vowel or consonant sounds; what they cannot hear, they cannot write. Dysgraphia is the inability to write legibly. The basis for this problem is a lack of the hand-eye coordination required to write legibly.

Usually, a child who suffers from visual dyslexia also exhibits elements of auditory dyslexia. This complicates the issue of teaching such a student, because only one type of dyslexic symptom can be treated at a time. Also, dyslexia appears to be a sex-linked disorder; three to four times as many boys have it as do girls. In all cases, early diagnosis and treatment of dyslexia are essential to its eventual correction. For example, if treatment begins before the third grade, there is an 80 percent probability that dyslexia can be corrected. When dyslexia remains undiscovered until the fifth grade, this probability is halved. If treatment does not begin until the seventh grade, the probability of successful treatment is only 3

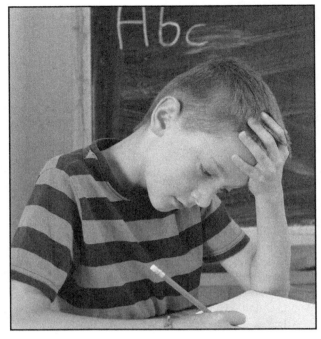

Photo: iStock

to 5 percent.

ASSESSMENT METHODS AND TREATMENT

Preliminary identification of the dyslexic child often can be made from symptoms that include poor written schoolwork, easy distractibility, clumsiness, poor coordination and spatial orientation, confused writing and/or spelling, and poor left-right orientation. Because non-dyslexic children can also show many of these symptoms, the second step of such identification is the use of written tests designed to pick out dyslexic children. These include the Peabody Individual Achievement Test, the Halstead-Reitan Neuropsychological Test Battery, and the SOYBAR Criterion Tests. Many more personalized tests are also available.

Once conclusive identification of a dyslexic child has been made, it becomes possible to begin a corrective treatment program. Most such programs are carried out by special-education teachers in school resource rooms, in special classes limited to children with reading disabilities, and in schools that specialize in treating the disorder.

One often-cited method is that of Grace Fernald, which utilizes kinesthetic imprinting, based on a combination of "language experience" and tactile stimulation. In this popular method, the child relates a spontaneous story to the teacher, who transcribes it. Next, each word unknown to the child is written down by the teacher, and the child traces its letters over and over until he or she can write that word without using the model. Each word learned becomes part of the child's word file. A large number of stories are handled this way. Many variants of the method are in use. Though it is quite slow, many anecdotal reports praise its results. (Despite this, Donald K. Routh pointed out in 1987 that the method had never been subjected to a rigorous, controlled study of its efficacy.)

A second common method utilized by special educators is the Orton-Gillingham-Stillman method, developed in a collaboration by teachers Anna Gillingham and Essie Stillman and the pediatric neurologist Samuel T. Orton. The method evolved from Orton's conceptualization of language as developing from a sequence of processes in the nervous system that end in unilateral control by the left cerebral hemisphere. He proposed that dyslexia arises from conflicts, which need to be corrected, between this hemisphere and the right cerebral hemisphere, usually involved in the handling of nonverbal, pictorial, and spatial stimuli.

Consequently, the method used is multisensory and kinesthetic, like Fernald's; however, it begins with the teaching of individual letters and phonemes, and progresses to dealing with syllables, words, and sentences. Children taught by this method are drilled systematically to imprint a mastery of phonics and the sounding out of unknown written words. They are encouraged to learn how the elements of written language look, how they sound, how it feels to pronounce them, and how it feels to write them down. Routh has pointed out that the Orton-Gillingham-Stillman method is as laborious as that of Fernald. It is widely used and appreciated, however, and believed to work well.

Another method that merits brief discussion is the use of therapeutic drugs in the treatment of dyslexia. Most physicians and educators propose the use of these drugs as a useful adjunct to the training of dyslexic children who are easily distracted and restless or who have low morale because of embarrassment resulting from peer pressure. The drugs used most often are the amphetamine Dexedrine and methylphenidate (Ritalin).

These stimulants, taken in appropriate doses, lengthen the time period during which some dyslexic children function well in the classroom and also produce feelings of self-confidence. Side effects of overdose, however, include lost appetite, nausea, nervousness,

and sleeplessness. Furthermore, there is the potential problem of drug abuse. Despite this, numerous sources (including both Valett and Jordan) indicate that stimulant benefits far outweigh any possible risks when the drugs are utilized carefully and under close medical supervision. Other, less dependable therapies sometimes attempted include special diets and the use of vitamins and minerals.

One other important aspect of the treatment of dyslexia is good parental emotional support, which helps children cope with their problems and with peer pressure. Useful aspects of this support include a positive attitude toward the afflicted child; appropriate home help for the child that complements efforts undertaken at school; encouragement and praise for achievements, without recrimination when repeated mistakes are made; and good interaction with special-education teachers assigned to a child.

RESEARCH

The identification of dyslexia more than one hundred years ago, which resulted from the endeavors of the German physician Berlin and of W. A. Morgan, in England, launched efforts to find a cure for this unfortunate disorder. In 1917, the Scottish eye surgeon James Hinshelwood published a book on dyslexia, which he viewed as being a hereditary problem, and the phenomenon became better known to physicians. Attempts at educating dyslexics, as recommended by Hinshelwood and other physicians, were highly individualized until the endeavors of Orton and coworkers and of Fernald led to more standardized and soon widely used methods.

Furthermore, with the development of a more complete understanding of the brain and its many functions, better counseling facilities, and the conceptualization and actualization of both parent-child and parent-counselor interactions, the prognosis for successful dyslexic training has improved significantly. Also, a number of extensive studies of dyslexic children have been carried out and have identified dyslexia as a complex syndrome composed of numerous associated behavioral dysfunctions related to visual-motor brain immaturity. These include poor memory for details, easy distractibility, poor motor skills, letter and word reversal, and the inability to distinguish between important elements of the spoken language.

A particularly extensive and useful study was carried out by Edith Klasen and described in her book *The Syndrome of Specific Dyslexia: With Special Consideration* of Its Physiological, Psychological, Testpsychological, and Social Correlates (1972). The Klasen study identified the role of psychoanalytical interventions in the treatment of some dyslexic subjects, and it pointed out that environmental and socioeconomic factors contribute relatively little to the occurrence of dyslexia but affect the outcomes of its treatment.

It is the endeavors of special education that have made the greatest inroads into treatment of dyslexia. Further advances in the area will undoubtedly be made, as the science of the mind grows and diversifies and as the contributions of the psychologist, physician, physiologist, and special educator mesh together more effectively.

FURTHER READING

Hoien, Torliev, and Ingvar Lundberg. *Dyslexia: From Theory to Intervention*. Norwell, Mass.: Kluwer, 2000. Presents European research in the causes and treatment of dyslexia, much of it presented in English for the first time.

Nicolson, Roderick I., and Angela Fawcett. *Dyslexia, Learning, and the Brain*. Cambridge, Mass.: MIT Press, 2008. Leading dyslexia researchers theorize that the source of this disability may be rooted in the procedural learning system, in the cortical and subcortical regions of the brain.

Reid, Gavin. *Dyslexia: A Practitioner's Handbook*. 4th ed. New York: John Wiley & Sons, 2008. A review of dyslexia research and teaching practices for educators. Includes a review of resources for classroom strategies.

Reid, Gavin, and Janice Wearmouth. Dyslexia and Literacy: An Introduction to Theory and Practice. New York: John Wiley & Sons, 2002. Covers recent theoretical and practical approaches to dyslexia in both psychological and pedagogical contexts.

Snowling, Margaret J. *Dyslexia: A Cognitive Developmental Perspective*. 2d ed. New York: Basil Blackwell, 2000. Covers many aspects of dyslexia, including its identification, associated cognitive defects, the basis for development of language skills, and the importance of phonology. In addition, it contains many references.

West, Thomas G. *In the Mind's Eye: Visual Thinkers, Gifted People with Dyslexia and Other Learning Difficulties, Computer Images, and the Ironies of Creativity*. Updated ed. Amherst, N.Y.: Prometheus Press, 1997. Argues that the rise of computer technology favors visual over verbal thinkers, decreasing the difficulties faced by dyslexics and others with verbal learning disorders.

Sanford S. Singer

SEE ALSO: Brain, The

Eating disorders

Eating disorders include a group of eating and weight disturbances, including anorexia nervosa, bulimia nervosa, and binge eating disorder, associated with underlying psychological problems.

INTRODUCTION

Eating disorders were identified as early as ancient Rome, when banqueters gorged themselves, then induced vomiting. Some of the early female Christian saints were anorexic. However, eating disorders only emerged as an area of social and medical concern in the second half of the twentieth century.

Persons with eating disorders have a distorted body image and unrealistic ideas about weight. Although they are found primarily among young, middle- to upper-middle-class, well-educated Caucasian women, eating disorders increasingly affect and may be overlooked in men, older women, and persons of color. No single factor appears to be the cause of eating disorders, with social, cultural, psychological, genetic, biological, and physical factors all playing a part. Treatment may include hospitalization for nutritional monitoring and for stabilization in persons with serious medical complications or who are at risk for suicide. Regardless of the setting, treatment is best carried out by a multidisciplinary team, including a primary care physician or psychiatrist, a psychotherapist, a nutritionist, and, if appropriate, a family therapist.

Eating disorders are best thought of as problems involving body weight and distorted body image on a continuum of severity. The most serious is anorexia nervosa, a disorder characterized by weight loss greater than or equal to 15 percent of the body weight normal for the person's height and age. Bulimia nervosa is usually found in persons of normal weight and is characterized by consumption of large amounts of food followed by self-induced vomiting, purging with diuretics or laxatives, or excessive exercise. Binge eating disorder, found usually in persons with some degree of overweight, is characterized by the consumption of large amounts of food without associated vomiting or purging. Other, milder, forms of eating disorders are at the least serious end of the continuum. Obesity may or may not be part of this continuum, depending on the presence or absence of underlying psychological problems. About one-third of obese persons have binge eating disorder.

POPULATION AT RISK

Women constitute 90 percent of people diagnosed with eating disorders—eight million adolescent and young adult women in the United States alone. The majority of these are Caucasian (95 percent) and from middle- to upper-middle-class backgrounds. Research in the latter part of the twentieth century indicated that adolescent and young adult women were most likely to be affected; however, these disorders are now found in girls as young as nine and in older women. By the end of the twentieth century, eating disorders were also increasingly identified in women from other ethnic and socioeconomic groups. These disorders are most likely underreported in men and seem to affect gay men disproportionately. Also at risk are men with certain professions or avocations such as jockeys, dancers, body builders, and wrestlers, in which weight and body shape are an issue.

CAUSES OF EATING DISORDERS

No single cause has been identified for eating disorders. However, it is important to note that nearly all eating disorders begin with dieting to lose weight. Because these disorders are found almost exclusively in the developed world, where food is plentiful and where thinness in women is idealized, it appears that social and cultural factors are important contributors. Some theorists believe that cultural values of independence and personal autonomy rather than interdependence and the importance of human relationships contribute to eating pathology. Still others point to the changing and contradictory societal expectations about the roles of women as a contributing factor.

Studies suggest a genetic predisposition to eating disorders, particularly in those persons who engage in binge eating and purging behaviors. Their family histories typically include higher than expected numbers of persons with mood disorders and substance abuse disorders problems. Dysfunctions in the pathways for the substances that transmit messages in the brain, the neurotransmitters, are thought to play a role in the development and maintenance of eating disorders, although these dysfunctions are not sufficient to explain the entire problem by themselves. The psychological theories about the causes of eating disorders postulate that individuals with underlying feelings of powerlessness or personal inadequacy attempt to cope by becoming preoccupied

with their body's shape and size. Finally, the incidence of sexual abuse is higher among persons with eating disorders, particularly bulimia nervosa, than among those in the general population.

Eating disorders seem to develop in three stages. Stage 1 involves the period from the time a child is conceived until the onset of a particular behavior that precipitates the eating disorder. During this stage, individual psychological, personal, and physical factors, plus family, social, and cultural factors, place the person at increased risk. Individual risk factors include a personal history of depression, low self-esteem, perfectionism, an eagerness to please others, obesity, and physical or sexual abuse. Family risk factors include a family member with an eating disorder or a mood disorder and excessive familial concern for appearance and weight. Social and cultural issues include emphasis on the cultural ideal of excessive thinness, leading to dissatisfaction with the body and dieting for weight loss. Young women who are dancers, runners, skaters, gymnasts, and the like may be particularly susceptible to this kind of cultural pressure.

Stage 2 involves the factors that precipitate the eating disorder. Some identified precipitating factors include onset of puberty, leaving home, new relationships, death of a relative, illness, adverse comments about weight and body appearance, fear of maturation, the struggle for autonomy during the midteen years, and identity conflicts.

Stage 3 involves the factors that perpetuate the eating disorder. These can be cognitive distortions, interpersonal events, or biological changes related to starvation.

ASSOCIATED MEDICAL PROBLEMS

Women with anorexia nervosa stop menstruating. Anorexics may also have abdominal pain, constipation, and increased urination. The heart rate may be slow or irregular. Many develop downy, dark body hair (lanugo) over normally hairless areas. They may have bloating after eating and swelling of the feet and lower legs. Low levels of potassium and sodium and other imbalances in the body's electrolytes can lead to cardiac arrest, kidney failure, weakness, confusion, poor memory, disordered thinking, and mood swings. The death rate for anorexics is high: About 5 percent will die within eight years of being diagnosed and 20 percent within twenty years.

Self-induced vomiting can lead to erosion of tooth enamel, gum abscesses, and swelling of the parotid glands in front of the ear and over the angle of the jaw. About one-third of women with bulimia have abnormal changes in their menstrual cycles. Some bulimics consume so much food in such a short period of time that their stomachs rupture. More than 75 percent of these individuals die. Use of ipecac and laxatives can lead to heart damage. Symptoms include chest pain, skipped heartbeats, and fainting, and these heart problems can lead to death. In addition, bulimics are at increased risk for ulcers of the stomach and small intestine and for inflammation of the pancreas.

One commonly overlooked problem is the female athletic triad,Athletes, eating disorders a combination of disordered eating, loss of menstruation, and osteoporosis. This can lead to fractures and permanent loss of bone minerals.

ANOREXIA NERVOSA

The diagnosis of Anorexia nervosa is made for persons who have lost 15 percent or more of the body weight that is considered normal for their height and age and who have an intense and irrational fear of gaining weight. Even with extreme weight loss, anorexics perceive themselves as overweight. Their attitude toward food and weight control becomes obsessive and they frequently develop bizarre or ritualistic behaviors around food, such as chewing each bite a specific number of times. Anorexics minimize the seriousness of their weight loss and are highly resistant to treatment.

The two basic types of anorexia nervosa are the restricting type and the binge eating/purging type. The restricting type is characterized by an extremely limited diet, often without carbohydrates or fats. This may be accompanied by excessive exercising or hyperactivity. Up to half of anorexics eventually lose control over their severely restricted dieting and begin to engage in binge eating. They then induce vomiting, use diuretics or laxatives, or exercise excessively to control their weight. People who are in the binge eating/purging group are at greater risk for medical complications.

As the weight loss in either type reaches starvation proportions, anorexics become more and more preoccupied with food; they may hoard food or steal. They also experience sleep abnormalities, loss of interest in sex, and poor concentration and attention. In addition, they slowly restrict their social contacts and become more and more socially isolated. In general, anorexics of the binge eating/purging type are likely to have problems with impulse control and may engage in substance abuse, excessive spending, sexual promiscuity, and other forms of compulsive behavior. This group is also more likely to

attempt suicide or to hurt themselves than others with eating disorders.

BULIMIA NERVOSA

Persons who have Bulimia nervosa are similar in behavior to the subset of anorexics who binge and purge, but they tend to maintain their weight at or near normal for their age and height. They intermittently have an overwhelming urge to eat, usually associated with a period of anxiety or depression, and can consume as many as 15,000 calories in a relatively short period of time, typically one to two hours. Binge foods are usually high calorie and easy to digest, such as ice cream. The binge eating provides a sense of numbing of the anxiety or relief from the depression. Failing to recognize that they are full, bulimics eventually stop eating because of abdominal pain, nausea, being interrupted, or some other non-hunger-related reason. At that point, psychological stress again increases as they reflect on the amount they have eaten. Most bulimics then induce vomiting, but some use laxatives, diuretics, severe food restriction, fasting, or excessive exercise to avoid gaining weight.

Bulimics tend to be secretive, binge eating and purging when alone. These episodes may occur only a few times a week or as often as several times a day. As with binge eating/purging anorexics, bulimics are likely to abuse alcohol and other drugs, make suicidal gestures, and engage in other kinds of impulsive behavior such as shoplifting. Because of the electrolyte imbalances and other adverse consequences of repeated vomiting or the use of laxatives or diuretics, bulimics are at risk for multiple serious medical complications which, if uncorrected, can lead to death.

BINGE EATING DISORDER

The American Psychiatric Association has developed provisional criteria for Binge eating disorder to study this disorder more completely. The criteria include compulsive and excessive eating at least twice a week for six months without self-induced vomiting, purging, or excessive exercise. That is, binge eating disorder is bulimia nervosa without the compensatory weight-loss mechanisms. For this reason, most binge eaters are slightly to significantly overweight. In addition to the eating problems, many binge eaters experience relationship problems and have a history of depression or other psychiatric disorders.

OTHER EATING DISORDERS

Anorexia and bulimia nervosa and binge eating disorder have strict diagnostic criteria set forth by the American Psychiatric Association. However, these three do not cover the entire spectrum of disordered eating patterns. Those people who induce vomiting after consuming only a small amount of food, for example, or those who chew large amounts of food and spit it out rather than swallow it, do not fit the diagnosis of bulimia. For such persons, a diagnosis of "eating disorder, not otherwise specified" is used.

PREVALENCE OF EATING DISORDERS

Anorexia nervosa is the rarest of the eating disorders, affecting fewer than 1 percent of adolescent and young women (that is, women ages thirteen to twenty-five) and a tiny proportion of young men. Bulimia nervosa, on the other hand, affects up to 3 percent of teenage and young adult women and about 0.2 percent of men. Even more of this age group, probably 5 percent, suffer from binge eating disorder. In obese patients, fully one-third meet the criteria for this disorder. Binge eating is the most common eating disorder in men, although more women actually have this disorder. Eating disorders, not otherwise specified, are even more common.

TREATMENT

Treatment of persons with eating disorders can take place in an inpatient or an outpatient setting. Hospitalization is indicated for patients with severe malnutrition, serious medical complications, an increased risk of suicide, and those who are unable to care for themselves or have failed outpatient treatment.

The first step in the treatment of anorexics must be restoring their body weight. This may require hospitalization. A system of carefully structured rewards for weight gain is often successful. For example, the gain of a target amount of weight may be tied to being allowed to go outside or having visits from friends. Once the anorexic is nutritionally stabilized, individual, family, Cognitive behavior therapy, and other therapies are indicated to address issues specific to the individual.

The first step in the treatment of bulimics is a comprehensive medical evaluation. Bulimics are less likely than anorexics to require hospitalization. As with anorexia nervosa, treatment includes individual, family, and cognitive behavior therapies. In addition, group therapy may be helpful. Cognitive behavior therapies are effective in the treatment of bulimia nervosa. Patients are taught to recognize and analyze cues that trigger the binge-purge cycle. Once analyzed, they are taught to reframe these thoughts, feelings, and beliefs to more adaptive and less destructive ones, thus altering the cycle.

Outpatient care should be carefully coordinated among a multidisciplinary team: an experienced health care practitioner to monitor the patient's medical condition, a therapist to address psychological and emotional issues, a family therapist to deal with control and other issues within the family, and a nutritionist to develop and monitor a sensible meal plan.

Medications may be a helpful adjunct in some cases, particularly in those eating-disordered patients who have an additional psychiatric diagnosis such as major depression or obsessive-compulsive disorder. Simply gaining weight usually improves mood in anorexics, but antidepressants (particularly the selective serotonin-reuptake inhibitors or SSRIs) may help not only with depression but also with the obsessive-compulsive aspects of the anorexic's relationship with food.

Several different antidepressants (including monoamine oxidase inhibitors, the tricyclics amitriptyline and desipramine, and high-dose fluoxetine, an SSRI) are associated with fewer episodes of binge eating and purging in bulimic patients, in addition to treating anxiety and depression. These drugs have not been studied extensively in the treatment of binge eating disorder, however.

PREVENTION OF EATING DISORDERS

Prevention measures should include education about normal body weight for height and techniques used in advertising and the media to promote an unrealistic body image. Parents, teachers, coaches, and health care providers all play a role in prevention. Parents, coaches, and teachers need to be educated about the messages they give to growing children about bodies, body development, and weight. In addition, they need to be aware of early signs of risk. Health care providers need to include screening for eating disorders as a routine part of care. Specific indicators include dieting for weight loss associated with unrealistic weight goals, criticism of the body, social isolation, cessation of menses, and evidence of vomiting or laxative or diuretic use.

BIBLIOGRAPHY

Arenson, Gloria. *A Substance Called Food*. 2d ed. Boston: McGraw-Hill, 1989. Presents a variety of perspectives on eating, including the physiological and the transpersonal. Particularly useful in providing self-help advice and treatment modalities. Examines the compulsiveness of food addiction and sees behavior modification as a means of addressing the addictive behavior.

Battegay, Raymond. *The Hunger Diseases*. Northvale, N.J.: Jason Aronson, 1997. Addresses the emotional hunger that, the author contends, underlies all eating disorders, from anorexia to obesity.

Bruch, Hilde. *The Golden Cage: The Enigma of Anorexia Nervosa*. Reprint. Cambridge, Mass.: Harvard University Press, 2001. A classic work by a pioneer in the field of eating disorders. Portrays the development of anorexia nervosa as an attempt by a young woman to attain a sense of control and identity. Discusses the etiology and treatment of anorexia from a modified psychoanalytic perspective.

Brumberg, Joan J. *Fasting Girls: The History of Anorexia Nervosa*. Rev. ed. New York: Vintage, 2000. Outlines the history of anorexia nervosa. Examines the syndrome from multiple perspectives while leaning toward a cultural and feminist perspective. A well-researched and very readable work.

Fairburn, Christopher G. *Cognitive Behavior Therapy and Eating Disorders*. New York: Guilford Press, 2008. This treatment guide offers information on eating disorders that cover a range of severity, even those that may fall outside the usual diagnoses. Especially helpful to clinicians treating those suffering from eating disorders.

Gordon, Richard. Eating Disorders: Anatomy of a Social Epidemic. 2d rev. ed. New York: Blackwell, 2000. A survey of clinical practice in dealing with eating disorders, as well as thorough coverage of their history and social context.

Gura, Trisha. *Lying in Weight: The Hidden Epidemic of Eating Disorders in Adult Women*. New York: Harper, 2008. Science writer Gura contends that the figure for those with an eating disorder—25 to 30 million—is woefully short. Millions more, she claims, have "subthreshold" eating disorders, those that do not rise to the standard set by the American Psychiatric Association's *Diagnostic and Statistical Manual of Mental Disorders*. While these girls may be dangerously obsessed with their bodies and exercise excessively, doctors often overlook their problem.

Hirschmann, Jane R., and Carol H. Munter. *When Women Stop Hating Their Bodies: Freeing Yourself from Food and Weight Obsessions*. New York: Fawcett, 1997. A follow-up to the authors' *Overcoming Overeating* (1988), reviews the psychological basis for compulsive eating and provides alternative strategies to persons who have an addictive relationship with food. Presents convincing arguments against dieting and proposes that self-acceptance, physical activity, and health are more appropriate long-term solutions to the problem of overeating.

Martin, Courtney E. *Perfect Girls, Starving Daughters: The Frightening New Normalcy of Hating Your Body*. New York: Free Press, 2008. Using more than one hundred interviews with women and girls from ages nine to twenty-nine, the writer concludes that perfection is the goal for them all, especially in their bodies. Includes coverage of such topics as the role fathers play in influencing their daughter's self-esteem, athletes' eating disorders, and the depiction of women in hip-hop.

Sacker, Ira M., and Marc A. Zimmerman. *Dying to Be Thin: Understanding and Defeating Anorexia Nervosa and Bulimia*. Updated ed. New York: Warner Books, 2001. A practical approach, written by two medical doctors, to understanding the sources and causes of eating disorders and how to overcome them. Includes a guide to resources, treatment clinics, and support groups.

Schwartz, Hillel. *Never Satisfied: A Cultural History of Diets, Fantasies, and Fat*. New York: Anchor Books, 1990. Schwartz, a historian, looks at diets and eating from the perspective of American social and cultural history. Begins with the first weight watchers, in the early nineteenth century; examines how "shared fictions" about the body fit with various reducing methods and fads in different eras.

Rebecca Lovell Scott

SEE ALSO: Anorexia Nervosa and Bulimia Nervosa

Eczema

An inflammation of the skin.

CAUSES AND SYMPTOMS

The term eczema refers to a noncontagious inflammation of the skin. Several types of eczema exist, resulting in a range of symptoms that vary in appearance, duration, and severity. The common characteristic, however, is red, dry, and itchy skin. Other symptoms may include scaling, thickening, or cracking of the skin, leading to infections and severe discomfort.

INFORMATION ON ECZEMA

Causes: Genetic sensitivity to irritants (soaps, detergents, rough clothes), allergens (certain foods, pollen, animal dander), and climate or temperature changes

Symptoms: Red, dry, and itchy skin; scaling, thickening, or cracking of skin

Duration: Often chronic

Treatments: Minimal exposure to irritants, drugs (corticosteroid creams and ointments, antihistamines, antibiotics); in severe cases, oral corticosteroids or phototherapy

---

Atopic dermatitis, the most common form of eczema, is characterized by itchy and cracked skin of the cheeks, arms, and legs. The onset of this chronic type of eczema occurs most often during infancy or childhood, although symptoms may continue into adulthood. The cause of atopic dermatitis is thought to be a hereditary predisposition to skin sensitivities to various environmental factors. These factors include irritants such as soaps, detergents, and rough clothes; allergens such as certain foods, pollen, or animal dander; and changes in climate or temperature. Other forms of eczema, such as contact dermatitis, have similar environmental causes. Seborrheic eczema, nummular eczema, and dishydrotic eczema may result from a combination of several possible causes. Emotional factors, such as stress or frustration, may aggravate the symptoms.

The diagnosis of eczema requires a careful and detailed observation of symptoms. Family and personal medical histories are often useful to determine the presence of allergies or exposure to allergens or irritants. Dermatologists may also use skin biopsies or blood tests to determine a tendency toward elevated allergic or immune response.

TREATMENT AND THERAPY

The treatment of eczema involves minimizing exposure to possible causes while at the same time managing symptoms to maintain a high quality of life. Identifying known allergens and irritants specific to the individual is an important first step. Lifestyle changes aimed at avoiding exposure to these possible causes can lower the frequency and duration of symptoms dramatically. Proper skin care to avoid excessive drying of the skin, including the use of moisturizers or creams and minimizing exposure to water, may also help reduce skin irritation. Avoiding scratching of existing irritations and eliminating sources of emotional stress are other ways that patients can lessen the severity of their symptoms. Dermatologists may prescribe additional treatments, such as corticosteroid creams and ointments, antihistamines, or antibiotics. In more severe cases, systemic corticosteroid treatments or phototherapy, the use of ultraviolet (UV) light, may be tried.

The approval of a new type of treatment for eczema called topical immunomodulators has changed the way eczema is treated in recent years. This new class of drug counteracts the inflammation of the skin without interfering in the body's normal immune response. This treatment has been successful in preventing and even eliminating symptoms of eczema.

FURTHER READING

Fry, Lionel. *An Atlas of Atopic Eczema.* New York: Parthenon, 2004.

Hellwig, Jennifer. "Eczema." *Health Library,* Mar. 11, 2013.

MedlinePlus. "Eczema." *MedlinePlus,* May 6, 2013.

National Eczema Society. *National Eczema Society,* n. d.

Rakel, Robert E., and Edward T. Bope, eds. *Conn's Current Therapy.* Philadelphia: Saunders, 2007.

Ring, J., B. Przybilla, and T. Ruzicka, eds. *Handbook of Atopic Eczema.* 2d ed. New York: Springer, 2006.

Turkington, Carol A., and Jeffrey S. Dover. *Skin Deep: An A-Z of Skin Disorders, Treatments, and Health.* 3d ed. New York: Checkmark, 2007.

Westcott, Patsy. *Eczema: Recipes and Advice to Provide Relief.* New York: Welcome, 2000.

Paul J. Frisch

SEE ALSO: Skin Disorders

Endometriosis

Growth of cells of the uterine lining at sites outside the uterus, causing severe pain and infertility.

CAUSES AND SYMPTOMS

Endometriosis is the presence of endometrial tissue outside its normal location as the lining of the uterus . It can be asymptomatic, mild, or a disabling disease causing severe pain. The classic symptoms of endometriosis are very painful menstruation (dysmenorrhea), painful intercourse (dyspareunia), and infertility. Some other common endometriosis symptoms include nausea, vomiting, diarrhea, and fatigue.

It has been estimated that endometriosis affects between five million and twenty-five million American women. Often, it is incorrectly stereotyped as being a disease of upwardly mobile, professional women. According to many experts, the incidence of endometriosis worldwide and across most racial groups is probably very similar. They propose that the reported occurrence rate difference for some racial groups, such as a lower incidence in African Americans and a higher diagnosis rate among Caucasians, has been a socioeconomic phenomenon attributable to the social class of women who seek medical treatment for the symptoms of endometriosis and to the highly stratified responses of many health care professionals who have dealt with the disease.

The symptoms of endometriosis arise from abnormalities in the effects of the menstrual cycle on the endometrial tissue lining the uterus. The endometrium normally thickens and becomes engorged (swollen with blood) during the cycle, a process controlled by female hormones called "estrogens" and "progestins." This engorgement is designed to prepare the uterus for conception by optimizing conditions for implantation in the endometrium of a fertilized egg, which enters the uterus via one of the Fallopian tubes leading from the ovaries.

By the middle of the menstrual cycle, the endometrial lining is normally about ten times thicker than at its beginning. If the egg that is released into the uterus is not fertilized, pregnancy does not occur and decreases in production of the female sex hormones result in the breakdown of the endometrium. Endometrial tissue mixed with blood leaves the uterus as the menstrual flow, and a new menstrual cycle begins. This series of uterine changes occurs repeatedly, as a monthly cycle, from puberty (which usually occurs between the ages of twelve and fourteen) to menopause (which usually occurs between the ages of forty-five and fifty-five).

In women who develop endometriosis, some endometrial tissue begins to grow ectopically (in an abnormal position) at sites outside the uterus. The ectopic endometrial growths may be found attached to the ovaries, the Fallopian tubes, the urinary bladder, the rectum, other abdominal organs, and even the lungs. Regardless of body location, these implants behave as if they were still in the uterus, thickening and bleeding each month as the menstrual cycle proceeds. Like the endometrium at its normal uterine site, the ectopic tissue responds to the hormones that circulate through the body in the blood. Its inappropriate position in the body prevents this ectopic endometrial tissue from leaving the body as menstrual flow; as a result, some implants grow to be quite large.

In many cases, the endometrial growths that form between two organs become fibrous bands called "adhesions." The fibrous nature of adhesions is attributable to the alternating swelling and breakdown of the ectopic tissue, which yields fibrous scar tissue. The alterations in size of living portions of the adhesions and other endometrial implants during the monthly menstrual cycle cause many afflicted women considerable pain. Because the body location of implants varies, the site of the pain may be almost anywhere, including the back, chest, thighs, pelvis, rectum, or abdomen. For example, dyspareunia occurs when adhesions hold a uterus tightly to the abdominal wall, making its movement during intercourse painful. Many women report significant pain on a monthly basis with ovulation as well.

The presence of endometriosis is usually confirmed by laparoscopy, viewed as being the most reliable method for its diagnosis. Laparoscopy is carried out after a physician makes an initial diagnosis of probable endometriosis from a combined study including an examination of the patient's medical history and careful exploration of the patient's physical problems over a period of at least six months. During prelaparoscopy treatment, the patient is very often maintained on pain medication and other therapeutic drugs that will produce symptomatic relief.

For laparoscopy, the patient is anesthetized with a general anesthetic, a small incision is made near the navel, and a laparoscope (flexible lighted tube) is inserted into this incision. The laparoscope, equipped with fiber optics, enables the examining physician to search the patient's abdominal organs for endometrial implants. Visibility of the abdominal organs in laparoscopic

---

INFORMATION ON ENDOMETRIOSIS

Causes: Unknown
Symptoms: Painful menstrual periods, discomfort during sexual intercourse, localized pain, infertility
Duration: Chronic
Treatments: Chemotherapy, surgery

examination can be enhanced by pumping harmless carbon dioxide gas into the abdomen, causing it to distend. Women who undergo laparoscopy usually require a day of postoperative bed rest, followed by seven to ten days of curtailed physical activity. After a laparoscopic diagnosis of endometriosis is made, a variety of surgical and therapeutic drug treatments can be employed to manage the disease.

Between 30 and 50 percent of all women who have endometriosis are infertile; contemporary wisdom evaluates this relationship as one of cause and effect, which should make this disease the second most common cause of fertility problems. The actual basis for this infertility is not always clear, but it is often the result of damage to the ovaries and Fallopian tubes, scar tissue produced by implants on these and other abdominal organs, and hormone imbalances.

Because the incidence of infertility accompanying endometriosis increases with the severity of the disease, all potentially afflicted women are encouraged to seek early diagnosis. Many experts advise all women with abnormal menstrual cycles, dysmenorrhea, severe menstrual bleeding, abnormal vaginal bleeding, and repeated dyspareunia to seek the advice of a physician trained in identifying and dealing with endometriosis. Because the disease can begin to present symptoms at any age, teenagers are also encouraged to seek medical attention if they experience any of these symptoms.

John Sampson coined the term "endometriosis" in the 1920s. Sampson's theory for its causation, still widely accepted, is termed "retrograde menstruation." Also called "menstrual backup," this theory proposes that the backing up of some menstrual flow into the Fallopian tubes and then into the abdominal cavity, forms the endometrial implants. Evidence supporting this theory, according to many physicians, is the fact that such backup is common. Others point out, however, that the backup is often found in women who do not have the disease. A

IN THE NEWS:
LINK BETWEEN ENDOMETRIOSIS AND OTHER DISEASES

In the October, 2002, issue of Human Reproduction, the Endometriosis Association and the National Institutes of Health (NIH) announced the results of a study involving 3,680 women who were members of the Endometriosis Association and who had been diagnosed with endometriosis. The study suggested that women with endometriosis are significantly more likely than other women to contract a number of serious autoimmune diseases including lupus, Sjögren's syndrome, rheumatoid arthritis, and multiple sclerosis.

Although a study conducted in 1980 established a link between endometriosis and immune dysfunctions, the new study sought to identify specific diseases for which women with endometriosis are at higher risk. In addition to the connection between endometriosis and autoimmune diseases, researchers found that the women in the study were more than one hundred times more likely than women in the general population to suffer from chronic fatigue syndrome; twice as likely to suffer from fibromyalgia (recurrent debilitating pain in the muscles, tendons, and ligaments), and seven times as likely to suffer from hypothyroidism (which can also be an autoimmune disorder). Researchers also found that the women studied reported higher rates of allergies and asthma than women in the general population.

Researchers warn that the study may not be representative of all patients with endometriosis, both because members of the Endometriosis Association are most probably those patients suffering pain from their condition and because the survey was completed predominantly by white, educated women. Even so, this new information provides more light on an enigmatic disease and should help health care professionals treat patients.

—*Cassandra Kircher, Ph.D*

---

surgical experiment was performed on female monkeys to test this theory. Their uteri were turned upside down so that the menstrual flow would spill into the abdominal cavity. Sixty percent of the animals developed endometriosis postoperatively—an inconclusive result.

Complicating the issue is the fact that implants are also found in tissues (such as in the lung) that cannot be reached by menstrual backup. It has been theorized that the presence of these implants results from the entry of endometrial cells into the lymphatic system, which returns body fluid to the blood and protects the body from many other diseases. This transplantation theory is supported by the occurrence of endometriosis in various portions of the lymphatic system and in tissues that could not otherwise become sites of endometriosis.

A third theory explaining the growth of implants is the iatrogenic, or nosocomial, transmission of endometrial tissue. These terms both indicate an accidental creation of the disease through the actions of physicians. Such implant formation is viewed as occurring most often after cesarean delivery of a baby when passage through the birth canal would otherwise be fatal to mother and/or child. Another proposed cause is episiotomy—widening of the birth canal by an incision between the anus and vagina—to ease births.

Any surgical procedure that allows the spread of endometrial tissue can be implicated, including surgical procedures carried out to correct existing endometriosis, because of the ease with which endometrial tissue implants itself anywhere in the body. Abnormal endometrial tissue growth, called "adenomyosis," can also occur in the uterus and is viewed as a separate disease entity.

Other theories regarding the genesis of endometriosis include an immunologic theory, which proposes that women who develop endometriosis are lacking in antibodies that normally cause the destruction of endometrial tissue at sites where it does not belong, and a hormonal theory, which suggests the existence of large imbalances in hormones such as the prostaglandins that serve as the body's messengers in controlling biological processes. Several of these theories—retrograde menstruation, the transplantation theory, and iatrogenic transmission—all have support, but none has been proved unequivocally. Future evidence will identify whether one cause is dominant, whether they all interact to produce the disease, or whether endometriosis is actually a group of diseases that simply resemble one another in the eyes of contemporary medical science.

TREATMENT AND THERAPY

Laparoscopic examination most often identifies endometriosis as chocolate-colored lumps (chocolate cysts) ranging from the size of a pinhead to several inches across or as filmy coverings over parts of abdominal organs and ligaments. Once a diagnosis of the disease is confirmed by laparoscopy, endometriosis is treated by chemotherapy, surgery, or a combination of both methods. The only permanent contemporary cure for endometriosis, however, is the onset of the biological menopause at the end of a woman's childbearing years. As long as menstruation continues, implant development is likely to recur, regardless of its cause. Nevertheless, a temporary cure of endometriosis is better than no cure at all.

The chemotherapy that many physicians use to treat mild cases of endometriosis (and for prelaparoscopy periods) is analgesic painkillers, including aspirin, acetaminophen, and ibuprofen. The analgesics inhibit the body's production of prostaglandins, and the symptoms of the disease are merely covered up. Therefore, analgesics are of quite limited value except during a prelaparoscopy diagnostic period or with mild cases of endometriosis. In addition, the long-term administration of aspirin will often produce gastrointestinal bleeding, and excess use of acetaminophen can lead to severe liver damage. In some cases of very severe endometriosis pain, narcotic painkillers are given, such as codeine, Percodan (oxycodone and aspirin), or morphine. Narcotics are addicting and should be avoided unless absolutely necessary.

More effective for long-term management of the disease is hormone therapy. Such therapy is designed to prevent the monthly occurrence of menstruation—that is, to freeze the body in a sort of chemical menopause. The hormone types used, made by pharmaceutical companies, are chemical cousins of female hormones (estrogens and progestins), male hormones (androgens), and a brain hormone that controls ovulation (gonadotropin-releasing hormone, or GnRH). Appropriate hormone therapy is often useful for years, although each hormone class produces disadvantageous side effects in many patients.

The use of estrogens stops ovulation and menstruation, freeing many women with endometriosis from painful symptoms. Numerous estrogen preparations have been prescribed, including the birth control pills that contain them. Drawbacks of estrogen use can include weight gain, nausea, breast soreness, depression, blood-clotting abnormalities, and elevated risk of vaginal cancer. In addition, estrogen administration may cause endometrial implants to enlarge.

The use of progestins arose from the discovery that pregnancy—which is maintained by high levels of a natural progestin called progesterone—reversed the symptoms of many suffering from endometriosis. This realization led to the utilization of synthetic progestins to cause prolonged false pregnancy. The rationale is that all endometrial implants will die off and be reabsorbed during the prolonged absence of menstruation. The method works in most patients, and pain-free periods of up to five years are often observed. In some cases, however, side effects include nausea, depression, insomnia, and a very slow resumption of normal menstruation (such as lags of up to a year) when the therapy is stopped. In addition, progestins are ineffective in treating large implants; in fact, their use in such cases can lead to severe complications.

In the 1970s, studies showing the potential for heart attacks, high blood pressure, and strokes in patients receiving long-term female hormone therapy led to a search for more advantageous hormone medications. An alternative developed was the synthetic male hormone danazol (Danocrine), which is very effective. Danazol works by decreasing the amount of estrogen that is produced by the ovaries on a monthly basis to close to that which is present at menopause. The lack of estrogen prevents endometrial cells from growing, thereby eliminating most of the symptoms associated with endometriosis. One of its advantages over female hormones is the ability to shrink large implants and restore fertility to those patients whose problems arise from nonfunctional ovaries or Fallopian tubes. Danazol has become the drug of choice for treating millions of endometriosis sufferers. Problems associated with danazol use, however, can include weight gain, masculinization (decreased bust size, increased muscle mass, muscle cramping, facial hair growth, and deepened voice), fatigue, depression, and baldness. Those women contemplating danazol use should be aware that it can also complicate pregnancy.

Because of the side effects of these hormones, other chemotherapy was sought. Another valuable drug that has become available is GnRH, which suppresses the function of the ovaries in a fashion equivalent to surgical oophorectomy (removal of the ovaries). This hormone produces none of the side effects of the sex hormones, such as weight gain, depression, or masculinization, but some evidence indicates that it may lead to osteoporosis.

Thus, despite the fact that hormone therapy may relieve or reduce pain for years, contemporary chemotherapy is flawed by many undesirable side effects. Perhaps more serious, however, is the high recurrence rate of endometriosis that is observed after the therapy is stopped. Consequently, it appears that the best treatment of endometriosis combines chemotherapy with surgery.

The extent of the surgery carried out to combat endometriosis is variable and depends on the observations made during laparoscopy. In cases of relatively mild endometriosis, conservative laparotomy surgery removes endometriosis implants, adhesions, and lesions. This type of procedure attempts to relieve endometriosis pain, to minimize the chances of postoperative recurrence of the disease, and to allow the patient to have children.

Even in the most severe cases of this type, the uterus, an ovary, and its associated Fallopian tube are retained. Such surgery will often include removal of the appendix, whether diseased or not, because it is very likely to develop implants. The surgical techniques performed are the conventional excision of diseased tissue or the use of lasers to vaporize it. Many physicians prefer lasers because it is believed that they decrease the chances of recurrent endometriosis resulting from retained implant tissue or iatrogenic causes. In a new procedure, following the removal of endometrial tissue by surgical means, an intrauterine device containing levonogestrel (a hormone that will decrease estrogen levels) is placed in order to prevent recurrence of endometriosis.

In more serious cases, hysterectomy is carried out. All visible implants, adhesions, and lesions are removed from the abdominal organs, as in conservative surgery. In addition, the uterus and cervix are taken out, but one or both ovaries are retained. This allows female hormone production to continue normally until the menopause. Uterine removal makes it impossible to have children, however, and may lead to profound psychological problems that require psychiatric help. Women planning to elect for hysterectomy to treat endometriosis should be aware of such potential difficulties. In many cases of conservative surgery or hysterectomy, danazol is used, both preoperatively and postoperatively, to minimize implant size.

The most extensive surgery carried out on the women afflicted with endometriosis is radical hysterectomy, also called "definitive surgery," in which the ovaries and/or the vagina are also removed. The resultant symptoms are menopausal and may include vaginal bleeding atrophy (when the vagina is retained), increased risk of heart disease, and the development of osteoporosis. To counter the occurrence of these symptoms, hormone replacement therapy is suggested. Paradoxically, this hormone therapy can lead to the return of endometriosis by stimulating the growth of residual implant tissue.

Recently, more women have turned to complementary and alternative medicine in an attempt to relieve the symptoms of endometriosis. Acupuncture, homeopathy, and herbal therapy are currently being explored as means of treatment for endometriosis.

PERSPECTIVE AND PROSPECTS
Modern treatment of endometriosis is viewed by many physicians as beginning in the 1950s. A landmark development in this field was the accurate diagnosis of endo-

metriosis via the laparoscope, which was invented in Europe and introduced into the United States in the 1960s. Medical science has progressed greatly since that time. Physicians and researchers have recognized the wide occurrence of the disease and accepted its symptoms as valid; realized that hysterectomy will not necessarily put an end to the disease; utilized chemotherapeutic tools, including hormones and painkillers, as treatments and as adjuncts to surgery; developed laser surgery and other techniques that decrease the occurrence of formerly ignored iatrogenic endometriosis; and understood that the disease can ravage teenagers as well and that these young women should be examined as early as possible.

Research into endometriosis is ongoing, and the efforts and information base of the proactive American Endometriosis Association, founded in 1980, have been very valuable. As a result, a potentially or presently afflicted woman is much more aware of the problems associated with the disease. In addition, she has a source for obtaining objective information on topics including state-of-the-art treatment, physician and hospital choice, and both physical and psychological outcomes of treatment.

Many potentially viable avenues for better endometriosis diagnosis and treatment have become the objects of intense investigation. These include the use of ultrasonography and radiology techniques, such as magnetic resonance imaging (MRI), for the predictive, nonsurgical examination of the course of growth or the chemotherapeutic destruction of implants; the design of new drugs to be utilized in the battle against endometriosis; endeavors aimed at the development of diagnostic tests for the disease that will stop it before symptoms develop; and the design of dietary treatments to soften its effects.

Regrettably, because of the insidious nature of endometriosis—which has the ability to strike almost anywhere in the body—some confusion about the disease still exists. New drugs, surgical techniques, and other aids are expected to be helpful in clarifying many of these issues. Particular value is being placed on the study of the immunologic aspects of endometriosis. Scientists hope to explain why the disease strikes some women and not others, to uncover its etiologic basis, and to solve the widespread problems of iatrogenic implant formation and other types of endometriosis recurrence.

FOR FURTHER INFORMATION:

American Society for Reproductive Medicine. "Endometriosis and Infertility: Can Surgery Help?" *ReproductiveFacts.org*, 2012.

Berek, Jonathan S., ed. *Berek and Novak's Gynecology*. 14th ed. Philadelphia: Lippincott Williams & Wilkins, 2007.

Endometriosis.org. http://www.endometriosis.org. "Endometriosis." *Mayo Foundation for Medical Education and Research*, April 2, 2013.

Fernandez, I., C. Reid, and S. Dziurawiec. "Living with Endometriosis: The Perspective of Male Partners." *Journal of Psychosomatic Research* 61, no. 4 (October, 2006): 433–438.

Henderson, Lorraine, and Ros Wood. *Explaining Endometriosis*. 2d ed. St. Leonards, N.S.W.: Allen and Unwin, 2000.

National Institute of Child Health and Human Development. "Endometriosis: Condition Information." *National Institutes of Health*, April 3, 2012.

Phillips, Robert H., and Glenda Motta. *Coping with Endometriosis*. New York: Avery, 2000. Physicians" Desk Reference. 64th ed. Montvale, N.J.: PDRNetwork, 2009.

Shaw, Michael, ed. *Everything You Need to Know about Diseases*. Springhouse, Pa.: Springhouse Press, 1996.

Sherwood, Lauralee. *Human Physiology: From Cells to Systems*. 7th ed. Pacific Grove, Calif.: Brooks/Cole, 2010.

Weinstein, Kate. *Living with Endometriosis*. Reading, Mass.: Addison-Wesley, 1991.

Weschler, Toni. *Taking Charge of Your Fertility*. Rev. ed. New York: Collins, 2001.

Wood, Debra, and Andrea Chisholm. "Endometriosis." *Health Library*, September 10, 2012

Sanford S. Singer,
updated by Robin Kamienny Montvilo

SEE ALSO: Infertility, Female; Lupus; Multiple Sclerosis; Reproductive System, The

Gender identity disorder

Gender identity disorder is the diagnosis for individuals who are highly uncomfortable with the sex of their bodies and who wish to behave, think, and be members of the opposite sex. This diagnosis is the subject of considerable controversy among psychiatrists. The causes for this disorder remain speculative, and treatment typically aims to diminish associated symptoms of anxiety, depression, or other social interactional difficulties. In severe cases, psychiatrists may recommend sex changes.

INTRODUCTION

Gender identity disorder is an artifact of psychiatric politics in the 1970's and 1980's. To understand this diagnosis and contemporary debates, some awareness of the past is essential. The American Psychiatric Association (APA), one of the major professional organizations for medical practitioners and therapists dealing with mental health, was the obvious organizational choice when there was a need to create a list of mental illnesses to provide some unity of medical diagnoses across the United States. The early *Diagnostic and Statistical Manual of Mental Disorders* (1952, DSM) and the second edition, published in 1968, provided brief definitions of psychiatric ailments, although they typically lacked clear diagnostic criteria, posing dilemmas for practitioners.

During the 1950's and 1960's, American psychiatrists were strongly influenced by the Austrian psychologist Sigmund Freud, who popularized psychoanalysis. Freud's work encouraged the view that adult mental maladies often were the result of stunted or misdirected sexual desires in childhood. This emphasis on the importance of sexuality meant that psychiatrists paid a tremendous amount of attention to activities in the nation's bedrooms, although little research data supported many contentions about sexual practices.

One of the early outcomes of this history was that the first edition of the manual listed homosexuality as a sociopathic personality disturbance and the second edition moved it into the category of nonpsychotic mental ailments, including a variety of other supposedly unhealthy sexual practices. Some psychiatrists argue that this inclusion of homosexuality paved the way for the later conceptualized gender identity disorder, while others would dispute this contention. Certainly, many of the same objections to the earlier inclusion of homosexuality as a mental illness also plague later supporters of gender identity disorder. For this reason, it is important to revisit some of this early history.

During the 1950's and 1960's, research evidence provided some challenges to the view that homosexuality was a mental illness. Sexual researcher Alfred Kinsey of Indiana University demonstrated that homosexual behavior was more common in the general population than typically recognized. Evelyn Hooker, who conducted research in the psychology department at the University of California, Los Angeles, and worked with homosexual individuals from outside therapeutic groups, showed that they displayed the same range of mental health issues as members of the general nonhomosexual population. In addition, cross-cultural anthropologists wrote about other societies with very different understandings of mental illness and sexuality, casting doubt on the universality and applicability of American beliefs and norms about mental well-being and sexual behaviors. These findings suggested that homosexuality might not be a mental illness, in direct opposition to the information published by the APA. Increasingly, organization members were challenged on this issue, and several association annual conferences in the early 1970's were disrupted by protests, fueled by the growth of civil rights and gay rights activism. By this time, the Association of Gay and Lesbian Psychiatrists (AGLP), informally founded in the late 1960's, was also active within the ranks of the APA, contributing to the impetus for change. Eventually after considerable internal dispute and political maneuvering, in 1973, the Board of Trustees of the APA (followed by the full membership in 1974) agreed to remove homosexuality from the list of mental illnesses in the next edition of the DSM. This history assists in understanding contemporary disputes about gender identity disorder.

CAUSES AND DIAGNOSTIC CRITERIA

The term "gender identity disorder" was first included in the DSM-III (1980) and appeared in the fourth edition in 1994 and the fourth revised edition in 2000, with its operational definition. An individual suffering from gender identity disorder was a person who felt strongly that he or she was living in an incorrectly sexed body. For example, boys or men would feel their gender, behavior, and feelings were feminine, and their physique should be female to reflect this identity, while girls or women would feel the opposite.

Despite the fact that gender identity disorder has been considered to be a problem for both adults and children for several decades, there are limited data about causation. It has been suggested that biology may play a role, with possible proposals including intrauterine development of the fetus and hormonal influences. Other hypotheses uphold cultural influences, with parental behavior, socialization by peers, or the presence of other social norms providing a causal link. Most likely, the answer lies in some combination of these or other factors.

Although the causes of gender identity disorder remain unclear, distinct diagnostic criteria are presented in the fourth revised edition of the manual. The diagnosis

DSM-IV-TR CRITERIA FOR GENDER IDENTITY DISORDER

Strong and persistent cross-gender identification, not merely a desire for any perceived cultural advantages of being the other sex

In children, disturbance manifested by four or more of the following:
- repeatedly stated desire to be, or insistence that he or she is, the other sex
- in boys, preference for cross-dressing or simulating female attire; in girls, insistence on wearing only stereotypically masculine clothing
- strong and persistent preferences for cross-sex roles in make-believe play or persistent fantasies of being the other sex
- intense desire to participate in the stereotypical games and pastimes of the other sex
- strong preference for playmates of the other sex; in adolescents and adults, symptoms such as stated desire to be the other sex, frequent passing as the other sex, desire to live or be treated as the other sex, conviction that he or she has the typical feelings and reactions of the other sex

Persistent discomfort with his or her sex or sense of inappropriateness in the gender role of that sex

In children, disturbance manifested by any of the following:
- in boys, assertion that his penis or testes are disgusting or will disappear or assertion that it

would be better not to have a penis, or aversion toward rough-and-tumble play and rejection of male stereotypical toys, games, and activities
- in girls, rejection of urinating in a sitting position, assertion that she has or will grow a penis, or assertion that she does not want to grow breasts or menstruate, or marked aversion toward normative feminine clothing

In adolescents and adults, disturbance manifested by symptoms such as preoccupation with getting rid of primary and secondary sex characteristics (request for hormones, surgery, or other procedures to physically alter sexual characteristics to simulate the other sex) or belief that he or she was born the wrong sex

Disturbance not concurrent with a physical intersex condition

Disturbance causes clinically significant distress or impairment in social, occupational, or other important areas of functioning

DSM code based on current age:
- Gender Identity Disorder in Children (DSM code 302.6)
- Gender Identity Disorder in Adolescents or Adults (DSM code 302.85)

For sexually mature individuals, specify if Sexually Attracted to Males, Sexually Attracted to Females, Sexually Attracted to Both, or Sexually Attracted to Neither

requires the presence of a minimum of four behaviors or beliefs, all of which must be strongly expressed on a variety of occasions over some time period. The criteria include identification with a different sex, cross-dressing, occupying cross-sex roles while playing or daydreaming, stating the strongly expressed goal to perform as the other sex, and expressing the desire to play or interact with members of the different sex, or live as a member of the opposite sex. In addition, individuals are distressed by the presence of their female or male external genitalia and secondary sexual characteristics, such as breasts. Generally, they do not want to behave according to the

norms of their socially ascribed gender, and their reactions are not simply based on awareness of gender inequities in society, but on strong feelings of revulsion for the sex of their bodies. These individuals are not physically intersexed, and their sense of distress is so strong that they function poorly in their daily lives.

PROBLEMS WITH THE DIAGNOSIS AND TREATMENT OPTIONS

Several different concerns have been expressed about applying a diagnosis of gender identity disorder. One issue is that gender identity disorder is not diagnosed in the same manner internationally, and if it is assumed that all human minds operate in a similar manner, this is problematic. In addition, the history of the APA and the battles over homosexuality foreshadow many of the current debates over gender identity disorder. Certainly, the pathologization of cross-dressing, transgender, and transsexual community members is in striking opposition to greater knowledge about gender and sexual diversity around the world, the relaxing of sexual norms in the United States, and an increasingly activist and rights-conscious society. For these reasons, the diagnosis of gender identity disorder and its inclusion in the APA's manual is not accepted by all of the association's members, mental health workers, or members of the general public.

Additional questions surround the practice of applying the diagnosis of gender identity disorder to children. One issue is that some individuals may be diagnosed as gender identity disordered when in fact they are merely expressing their dissatisfaction with contemporary gender inequities, and desiring to behave and be treated in the manner accorded to the more dominant sex. This issue would most likely pertain more to girls. Another development is that girls seem to be diagnosed with gender identity disorder at lower rates than boys, and the underlying reason is unclear. It may relate to hormonal or other factors of the ailment, or it may relate to social comfort with girls cross-dressing and demonstrating "tough boy" behavior. This gender difference in the disorder has been used by some social scientists to argue that gender identity disorder is more a function of American culture rather than a real mental illness.

People who are comfortable with their experiences cross-dressing and who live in locations where others are comfortable with their identities are unlikely to seek help from psychiatrists. It is those adults who are uncomfortable with their cross-gender identities and their inability to fit social expectations who often feel depression or anxiety, and consequently may seek treatment at clinical outpatient facilities. Gender identity disorder can feel overwhelmingly difficult for people. In these cases, initially, the accompanying anxiety or depression may be treated, possibly by pharmaceutical interventions in combination with talk therapies. The type of treatment will vary depending on the patient's symptoms. A similar treatment trajectory is often experienced by children or adolescents, although in their cases, parental intervention may play a greater role in moving them into treatment.

Once some of the accompanying issues are under control, individuals may then become more comfortable with their sex and gender disjunction. If this does not occur, people may request psychiatric and medical assistance in changing their bodies and becoming transsexuals. This is a slow process, with individuals first living as the opposite sex for a period of time, often with hormonal prescriptions helping them look more like their desired sex. Ultimately, with medical approval, they may be offered sex change surgeries of various kinds, which allow them to live permanently as the opposite sex.

FURTHER READING

Bartlett, Nancy H., et al. "Is Gender Identity Disorder in Children a Mental Disorder?" *Sex Roles* 43, nos. 11/12 (December, 2000): 753-785. Consideration of gender identity disorder and its diagnosis in children.

Bayer, Ronald. *Homosexuality and American Psychiatry: The Politics of Diagnosis.* Princeton, N.J.: Princeton University Press, 1987. Discussion of the 1970's disputes among members of the American Psychiatric Association, which can be argued to underlie the creation of the diagnosis of gender identity disorder in DSM-III.

Besnier, Niko. "Polynesian Gender Liminality Through Time and Space." *In Third Sex, Third Gender: Beyond Sexual Dimorphism in Culture and History,* edited by Gilbert Herdt. New York: Zone Books, 1993. Provides cross-cultural data on gender and sexuality that suggests that the diagnosis of gender identity disorder may be a product of specific cultural, geographic, and temporal conditions, rather than a psychiatric illness identifiable in all social groups. Other chapters in the volume contribute to this theme.

Giordano, Simona. "Gender Atypical Organization in Children and Adolescents: Ethico-Legal Issues and a Proposal for New Guidelines." *International Journal of Children's Rights* 15, nos. 3/4 (July, 2007): 365-390. Consideration of gender identity disorder in youth, ethics, legal rights, and a comparison of the situation in the United Kingdom with the United States.

McHugh, Paul R., et al. *The Perspectives of Psychiatry.* 2d ed. Baltimore: Johns Hopkins University Press, 1998. History of psychiatry, with information about how disorders are conceptualized and researched.

Wilson, Mitchell. "DSM-III and the Transformation of American Psychiatry: A History." *American Journal of Psychiatry* 150, no. 3 (March, 1993): 399-410. History of the DSM and the conceptualizations underlying new editions.

Zucker, Kenneth J. "Commentary on Langer and Martin's 2004 'How Dresses Can Make You Mentally Ill: Examining Gender Identity Disorder in Children.'" *Child and Adolescent Social Work Journal* 23, nos. 5/6 (December, 2006): 533-555. Detailed discussion about gender differences in the diagnosis of gender identity disorder, including the history of the disorder.

Susan J. Wurtzburg

Hemophilia

A genetic disorder characterized by the blood's inability to form clots as a result of the lack or alteration of certain trace plasma proteins.

CAUSES AND SYMPTOMS

The circulatory system must be self-healing; otherwise, continued blood loss from even the smallest injury would be lifethreatening. Normally, all except the most catastrophic bleeding is rapidly stopped in a process known as hemostasis. Hemostasis takes place through several sequential steps or processes. First, an injury stimulates platelets (unpigmented blood cells) to adhere to the damaged blood vessels and then to one another, forming a plug that can stop minor bleeding. This association is mediated by what is called the von Willebrand factor, a protein that binds to the platelets. As the platelets aggregate, they release several substances that stimulate vasoconstriction, or a reduction in size of the blood vessels. This reduces the blood flow at the injury site. Finally, the aggregating platelets and damaged tissue initiate blood clotting, or coagulation. Once bleeding has stopped, the firmly adhering clot slowly contracts, drawing the edge of the wounds together so that tough scar tissue can form a permanent repair on the site.

Formation of a blood clot involves the participation of nearly twenty different substances, most of which are proteins synthesized by plasma. All but two of these substances, or factors, are designated by a roman numeral and a common name. A blood clot will be defective if one of the clotting factors is absent or deficient in the blood, and clotting time will be longer. The clotting factors, with some of their alternative names, are factor I (fibrinogen), factor II (prothrombin), factor III (tissue factor or thromboplastin), factor IV (calcium), factor V (proaccelerin),

factor VII (proconvertin), factor VIII (antihemophilic factor), factor IX (Christmas factor), factor X (Stuart factor), factor XI (plasma thromboplastin antecedent), factor XII (Hageman factor), and factor XIII (fibrin stabilizing factor).

Several of the clotting factors have been discovered by the diagnosis of their deficiencies in various clotting disorders. The inherited coagulation disorders are uncommon conditions with an overall incidence of probably no more than 10 to 20 per 100,000 of the population. Hemophilia A, the most common or classic type of coagulation disorder, is caused by factor VIII deficiency. Hemophilia B (or Christmas disease) is the result of factor IX deficiency. It is quite common for severe hemophilia to manifest itself during the first year of life. Hazardous bleeding occurs in areas such as the central nervous system, the retropharyngeal area, and the retroperitoneal area. Bleeding in these areas requires admission to the hospital for observation and therapy. Joint lesions are very common in hemophilia because of acute spontaneous hemorrhage in the area, especially in weight-bearing joints such as ankles and knees. Urinary bleeding is often present at some time. The appearance of pseudotumors, caused by swelling involving muscle and bone produced by recurrent bleeding, is also common.

Hemophilia is transmitted entirely by unaffected women (carriers) to their sons in a sex-linked inheritance deficiency. Congenital deficiencies of the other coagulation factors are well recognized, even though bleeding episodes in these cases are uncommon. Deficiency of more than one factor is also possible, although documentation of such cases is rare, perhaps because only patients with milder variations of the disease survive.

Von Willebrand's disease, unlike the hemophilias that mainly involve bleeding in joints and muscles, involves mainly bleeding of mucocutaneous tissues or skin. It affects both men and women. This disease shares clinical characteristics with hemophilia A, or classic hemophilia, including decreasedlevels of clotting factor VIII. This similarity made the differentiation between the two diseases very difficult for a long time. It has been established that there are two different factors involved in von Willebrand's disease, each with a different function. The von Willebrand factor is involved in the adhesion of platelets to the injured blood vessel wall and to one another and, together with factor VIII, circulates in plasma as a complex held by electrostatic and hydrophobic forces. The von Willebrand factor is a very large molecule, consisting of a series of possible multimeric structures. The bigger and heavier the multimer, the better it works against bleeding. Von Willebrand's disease is one of the least understood clotting disorders. Three types have been identified, with at least twenty-seven variations. With type I, all the multimers needed for successful clotting are present in the blood, but in lesser amounts than in healthy individuals. In type II, the larger multimers, which are more active in hemostasis, are lacking, and type III patients exhibit a severe lack of all multimers.

TREATMENT AND THERAPY

The normal body is continually producing clotting factors in order to keep up with natural loss. Sometimes the production is stepped up to cover a real or anticipated increase in the need for these factors, such as in childbirth. Hemophiliacs, lacking some of these clotting factors, may lose large amounts of blood from even the smallest injury and sometimes hemorrhage without any apparent cause. The symptoms of their diseases may be alleviated by the intravenous administration of the deficient clotting factor. How this is done depends on the specific factor deficiency and the magnitude of the bleeding episode, the age and size of the patient, convenience, acceptability, cost of product, and method and place of delivery of care.

There are many sources for clotting factors. Fresh frozen plasma contains all the clotting factors, but since the concentration of the factors in plasma is relatively low, a large volume is required for treatment. Therefore, it can be used only when small amounts of clotting factor must be delivered. Its use is the only therapy for deficiencies of factors V, XI, and XII. Plasma is commonly harvested from single donor units to minimize the risk of infection by the hepatitis virus or human immunodeficiency

virus (HIV), thus eliminating the risk involved in using pooled concentrates from many donors. Cryoprecipitates are the proteins that precipitate in fresh frozen plasma thawed at 4 degrees Celsius. The precipitate is rich in factors VIII and XIII and in fibrinogen, and carries less chance of infection with hepatitis. Its standardization is diffi-cult, however, and is not required by the Food and Drug Administration. As a result, dosage calculation can be a problem. In addition, there is no method for the control of viral contamination. Therefore, cryoprecipitates are not commonly used unless harvested from a special known and tested donor pool. Clotting factor concentrates present many advantages. They are made from pooled plasma obtained from plasmapheresis or a program of total donor unit fractionation and are widely available. Factors VIII and IX can also be produced from plasma using monoclonal methods. Porcine factor VIII presents an alternative to patients with a naturally occurring antibody to human factor VIII.

Other substances can replace missing clotting factors as well. The synthetic hormone desmopressin acetate (also known by the letters DDAVP) has been used to stimulate the release of factor VIII and vonWillebrand factor from the endothelial cells lining blood vessels. It is commonly used for patients with mild hemophilia and vonWillebrand's disease. DDAVP has no effect on the concentration of the other factors, and aside from the common side effect of water retention, it is a safe drug. Antifibrinolytic drugs prevent the natural breakdown of blood clots that have already been formed. Although such drugs are not useful for the primary care of hemophiliacs, they are useful for use after dental extractions and in the treatment of other open wounds, after a clot has formed.

Between 10 and 15 percent of the patients affected with severe hemophilia develop factor VIII inhibitors (antibodies), which prevents their treatment with the usual methods. Newer therapeutic approaches have provided additional options for the management and control of bleeding episodes. The use of prothrombin complex concentrates or porcine factor VIII concentrates is indicated for low responders (those with a low amount of antibodies present in their system). An option for high responders is to try to eradicate the inhibitor present in their systems. One way to do this is with a regimen of immunosuppressive drugs. These are very limited in value, however, and cannot be used with HIV-positive hemophiliacs. The drugs used in this approach include substances such as cyclophosphamide, vincristine, azathioprine, and corticosteroids. Another approach utilizes intravenous doses of gamma globulin to suppress, but not eradicate, the inhibitors. Yet another strategy is an immune tolerance regimen, in which factor VIII is administered daily in small amounts. This method causes the inhibitors to decrease and, in some cases, disappear. The regimen can also involve the prophylactic use of factor VIII (or factor VIII in combination with immunosuppressive drugs).

The introduction of plasma clotting factor concentrates has changed the treatment of patients with clotting factor deficiencies. It has brought about a remarkable change in the longevity of these patients and their quality of life. The availability of cryoprecipitates and concentrates of factors II, VII, VIII, IX, X, and XIII has made outpatient treatment for bleeding episodes routine and home infusion or self-infusion a possibility for many patients. Hospitalization for inpatient treatment is rare, and early outpatient therapy of bleeding episodes has decreased the severity of joint deformities.

Nevertheless, other problems are apparent in hemophiliac patients. Viral contamination of the factor concentrates has allowed the development of chronic illnesses, infection with HIV, immunologic diseases, liver and renal diseases, joint disorders, and cardiovascular diseases. While the use of heat for virus inactivation, beginning in 1983, resulted in a reduction in HIV infections, the majority of patients exposed to the virus had already been infected. The strategies to prevent contraction of hepatitis from these concentrates include vaccination against the contaminating viruses and the elimination of viruses from the factor replacement product. The non-A, non-B hepatitis virus is difficult to remove, however, and the use of monoclonal factors seems to be the only solution to this problem. In general, difficulties associated with treatment have been largely eliminated through the production of the required clotting factors using recombinant DNA techniques, a process performed independent of human blood.

Treatment of von Willebrand's disease also includes pressure dressing, suturing, and oral contraceptives. A pasteurized antihemophiliac concentrate that contains substantial amounts of von Willebrand factor is used in severe cases.

Hematomas, or hemorrhages under the skin and within muscles, can frequently be controlled by application of elastic bandage pressure and ice. The ones that cannot be controlled easily within a few hours may cause muscle contraction and require factor replacement

therapy. Exercise is recommended for joints after bleeding, as it helps protect joints by increasing muscle bulk and power and can also help relieve stress. Devices to protect joints, such as elastic bandages and splints, are commonly used. In extreme cases, orthopedic surgical procedures are readily available.

Analgesics, or painkillers, play an important part in the alleviation of chronic pain. Because patients cannot use products with aspirin and/or antihistamines, which inhibit platelet aggregation and prolong bleeding time, substances such as acetaminophen, codeine, and morphine are used. Chronic joint inflammation is reduced by the use of anti-inflammatory agents such as ibuprofen and drugs used with rheumatoid arthritis patients.

The need for so many specialties and disciplines in the management of hemophilia has led to the development of multidisciplinary hemophilia centers. Genetic education (information on how the disease is transmitted), genetic counseling (the discussion of an individual's genetic risks and reproductive options), and genetic testing have provided great help to patients and affected families. Early and prenatal diagnosis and carrier detection have provided options for family planning.

PERSPECTIVE AND PROSPECTS

Descriptions of hemophilia are among the oldest known accounts of genetic disease. References to a bleeding condition highly suggestive of hemophilia go back to the fifth century, in the Babylonian Talmud. The first significant report in medical literature appeared in 1803 when John C. Otto, a Philadelphia physician, described several bleeder families with only males affected and with transmission through the mothers. The literature of the nineteenth century contains many descriptions of the disease, particularly the clinical characteristics of the hemorrhages and family histories. The disease was originally called haemorrhaphilia, or "tendency toward hemorrhages," but the name was later contracted through usage to hemophilia ("tendency toward blood"), the accepted name since around 1828.

Transfusion therapy was proposed as early as 1832, and the first successful transfusion for the treatment of a hemophiliac patient was reported in 1840 by Samuel Armstrong Lane. The use of blood from cows and pigs in the transfusions was explored but abandoned because of the numerous side effects. It was not until the beginning of the twentieth century that serious studies on clotting in hemophilia were started. Attention was directed to the use of normal human serum for treatment of bleeding episodes. Some of the patients responded well, while others did not. This result is probably attributable to the fact that some had hemophilia A—these patients did not respond because factor VIII, in which they are deficient, is not present in serum—while some others had hemophilia B, for which the therapy worked. In 1923, harvested blood plasma was used in transfusion, and it was shown to work as well as whole blood. With blood banking becoming a reality in the 1930s, transfusions were performed more frequently as a treatment for hemophilia.

The history of the fractionation of plasma began around 1911 with a Dr. Addis, who prepared a very crude fraction by acidification of plasma. In 1937, Drs. Patek and Taylor produced a crude fraction which, on injection, lowered the blood-clotting time in hemophiliacs. In the period from 1945 to 1960, a number of plasma fractions with antihemophiliac activity were developed. The use of fresh frozen plasma increased as a result of advances in the purification of the fractions. Some milestones can be identified in the production of the plasma fractions: the development of quantitative assays for antihemophiliac factors, the discovery of cryoprecipitation, and the development of glycine and polyethylene precipitation.

In 1952, four significant and independent publications indicated that there is a plasma-clotting activity separate from that concerned with classic hemophilia—in other words, that there are two types of hemophilia. One (hemophilia A) is characterized by a deficiency in factor VIII, while the other (hemophilia B) is characterized by deficiency in factor IX. Carriers of hemophilia A can have a mean factor VIII level that is 50 percent lower than that of normal females, while carriers of hemophilia B show levels of factor IX that are 60 percent below normal. The two diseases have the same pattern of inheritance, are similar in clinical appearance, and can be distinguished only by laboratory tests.

Hemophilias are caused by a disordered and complex biological mechanism that continues to be explored. Recombinant DNA techniques have now revealed the molecular defect in factor VIII or factor IX deficiencies in some families, demonstrating that a variety of gene defects can produce the classic phenotype of hemophilia. These techniques have also provided new tools for carrier detection and prenatal diagnosis.

Current treatment of hemophilia has converted the hemophiliac from an in-hospital patient to an individual with more independent status. Crucial in this development has been the creation of comprehensive care centers and of the National Hemophilia Foundation, which provide comprehensive treatment for the hemophilia patient. Home treatment with replacement therapy has become common. With the advancement of recombinant DNA technology, the future looks brighter for the sufferers of this disease.

FOR FURTHER INFORMATION:

Bloom, Arthur L., ed. *The Hemophilias*. New York: Churchill Livingstone, 1982.

Hilgartner, Margaret W., and Carl Pochedly, eds. *Hemophilia in the Child and Adult*. 3d ed. New York: Raven Press, 1989.

Hoffman, Ronald, et al. *Hematology: Basic Principles and Practice*. Philadelphia: Saunders/Elsevier, 2013.

Jones, Peter. *Living with Haemophilia*. 5th ed. New York: Oxford University Press, 2002.

Judd, Sandra J., ed. *Genetic Disorders Sourcebook: Basic Consumer Information About Hereditary Diseases and Disorders*. 4th ed. Detroit, Mich.: Omnigraphics, 2010.

King, Richard A., Jerome I. Rotter, and Arno G. Motulsky, eds. *The Genetic Basis of Common Diseases*. 2d ed. New York: Oxford University Press, 2002.

Leenhardt, Christine, Erik E. Berntorp, and Keith W. Hoots. *Textbook of Hemophilia*. 2d ed. Hoboken, N.J.: Wiley-Blackwell, 2010.

Ma, Alice D., Harold Ross Roberts, and Miguel A. Escobar. *Hemophilia and Hemostasis: A Case-Based Approach to Management*. Hoboken, N.J.: John Wiley & Sons, 2013.

Makris, M., and C. Kasper. "The World Federation of Hemophilia Guideline on Management of Haemophilia." *Haemophilia* 19, no. 1 (December, 2012): 1ff.

National Hemophilia Foundation. http://www.hemo philia.org.

Parker, James N., and Philip M. Parker, eds. *The Official Patient's Sourcebook on Hemophilia: A Revised and Updated Directory for the Internet Age*. San Diego, Calif.: Icon Health, 2005.

Rodak, Bernadette, ed. *Hematology: Clinical Principles and Applications*. 4th ed. St. Louis, Mo.: Saunders/ Elsevier, 2012.

Voet, Donald, and Judith G. Voet. *Biochemistry*. 4th ed. Hoboken, N.J.: John Wiley & Sons, 2011.

Maria Pacheco

SEE ALSO: Circulation

Infertility, female

The inability to achieve a desired pregnancy as a result of dysfunction of female reproductive organs.

CAUSES AND SYMPTOMS

Infertility is defined as the failure of a woman to conceive despite regular sexual activity over the course of at least one year. Studies have estimated that in the United States, 10 to 15 percent of couples are infertile. In about half of these couples, it is the woman who is affected.

Female infertility may be caused by hormonal problems, or it may originate in the reproductive organs: the ovaries, oviducts, uterus, cervix, and vagina. The frequency of specific problems among infertile women is as follows: ovarian problems, 20 percent to 30 percent; damage to the Fallopian tubes, 30 percent to 50 percent; uterine problems, 5 percent to 10 percent; and cervical or vaginal abnormalities, 5 percent to 10 percent. Another 10 percent of women have unexplained infertility. Behavioral factors, such as diet and exercise and the use of tobacco, alcohol, or drugs, also play a role in infertility.

The ovaries have two important roles in conception: the production of ova (egg cells), culminating in ovulation, and the production of hormones. Ovulation usually occurs halfway through a woman's four-week menstrual cycle. In the two weeks preceding ovulation, follicle-stimulating hormone (FSH) from the pituitary gland causes follicles in the ovaries to grow and the ova within them to mature. As the follicles grow, they produce increasing amounts of estrogen. Near the middle of the cycle, the estrogen causes the pituitary gland to release a surge of luteinizing hormone (LH), which causes ovulation of the largest follicle in the ovary.

Anovulation (lack of ovulation) can result either directly, from an inability to produce LH, FSH, or estrogen, or indirectly, because of the presence of other hormones that interfere with the signaling systems between the pituitary and ovaries. For example, the woman may have an excess production of androgen (testosterone-like) hormones, either in her ovaries or in her adrenal glands, or her pituitary may produce too much prolactin, a hormone that is normally secreted in large amounts only after the birth of a child.

Besides ovulation, the ovaries have another critical role in conception, since they produce hormones that act on the uterus to allow it to support an embryo. In the first two weeks of the menstrual cycle, the uterine lining is prepared for a possible pregnancy by estrogen from the ovaries. Following ovulation, the uterus is maintained in a state that can support an embryo by progesterone, which is produced in the ovary by the follicle that just ovulated, now called a corpus luteum. Because of the effects of hormones from the corpus luteum on the uterus, the corpus luteum is essential to the survival of the embryo. If conception does not occur, the corpus luteum disintegrates and stops producing progesterone. As progesterone levels decline, the uterine lining can no longer be maintained and is shed as the menstrual flow.

Failure of the pregnancy can result from improper function of the corpus luteum, such as an inability to produce enough progesterone to sustain the uterine lining. The corpus luteum may also produce progesterone initially but then disintegrate too early. These problems in corpus luteum function, referred to as luteal phase insufficiency, may be caused by the same types of hormonal abnormalities that cause lack of ovulation. Some cases of infertility may be associated with an abnormally shaped uterus or vagina. Such malformations of the reproductive organs are common in women whose mothers took diethylstilbestrol (DES) during pregnancy. DES was prescribed to many pregnant women from 1941 to about 1970 as a protection against miscarriage; infertility and other problems have occurred in the offspring of these women.

Conception depends on normal function of the oviducts (or Fallopian tubes), thin tubes with an inner diameter of only a few millimeters; they are attached to the top of the uterus and curve upward toward the ovaries. The inner end of each tube, located near one of the ovaries, waves back and forth at the time of ovulation, drawing the mature ovum into the opening of the oviduct. Once in the oviduct, the ovum is propelled along by movements of the oviduct wall. Meanwhile, if intercourse has occurred recently, the man's sperm will be moving upward in the female system, swimming through the uterus and the oviducts. Fertilization, the union of the sperm and ovum, will occur in the oviduct, and then the fertilized ovum will pass down the oviduct and reach the uterus about three days after ovulation.

Infertility can result from scar tissue formation inside the oviduct, resulting in physical blockage and inability to transport the ovum, sperm, or both. The most common cause of scar tissue formation in the reproductive organs is pelvic inflammatory disease (PID), a condition characterized by inflammation that spreads throughout the female reproductive tract. PID may be initiated by a sexually transmitted disease such as gonorrhea or chlamydia. Physicians in the United States have documented an increase in infertility attributable to tubal damage caused by sexually transmitted infections.

Damage to the outside of the oviduct can also cause infertility, because such damage can interfere with the mobility of the oviduct, which is necessary to the capture of the ovum at the time of ovulation. External damage to the oviduct may occur as an aftermath of abdominal surgery, when adhesions induced by surgical cutting are likely to form. An adhesion is an abnormal scar tissue connection between adjacent structures.

Another possible cause of damage to the oviduct that can result in infertility is the presence of endometriosis. Endometriosis refers to a condition in which patches of the uterine lining implant outside the uterus, in or on the surface of other organs. These patches are thought to arise during menstruation, when the uterine lining (endometrium) is normally shed from the body through the cervix and vagina; in a woman with endometriosis, for unknown reasons, the endometrium is carried to the interior of the pelvic cavity by passing up the oviducts. The endometrial patches can lodge in the oviduct itself, causing blockage, or can adhere to the outer surface of the oviducts, interfering with mobility.

Endometriosis can cause infertility by interfering with organs other than the oviducts. Endometrial patches on the outside of the uterus can cause distortions in the shape or placement of the uterus, interfering with embryonic implantation. Ovulation may be prevented by the presence of the endometrial tissues on the surface of the ovary. The presence of endometriosis, however, is not always associated with infertility: Thirty percent to forty percent of women with endometriosis cannot conceive, but the remainder appear to be fertile.

Another critical site in conception is the cervix. The cervix, the entryway to the uterus from the vagina, represents the first barrier through which sperm must pass on their way to the ovum. The cervix consists of a ring of strong, elastic tissue with a narrow canal. Glands in the cervix produce the mucus that fills the cervical canal and through which sperm swim en route to the ovum. The amount and quality of the cervical mucus change throughout the menstrual cycle, under the influence of hormones from the ovary. At ovulation, the mucus is in a state that is most easily penetrated by sperm; after ovulation, the mucus becomes almost impenetrable.

Cervical problems that can lead to infertility include production of a mucus that does not allow sperm passage at the time of ovulation (hostile mucus syndrome) and interference with sperm transport caused by narrowing of the cervical canal. Such narrowing may be the result of a developmental abnormality or the presence of an infection, possibly a sexually transmitted disease.

TREATMENT AND THERAPY

The diagnosis of the exact cause of a woman's infertility is crucial to successful treatment. A complete medical history should reveal any obvious problems of previous infection or menstrual cycle irregularity. Adequacy of ovulation and luteal phase function can be determined from records of menstrual cycle length and changes in body temperature (body temperature is higher after ovulation). Hormone levels can be measured with tests of blood or urine samples. If damage to the oviducts or uterus is suspected, a hysterosalpingography will be performed. In this procedure, the injection of a special fluid into the uterus is followed by x-ray analysis of the fluid movement to reveal the shape of the uterine cavity and the oviducts. Cervical functioning can be assessed with the postcoital test, in which the physician attempts to recover sperm from the woman's uterus some hours after she has had intercourse with her partner. If a uterine problem is suspected, the woman may have an endometrial biopsy, in which a small sample of the uterine lining is removed and examined for abnormalities. Sometimes, exploratory surgery is performed to pinpoint the location of scar tissue or the location of endometrial patches.

Surgery may be used for treatment as well as diagnosis. Damage to the oviducts can sometimes be repaired surgically, and surgical removal of endometrial patches is a standard treatment for endometriosis. Often, however, surgery is a last resort because of the likelihood of the development of postsurgical adhesions, which can further complicate the infertility. Newer forms of surgery using lasers and freezing offer better success because of a reduced risk of adhesions.

Some women with hormonal difficulties can be treated successfully with so-called fertility drugs, which are intended to stimulate ovulation. There are several different drugs and hormones that fall under this heading: Clomiphene citrate (Clomid), human menopausal gonadotropin (hMG), gonadotropin-releasing hormone (GnRH), and bromocriptine mesylate (Parlodel) are among the medications commonly used, with the exact choice depending on the woman's particular problem. One problem with some of the drugs is the risk of multiple pregnancy (more than one fetus in the uterus). Other possible problems include nausea, dizziness, headache, and general malaise.

Aside from fertility drugs, there are a variety of methods in use to try to achieve pregnancy with external assistance, known collectively as assisted reproductive technology (ART). One example of this, artificial insemination, also known as intrauterine insemination (IUI), is an old technique that is still useful in various types of infertility. A previously collected sperm sample is placed in the woman's vagina or uterus using a special tube. Artificial insemination is always performed at the time of ovulation, in order to maximize the chance of conception. The ovulation date can be determined with body temperature records or by hormone measurements. In some cases, this procedure is combined with fertility drug treatment. Since the sperm can be placed directly in the uterus, it is useful in treating hostile mucus syndrome and certain types of male infertility. The sperm sample can be provided either by the woman's partner or by a donor. The pregnancy rate after artificial insemination is highly variable (anywhere from 10 to 70 percent), depending on the particular infertility problem in the couple.

Another assisted reproductive technology is gamete intrafallopian transfer (GIFT), the surgical placement of ova and sperm directly into the woman's oviducts. To be a candidate for this procedure, the woman must have at least one partially undamaged oviduct and a functional uterus. Ova are collected surgically from the ovaries after stimulation with a fertility drug, and a semen sample is collected from the male. The ova and the sperm are introduced into the oviducts through the same abdominal incision used to collect the ova. This procedure is useful in certain types of male infertility, if the woman produces an impenetrable cervical mucus, or if the ovarian ends of the oviducts are damaged. The range of infertility problems that may be resolved with GIFT can be extended by using donated ova or sperm. The pregnancy rate is about 33 percent overall, but the rate varies with the type of infertility present.

The most common assisted reproductive technology is in vitro fertilization (IVF), or the fertilization of the sperm and egg outside the woman's body, followed by implantation of the fertilized egg in the woman's uterus. In this procedure, ova are collected surgically after stimulation with fertility drugs and then placed in a laboratory dish and combined with sperm from the man. The actual fertilization, when a sperm penetrates the ovum, will occur in the dish. The resulting embryo is allowed to remain in the dish for two days, during which time it will have grown to two to four cells. Then, the embryo is placed in the woman's uterine cavity using a flexible tube. In vitro fertilization can be used in women who are infertile because of endometriosis, damaged oviducts, impenetrable cervical mucus, or ovarian failure. As with GIFT, in vitro fertilization may utilize donated ova or donated sperm, or extra embryos that have been produced by one couple may be implanted in a second woman. Embryos created through IVF can either be used immediately or frozen for later implantation. Success rates for in vitro fertilization have improved greatly over time, and in the United States in 2010, the proportion of IVF procedures that resulted in live births was about 56 percent for fresh embryos and 35 percent for frozen embryos, according to the Centers for Disease Control and Prevention.

Some women may benefit from nonsurgical embryo transfer. In this procedure, a fertile woman is artificially inseminated at the time of her ovulation; five days later, her uterus is flushed with a sterile solution, washing out the resulting embryo before it implants in the uterus. The retrieved embryo is then transferred to the uterus of another woman, who will carry it to term. Typically, the sperm provider and the woman who receives the embryo are the infertile couple who wish to rear the child, but the technique can be used in other circumstances as well. Embryo transfer can be used if the woman has damaged oviducts or is unable to ovulate, or if she has a genetic disease that could be passed to her offspring, because in this case the baby is not genetically related to the woman who carries it.

Some infertile women who are unable to achieve a pregnancy themselves turn to the use of a surrogate, a woman who will agree to bear a child and then turn it over to the infertile woman to rear as her own. In the typical situation, the surrogate is artificially inseminated with the sperm of the infertile woman's husband. The surrogate then proceeds with pregnancy and delivery as normal, but relinquishes the child to the infertile couple after its birth.

PERSPECTIVE AND PROSPECTS

One of the biggest problems that infertile couples face is the emotional upheaval that comes with the diagnosis of infertility, as bearing and rearing children is an experience that most people treasure. In addition to the emotional difficulty that may come with the recognition of infertility, more stress may be in store as the couple proceeds through treatment. The various treatments can cause embarrassment and sometimes physical pain, and fertility drugs themselves are known to cause emotional swings. For these reasons, a couple with an infertility problem is often advised to seek help from a private counselor or a support group.

Along with the emotional and physical challenges of infertility treatment, there is a considerable financial burden. Infertility treatments, in general, are expensive, especially for more sophisticated procedures such as in vitro fertilization and GIFT. Since the chances of a single procedure resulting in a pregnancy are often low, the couple may be faced with submitting to multiple procedures repeated many times. The cost over several years of treatment—a realistic possibility—can be very high. Many health insurance companies in the United States refuse to cover the costs of such treatment and are required to do so in only a few states.

Some of the treatments are accompanied by unresolved legal questions. In the case of nonsurgical embryo transfer, is the legal mother of the child the ovum donor or the woman who gives birth to the child? The same question of legal parentage arises in cases of surrogacy. Does a child born using donated ovum or sperm have a legal right to any information about the donor, such as medical history? How extensive should governmental regulation of infertility clinics be? For example, should there be standards for ensuring that donated sperm or ova are free from genetic defects? In the United States, some states have begun to address these issues, but no uniform policies have been set at the federal level.

The legal questions are largely unresolved because American society is still involved in religious and philosophical debates over the propriety of various infertility treatments. Some religions hold that any interference in conception is unacceptable. To these denominations, even artificial insemination is wrong. Other groups approve of treatments confined to a husband and wife, but disapprove of a third party being involved as a donor or surrogate. Many people disapprove of any infertility treatment to help an individual who is not married. Almost all these issues stem from the fact that these reproductive technologies challenge the traditional definitions of parenthood.

FURTHER READING

American Society for Reproductive Medicine. http://www.asrm.org/.

"Assisted Reproductive Technology (ART) Report." *Centers for Disease Control and Prevention*, January 6, 2012.

"Female Infertility." *Mayo Clinic*, September 9, 2011.

Harkness, Carla. *The Infertility Book: A Comprehensive Medical and Emotional Guide*. Rev. ed. Berkeley, Calif.: Celestial Arts, 1996.

InterNational Council on Infertility Information Dissemination. http://www.inciid.org.

Phillips, Robert H., and Glenda Motta. *Coping with Endometriosis*. New York: Avery, 2000.

Quilligan, Edward J., and Frederick P. Zuspan, eds. *Current Therapy in Obstetrics and Gynecology*. 5th ed. Philadelphia: W. B. Saunders, 2000.

Riley, Julie. "Infertility in Women." *Health Library*, October 31, 2012.

Speroff, Leon, and Marc A. Fritz. *Clinical Gynecologic Endocrinology and Infertility*. 8th ed. Philadelphia: Lippincott Williams & Wilkins, 2011.

Turkington, Carol, and Michael M. Alper. *Encyclopedia of Fertility and Infertility*. New York: Facts On File, 2001.

Weschler, Toni. *Taking Charge of Your Fertility*. Rev. ed. New York: Collins, 2006.

Wisot, Arthur L., and David R. Meldrum. *Conceptions and Misconceptions: The Informed Consumer's Guide Through the Maze of In Vitro Fertilization and Other Assisted Reproduction Techniques*. 2d ed. Point Roberts, Wash.: Hartley & Marks, 2004.

Zouves, Christo. *Expecting Miracles: On the Path of Hope from Infertility to Parenthood*. New York: Berkley, 2003.

Marcia Watson-Whitmyre

Infertility, male

The inability to achieve a desired pregnancy as a result of dysfunction of male reproductive organs.

CAUSES AND SYMPTOMS

To create a baby requires three things: healthy sperm from a man, a healthy egg from a woman, and a healthy, mature uterus. Anything that blocks the availability of the sperm, egg, or uterus can cause infertility. Infertility can be thought of as an abnormal, unwanted form of contraception.

Many different factors may be responsible for infertility. In general, these factors may be infectious, chemical (from inside or outside the body, such as pharmaceuticals, toxins, or illegal drugs), or anatomical. Genetic factors may be responsible as well, since genes control the formation of body chemicals (such as hormones and antibodies) and body structures (one's anatomy). The way that these factors work is illustrated by male infertility.

Sperm are made in a man's testes (or testicles). Because the creation of sperm is controlled by genes and hormones, abnormalities in these can cause infertility. Sperm are initially formed in the seminiferous tubules, extremely narrow, tightly coiled tubes in the main body of the testes; from there, sperm are released into another set of tubes to the rear of the testes called the epididymis, where they become mature. Sperm are stored in the epididymis until being released into the vas deferens and then the urethra before leaving the body during intercourse. A blockage of any part of this reproductive tract, or premature release of sperm from the epididymis, can cause infertility.

A blockage of reproductive ducts can occur as a result of a bodily enlargement, such as swollen tissue, a tumor, or cancer. An infection usually causes tissue swelling and can leave ducts permanently scarred, narrowed, or blocked. Infection can have a direct detrimental effect on the production of normal sperm. Cancer and the drugs or chemicals used to treat cancer can also damage a man's reproductive tract.

Another factor that may be important to male fertility is scrotal temperature. The temperature in the scrotum, the sac that holds the testes, is somewhat lower than body temperature. The normal production of sperm seems to be dependent upon a cool testicular environment.

One cause of male infertility is varicoceles—basically varicose veins of the testes—which occur when one-way

INFORMATION ON MALE INFERTILITY

Causes: Low sperm count, infection, blockage of sperm ducts (from swollen tissue or tumor), premature release of sperm from epididymis, improper scrotal temperature, varicoceles
Symptoms: Typically asymptomatic
Duration: Short-term to chronic
Treatments: Surgery, hormonal therapy, fertility procedures (e.g., artificial insemination)

valves fail in the veins that take blood away from the testicles. When these venous valves become leaky, blood flow becomes sluggish and causes the veins to swell. Many men with varicoceles are infertile, but the exact reason for this association is unknown. The reasons sometimes given are increased scrotal temperature and improper removal of materials (hormones) from the testis.

Mature sperm capable of fertilizing an egg are normally placed in the female reproductive tract by the ejaculation phase of sexual intercourse. The sperm are accompanied by fluid called seminal plasma; together, they form semen. A blockage of the ducts that transport the semen into the woman or toxic chemicals, including antibodies, in the semen can cause infertility.

For conception to take place—that is, for an egg to be fertilized after sperm enters the female tract—a healthy egg must be present in the portion of the female reproductive tract called the Fallopian tube, and sperm must move through the female tract to that egg. If the egg is absent or is abnormal, or if healthy sperm cannot reach the egg, failure to conceive will result. The female factors that determine whether sperm fertilize an egg are the same as the male factors: anatomy, chemicals, infection, and genes.

For those who seek help with fertility issues, there are many methods available. Female infertility may be treated, depending upon the cause, by surgery, hormone therapy, or in vitro fertilization. Treatment of male infertility may be by surgery, hormone therapy, or artificial insemination. Artificial insemination is often performed when the couple is composed of a fertile woman and an infertile man.

The first step for artificial insemination is for a physician to determine when the woman ovulates or releases an egg into the Fallopian tube. At the time of ovulation, semen is placed with medical instruments in the woman's reproductive tract, either on her cervix or in her uterus.

The semen used by the physician is obtained through masturbation by either the infertile man (the patient) or a fertile man (a donor), depending on the cause of the man's infertility. The freshly produced semen from either source usually undergoes laboratory testing and processing. Tests are used to evaluate the sperm quality. An effort may be made to enhance the sperm from an infertile patient and then to use these sperm for artificial insemination or in vitro fertilization. Other tests evaluate semen for transmissible diseases. During testing, which may require many days, the sperm can be kept alive by cryopreservation, or freezing. Freshly ejaculated sperm remains fertile for only a few hours in the laboratory if it is not cryopreserved.

There are several processes that might enhance sperm from an infertile man. If the semen is infertile because it possesses too few normal sperm, an effort can be made to eliminate the abnormal sperm and to increase the concentration of normal sperm. Sperm may be abnormal in four basic ways: They may have abnormal structure, they may have abnormal movement, they may be incapable of fusing with an egg, or they may contain abnormal genes or chromosomes. Laboratory processes can often eliminate from semen those sperm with abnormal structure or abnormal movement. These processes usually involve replacing the seminal plasma with a culture medium. Removing the seminal plasma gets rid of substances that may be harmful to the sperm. After the plasma is removed, the normal sperm can be collected and concentrated. Pharmacologic agents can be added to the culture medium to increase sperm movement.

Testing for transmissible diseases is especially important if donor semen is used; these diseases may be genetic or infectious. There are many thousand genetic disorders. Most of these disorders are very rare and can be transmitted to offspring only if the sperm and the egg both have the same gene for the disorder. It is impossible, therefore, to test a donor for every possible genetic disorder; he is routinely tested only for a small group of troublesome disorders that are especially likely to occur in offspring. Tests for other disorders that the donor might transmit can be performed at the woman's request, usually based upon knowledge of genetic problems in her own family.

Much of the genetic information about a person is based on family history. Special laboratory procedures allow the genetic code inside individual cells to be interpreted. For this reason, it is important to store a sample of donor cells, not necessarily sperm, for many years after the procedure. These cells provide additional genetic information that might be important to the donor's offspring but not known at the time of insemination.

Semen can also be the source of some infectious diseases. Syphilis, gonorrhea, chlamydia, and acquired immunodeficiency syndrome (AIDS) are examples of sexually transmitted infections (STIs) that can be transmitted by donor semen. Screening history and testing are done on donors, but they cannot ensure that there will be no chance of infection. For example, the human immunodeficiency virus (HIV) may be newly present from recently acquired infection, but screening tests depend on the presence of antibodies, which do not show up immediately after someone is infected.

Cryopreservation of sperm is important to artificial insemination for two major reasons. First, it gives time to complete all necessary testing. Second, it allows an inventory of sperm from many different donors to be kept constantly available for selection and use by patients. Sperm have been cryopreserved for over twenty years and then thawed and used successfully.

Cryopreservation involves treating freshly ejaculated sperm with a cryoprotectant pharmaceutical that enables the sperm to survive when frozen; the cryoprotectant for sperm is usually glycerol. Survival of frozen sperm is also dependent upon the rate of cooling, the storage temperature, and the rate of warming at the time of thawing. Sperm treated with a cryoprotectant have the best chance of survival if they are cooled at a rate of about 1 degree Celsius per minute and stored at a temperature of −150 degrees Celsius (about −240 degrees Fahrenheit) or colder. An environment of liquid nitrogen is often used to attain these storage temperatures. The storage temperature must be kept constant to avoid the damaging effects of recrystallization.

Human sperm can be shipped to almost any location for artificial insemination. Sperm is usually cryopreserved before shipment and thawed at the time of insemination.

TREATMENT AND THERAPY

The use of artificial insemination to treat two kinds of male infertility will be considered here. The first example is male infertility that cannot be treated by other means. The second example is a fertile man at high risk for becoming infertile because of his lifestyle or because he is receiving treatment for a life-threatening disease.

The first example might occur when a heterosexual couple, having used no contraception for a year or longer, has been unsuccessful in conceiving a baby. In 40 percent of infertility cases, the woman has the major, but not necessarily the only, problem preventing the pregnancy. In 40 percent of the cases, the man is the major factor. In 20 percent, each person makes a contribution to the problem, or the problem is unidentified. Therefore, both partners must deal with the infertility and be involved in the treatment.

The solution to a couple's infertility involves evaluation and therapy. The couple will be evaluated in regard to their present sexual activity and history, such as whether either one has ever contributed to a pregnancy. The medical evaluation of both partners will include a physical examination, laboratory tests, and even imaging techniques such as x-rays, ultrasonography, or magnetic resonance imaging (MRI). For the man, the physical examination will include a search for the presence of varicoceles, and the laboratory tests will include a semen analysis.

Varicoceles are probably the most readily detected problem that may cause male infertility. They are three times more common in infertile men than in men with proven fertility. This association does not prove that varicoceles cause infertility, however, because surgery that corrects a varicocele does not always correct infertility.

If the medical evaluation determines that the female partner has a normal reproductive tract and is ovulating on a regular basis, and if it determines that the male partner has too few normal sperm to make a pregnancy likely, the couple may be asked to consider adopting a baby or undergoing artificial insemination. With artificial insemination using a sperm donor, if the woman becomes pregnant, half of the baby's genes come from the mother, and the other half of the genes come from the donor, usually a person unknown to the couple. The physician performing artificial insemination may provide the couple with extensive information on several possible donors. Such information might include race, ethnic origin, blood type, physical characteristics, results of medical and genetic tests, and personal information, but the donor usually remains anonymous. The semen from each donor has undergone laboratory testing and cryopreservation. The frozen semen is then thawed at the time of insemination.

Although the idea of artificial insemination is simple, it usually involves some very complicated emotions. Although a couple may be very happy about all other aspects of their lives together, they may be disturbed to learn of the man's infertility. If the couple chooses artificial insemination using a sperm donor, later, they must decide whether to tell the child about the circumstances of his or her birth. Sometimes, a child who originated through artificial insemination may try to learn the identity of the donor.

Although male-factor infertility is the situation that benefits most from insemination and semen cryopreservation procedures, these procedures might be requested by a fertile couple that is at risk for male-factor infertility. Such couples may fear that the man's lifestyle, such as working with hazardous materials (solvents, toxins, radioisotopes, or explosives), may endanger his ability to produce sperm or may harm his genetic information. The man could be facing medical therapy that will cure a malignancy, such as Hodgkin's disease or a testicular tumor, but may render him sterile. A man facing such a situation may benefit from having some of his semen cryopreserved for his own future use, in the event that he does become infertile.

There are ways to compensate for decreased semen quality. The semen may be processed in ways to increase the concentration of normal sperm. The processed semen may be placed directly into the woman's uterus (intrauterine insemination) rather than on her cervix, or in vitro fertilization (IVF) may be used. In this procedure, the sperm and eggs are mixed in a laboratory and the resulting embryo is implanted in the woman. For men with difficulties in sperm production, IVF may be achieved using intracytoplasmic sperm injection (ICSI), which involves the implantation of one sperm directly into an ovum, thus avoiding the need for large numbers of sperm. All these techniques have proved helpful to infertile couples wanting children.

PERSPECTIVE AND PROSPECTS

Studies have shown that about 15 percent of American couples are unable to conceive after one year of unprotected sex, and 10 percent do not conceive after two years. By the early 1990s, artificial insemination produced more than thirty thousand American babies yearly. This procedure advanced in the United States during the latter half of the twentieth century in large measure because of changes in attitudes, more than new medical knowledge.

The medical knowledge to treat male infertility has been available for several centuries, even when the biological basis for pregnancy was not understood. The

Bible records stories of patriarchal families that knew the problem of infertility (Abraham and Sarah, Jacob and Rachel) and even indicates, in the story of Onan and Tamar (Genesis 38:9), that semen was understood to be important to reproduction. The possibility of therapeutic insemination was mentioned in the fifth century Talmud. Arabs used insemination in horse breeding as early as the fourteenth century, and Spaniards used it in human medicine during the fifteenth century.

The presence of sperm in semen was first observed by the Dutch scientist Antoni van Leeuwenhoek in the seventeenth century, but their importance and function in the fertilization process was not recognized until the nineteenth century. In 1824, Jean Louis Prévost and J. A. Dumas correctly guessed the role of sperm in fertilization, and in 1876, Oskar Hertwig and Hermann Fol proved that the union of sperm and egg was necessary to create an embryo.

Artificial insemination became an established but clandestine procedure in the late nineteenth century in the United States and England. Compassionate physicians pioneering artificial insemination encouraged secrecy to protect the self-esteem of the infertile man, his spouse, the offspring, and the donor. In an uncertain legal climate, the offspring might have been viewed as the illegitimate product of an adulterous act. Even by the beginning of the twenty-first century, many Americans continued to stigmatize masturbation and artificial insemination. Social attitudes, especially traditional notions of masculinity, have limited the acceptability of artificial insemination to many infertile couples worldwide.

Cryopreservation of sperm became practical with the discovery of chemical cryoprotectants, reported in 1949 by Christopher Polge, Audrey Smith, and Alan Parkes of England. In 1953, American doctors R. G. Bunge and Jerome Sherman were the first to use this procedure to produce a human baby. Cryopreservation made possible the establishment of sperm banks; prior to this development, sperm donors had to provide the physician with semen immediately before insemination was to take place.

Researchers continue to theorize about new fertility-enhancing techniques using sperm. In 2003, scientists discovered that sperm have a type of chemical sensor that causes the sperm to swim vigorously toward concentrations of a chemical attractant. While researchers long have known that chemical signals are an important component of conception, the 2003 findings were the first to demonstrate that sperm will respond in a predictable and controllable way. The findings provided strong evidence that the egg signals its location to the sperm and the sperm respond by swimming toward the egg, a process which could prove promising for future contraception and infertility research. Scientists note that these findings might allow specific tests to be developed to determine if the egg is making the attractant or if the sperm have the receptor, thus helping in identifying those couples who are infertile because of poor signaling between the sperm and egg.

Artificial insemination and other alternative means of reproduction give rise to thorny issues of personal rights of various "parents" (social, birth, and genetic) and their offspring. In the United States, a few states have addressed these issues by enacting laws, usually to grant legitimacy to offspring of donor insemination. In the United Kingdom, Parliament established a central registry of sperm and egg donors. Offspring in the United Kingdom have access to nonidentifying donor information; these children are even able to learn whether they are genetically related to a prospective marriage partner.

FURTHER READING

American Society for Reproductive Medicine. http://www.asrm.org/

Doherty, C. Maud, and Melanie M. Clark. *The Fertility Handbook: A Guide to Getting Pregnant.* Omaha, Nebr.: Addicus Books, 2002.

Fisch, Harry, and Stephen Braun. *The Male Biological Clock: The Startling News About Aging, Sexuality, and Fertility in Men.* New York: Free Press, 2005.

Glover, Timothy D., and C. L. R. Barratt, eds. *Male Fertility and Infertility.* New York: Cambridge University Press, 2003.

InterNational Council on Infertility Information Dissemination. http://www.inciid.org.

"Male Infertility." *Mayo Clinic*, September 15, 2012.

"Male Infertility." *Urology Care Foundation*, March, 2013.

Riley, Julie. "Infertility in Men." *Health Library*, September 26, 2012.

Schover, Leslie R., and Anthony J. Thomas. *Overcoming Male Infertility: Understanding Its Causes and Treatments.* New York: John Wiley & Sons, 2000.

Taguchi, Yosh, and Merrily Weisbord, eds. *Private Parts: An Owner's Guide to the Male Anatomy.* 3d ed. Toronto, Ont.: McClelland & Stewart, 2003.

Armand M. Karow, updated by Paul Moglia

Muscular dystrophy

A group of related diseases that attack different muscle groups, are progressive and genetically determined, and have no known cure.

CAUSES AND SYMPTOMS

Muscles, attached to bones through tendons, are responsible for movement in the human body. In muscular dystrophy, muscles become progressively weaker. As individual muscle fibers become so weak that they die, they are replaced by connective tissue, which is fibrous and fatty rather than muscular. These replacement fibers are commonly found in skin and scar tissue and are not capable of movement, and the muscles become progressively weaker. There are several different recognized types of muscular dystrophy. These have in common degeneration of muscle fibers and their replacement with connective tissue. They are distinguished from one another on the basis of the muscle group or groups involved and the age at which individuals are affected.

The most common type is Duchenne muscular dystrophy. In this disease, the muscles involved are in the upper thigh and pelvis. The disease strikes in early childhood, usually between the ages of four and seven. It is known to be genetic and occurs only in boys. Two-thirds of affected individuals are born to mothers who are known to carry a defective gene; one-third are simply new cases whose mothers are genetically normal. Individuals afflicted with Duchenne muscular dystrophy suffer from weakness in their hips and upper thighs. Initially, they may experience difficulty in sitting up or standing. The disease progresses to involve muscle groups in the shoulder and trunk. Patients lose the ability to walk during their early teens. As the disease progresses, portions of the brain become affected, and intelligence is reduced. Muscle fibers in the heart are also affected, and most individuals die by the age of twenty.

The dystrophin gene normally produces a very large protein called dystrophin that is an integral part of the muscle cell membrane. In Duchenne muscular dystrophy, a defect in the dystrophin gene causes no dystrophin or defective dystrophin to be produced, and the protein will be absent from the cell membrane. As a result, the muscle fiber membrane breaks down and leaks, allowing fluid from outside the cell to enter the muscle cell. In turn, the contents of affected cells are broken down by other chemicals called proteases that are normally stored in the muscle cell. The dead pieces of muscle fiber are removed by scavenging cells called macrophages. The result of this process is a virtually empty and greatly weakened muscle cell.

A second type is Becker's muscular dystrophy, which is similar to the Duchenne form of the disease. Approximately three in two hundred thousand people are affected, and it too is found only among males. The major clinical difference is the age of onset. Becker's muscular dystrophy typically first appears in the early teenage years. The muscles involved are similar to those of Duchenne muscular dystrophy, but the course of the disease is slower. Most individuals require the use of a wheelchair in their early thirties and eventually die in their forties.

Myotonic dystrophy is a form of muscular dystrophy that strikes approximately five out of one hundred thousand people in a population. Myotonia is the inability of a muscle group to relax after contracting. Individuals with myotonic dystrophy experience this difficulty in their hands and feet. On average, the disease first appears at the age of nineteen. The condition is benign, in that it does not shorten an affected person's life span. Rather, it causes inconveniences to the victim. Affected persons also experience a variety of other problems, including baldness at the front of the head and malfunction of the ovaries and testes. The muscles of the stomach and intestines can become involved, leading to a slowing down of intestinal functions and diarrhea.

Another type is limb girdle muscular dystrophy. The muscles of both upper and lower limbs—the shoulders and the pelvis—are involved. The onset of this dystrophy form is variable, from childhood to middle age. While the disorder is not usually fatal, it does progress, and victims experience severe disability about twenty years after the

---

INFORMATION ON MUSCULAR DYSTROPHY

Causes: Genetic defect
Symptoms: Ranges widely; may include progressive muscle weakness, loss of coordination, impaired gait, reduced intelligence, malfunction of ovaries or testes, slowed intestinal functions, impaired swallowing, impaired eye movement
Duration: Chronic
Treatments: None; supportive care (physical therapy, braces, orthopedic surgery, drug therapy)

disease first appears. While this variant is also genetically transmitted, men and women are about equally affected.

One type of muscular dystrophy found almost exclusively among individuals of Scandinavian descent is called distal dystrophy. It first appears relatively early in adult life, between the thirties and fifties. The muscles of the forearm and hand become progressively weaker and decrease in size. Eventually, the muscles of the lower leg and foot also become involved. This form of muscular dystrophy is not usually fatal.

Oculopharyngeal muscular dystrophy is a particularly serious form that involves the muscles of the eyes and throat. In this disease, victims are affected in their forties and fifties. There is progressive loss of control of the muscles that move the eyes and loss of the ability to swallow. Death usually results from starvation or from pneumonia acquired when the affected individual accidentally inhales food or drink.

A type of muscular dystrophy for which the location of the genetic abnormality is known is facioscapulohumeral muscular dystrophy; the defect is confined to the tip of the fourth chromosome. This disease initially involves the muscles of the face and later spreads to the muscles of the posterior or back of the shoulder. Eventually, muscles in the upper thigh are involved. The affected person loses the ability to make facial expressions and assumes a permanent pout as a result of loss of muscle function. As the condition advances, the shoulder blades protrude when the arms are raised.Weakness and difficulty walking are eventually experienced. Aswith other forms of muscular dystrophy, there is some variability in the degree to which individuals are affected. Occasionally, a variety of deafness occurs involving the nerves that connect the inner ear and the brain. Less commonly, victims become blind.

There are other variants of muscular dystrophy that have been recognized and described. These forms of the disease, however, are rare. The main problem facing physicians is differentiating accurately the variety of muscular dystrophy seen in a particular patient so as to arrive at a correct diagnosis.

TREATMENT AND THERAPY

The diagnosis of muscular dystrophy is initially made through observation. Typically, parents notice changes in their affected children and bring these concerns to the attention of a physician. The physician takes a careful family history and then examines a suspected victim to make a tentative or working diagnosis. Frequently, knowledge of other family members with the condition and observations are sufficient to establish a firm diagnosis. Occasionally, a physician may elect to order physiological or genetic tests to confirm the tentative diagnosis. As Duchenne muscular dystrophy is the most common form of muscular dystrophy, it provides a convenient example of this process.

A diagnosis of Duchenne or any other form of muscular dystrophy is rarely made before the age of three. This form of the disease almost always occurs in boys. (Variants, rather than true Duchenne muscular dystrophy, are seen in girls, but this situation is extremely rare.) The reason for this finding is that the genetic defect occurs on the X chromosome, of which males only possess one. Approximately two-thirds of all victims inherit the defective chromosome from their mothers, who are asymptomatic carriers; thus, the condition is recessive and said to be X-linked. The disease occurs in the remaining one-third of victims as a result of a fresh mutation, in which there is no family history of the disease and the parents are not carriers.

Victims usually begin to sit, walk, and run at an older age than normally would be expected. Parents describe walking as waddling rather than the usual upright posture. Victims have difficulty climbing stairs. They also have apparently enlarged calf muscles, a finding called muscular hypertrophy. While the muscles are initially strong, they lose their strength when connective and fatty tissues replace muscle fibers. The weakness of muscles in the pelvis is responsible for difficulties in sitting and the unusual way of walking. Normal children are able to go directly from a sitting position to standing erect.Victims of Duchenne muscular dystrophy first roll onto their stomachs, then kneel and raise themselves up by pushing their hands against their shins, knees, and thighs; they literally climb up themselves in order to stand. These children also have a pronounced curvature of their lower backs, an attempt by the body to compensate for the weakness in the muscles of the hips and pelvis.

There is frequently some weakness in the muscles of the shoulder. This finding can be demonstrated by a physician, but it is not usually seen by parents and is not an early problem for the victim. A physician tests for this weakness by lifting the child under the armpits. Normal children will be able to support themselves using the muscles of the shoulder. Individuals with Duchenne muscular dystrophy are unable to hold themselves up and will slip through the physician's hands. Eventually, these children will be unable to lift their arms over their heads. Most victims of Duchenne muscular dystrophy are unable to walk by their teen years. The majority die before the age of twenty, although about one-quarter live for a few more years. Most victims also have an abnormality in the muscles of the heart that leads to decreased efficiency of the heart and decreased ability to be physically active; in some cases, it also causes sudden death. Most victims of Duchenne muscular dystrophy suffer mental impairment. As their muscles deteriorate, their measured intelligence quotient (IQ) drops approximately twenty points below the level that it was at the onset of the disease. Serious mental handicaps are experienced by about one-quarter of victims.

Other forms of muscular dystrophy are similar to Duchenne muscular dystrophy. Their clinical courses are also similar, as are the methods of diagnosis. The critical differences are the muscles involved and the age of onset.

Laboratory procedures used to confirm the diagnosis of muscular dystrophy include microscopic analysis of muscle tissue, measurement of enzymes found in the blood, and measurement of the speed and efficiency of nerve conduction, a process called electromyography. Some cases have been diagnosed at birth by measuring a particular enzyme called creatinine kinase. It is possible to diagnose some types of muscular dystrophy before birth with chorionic villus sampling or amniocentesis.

There is no specific treatment for any of the muscular dystrophies. Physical therapy is frequently ordered and used to prevent the remaining unaffected muscles from losing their tone and mass. In some stages of the disease, braces, appliances, and orthopedic surgery may be used. These measures do not reverse the underlying pathology, but they may improve the quality of life for a victim. The cardiac difficulties associated with myotonic dystrophy may require treatment with a pacemaker. For victims of myotonic dystrophy, some relief is obtained by using drugs; the most commonly used pharmaceuticals are phenytoin and quinine. The inability to relax muscles once they are contracted does not usually present a major problem for sufferers of myotonic dystrophy.

More useful and successful is prevention, which involves screening individuals in families or kinship groups who are potential carriers. Carriers are persons who have some genetic material for a disease or condition but lack sufficient genes to cause an apparent case of a disease or condition; in short, they appear normal. When an individual who is a carrier conceives a child, however, there is an increased risk of the offspring having the disease.

Genetic counseling should be provided after screening, so that individuals who have the gene for a disease can make more informed decisions about having children.

Chemical tests are available for use in diagnosing some forms of muscular dystrophy. Carriers of the gene for Duchenne muscular dystrophy can be detected by staining a muscle sample for dystrophin; a cell that is positive for Duchenne muscular dystrophy will have no stained dystrophin molecules. The dystrophin stain test is also used to diagnose Becker's muscular dystrophy, but the results are not quite as consistent or reliable. Approximately two-thirds of carriers and fetuses at risk for both forms of muscular dystrophy can be identified by analyzing DNA. Among individuals at risk for myotonic dystrophy, nine out of ten who carry the gene can be identified with DNA analysis before they experience actual symptoms of the disease.

PERSPECTIVE AND PROSPECTS

Muscular dystrophy has been recognized as a medical entity for several centuries. Initially, it was considered to be a degenerative disease only of adults, and it was not until the nineteenth century that the disease was addressed in children with Guillaume-Benjamin-Amand Duchenne's description of progressive weakness of the hips and upper thighs. An accurate classification of the various forms of muscular dystrophy depended on accurate observation and on the collection of sets of cases. Correct diagnosis had to wait for the development of accurate laboratory methods for staining muscle fibers. The interpretation of laboratory findings depended on the development of biochemical knowledge. Thus, much of the integration of knowledge concerning muscular dystrophy is relatively recent.

Genes play an important role in the understanding of muscular dystrophy. All forms of muscular dystrophy are hereditary, although different chromosomes are involved in different forms of the disease. The development of techniques for routine testing and diagnosis has also occurred relatively recently. Specific chromosomes for all forms of muscular dystrophy have not yet been discovered. Considering initial successes of the Human Genome Project, an effort to identify all human genes, it seems likely that more precise genetic information related to muscular dystrophy will emerge.

There still are no cures for muscular dystrophies, and many forms are relentlessly fatal. Cures for many communicable diseases caused by bacteria or viruses have been discovered, and advances have been made in the treatment of cancer and other degenerative diseases by identifying chemicals that cause the conditions or by persuading people to change their lifestyles. Muscular dystrophy, however, is a group of purely genetic conditions. Many of the particular chromosomes involved are known, but no techniques are yet available to cure the disease once it is identified.

The availability of both a mouse model and a dog model of Duchenne muscular dystrophy, however, has facilitated the testing of gene therapy for this disease. Dystrophic mouse early embryos have been cured by injection of a functional copy of the dystrophin gene; however, this technique must be performed in embryos and is not useful for human therapy. Two avenues of research under way in these animal models are the introduction of normal muscle-precursor cells into dystrophic muscle cells and the direct delivery of a functional dystrophin gene into dystrophic muscle cells. It is hoped that these studies will lead to a cure for the disease.

In the meantime, muscular dystrophy continues to cause human suffering and to cost victims, their families, and society large sums of money. The disease is publicized on an annual basis via efforts to raise money for research and treatment, but there is little publicity on an ongoing basis. For these reasons, muscular dystrophy remains an important medical problem in contemporary society.

FURTHER READING

Alan, Rick. "Muscular Dystrophy." *Health Library,* September 20, 2011.

Beers, Mark H., et al., eds. *The Merck Manual of Diagnosis and Therapy.* 19th ed. Whitehouse Station, N.J.: Merck Research Laboratories, 2011.

Behrman, Richard E., Robert M. Kliegman, and Hal B. Jenson, eds. *Nelson Textbook of Pediatrics.* 18th ed. Philadelphia: Saunders/Elsevier, 2007.

Brown, Susan S., and Jack A. Lucy, eds. *Dystrophin: Gene, Protein, and Cell Biology.* New York: Cambridge University Press, 1997.

Emery, Alan E. H. *Muscular Dystrophy: The Facts.* 3rd ed. New York: Oxford University Press, 2008.

"Facts about Muscular Dystrophy." *Centers for Disease Control and Prevention,* April 6, 2012.

Goldman, Lee, and Dennis Ausiello, eds. *Cecil Textbook of Medicine.* 23d ed. Philadelphia: Saunders/Elsevier, 2007.

Kumar, Vinay, Abul K. Abbas, and Nelson Fausto, eds. *Robbins and Cotran Pathologic Basis of Disease.* 8th ed. Philadelphia: Saunders/Elsevier, 2010.

"Muscular Dystrophy: Hope Through Research." *National Institute of Neurological Disorders and Stroke.* February 14, 2013.

Tierney, Lawrence M., Stephen J. McPhee, and Maxine A. Papadakis, eds. *Current Medical Diagnosis and Treatment 2007.* New York: McGraw-Hill Medical, 2006.

Wolfson, Penny. *Moonrise: One Family, Genetic Identity, and Muscular Dystrophy.* New York: St. Martin's Press, 2003.

L. Fleming Fallon, Jr.; updated by Karen E. Kalumuck

SEE ALSO: Genetics and Inheritance; Muscles

Obsessive-compulsive disorder

Obsessions and compulsions are the cardinal features of a chronic anxiety disorder known as obsessive-compulsive disorder. The identification of repetitive, anxiety-provoking thoughts known as obsessions and of associated compulsive, ritualistic behaviors is critical in the diagnosis and assessment of this debilitating condition.

INTRODUCTION

Obsessive thinking and urges to engage in ritualistic compulsive behaviors are common phenomena that most individuals experience to some extent throughout their lives. It is not uncommon, for example, for a person to reexperience in his or her mind involuntary, anxiety-provoking images of circumstances surrounding a traumatic accident or embarrassing moment. Similarly, behaviors such as returning home to make sure the iron is turned off or refusing to eat from a spoon that falls on a clean floor represent mild compelling rituals in which many persons engage from time to time. It is only when these patterns of obsessive thinking and behaving become either too frequent or too intense that they may escalate into a distressing clinical condition known as obsessive-compulsive disorder.

According to the American Psychiatric Association's *Diagnostic and Statistical Manual of Mental Disorders: DSM-IV-TR* (rev. 4th ed., 2000), the primary feature of this disorder is the presence of distressing obsessions or severe compulsive behaviors that interfere significantly with a person's daily functioning. Although diagnosis requires only the presence of either obsessions or compulsions, they typically are both present in obsessive-compulsive disorder. In most cases, persons with this diagnosis spend more time on a daily basis experiencing obsessive thinking and engaging in ritualistic behaviors than other constructive activities, including those pertaining to occupational, social, and family responsibilities. Therefore, it is not uncommon for obsessive-compulsive patients also to experience severe vocational impairment and distraught interpersonal relationships.

OBSESSIONS

The word "obsession" comes from the Latin word obsidere ("to besiege") and can be defined as a recurrent thought, impulse, idea, or image that is intrusive, disturbing, and senseless. Among the most common types are themes of violence (for example, images of killing a loved one), contamination (for example, thoughts of catching a disease from a doorknob), and personal injury or harm (for example, impulses to leap from a bridge). Obsessional doubting is also characteristic of most patients with obsessive-compulsive disorder, which leads to indecisiveness in even the most simple matters such as selecting a shirt to wear or deciding what to order at a restaurant. The basic content of obsessive thinking distinguishes it from simple "worrying." Worrying involves thinking about an event or occurrence that may realistically result in discomfort, embarrassment, or harm and has a likely probability of occurring; obsessive thinking is typically recognized by the patient as being senseless and not likely to occur. An example of a worry is thinking about an event that possesses a strong likelihood of occurring, such as failing a test when one has not studied. Imagining that one might leap from the third-floor classroom during the exam, a highly unlikely event, is considered an obsession. Furthermore, because the obsessive-compulsive patient is aware that these intrusive thoughts are senseless and continuously attempts to rid the thought from his or her mind, obsessive thinking is not delusional or psychotic in nature. Although both delusional and obsessive patients may experience a similar thought (for example, that they have ingested tainted food), the obsessive patient recognizes that the thought is unlikely and is a product of his or her mind and struggles to get rid of the thought. The delusional patient adheres to the belief with little to no struggle to test its validity.

COMPULSIONS

Most obsessive-compulsive patients also exhibit a series of repetitive, intentional, stereotyped behaviors known as compulsions, which serve to reduce the anxiety experienced from severe obsessive thinking. The most common forms include counting (for example, tapping a pencil three times before laying it down), cleaning (for example, hand washing after shaking another person's hand), checking (for example, checking pilot lights several times a day), and ordering (for example, arranging pencils from longest to shortest before doing homework). Compulsions are different from simple habits in that attempts to resist urges to engage in them result in a substantial increase in anxiety, eventually forcing the patient to engage in the compelling behavior to reduce the tension. Urges to engage in simple habits, on the other hand, can often be resisted with minimal discomfort. Furthermore, most habits result in deriving some degree of pleasure from the activity (for example, shopping, gambling, drinking), while engaging in compulsive behaviors is rarely enjoyable for the patient. Compulsions must also be distinguished from superstitious behaviors, such as an athlete's warm-up ritual or wearing the same "lucky" shoes for each sporting event. In contrast to superstitious people, who employ their rituals to enhance confidence, obsessive-compulsive patients are never certain their rituals will result in anxiety reduction. This typically forces these patients continually to expand their repertoire of ritualistic behaviors, searching for new and better ways to eliminate the anxiety produced by obsessive thinking.

It is estimated that approximately 2 percent of the adult population in the United States—a larger percentage than was once believed—has at some time experienced obsessive-compulsive symptoms severe enough to warrant diagnosis. Typically, obsessive-compulsive symptoms begin in adolescence or early adulthood, although most patients report symptoms of anxiety and nervousness as children. Regarding early developmental histories, many obsessive-compulsive patients report being reared in very strict, puritanical homes. The disorder occurs equally in males and females, although cleaning rituals occur more frequently among women. Although the course of the disorder is chronic, the intensity of symptoms fluctuates throughout life and it occasionally has been reported to remit spontaneously. Because of the unusual nature of the symptoms, obsessive-compulsive patients often keep their rituals hidden and become introverted and withdrawn; as a result, the clinical picture becomes complicated by a coexisting depressive disorder. It is typically the depression that forces the patient to seek psychological help.

ETIOLOGY AND TREATMENTS

Because of the distressing yet fascinating nature of the symptoms, several theoretical positions have attempted to explain how obsessive-compulsive disorder develops. From an applied perspective, each theoretical position has evolved into a treatment or intervention strategy for eliminating the problems caused by obsessions and compulsions. According to psychoanalytic theory, as outlined by Sigmund Freud in 1909, obsessive-compulsive rituals are the product of overly harsh toilet training that leaves the patient with considerable unconscious hostility, primarily directed toward an authoritarian caregiver. In a sense, as uncomfortable and disconcerting as the obsessions and compulsive behaviors are, they are preferable to experiencing the intense emotions left from these childhood incidents. Obsessions and compulsions permit the patient to avoid experiencing these emotions.

Furthermore, obsessive-compulsive symptoms force the patient to become preoccupied with anxiety-reduction strategies that prevent them from dealing with other hidden impulses, such as sexual urges and desires. Based on the psychoanalytic formulation, treatment involves identifying the original unconscious thoughts, ideas, or impulses and allowing the patient to experience them consciously. In his classic case report of an obsessive patient, Freud analyzed a patient known as the "rat man," who was plagued by recurrent, horrifying images of a bucket of hungry rats strapped to the buttocks of his girlfriend and his father. Although periodic case reports of psychoanalytic treatments for obsessive-compulsive disorder exist, there is very little controlled empirical work suggesting the effectiveness of this treatment approach.

Behavioral theorists, differing from the psychoanalytic tradition, have proposed that obsessive-compulsive disorder represents a learned habit that is maintained by the reinforcing properties of the anxiety reduction that occurs following ritualistic behaviors. It is well established that behaviors that are reinforced occur more frequently

---

DSM-IV-TR CRITERIA FOR OBSESSIVE-COMPULSIVE DISORDER (DSM CODE 300.3)

Either obsessions or compulsions

Obsessions defined by all of the following:
- recurrent and persistent thoughts, impulses, or images experienced, at some time during disturbance, as intrusive and inappropriate and cause marked anxiety or distress
- thoughts, impulses, or images not simply excessive worries about real-life problems
- attempts made to ignore or suppress thoughts, impulses, or images, or to neutralize them with some other thought or action
- recognition that thoughts, impulses, or images are product of his or her own mind (not imposed from without, as in thought insertion)

Compulsions defined by both of the following:
- repetitive behaviors (hand washing, ordering, checking) or mental acts (praying, counting, repeating words silently) that individual feels driven to perform in response to an obsession or according to rules that must be applied rigidly

- behaviors or mental acts aimed at preventing or reducing distress or preventing some dreaded event or situation; behaviors or mental acts either are not connected in a realistic way with what they are designed to neutralize or prevent or are clearly excessive

At some point, individual recognizes obsessions or compulsions as excessive or unreasonable; this does not apply to children

Obsessions or compulsions cause marked distress, are time-consuming, or interfere significantly with normal routine, occupational or academic functioning, or usual social activities or relationships

If another Axis I disorder is present, content of obsessions or compulsions not restricted to it

Disturbance not due to direct physiological effects of a substance or general medical condition

Specify if with Poor Insight (most of the time during current episode, obsessions and compulsions not recognized as excessive or unreasonable)

in the future. In the case of compulsive behaviors, the ritual is always followed by a significant reduction in anxiety, therefore reinforcing the compulsive behavior as well as the preceding obsessive activity. Based on the behavioral perspective, an intervention strategy called response prevention, or flooding, Flooding was developed to facilitate the interruption of this habitually reinforcing cycle. Response prevention involves exposing the patient to the feared stimulus (for example, a doorknob) or obsession (for example, an image of leaping from a bridge) to create anxiety. Rather than allowing the patient to engage in the subsequent compulsive activity, however, the therapist prevents the response (for example, the patient is not permitted to wash his or her hands). The patient endures a period of intense anxiety but eventually experiences habituation of the anxiety response. Although treatments of this nature are anxiety provoking for the patient, well-controlled investigations have reported significant reductions in obsessive thinking and ritualistic behavior following intervention. Some estimates of success rates with response prevention are as high as 80 percent, and treatment gains are maintained for several years.

Theories emphasizing the cognitive aspects of the obsessive-compulsive disorder have focused on information-processing impairments of the patient. Specifically, obsessive-compulsive patients tend to perceive harm (for example, contamination) when in fact it may not be present and to perceive a loss of control over their environment. Although most individuals perceive a given situation as safe until proved harmful, the obsessive-compulsive patient perceives situations as harmful until proved safe. These perceptions of harm and lack of control lead to increased anxiety; the belief that the patient controls his or her life or the perception of safety leads to decreased anxiety. Accordingly, compulsive rituals represent a patient's efforts to gain control over his or her environment. Cognitive interventions aim to increase the patient's perception of control over the environment and to evaluate realistically environmental threats of harm. Although cognitive approaches may serve as a useful adjunct to behavioral treatments such as response prevention, evidence for their effectiveness when used in treating obsessions and compulsions is lacking.

Finally, biological models of obsessive-compulsive disorder have also been examined. There is some indication that electrical activity in the brain during information processing, particularly in the frontal lobes, is somewhat slower for obsessive-compulsive patients in comparison with other people. For example, metabolic activity of the frontal brain regions measured using positron emission tomography (PET) scans differentiates obsessive-compulsive patients from both normal people and depressive patients. Further, a deficiency in certain neurotransmitters (for example, serotonin and norepinephrine) has been implicated in the etiology of the disorder. Several interventions based on the biological model have been employed as well. Pharmacotherapy, using antidepressantAntidepressantsobsessive-compulsive disorder medications that primarily act to facilitate neurotransmitter functioning (for example, clomipramine), has been shown to be effective in treating from 20 to 50 percent of obsessive-compulsive patients. More drastic interventions such as frontal lobotomies have been reported in the most intractable cases, with very limited success.

Among the interventions employed to rid patients of troublesome obsessions and compulsions, response prevention holds the most promise. Because of the intensity of this treatment approach, however, the cost may be substantial, and many patients may not immediately respond. A number of predictors of poor treatment response to behavioral interventions (characteristic of those most refractory to treatment) have been identified. These include a coexisting depression, poor compliance with exposure/response-prevention instructions, the presence of fears that the patient views as realistic, and eccentric superstition. In these cases, alternative forms of treatment are typically considered (for example, pharmacotherapy).

PREVALENCE AND RESEARCH

Obsessions and compulsions represent human phenomena that have been a topic of interest for several centuries; for example, William Shakespeare's characterization of the hand-washing Lady Macbeth has entertained audiences for hundreds of years. Prior to the first therapeutic analysis of obsessive-compulsive disorder, then called a neurosis—Freud's description of the "rat man"—obsessive thoughts were commonly attributed to demoniac influence and treated with exorcism. Freud's major contribution was delivering the phenomenon from the spiritual into the psychological realm. Although initial case reports employing psychoanalysis were promising, subsequent developments using behavioral and pharmacological formulations have more rapidly advanced the understanding of the phenomenology and treatment of this unusual condition. In addition, with the public revelation that certain prominent individuals such as the aircraft designer and film producer Howard Hughes suffered from this condition, the prevalence estimates of this disorder have steadily increased. Although a number of patients have sought help for this debilitating disorder since the time it was first clinically described, it has been confirmed that this problem is far more prevalent than initially thought. The increase is probably related not to an actual increase in incidence but to individuals becoming more willing to seek help for the problem. Because of the increasing number of individuals requesting help for problems relating to obsessions and compulsions, it is becoming more and more important to foster the maturation of appropriate treatment strategies to deal with this disorder.

Further, it has become increasingly important to understand the manifestation of obsessions and compulsions from a biological, psychological, and socio-occupational level. Ongoing investigations are examining the biological makeup of the nervous systems peculiar to this disorder. Research examining the specific information-processing styles and cognitive vulnerabilities of obsessive-compulsive patients is also being conducted. Both response-prevention and biochemical-intervention strategies (for example, clomipramine) are deserving of continued research, primarily in examining the characteristics of obsessive-compulsive patients that predict treatment efficacy with either form of intervention. Finally, early markers for this condition, including childhood environments, early learning experiences, and biological predispositions, require further investigation so that prevention efforts can be provided for individuals who may be at risk for developing obsessive-compulsive disorder. With these advances, psychologists will be in a better position to reduce the chronic nature of obsessive-compulsive disorder and to prevent these distressing symptoms in forthcoming generations.

FURTHER READING

American Psychiatric Association. *Diagnostic and Statistical Manual of Mental Disorders: DSM-IV-TR*. Rev. 4th ed. Washington, D.C.: Author, 2000. The DSM-IV-TR provides specific criteria for making psychiatric diagnoses of obsessive-compulsive disorder and other anxiety disorders. Brief summaries of research findings regarding each condition are also provided.

Clark, David A. *Cognitive-Behavioral Therapy for OCD*. New York: Guilford Press, 2007. This book offers guidelines on the assessment of obsessive-compulsive disorder and presents a variety of effective treatments, based on patient models.

Emmelkamp, Paul M. G. *Phobic and Obsessive Compulsive Disorders: Theory, Research, and Practice*. New York: Plenum, 1982. A somewhat dated but classic work outlining the importance of behavioral strategies in overcoming obsessive-compulsive, as well as phobic, conditions.

Hyman, Bruce M., and Troy Dufrene. *Coping with OCD: Practical Strategies for Living Well with Obsessive-Compulsive Disorder*. Oakland, Calif.: New Harbinger, 2008. This resource, designed for those who are struggling with obsesseive-compulsive disorder, describes the condition in layperson's terms and advises sufferers on how to deal with the depression, shame, and blame that usually accompanies it.

Jenike, Michael A., Lee Baer, and William E. Minichiello. *Obsessive-Compulsive Disorders: Theory and Management*. 2d ed. Littleton, Mass.: PSG, 1990. A comprehensive overview of the topic that does not burden the reader with intricate details of analysis. Readable by the layperson. Covers the topic thoroughly.

Mavissakalian, Matig, Samuel M. Turner, and Larry Michelson. *Obsessive-Compulsive Disorders: Psychological and Pharmacological Treatment*. New York: Plenum, 1985. An exceptionally well-written text based on a symposium held at the University of Pittsburgh. Issues pertaining to etiology, assessment, diagnosis, and treatment are covered in detail.

Rachman, S. J. "Obsessional-Compulsive Disorders." In *International Handbook of Behavior Modification and Therapy*, edited by Alan S. Bellack, Michel Hersen, and Alan E. Kazdin. 2d ed. New York: Plenum, 1990. Rachman's work using behavioral strategies with obsessive-compulsive patients is unparalleled. No bibliography would be complete without a contribution from Rachman, one of the most respected authorities in the field.

Steketee, Gail, and Andrew Ellis. *Treatment of Obsessive-Compulsive Disorder*. New York: Guilford, 1996. A comprehensive resource for mental health professionals. Covers behavioral and cognitive approaches, biological models, and pharmacological therapies.

Turner, S. M., and L. Michelson. "Obsessive-Compulsive Disorders." In *Behavioral Theories and Treatment of Anxiety*, edited by Samuel M. Turner. New York: Plenum, 1984. Summarizes information regarding diagnostic issues, assessment strategies, and treatment interventions for obsessive-compulsive disorder. Provides an excellent review of intervention efforts employing response prevention and clomipramine.

Kevin T. Larkin and Virginia L. Goetsch

SEE ALSO: Anxiety

Post-traumatic stress (PTS)

After an extreme psychological trauma, people tend to respond with stress symptoms that include reexperiencing the trauma through nightmares or unwanted thoughts, avoiding reminders of the traumatic event, loss of interest in daily life, and increased arousal; these symptoms can range from mild and temporary to severe, chronic, and psychologically disabling.

INTRODUCTION

It is common knowledge that there are psychological aftereffects from experiencing an intense psychological trauma. This discussion of post-traumatic stress symptoms will be organized around post-traumatic stress disorder (PTSD), one of the diagnostic categories of anxiety disorders recognized by the American Psychiatric Association. It should be realized at the outset, however, that it is normal for people to experience at least some of these symptoms after suffering a psychological trauma. The first step in understanding PTSD is to know its symptoms.

The first criterion for PTSD is that one has suffered a trauma. The American Psychiatric Association's definition of PTSD states that the trauma must be something that "is outside the range of usual human experience and that would be markedly distressing to almost anyone." It is not so much the objective event as one's perception of it that determines the psychological response. For example, the death of one's parents is not "outside the range of usual human experience," but it can result in some of the symptoms described later. Some of the traumatic experiences deemed sufficient to cause PTSD include threat to one's own life or the life of a close relative or friend, sudden destruction of one's home or community, seeing another person violently injured or killed, or being the victim of a violent crime. Specific experiences that often cause PTSD include combat, natural or man-made disasters, automobile accidents, airplane crashes, rape, child abuse, and physical assault. In general, the more traumatic the event, the worse the post-traumatic

symptoms. Symptoms of stress are often more severe when the trauma is sudden and unexpected. In addition, when the trauma is the result of intentional human action (for example, combat, rape, or assault), stress symptoms are worse than when the trauma is a natural disaster (flood or earthquake) or an accident (automobile crash). It has been found that combat veterans who commit or witness atrocities are more likely than their comrades to suffer later from PTSD.

The central symptom of post-traumatic stress disorder is that the person reexperiences the trauma. This can occur in a number of ways. The person can have unwanted, intrusive, and disturbing thoughts of the event or nightmares about the trauma. The most dramatic means of reexperiencing is through a flashback, in which the person acts, thinks, and feels as if he or she were reliving the event. Another way in which reexperiencing might be manifested is intense distress when confronted with situations that serve as reminders of the trauma. Vietnam veterans with combat-related PTSD will often become very upset at motion pictures about the war, hot and humid junglelike weather, or even the smell of Asian cooking. A person with PTSD often will attempt to avoid thoughts, feelings, activities, or events that serve as unwanted reminders of the trauma.

Another symptom that is common in people with PTSD is numbing of general responsiveness. This might include the loss of interest in hobbies or activities that were enjoyed before the trauma, losing the feeling of closeness to other people, an inability to experience strong emotions, or a lack of interest in the future. A final set of PTSD symptoms involves increased arousal. This can include irritability, angry outbursts, and problems with sleeping and concentrating. A person with PTSD may be oversensitive to the environment, always on the alert, and prone to startle at the slightest noise.

The paragraphs above summarize the symptoms that psychologists and psychiatrists use to diagnose PTSD; however, other features are often found in trauma survivors that are not part of the diagnosis. Anxiety and depression are common in people who have experienced a trauma. Guilt is common in people who have survived a trauma in which others have died. People will sometimes use alcohol or tranquilizers to cope with sleep problems, disturbing nightmares, or distressing, intrusive recollections of a trauma, and they may then develop dependence on the drugs.

Post-traumatic stress disorder is relatively common in people who suffer serious trauma. In the late 1980's, the most extensive survey on PTSD ever done was undertaken on Vietnam combat veterans. It found that more than half of all those who served in the Vietnam theater of operations had experienced serious post-traumatic stress at some point in their lives after the war. This represents about 1.7 million veterans. Even more compelling was the fact that more than one-third of the veterans who saw heavy combat were still suffering from PTSD when the survey was done—about fifteen years after the fall of Saigon. Surveys of crime victims are also sobering. One study found that 75 percent of adult females had been the victim of a crime, and more than one in four of these victims developed PTSD after the crime. Crime victims were even more likely to develop PTSD if they were raped, were injured during the crime, or believed that their lives were in danger during the crime.

Symptoms of post-traumatic stress are common after a trauma, but they often decrease or disappear over time.

DSM-IV-TR CRITERIA FOR POST-TRAUMATIC STRESS DISORDER (DSM CODE 309.81)

Person has been exposed to a traumatic event in which both of the following were present:
- person experienced, witnessed, or was confronted with event or events involving actual or threatened death or serious injury, or threat to physical integrity of self or others
- person's response involved intense fear, helplessness, or horror; in children, may be expressed instead by disorganized or agitated behavior

Traumatic event persistently reexperienced in one or more of the following ways:
- recurrent and intrusive distressing recollections of event, including images, thoughts, or perceptions; in young children, repetitive play may express themes or aspects of trauma
- recurrent distressing dreams of event; in children, frightening dreams without recognizable content may occur
- acting or feeling as if traumatic event were recurring (includes a sense of reliving the experience, illusions, hallucinations, and dissociative flashback episodes, including those occurring on awakening or when intoxicated); in young children, trauma-specific reenactment may occur
- intense psychological distress at exposure to internal or external cues that symbolize or resemble an aspect of traumatic event
- physiological reactivity on exposure to internal or external cues that symbolize or resemble an aspect of traumatic event

Persistent avoidance of stimuli associated with trauma and numbing of general responsiveness (not present before trauma), as indicated by three or more of the following:
- efforts to avoid thoughts, feelings, or conversations associated with trauma
- efforts to avoid activities, places, or people arousing recollections of trauma
- inability to recall an important aspect of trauma
- markedly diminished interest or participation in significant activities
- feeling of detachment or estrangement from others
- restricted range of affect (such as inability to have loving feelings)
- sense of a foreshortened future (such as not expecting to have career, marriage, children, or normal life span)

Persistent symptoms of increased arousal (not present before trauma), as indicated by two or more of the following:
- difficulty falling or staying asleep
- irritability or outbursts of anger
- difficulty concentrating
- hypervigilance
- exaggerated startle response

Duration of more than one month
Disturbance causes clinically significant distress or impairment in social, occupational, or other important areas of functioning
Specify Acute (duration less than three months) or Chronic (duration three months or more)
Specify if with Delayed Onset (onset at least six months after stressor)

A diagnosis of PTSD is not made unless the symptoms last for at least one month. Sometimes a person will have no symptoms until long after the event, when memories of the trauma are triggered by another negative life event. For example, a combat veteran might cope well with civilian life for many years until, after a divorce, he begins to have nightmares about his combat experiences.

FROM WAR TO EVERYDAY LIFE

Most of the theory and research regarding PTSD have been done on combat veterans, particularly veterans of the Vietnam War. One of the most exciting developments in this area, however, is that the theory and research are also being applied to victims of other sorts of trauma. This has a number of important implications. First, it helps extend the findings about PTSD beyond the combat-veteran population, which is mostly young and male. Second, information gathered from combat veterans can be used to assist in the assessment and treatment of anyone who has experienced a serious trauma. Because a large proportion of the general population experiences severe psychological trauma at some time, understanding PTSD is important to those providing mental health services.

An extended example will illustrate the application of theory and research findings on PTSD to a case of extreme psychological trauma. The case involves a woman who was attacked and raped at knifepoint one night while walking from her car to her apartment. Because of injuries suffered in the attack, she went to an emergency room for treatment. Knowledge about PTSD can help in understanding this woman's experience and could aid her in recovery.

First, research has shown that this woman's experience—involving rape, life threat, and physical injury—puts her at high risk for symptoms of post-traumatic stress. Risk is so great, in fact, that researchers have proposed that psychological counseling be recommended to all people who are the victims of this sort of episode. This suggestion is being implemented in many rape-recovery and crime-victim programs around the United States.

Knowing what symptoms are common following a traumatic event can help professionals counsel a victim about what to expect. This woman can expect feelings of anxiety and depression, nightmares and unwanted thoughts about the event, irritability, and difficulties in sleeping and concentrating. Telling a victim that these are normal responses and that there is a likelihood that the problems will lessen with time is often reassuring.

Since research has shown that many people with these symptoms cope by using drugs and alcohol, it may also help to warn the victim about this possibility and caution that this is harmful in the long run.

One symptom of PTSD—psychological distress in situations that resemble the traumatic event—suggests why combat veterans who experience their trauma in a far-off land often fare better than those whose trauma occurs closer to home. Women who are raped in their home or neighborhood may begin to feel unsafe in previously secure places. Some cope by moving to a different house, a new neighborhood, or even a new city—often leaving valued jobs and friends. If an attack occurred after dark, a person may no longer feel safe going out after dark and may begin living a restricted social life. Frequently, women who are raped generalize their fear to all men and especially to sexual relations, seriously damaging their interpersonal relationships. Given the problems that these post-traumatic symptoms can cause in so many areas of one's life, it may not be surprising that one study found that nearly one in every five rape victims attempted suicide.

The main symptoms of post-traumatic stress are phobialike fear and avoidance of trauma-related situations, thoughts, and feelings, and the most effective treatment for PTSD is the same as for a phobia. Systematic desensitization and flooding, which involve confronting the thoughts and feelings surrounding the traumatic event, are the treatments that appear to be most effective. It may seem paradoxical that a disorder whose symptoms include unwanted thoughts and dreams of a traumatic event could be treated by purposefully thinking and talking about the event; however, Mardi Horowitz, one of the leading theorists in traumatic stress, believes that symptoms alternate between unwanted, intrusive thoughts of the event and efforts to avoid these thoughts. Because intrusive thoughts always provoke efforts at avoidance, the event is never fully integrated into memory; it therefore retains its power. Systematic desensitization and flooding, which involve repeatedly thinking about the event without avoidance, allow time for the event to become integrated into the person's life experiences so that the memory loses much of its pain.

Another effective way to reduce the impact of a traumatic event is through social support. Social support People who have a close network of friends and family appear to suffer less from symptoms of trauma. After a traumatic experience, people should be encouraged to maintain and even increase their supportive social contacts, rather than withdrawing from people, as often happens. Support groups of people who have had similar experiences, such as Vietnam veteran groups or child-abuse support groups, also provide needed social support. These groups have the added benefit of encouraging people to talk about their experiences, which provides another way to think about and integrate the traumatic event.

Psychotherapy can help trauma victims in many ways. One way is to help the patient explore and cope with the way the trauma changes one's view of the world. For example, the rape victim may come to believe that "the world is dangerous" or that "men can't be trusted." Therapy can help this person learn to take reasonable precautions without shutting herself off from the world and relationships. Finally, symptoms of overarousal are common with PTSD. A therapist can address these symptoms by teaching methods of deep relaxation and stress reduction. Sometimes mild tranquilizers are prescribed when trauma victims are acutely aroused or anxious.

HISTORY

The concept of post-traumatic stress is very old and is closely tied to the history of human warfare. The symptoms of PTSD have been known variously as soldier's heart, combat neurosis, and battle fatigue. Stephen Crane's novel *The Red Badge of Courage*, first published in 1895, describes post-traumatic symptoms in a Civil War soldier. It was the postwar experiences of the Vietnam combat veteran, however, studied and described by scholars such as Charles Figley, that brought great attention to issues of post-traumatic stress. It was not until 1980 that the American Psychiatric Association recognized post-traumatic stress disorder in its manual of psychiatric disorders. Since then there has been an explosion of published research and books on PTSD, the creation of the Society for Traumatic Stress Studies in 1985, and the initiation of the quarterly *Journal of Traumatic Stress* in 1988. Since these developments, attention has also been directed toward post-traumatic symptoms in victims of natural disasters, violent crime, sexual and child abuse; Holocaust survivors; and many other populations. Surveys have found that more than 80 percent of college students have suffered at least one trauma potentially sufficient to cause PTSD, and many people seeking psychological counseling have post-traumatic stress symptoms. Thus, it is fair to say that the attention garnered by Vietnam veteran readjustment problems and by the recognition of PTSD as a disorder by the American Psychiatric Association has prompted the examination of many important issues related to post-traumatic stress.

Because research in this area is relatively new, many important questions remain unanswered. One mystery is that two people can have exactly the same traumatic experience, yet one will have extreme post-traumatic stress and one will have no problems. Some factors are known to be important; for example, young children and the elderly are more likely to suffer from psychological symptoms after a trauma. Much research is needed, however, to determine what individual differences will predict who fares well and who fares poorly after a trauma.

A second area of future development is in the assessment of PTSD. For the most part, it is diagnosed through a self-report of trauma and post-traumatic symptoms. This creates difficulty, however, when the person reporting the symptoms stands to gain compensation for the trauma suffered. Interesting physiological and cognitive methods for assessing PTSD are being explored. For example, researchers have found that Vietnam veterans with PTSD show high levels of physiological arousal when they hear combat-related sounds or imagine their combat experiences. Finally, the future will see more bridges built between post-traumatic stress and the more general area of stress and coping.

FURTHER READING

Crane, Stephen. *The Red Badge of Courage*. Reprint. New York: Pearson/Longman, 2008. This classic novel vividly portrays post-traumatic symptoms in Civil War soldiers, particularly in the main character, young Henry Fleming; first published in 1895, the book has been called the first modern war novel.

Figley, Charles R., ed. *Trauma and Its Wake: The Study and Treatment of Post-traumatic Stress Disorder*. New York: Brunner/Mazel, 1985. This book is one of the most often cited references in the field of PTSD and contains some of the most influential papers written on the subject. It is divided into sections on theory, research, and treatment; a second volume with the same title was published in 1986. It is part of the Brunner/Mazel Psychosocial Stress Series, the first volume of which was published in 1978; through 1990, this valuable series had published twenty-one volumes on many aspects of stress and trauma.

Figley, Charles R., and Seymour Leventman, eds. *Strangers at Home: Vietnam Veterans Since the War*. 1980. Reprint. New York: Brunner/Mazel, 1990.

Containing chapters by psychologists, sociologists, political activists, historians, political scientists, and economists, this book presents a look at the experience of the Vietnam veteran from different perspectives. Many of the authors were Vietnam veterans themselves, so the book has a very personal, sometimes stirring view of its subject.

Grinker, Roy Richard, and John P. Spiegal. *Men Under Stress*. Philadelphia: Blakiston, 1945. Long before the term "post-traumatic stress disorder" was coined, this classic book described the stress response to combat in Air Force flyers. It is written in jargon-free language by men who had unusual access to the flight crews.

Horowitz, Mardi Jon. *Stress Response Syndromes*. New York: Jason Aronson, 1976. Horowitz is one of the leading psychodynamic theorists in the area of post-traumatic stress. In this readable book, he describes his theory and his approach to treatment.

Kulka, Richard A. *Trauma and the Vietnam War Generation*. New York: Brunner/Mazel, 1990. Presents the results of the federally funded National Vietnam Veterans Readjustment Study. In contrast to Strangers at Home, which is a subjective view of the Vietnam veteran's plight, this book is very factual. It contains dozens of tables and figures filled with statistics about the mental and physical health of Vietnam veterans. The same authors published The National Vietnam Veterans Readjustment Study: Tables of Findings and Technical Appendices in 1990. This companion volume contains hundreds of tables of detailed results from this comprehensive study.

Schiraldi, Glenn. *The Post-Traumatic Stress Disorder Sourcebook: A Guide to Healing, Recovery, and Growth*. New York: McGraw-Hill, 2009. Designed as a self-help program for those suffering from post-traumatic stress disorder, this book discusses emotional triggers, drug addiction, and successful treatments.

Smyth, Larry. *Overcoming Post-Traumatic Stress Disorder—Therapist Protocol: A Cognitive-Behavioral Exposure-Based Protocol for the Treatment of PTSD and the Other Anxiety Disorders*. Oakland, Calif.: New Harbinger, 2008. Written for the therapist, this book outlines a protocol that has worked successfully with those who are experiencing post-traumatic stress disorder. The sessions involve assessment, goal setting, developing coping skills, and assimilation.

Scott R. Vrana

SEE ALSO: Anxiety; Military Families; Stress

Schizophrenia

Schizophrenia is a severe mental illness that interferes with a person's ability to think and to communicate. Researchers have studied the illness for decades, and while genetic factors contribute to the illness, the specific genetic mechanisms and how they interact with environmental factors remain unknown.

INTRODUCTION

According to the National Alliance on Mental Illness (NAMI) in 2013, approximately 1.1 US adults (about 2.4 million people) lived with schizophrenia. It is considered to be one of the most severe mental illnesses, because its symptoms can have a devastating impact on the lives of patients and their families. The patient's thought processes, communication abilities, and emotional expressions are disturbed. As a result, many patients with schizophrenia are dependent on others for assistance with daily life activities.

Schizophrenia is often confused, by the layperson, with dissociative identity disorder (commonly known as multiple personality disorder), is an illness defined as having two or more distinct personalities existing within the person. The personalities tend to be intact, and each is associated with its own style of perceiving the world and relating to others. Schizophrenia, in contrast, does not involve the existence of two or more personalities; rather, it is the presence of psychotic symptoms and characteristic deficits in social interaction that define schizophrenia.

The diagnostic criteria for schizophrenia have changed over the years; however, certain key symptoms for a diagnosis as noted by the *Diagnostic and Statistical Manual of Mental Disorders: DSM-5* (2013) include delusions, hallucinations, disorganized speech (such as frequent incoherence or connecting a sequence of unrelated ideas), completely disorganized or catatonic behavior, and such negative symptoms as diminished emotional expression or avolition (general lack of motivation or drive). The DSM-5 is published by the American Psychiatric Association and is periodically revised to incorporate changes in diagnostic criteria.

Of the five symptoms listed above and in the DSM-5, at least two of the symptoms must be present in an individual for at least one month. One of two of the symptoms must include delusions, hallucinations, or disorganized speech. Further, the presence of other disorders, such as drug reactions or organic brain disorders associated with aging, must be ruled out. Thus, the diagnosis of schizophrenia typically involves a thorough physical and mental assessment. Although no single individual symptom is necessary for a person to receive a diagnosis of schizophrenia, according to the DSM-5, the persistent and debilitating presence of hallucinations, a hallucinated voice commenting on the individual, or hallucinated conversations between two voices is a strong indication of schizophrenia. The presence of delusions or hallucinations and loss of contact with reality is referred to as psychosis and is often present in schizophrenia, but psychotic symptoms can be seen in other mental disorders (for example, bipolar disorder or substance-induced psychotic disorder), so the term "psychosis" is not synonymous with the diagnosis of schizophrenia. The DSM-5 also notes that not one single symptom denotes a diagnosis of schizophrenia. In other words, two individuals may be diagnosed with the disorder and have different symptoms, which then make them look and act completely different from one another.

Although not emphasized by the DSM-5, international and cross-cultural study of the symptoms of schizophrenia has noted that the most frequently observed symptom in schizophrenia is patients' lack of insight. That is, despite sometimes overwhelming evidence of gross abnormalities in perception and behavior, patients with schizophrenia are likely to deny that those problems are symptomatic of a disorder.

Each of these symptoms can take a variety of forms. Delusions are defined as false beliefs based on incorrect inferences about external reality. Delusions are classified based on the nature of their content. For example, grandiose delusions involve false beliefs about one's importance, power, or knowledge. The patient might express the belief that he or she is the most intelligent person in the world but that these special intellectual powers have gone unrecognized. As another example, persecutory delusions involve beliefs of being persecuted or conspired against by others. The patient might claim, for example, that there is a government plot to poison him or her.

Hallucinations are sensory experiences that occur in the absence of a real stimulus. In the case of auditory hallucinations, the patient may hear voices calling or conversing when there is no one in physical proximity. Visual hallucinations may involve seeing people who are deceased or seeing inanimate objects move on their own accord. Olfactory (smell) and tactile (touch) hallucinations are also possible.

The term "affect" is used to refer to observable behaviors that are the expression of an emotion. Affect is predominantly displayed in facial expressions. "Flat" affect describes a severe reduction in the intensity of emotional expressions, both positive and negative. Patients with flat affect may show no observable sign of emotion, even when experiencing a very joyful or sad event.

Among the symptoms of schizophrenia, abnormalities in the expression of thoughts are a central feature. When speech is incoherent, it is difficult for the listener to comprehend because it is illogical or incomplete. As an example, in response to the question "Where do you live?" one patient replied, "Yes, live! I haven't had much time in this or that. It is an area. In the same area. Mrs. Smith! If the time comes for a temporary space now or whatever." The term "loose associations" is applied to speech in which ideas shift from one subject to another subject that is completely unrelated. If the loosening of associations is severe, speech may be incoherent. As an illustration of loose associations, a patient described the meaning of "A rolling stone gathers no moss" by saying, "Inside your head there's a brain and it's round like a stone and when it spins around it can't make connections the way moss has little filaments."

With regard to speech, a variety of other abnormalities are sometimes shown by patients. They may use neologisms, which are new words invented by the patient to convey a special meaning. Some show clang associations, which involve the use of rhyming words in conversation: "Live and let live, that's my motto. You live and give and live-give." Abnormalities in the intonation and pace of speech are also common.

In addition to these symptoms, some patients manifest bizarre behaviors, such as odd, repetitive movements or unusual postures. Odd or inappropriate styles of dressing, such as wearing winter coats in the summer, may also occur in some patients. More deteriorated patients frequently show poor hygiene. To meet the diagnostic criteria for schizophrenia, the individual must show signs of disturbance for at least six months.

TYPES AND TREATMENT OF SCHIZOPHRENIA

Prior to the release of the DSM-5, clinicians recognized five subtypes of schizophrenia when making a diagnosis (the differentiation among these subtypes was based on the symptom profile, and the criteria for subtype designation were described in DSM-IV-TR). They were catatonic schizophrenia, disorganized schizophrenia, paranoid schizophrenia, residual schizophrenia, and undifferentiated schizophrenia. Because no one symptom is sufficient for a diagnosis of schizophrenia, patients vary in the numbers and the intensity of their symptoms. It was for this reason as well as the low reliability and poor validity in diagnosing and treating schizophrenics when using the subtypes that the subtypes were eliminated in the DSM-5.

In his writings shortly after the turn of the twentieth century, Eugen Bleuler often used the phrase "the group of schizophrenias," because he believed the disorder could be caused by a variety of factors. In other words, he believed that schizophrenia may not be a single disease entity. Today, some researchers and clinicians who work in the field take the same position. They believe that the differences among patients in symptom patterns and the course of the illness are attributable to differences in etiology.

Because schizophrenic symptoms have such a devastating impact on the individual's ability to function, family members often respond to the onset of symptoms by seeking immediate treatment. Clinicians, in turn, often respond by recommending hospitalization so that tests can be conducted and an appropriate treatment can be determined. Consequently, almost all patients who are diagnosed with schizophrenia are hospitalized at least once in their lives. The majority experience several hospitalizations.

Research on the long-term outcome of schizophrenia indicates that the illness is highly variable in its course. A minority of patients have only one episode of illness, then go into remission and experience no further symptoms. Unfortunately, however, the majority of patients have recurring episodes that require periodic rehospitalizations. The most severely ill never experience remission but instead show a chronic course of symptomatology. For these reasons, schizophrenia is viewed as having the poorest prognosis of all the major mental illnesses.

Prior to the 1950s, patients with schizophrenia were hospitalized for extended periods of time and frequently became institutionalized. There were only a few available somatic treatments, and those proved to be of little efficacy. Included among them were insulin coma therapy (the administration of large doses of insulin to induce coma), electroconvulsive therapy (the application of electrical current to the temples to induce a seizure), and prefrontal lobotomy (a surgical procedure in which the tracts connecting the frontal lobes to other areas of the brain are severed).

Also, in the 1950s, a class of drugs referred to as antipsychotic medications were discovered to be effective in treating schizophrenia. Antipsychotic drugs significantly reduce some of the symptoms of schizophrenia in many patients. The introduction of antipsychotic medications (also called neuroleptics) in combination with changes in public policy led to a dramatic decline in the number of patients in public mental hospitals. Antipsychotic medications have freed many patients from confinement in hospitals and have enhanced their chances for functioning in the community. Not all patients benefit from typical antipsychotic medications, and the discovery of new classes of medications has offered hope to patients and families. Despite the benefits of antipsychotic medications, they can also produce serious side effects, particularly tardive dyskinesia, a movement disorder associated in some patients with chronic use of typical antipsychotic medications.

The public policy that has contributed to the decline in the number of hospitalized patients with schizophrenia is the nationwide policy of deinstitutionalization. This policy, which has been adopted and promoted by most state governments in the years since 1970, emphasizes short-term hospitalizations, and it has involved the release of some patients who had been in institutions for many years. Unfortunately, the support services that were needed to facilitate the transition from hospital to community living were never put in place. Consequently, the number of homeless schizophrenic patients has increased dramatically. Some of these are patients whose family members have died or have simply lost touch with them. Other patients have withdrawn from contact with their families, despite efforts by concerned relatives to provide assistance. The plight of the homeless mentally ill is of great concern to mental health professionals.

HISTORY AND FUTURE DIRECTIONS

Writing in the late 1800s, the eminent physician Emil Kraepelin was among the first to document the symptoms and course of this illness, referring to it as dementia praecox (dementia of early life). Subsequently, Bleuler applied the term "schizophrenia," meaning splitting of the mind, to the disorder. Both Kraepelin and Bleuler assumed that organic factors were involved in developing schizophrenia. Contemporary research has confirmed this assumption; brain scans reveal that a significant proportion of schizophrenia patients do have organic abnormalities. The precise nature and cause of these abnormalities remain unknown.

In the majority of cases, the onset of schizophrenic symptoms occurs in late adolescence or early adulthood. The major risk period is between twenty and twenty-five years of age, but the period of risk extends well into adult life. The majority of individuals to not develop schizophrenia after the age of forty-five. For some patients, there are no readily apparent abnormalities prior to the development of illness. For others, however, the onset of schizophrenia is preceded by impairments in social, academic, or occupational functioning. Some are described by their families as having had adjustment problems in childhood. Childhood schizophrenia, which is defined as onset of schizophrenic symptoms prior to age thirteen, is relatively rare. It is estimated to occur in about one out of every ten thousand children. When schizophrenia is diagnosed in childhood, the same diagnostic criteria and treatments are applied.

Schizophrenia shows no clear pattern in terms of its distribution in the population. It occurs in both males and females, although it tends to have a slightly earlier onset in males than in females. The illness strikes individuals of all social, economic, and ethnic backgrounds. Some patients manifest high levels of intelligence and are excellent students prior to becoming ill; others show poor academic performance and signs of learning disability. Although the specific pathophysiology associated with schizophrenia remains obscure, the preponderance of evidence demonstrates a significant role for genetic factors in the risk for developing schizophrenia. According to the National Institute of Mental Health, schizophrenia occurs in roughly 1 percent of the general population, but it occurs in roughly 10 percent of individuals with a first-degree relative (parent, sibling) with the disorder. The risk increases when one has an identical twin with schizophrenia; that individual then has a 40–60 percent chance of developing the disorder.

Schizophrenia is an illness that has been recognized by medicine for more than a hundred years. During this time, only modest progress has been made in research on its etiology. Some significant advances have been achieved in treatment, however, and the prognosis for schizophrenia is better now than ever before. Moreover, there is reason to believe that the availability of new technologies for studying the central nervous system will speed the pace of further discovery.

FURTHER READING

Bleuler, Eugen. *Dementia Praecox: Or, The Group of Schizophrenias.* 1911. Albuquerque: American Institute for Psychological Research, 1990. Print.

Diagnostic and Statistical Manual of Mental Disorders: DSM-5. Washington: American Psychological Association, 2013. Print.

Duckworth, Ken. "Mental Illness Facts and Numbers." *NAMI.* National Alliance on Mental Illness, Mar. 2013. Web. 21 July 2014.

Gottesman, Irving I. *Schizophrenia Genesis: The Origins of Madness.* New York: W. H. Freeman, 1991. Print.

Herz, Marvin I., Samuel J. Keith, and John P. Docherty. *Psychosocial Treatment of Schizophrenia.* New York: Elsevier, 1990. Print.

Hirsch, Steven R., and Daniel R. Weinberger. *Schizophrenia.* Oxford: Blackwell Science, 2002. Print.

Kingdon, David G. , and Douglas Turkington. *Cognitive Therapy of Schizophrenia.* New York: Guilford Press, 2008. Print.

Kraepelin, Emil. *Clinical Psychiatry.* Translated by A. Ross Diefendorf. Delmar, N.Y.: Scholars' Facsimiles & Reprints, 1981. Print.

Maj, Mario, and Norman Sartorius. *Schizophrenia.* 2d ed. Hoboken, N.J.: John Wiley & Sons, 2003. Print.

Marder, Stephen R., and Vandra Chopra. *Schizophrenia.* New York: Oxford UP, 2014. Print.

Mueser, Kim T., and Dilip V. Jeste. *Clinical Handbook of Schizophrenia.* New York: Guilford Press, 2008. Print.

Neale, John M., and Thomas F. Oltmanns. *Schizophrenia.* New York: John Wiley & Sons, 1980. Print.

"Numbers of Americans Affected by Mental Illness." *NAMI.* National Alliance on Mental Illness, June 2014. Web. 20 July 2014..

Walker, Elaine F., ed. *Schizophrenia: A Life-Span Developmental Perspective.* San Diego, Calif.: Academic Press, 1991. Print.

"What is Schizophrenia?" *National Institute of Mental Health.* US Department of Health and Human Services, n.d. Web. 20 July 2014.

Elaine F. Walker; updated by Loring J. Ingraham

Seasonal affective disorder

Seasonal affective disorder is a form of major depressive disorder believed to exhibit two forms: winter depression, beginning in late fall or winter, and spring-onset, which continues through summer and fall.

INTRODUCTION

Seasonal affective disorder (SAD) became the focus of systematic scientific research in the early 1980's. Research originally focused on seasonal changes in mood that coincided with the onset of winter and became known as winter depression. Symptoms consistently identified by Norman Rosenthal and others as indicative of winter depression included hypersomnia, overeating, carbohydrate craving, and weight gain. Michael Garvey and others found the same primary symptoms and the following secondary ones: decreased libido, irritability, fatigue, anxiety, problems concentrating, and premenstrual sadness. Several researchers have found that winter depression is more of a problem at higher latitudes. Thomas Wehr and Rosenthal report on a description of winter depression by Frederick Cook during an expedition to Antarctica in 1898. While winter depression was the form of seasonal affective disorder that received the most initial attention, there is another variation that changes with the seasons.

Summer depression affects some people in the same way that winter depression affects others. Both are examples of seasonal affective disorder. According to Wehr and Rosenthal, symptoms of summer depression include agitation, loss of appetite, insomnia, and loss of weight. Many people with summer depression also have histories of chronic anxiety. As can be seen, the person with a summer depression experiences symptoms that are almost the opposite of the primary symptoms of winter depression.

To diagnose a seasonal affective disorder, there must be evidence that the symptoms vary according to a seasonal pattern. If seasonality is not present, the diagnosis of SAD cannot be made. In the Northern Hemisphere, the seasonal pattern for winter depression is for it to begin in November and continue unabated through March. Summer depression usually begins in May and continues through September. Siegfried Kasper and others reported that people suffering from winter depression outnumber those suffering from summer depression by 4.5 to 1. Wehr and Rosenthal reported that as people

come out of their seasonal depression they experience feelings of euphoria, increased energy, less depression, hypomania, and possibly mania.

Philip Boyce and Gordon Parker investigated seasonal affective disorder in Australia. Their interest was in determining whether seasonal affective disorder occurs in the Southern Hemisphere and, if so, whether it manifests the same symptoms and temporal relationships with seasons as noted in the Northern Hemisphere. Their results confirmed the existence of seasonal affective disorder with an onset coinciding with winter and remission coinciding with summer. Their study also provided evidence that seasonal affective disorder occurs independently of important holidays and celebrations, such as Christmas. There is also a subsyndromal form of seasonal affective disorder. This is usually seen in winter depression and represents a milder form of the disorder. It interferes with the person's life, although to a lesser degree than the full syndrome, and it is responsive to the primary treatment for seasonal affective disorder.

HYPOTHESES OF ETIOLOGY

Three hypotheses are being tested to explain seasonal affective disorder: the melatonin hypothesis, the circadian rhythm phase shift hypothesis, and the circadian rhythm amplitude hypothesis.

The melatonin hypothesis is based on animal studies and focuses on a chemical signal for darkness. During darkness, the hormone melatonin is produced in greater quantities; during periods of light, it is produced in lesser quantities. Increases in melatonin level occur at the onset of seasonal affective disorder (winter depression) and are thought to be causally related to the development of the depression.

The circadian rhythm phase shift hypothesis contends that the delay in the arrival of dawn disrupts the person's circadian rhythm by postponing it for a few hours. This disruption of the circadian rhythm is thought to be integral in the development of winter depression. Disruptions in the circadian rhythm are also related to secretion of melatonin.

The third hypothesis is the circadian rhythm amplitude hypothesis. A major tenet of this hypothesis is that the amplitude of the circadian rhythm is directly related to winter depression. Lower amplitudes are associated with depression and higher ones with normal mood states. The presence or absence of light has been an important determinant in the amplitude of circadian rhythms.

The melatonin hypothesis is falling out of favor. Rosenthal and others administered to volunteers in a double-blind study a drug known to suppress melatonin secretion and a placebo. Despite melatonin suppression, there was no difference in the degree of depression experienced by the two groups (drug and placebo). In addition, no difference was observed in melatonin rhythms when persons with SAD were compared with those not suffering from the disorder.

Nevertheless, scientists have continued to investigate the role played by neurological chemicals in the etiology of the disorder. Some of these studies have focused on the possible role of neurotransmitters such as serotonin, dopamine, and norepinephrine. It is known that these chemicals may play a role in some forms of depression. For example, low levels of serotonin have been linked with some disorders; similar depressed levels have been observed in SAD patients during the winter months. If at least some forms of SAD are linked to reduction in serotonin production or uptake, this would explain the craving for carbohydrates observed in some patients.

Association of SAD with reduced pharmacological agents does not exclude other possible causes. It is certainly possible that diagnosis of SAD encompasses a variety of disorders associated with several causes. Evidence for a genetic predisposition is also undergoing investigation and cannot be eliminated as a contributing factor. At least one study using adult twins has suggested that nearly 30 percent of SAD cases may have a genetic basis.

DIAGNOSIS OF SAD

Diagnosis is based on the description of the disorder as updated in the *Diagnostic and Statistical Manual of Mental Disorders: DSM-IV-TR* (rev. 4th ed., 2000). According to the manual, the presence of five specific symptoms typical of depression constitutes the criteria for diagnosis; these symptoms must have been present during a two-week interval prior to diagnosis. Symptoms include general daily depression, loss of interest in normal activities, significant loss of appetite, fatigue, insomnia, decreased ability in thinking or reasoning, and thoughts of suicide or death. To be diagnosed with SAD, the patient must exhibit among the symptoms either depression or loss of interest in normal activities. To differentiate SAD from other forms of depression, these symptoms must exhibit a seasonal pattern that has been experienced over a period of at least three years, with at least two of these periods occurring consecutively. Two forms of SAD have

been described. The more common type, affecting approximately 15 percent of the population at some period within their lifetime, is referred to as fall-onset or winter depression. Generally this form appears in late fall and lasts until the following spring. A less common form of SAD is typically a spring-onset form of depression. This form generally lasts throughout the summer into the following season.

Regardless of the form of SAD, for diagnostic purposes the depressed person must experience the beginning and ending of the depression during the sixty-day window of time at both the beginning and the ending of the seasons. The patient must not have been diagnosed with other forms of depression, though the incidence of SAD appears highest among patients with a history of mood disorders.

TREATMENT

Historically, light therapy or phototherapy has been the principal method of treatment for SAD. Studies have repeatedly shown that exposure of patients to bright light, at least 2,500 lux, has had some success in relieving the depression associated with the disorder. Such phototherapy sessions have generally consisted of two to four hours of exposure per day; similar results have been observed if the light intensity is increased to 10,000 lux, using treatment sessions as short as thirty minutes.

The major advantage of phototherapy is that it represents a nonpharmacological approach to treatment of the problem. However, as many as one-third of the patients exhibiting SAD do not respond to light therapy. Frequently, those patients who responded least well were those suffering from the highest degree of depression. The inclusion of negative air ionization in conjunction with light therapy has resulted in some degree of success with such patients.

A variety of pharmacological agents have been developed for treatment of SAD patients who show no response to conventional treatments. These includeSelective serotonin reuptake inhibitorsselective serotonin reuptake inhibitors (SSRIs) such as fluoxetine, paroxetine, and sertraline. Trials have been most successful when using these agents in combination with phototherapy, rather than either treatment alone.

EPIDEMIOLOGY OF SAD

Boyce and Parker, two Australian scientists, studied SAD in the Southern Hemisphere. Since the Southern Hemisphere has weather patterns reversed from those in the

Northern Hemisphere, and since holidays occurring during the winter in the Northern Hemisphere occur during the summer in the Southern Hemisphere, these researchers were able to reproduce Northern Hemisphere studies systematically while eliminating the possible influence of holidays, such as Christmas. Their findings support those of their colleagues in the Northern Hemisphere. There is a dependable pattern of depression beginning during autumn and early winter and ending in the late spring and early summer. The incidence of SAD is significantly greater in North America than in Europe, suggesting a possible genetic or climatic influence on appearance of the disorder.

It is important to study the prevalence of SAD to understand how many people are affected by it. Kasper and others investigated the prevalence of SAD in Montgomery County, Maryland, a suburb of Washington, D.C. The results of their study suggested that between 4.3 percent and 10 percent of the general population is affected to some extent. Mary Blehar and Rosenthal report data from research in New York City that between 4 percent and 6 percent of a clinical sample met the criteria for SAD. More significantly, between 31 percent and 50 percent of people responding to a survey reported changes to their life that were similar to those reported by SAD patients. There are strong indications that the overall prevalence rate for SAD is between 5 percent and 10 percent of the general population. As much as 50 percent of the population may experience symptoms similar to but less intense than those of SAD patients.

Prevalence studies have found that the female-to-male ratio for SAD is approximately 4 to 1. Gender differencesseasonal affective disorder The age of onset is about twenty-two. The primary symptoms of SAD overlap with other diagnoses that have a relatively high female-to-male ratio. For example, people diagnosed with winter depression frequently crave carbohydrate-loaded foods. In addition to carbohydrate-craving obesity, there is another serious disorder, bulimia nervosa, which involves binging on high-carbohydrate foods and has a depressive component. Bulimia nervosa is much more common in females than it is in males.

While most of the research has focused on SAD in adults, it has also been found in Childrenseasonal affective disorderchildren. Children affected with SAD seem to experience a significant decrease in their energy level as their primary symptom rather than the symptoms seen in adults. This is not unusual; in many disorders, children and adults experience different symptoms.

The winter variant of SAD is much more common than the summer variant. It appears that winter depression is precipitated by the reduction in light that accompanies the onset of winter. As a result, it is also quite responsive to phototherapy. Summer depression, the summer variant of SAD, is precipitated by increases in humidity and temperature associated with the summer months. This suggests a different (and currently unknown) mechanism of action for the two variations.

The importance of light in the development and treatment of the winter variant of SAD has been demonstrated in a variety of studies worldwide. The general finding is that people living in the higher latitudes are increasingly susceptible to SAD in the winter.

EARLY HISTORY OF SAD

The observation that seasons affect people's moods is not new. Hippocrates, writing in 400 b.c.e., noted in section 3 of his "Aphorisms" that, "Of natures (temperaments?), some are well- or ill-adapted for summer, and some for winter." What Hippocrates noticed (and many others since have noticed) is that there are differences in the way people experience the various seasons. Summer and winter are the most extreme seasons in terms of both light and temperature and, not surprisingly, are the seasons in which most people have problems coping.

As noted above, the physician Cook, on an expedition to Antarctica in 1898, noted that the crew experienced symptoms of depression as the days grew shorter. This same report (mentioned by Wehr and Rosenthal) revealed that "bright artificial lights relieve this to some extent." Emil Kraepelin reported in 1921 that approximately 5 percent of his patients with manic-depressive illness (bipolar disorder) also had a seasonal pattern to their depressions. The data from antiquity to the present strongly favor the existence of a form of mood disturbance associated with seasonal variation. Just as the observation of seasonal variations in mood and behavior dates back to antiquity, so does the use of light as a treatment. Wehr and Rosenthal report that light was used as a treatment nearly two thousand years ago. Not only was light used but also it was specified that the light was to be directed to the eyes.

In summary, seasonal affective disorder seems to have some degree of relationship to carbohydrate-craving obesity, bulimia nervosa, bipolar disorder, and premenstrual syndrome. It affects women more often than men and is more frequently seen covarying with winter than with summer. The winter variant is probably caused by changes in light; it is more severe in the higher latitudes. The summer variant seems to be attributable to intolerance of heat and humidity and would be more prevalent in the lower latitudes. Whether the cause is related to variation in circadian rhythms, abnormal levels of neurotransmitters, genetics, or combinations of these, reduced exposure to sunlight appears to be a major contributor.

FURTHER READING

Boyce, Philip, and Gordon Parker. "Seasonal Affective Disorder in the Southern Hemisphere." *American Journal of Psychiatry* 145, no. 1 (1988): 96-99. This study surveyed an Australian sample to determine the extent to which the people experienced symptoms of seasonal affective disorder and to see if the pattern was similar to that of people in the Northern Hemisphere. The results are presented as percentages and are easily understood. Addresses the issue of separating holidays from climatic changes and presents a table of symptoms for seasonal affective disorder.

Kasper, Siegfried, Susan L. Rogers, Angela Yancey, Patricia M. Schulz, Robert A. Skwerer, and Norman E. Rosenthal. "Phototherapy in Individuals with and Without Subsyndromal Seasonal Affective Disorder." *Archives of General Psychiatry* 46, no. 9 (1989): 837-844. This study extends research into seasonal variants of affective disorder to people who have less intense forms. Addresses issues of the difficulty of establishing adequate experimental control and practical implications for people with these disorders.

Kasper, Siegfried, Thomas A. Wehr, John J. Bartko, Paul A. Gaist, and Norman E. Rosenthal. "Epidemiological Findings of Seasonal Changes in Mood and Behavior." *Archives of General Psychiatry* 46, no. 9 (1989): 823-833. A thorough description of the major prevalence study on seasonal affective disorder. The statistics are fairly advanced, but the authors' use of figures and tables makes the results understandable. An extensive reference list is provided.

Lam, R. W. "An Open Trial of Light Therapy for Women with Seasonal Affective Disorder and Comorbid Bulimia Nervosa." *Journal of Clinical Psychiatry* 62, no. 3 (2001): 164-168. A discussion of the use of light therapy in the treatment of two of the more common psychiatric/mood disorders.

Partonen, Timo, ed. *Seasonal Affective Disorder: Practice and Research.* New York: Oxford University Press, 2001. Emphasis is on the clinical disorder of SAD. The first portion of the book deals primarily with presentation of the illness in a clinical situation; the second half of the text addresses research into SAD, including evidence for its physiological basis.

Rohan, Kelly J. *Coping with the Seasons: A Cognitive Behavioral Approach to Seasonal Affective Disorder Workbook.* New York: Oxford University Press, 2009. For the layperson, a simple but thorough description of "winter blues" and guidelines on how to deal with SAD symptoms.

Rosenthal, Norman E. *Winter Blues: Seasonal Affective Disorder—What It Is and How to Overcome It.* Rev. ed. New York: Guilford Press, 2006. A thorough description of SAD by an expert in the field. The author describes the clinical patterns associated with various degrees of the disorder.

Singer, Ethan. "Seasonal Affective Disorder: Autumn Onset, Winter Gloom." *Clinician Reviews*, November, 2001. The author provides an updated overview of the condition. In addition to epidemiological references, various physiological explanations for the disorder are discussed, as well as alternative treatments.

Wileman, S., et al. "Light Therapy for Seasonal Affective Disorder in Primary Care." *British Journal of Psychiatry* 178 (2001): 311-316. A clinical description of the disorder that includes a summary of the most popular method of treatment as well as a discussion of the efficacy of light therapy.

Wurtman, Richard J., and Judith J. Wurtman. "Carbohydrates and Depression." *Scientific American* 260 (January, 1989): 68-75. The authors provide a good review of seasonal affective disorder and the relationships that may exist between it and maladaptive behaviors. They also review the more important theories about the cause and treatment of seasonal affective disorder.

James T. Trent; updated by Richard Adler

SEE ALSO: Depression

Shingles

Reactivation of a viral infection within a nerve cell that causes a characteristic skin rash.

CAUSES AND SYMPTOMS

Shingles results from the same virus (varicella zoster) that causes chickenpox. All individuals who have had chickenpox are at risk for shingles. The disease most commonly affects those over fifty but can develop at any age. After initial manifestations of chickenpox, the virus remains dormant in sensory dorsal root ganglia. Each dorsal root receives sensation from a strip of skin on only one side of the body in a particular distribution called dermatome (map of the skin). Shingles outbreaks occur most commonly on the back, along the distribution of a single dermatome wrapping around one side to the chest or abdomen. They may travel from the upper back to the arm or from the lower back to the leg. Shingles can also occur on the face and rarely can involve the optic nerve of the eye.

The virus can stay inactive in the nerve root for decades. It is reactivated by stress, illness, decrease in immune function, or aging. The first symptom is often a sensation of tingling, burning, or sharp pain over the skin area supplied by the affected nerve root. Within several days, a rash appears, characterized by a cluster of blisters with surrounding redness spreading along the dermatomal pattern. The rash typically does not cross the midline. The blisters scab over in about three days and clear within several weeks. Until the blisters are completely scabbed over, the fluid within the blisters can be contagious via contact. Shingles cannot be acquired from contact exposure, but people who have never had chickenpox can develop chickenpox following exposure to the shingles rash.

The fluid within the blister may be sampled for viral culture to obtain an accurate diagnosis. The diagnosis can usually be made clinically by the characteristic rash. In rare cases, generally in the elderly, nerve pain may persist for months to years after disappearance of the rash, a condition called postherpetic neuralgia.

TREATMENT AND THERAPY

If shingles is diagnosed within three days of appearance of the rash, then antiviral medications (acyclovir, famciclovir, or valacyclovir) can be used to stop viral replication and help shorten the course of the illness. Treatment

---

INFORMATION ON SHINGLES

Causes: Viral infection with varicella zoster; triggered by stress, illness, decrease in immune function, aging
Symptoms: Tingly, burning, or sharp pain; rash with blisters
Duration: Three days to several weeks
Treatments: Antiviral medications (acyclovir, famciclovir, valacyclovir); pain relief (cool compresses, anti-inflammatory drugs, mild narcotics)

---

also involves pain control with local cool compresses, anti-inflammatory medications, or even mild narcotics. Gabapentin, a drug similar in structure to an inhibitory neurotransmitter, gammaaminobutyric acid (GABA), is useful against pain experienced in postherpetic neuralgia.

In 2006, Zostavax (zoster vaccine live) was approved for use in the United States to reduce the risk of shingles in older adults. The vaccine is only a preventive measure and does not treat ongoing shingles.

PERSPECTIVE AND PROSPECTS

The association between chickenpox and shingles was first made in 1888. The virus belongs to a family of viruses called herpes, which is derived from the Greek word herpein, meaning "to creep."

Because more than 90 percent of adults in the United States harbor the varicella zoster virus, diseases caused by the virus remain significant clinical problems, particularly in the elderly and those with compromised immune systems. Although vaccination, antiviral therapy, and symptomatic therapies provide effective prevention and treatment to many patients, further research on varicella virus and improved therapies continues.

FURTHER READING

Chen, T., S. George, C. Woodruff, and S. Hsu. "Clinical Manifestations of Varicella-Zoster Virus Infection." *Dermatology Clinics* 20, no. 2 (April 1, 2002): 267-282.

Gnann J. W., Jr., and R. J. Whitley. "Herpes Zoster." *New England Journal of Medicine* 347 (August 1, 2002): 340-346.

Goldman, Lee, and Dennis Ausiello, eds. *Cecil Textbook of Medicine*. 23d ed. Philadelphia: Saunders/Elsevier, 2007.

Mandell, Gerald L., John E. Bennett, and Raphael Dolin, eds. *Mandell, Douglas, and Bennett's Principles and Practice of Infectious Diseases*. 7th ed. New York: Churchill Livingstone/Elsevier, 2010.

Stankus, S. "Management of Herpes Zoster (Shingles) and Postherpetic Neuralgia." *American Family Physician* 61, no. 8 (April 15, 2000): 2437-2444, 2447-2448.

VZV Research Foundation. http://www.vzvfoundation.org.

Veronica N. Baptista, updated by W. Michael Zawada

SEE ALSO: Rashes; Skin Disorders

Skin disorders

Diseases and conditions that affect the skin, ranging from harmless to life-threatening.

ANATOMY OF THE SKIN

The skin is the largest organ of the body. It provides a barrier between the external world and the internal world: It protects against external contamination and helps to maintain the sterility of the internal body. The skin also assists in temperature regulation; humans can survive only within a narrow temperature range. The skin has nerve receptors that supply the brain with information, providing an interface with the world. There are specialized receptors for touch, temperature, vibration, and position in space (proprioception).

Appendages to the skin are fingernails, toenails, and hair. They are mainly of psychological importance. Nails protect the tips of fingers and toes in humans but are not needed for protection as claws are in lower animals. Hair is analogous to feathers. In birds, tiny muscles attached to the base of each feather cause them to be ruffled; this creates air pockets and allows birds to conserve heat and keep warm. The same muscles persist in humans, causing "goose flesh," but they do not serve any other function. The main importance of these appendages is cosmetic. For example, people spend billions of dollars on hair care products each year. The motivation for this activity is psychological.

The two main layers in skin are the epidermis and dermis. The epidermis is the upper or outermost layer, and cells are continually formed at its base. As new cells are formed, existing cells are pushed toward the surface of the skin. These cells gradually lose their watery central contents, causing them to dry out (desiccate) and become flattened. This process normally spans approximately a month. Thus, the surface of the body is largely composed of dead cells that have become flattened. These cells are normally lost on a continual basis and create dandruff when shed from the scalp. On other parts of the body, sloughed cells provide excellent conditions for bacterial growth, accounting for the unpleasant odors that accompany poor hygiene habits. Two other important types of cells are found in the epidermis: melanocytes and Langerhans cells. Melanocytes contain melanin and provide all the variations of pigmentation found in the human species. They multiply when stimulated by the ultraviolet radiation in sunlight. This causes the skin to become darker, a protective mechanism against damage from ultraviolet radiation. Langerhans cells contain surface receptors for immunoglobulins. They play a central role in allergic reactions of the skin, such as contact dermatitis or delayed hypersensitivity reaction.

The dermis is an inner layer of skin located beneath the epidermis. Its main function is protection. Within the dermis are highly specialized cells containing microscopic filaments. These cells impart tensile strength to the skin in much the same way that fibers strengthen fiberglass or reinforcing steel mesh strengthens concrete. Because they are so dense, they also serve as a barrier to the entry of most pathogens and many chemicals. Eccrine sweat glands are found in the dermis throughout the entire body. These produce a salty secretion (essentially salt water) that assists in thermoregulation through evaporative cooling. They are also sensitive to emotional stress. Apocrine sweat glands are primarily in the armpits (axilla) and groin and produce a milky secretion. When these secretions are broken down by bacteria on the surface of the skin, a characteristic odor is produced. The bases of hair follicles are also found in the dermis. The small sebaceous, or oil-secreting, gland associated with most hair follicles has the function of softening and moisturizing the hair.

Hair is found on most surfaces of the body; exceptions are the palms of the hands, the soles of the feet, and the glans penis in men. The texture and length of the hair vary with location on the body, gender, genetic heritage, and age. Dramatic increases in the growth and distribution of hair occur at puberty. With increasing age, hair is typically lost from the scalp and other body parts. It also changes color, assuming a gray or white color because of the loss of melanin at the base of the hair follicle.

COMPLICATIONS AND DISORDERS

When normal skin anatomy and physiology are upset, several common diseases or disorders result. When the barrier provided by the skin is broken, bacteria, viruses, fungi, and other pathogens can invade the body, leading to infections. Locally, these infections can cause inflammation (redness and pain) of the skin; if widespread, they can lead to systemic infections. When the cells and other substances found in the skin become irregular or are abnormal, skin disorders or conditions result.

Skin disorders and conditions. Pigmentation of the skin results from the presence of melanocytes, cells that manufacture and contain melanin. Most humans have pigmentation over their entire bodies; the degree of pigmentation varies with different racial and ethnic groups. Local areas of increased color have a range of names depending on the size of the pigmented area. A freckle is small and discrete. A nevus is a larger area of hyperpigmentation. These conditions are attributable to underlying variations in the distribution of melanocytes. They are genetic in origin and permanent; they are also accentuated by exposure to sunlight. Melasmas are irregular, flat, light brown areas on the neck, cheeks, or forehead. They are caused by hormonal changes associated with pregnancy or contraceptive pills and by exposure to sunlight. Melasmas fade with the reduction of excess hormones. There are also color changes in the labia of females during pregnancy; these changes are both harmless and permanent.

Generalized increases in skin coloration can occur with some metabolic diseases. Addison's disease involves an increase in melanocyte-stimulating hormone. This leads to an overall bronzing of the body, with accentuation in creases of the palms and soles. The condition subsides with treatment of the underlying cause of the disease. Similar pigment increases are associated with some forms of lung cancer, hemochromatosis, and chronic arsenic exposure. The latter two conditions are caused by the deposition of iron (hemochromatosis) and arsenic in the skin.

Generalized decreases in skin coloration can also occur. If melanocytes fail to migrate to the skin during embryologic development, hair follicles will lack color, resulting in a condition called piebaldism. Characteristically, this is a white patch in the hair of the forehead. Vitiligo is caused by an immunologically mediated loss of melanocytes. Individuals with phenylketonuria (PKU) experience a generalized depigmentation of hair and eye color, in addition to mental retardation, if the condition is not adequately and promptly treated. An individual totally lacking melanocytes is called an albino; because melanin is also responsible for eye color, albinos have red eyes. The loss of hair is called alopecia. It can occur because of aging, sustained pulling on the hair with some hairstyles, and genetics. Women do not usually experience much alopecia until after the menopause. Conversely, some men start to lose their hair during their twenties.

Skin diseases. Eczema or dermatitis is a general term that describes a skin disease involving vesicles that ooze fluid. These conditions are usually characterized by a rash; they are inflammatory reactions, commonly caused by contact with a chemical or plant material. They can be caused by an adverse reaction to a drug or by sunlight. Bacteria, yeasts, or other fungi on the skin can cause eczema. Most rashes itch or burn; they can be spread by scratching. Athlete's foot is a common example of an eczematous dermatitis.

Maculopapular diseases encompass several common skin conditions, such as red measles (rubeola), German measles (rubella), and scarlet fever. Viruses that land on the skin cause these diseases. They are characterized by relatively large, localized areas of changed skin color (macules) that are also raised (papules) but not fluid-filled. After their clinical course is run, they disappear without leaving a scar. The more dangerous toxic shock syndrome also belongs to this group of diseases; it is caused by toxin from the bacteria *Staphylococcus aureus*.

Thickening of the skin and the formation of red to purple areas having sharply defined borders characterize papulosquamous skin diseases. The most common example is psoriasis. Other examples are pityriasis and ichthyosis. The pathology responsible for psoriasis is an alteration in the normal development of skin cells. In individuals with psoriasis, new skin cells develop and migrate to the surface in only five days instead of the usual thirty. This fact alone explains the flaking (rapid cell turnover), redness (thinner skin and a rich blood supply for new skin), and pain and itching (less protection for sensory nerve endings) experienced. Pityriasis includes a group of different conditions caused by different viruses. Patches or large spots develop on the skin. They usually resolve within a few weeks. Aside from being locally photosensitive, they usually are not serious. Ichthyosis describes a group of genetic conditions characterized by extreme scaling of the skin.

Vesiculobullous diseases have fluid-filled blisters that can vary in size from relatively small (vesicles) to

---

INFORMATION ON SKIN DISORDERS

Causes: Infection, disease, allergies, environmental factors (e.g., ultraviolet radiation), hormonal changes, irritation, clogged sweat glands, eczema
Symptoms: May include inflammation, infection, flaking, pain, itching, redness, rashes, lesions, bleeding
Duration: Acute to chronic
Treatments: Topical ointments, antibiotics, corticosteroids, surgery, chemotherapy, radiation therapy

---

relatively large (bullae). Insect bites, herpes, and some bacterial infections lead to the formation of vesicles or bullae. Such conditions are attributable to an immune reaction that leads to the formation of blisters at the junction between epidermis and dermis. They can be accompanied by intense pruritus (itching); scratching often leads to scarring.

Pustular diseases of the skin include acne, folliculitis, and candidiasis. They are characterized by the inflammation of hair follicles caused by surface bacteria or yeasts. Adequate personal hygiene is the most effective method of prevention. These diseases are usually not serious, but prolonged or repeated attacks can result in scarring and disfigurement. The sebaceous glands, which secrete oil at the base of hair follicles, can increase in size. The subsequent increase in oil output worsens the condition.

Clogged sweat glands can lead to acne. While this is primarily a problem for teenagers, it can affect individuals of any age. Exposure to cutting oils and other hydrocarbons such as gasoline and paint thinners can cause a similar condition called chloracne, which is inflammation in the base of hair follicles found on exposed skin in areas such as the nape of the neck, forearms, and face. The inability to sense temperature and regulate body heat through sweating is called anhidrosis, a condition that can cause shock and potentially death.

Other diseases that can affect the skin. Five such diseases are worthy of mention: leprosy, scleroderma, lupus, atherosclerosis, and diabetes mellitus. Leprosy, or Hansen's disease, is caused by infection by *Mycobacterium leprae*, a relative of the bacteria that cause tuberculosis. In leprosy, the causative organism accumulates in the skin and peripheral nerves. This causes disfigurement and loss of sensation, the latter being similar to that experienced by an uncontrolled diabetic.

Disfigurement is responsible for the stigma associated with leprosy since ancient times: loss of fingers and toes, as well as mutilation of the nose and ears. Leprosy is caused by long-term association with the organism and can be adequately treated with appropriate antibiotics.

Scleroderma (literally, "hard skin") is an uncommon disease characterized by fibrosis of the skin and involvement of visceral organs. The skin involvement can range from an isolated, hardened patch to a life-threatening, generalized condition described as an ever-tightening case of steel. The skin becomes stretched tightly over the underlying skeleton. Skin tone is lost with restriction of movement.

Systemic lupus erythematosus is a disease of unknown etiology that is characterized by inflammation in many different organ systems. The skin is usually involved, as nearly all individuals with lupus develop a characteristic butterflyshaped rash on their faces. This red coloration covers the cheeks and nose. Persons with lupus are also sensitive to sunlight, and many develop alopecia. Most of those affected are female. The disease waxes and wanes; treatment depends on the particular organs involved.

Atherosclerosis and diabetes can block the arteries supplying the nerves of the skin, leading to a loss of sensory input. When the patient is unable to experience pain, cuts and other abrasions on the skin are not noticed. Untreated, these lesions can lead to gangrene, sometimes requiring amputation of a body part.

Skin cancer. The most commonly diagnosed form of cancer is that involving the skin. It is not the most fatal form, but millions of cases are discovered annually. The origin of most skin cancers can be traced to excessive exposure to radiation from the sun. They can occur on any surface of the body, although they are more common on areas that are usually exposed to the sun, such as the face, the backs of the hand, and the neck. Skin cancers can arise in the epidermis or dermis. The majority are noncancerous, or benign. Epidermal nodules are characterized by local thickening of the epidermis, often accompanied by scaling of the skin in the affected area. Nodules in the dermis may appear as lumps with no alteration of the epidermis above them.

There are three malignant forms of skin cancer. Basal cell carcinoma arises from cells deep in the epidermis. This form of tumor rarely spreads (metastasizes), but it can be extensive and destructive locally. Squamous cell carcinoma is less common but can be invasive (involving adjacent tissues) and can metastasize. Melanoma is relatively uncommon but can grow extremely rapidly; it has the potential to be fatal in a matter of months. It involves the uncontrolled growth of melanocytes. Melanomas have irregular borders and color or pigmentation. Any pigmented lesion or suspicious change in the skin should be evaluated by a medical professional in a timely manner.

Prevention is the preferred method of dealing with skin cancer. When outside, loose-fitting clothing can provide protection from the sun, and a hat can protect the head. When exposure is unavoidable, a product with a sun-blocking agent will reduce exposure. Limiting the time of exposure to the sun until the body has reacted by producing additional melanocytes (tanned) is recommended.

Prolonged exposure to the sun also accelerates changes in the skin associated with aging. Collagen fibers provide the characteristic firm feel to the skin of a young person. With aging the skin becomes less firm, losing some of its tone, and begins to sag. Inadequate moisture also contributes to the loss of skin tone. Excessive exposure to the sun hastens both of these processes.

FURTHER READING

Burns, Tony, et al., eds. *Rook's Textbook of Dermatology.* 7th ed. Malden, Mass.: Blackwell Science, 2004. This is a core text in dermatology that will appeal to professionals and members of the general public who want a concise introduction to the subject. The aim of the book is to integrate basic science with clinical practice.

Frankel, David H., ed. *Field Guide to Clinical Dermatology.* 2d ed. Philadelphia: Lippincott Williams & Wilkins, 2006. Frankel, a noted internist and dermatologist, has enlisted widely respected and talented colleagues to help in the production of this book. It is a uniquely organized and easily readable field guide complete with 220 pages of excellent color illustrations.

Freinkel, Ruth K., and David T. Woodley, eds. *Biology of the Skin.* New York: Parthenon, 2001. Covers the basic biology of the skin, how the skin functions, effects of the environment, the molecules that direct cutaneous function, genetic influences, and methods in cutaneous research.

Goldsmith, Lowell A., Gerald S. Lazarus, and Michael D. Tharp. *Adult and Pediatric Dermatology: A Color Guide to Diagnosis and Treatment.* Philadelphia: F. A. Davis, 1997. This book provides excellent pictures to accompany good descriptions of dermatologic diseases.

Grob, J. J., et al., eds. *Epidemiology, Causes, and Prevention of Skin Diseases.* Cambridge, Mass.:

Blackwell Science, 1997. This well written book presents data on large groups of people. The sections on skin cancer are especially noteworthy.

Kenet, Barney, and Patricia Lawler. *Saving Your Skin: Prevention, Early Detection, and Treatment of Melanoma and Other Skin Cancers.* 2d ed. Chicago: FourWalls EightWindows, 1998. Skin cancer is the focus of this title, which reviews the early symptoms of melanoma, its causes, and its treatment. Very few skin care titles do more than offer a chapter on the problem.

Sams, W. Mitchell, Jr., and Peter J. Lynch, eds. *Principles and Practice of Dermatology.* 2d ed. London: Churchill Livingstone, 1996. This is a new edition of a dermatology reference guide and text emphasizing accurate diagnosis by succinct discussions in eighty-five presentations featuring color photographs.

Weedon, David. *Skin Pathology.* 3d ed. New York: Churchill Livingstone/Elsevier, 2010. Text with extensive photographs, covering tissue reaction patterns; the epidermis, dermis, and subcutis; the skin in systemic and miscellaneous diseases; infections and infestations; and tumors, among other topics.

L. Fleming Fallon, Jr.

SEE ALSO: Acne; Allergies; Blisters; Eczema; Rashes; Psoriasis

Sleep disorders

Sleep disorders are a group of disorders that affect the quantity or quality of sleep. They often cause severe daytime consequences including chronic sleepiness, fatigue, impairments in cognitive functioning such as attention, concentration and memory, and mood difficulties including depression and anxiety. Sleep disorders may be physiological or psychological in nature.

INTRODUCTION

Although most individuals have experienced a bad night of sleep, individuals with a sleep disorder regularly have a disturbance in either or both, their sleep quality and quantity, and consequently suffer from severe daytime impairments. Certain sleep disorders have well-determined causes and evidence-based treatments that are highly effective, while others have causes that are less clear and treatments dependent on the individual's experience. The following presents information regarding five of the most common sleep disorders: insomnia, sleep-disordered breathing, narcolepsy, restless legs syndrome, and circadian rhythm disorders.

INSOMNIA

Insomnia has been commonly defined as the experience of having difficulty falling asleep, staying asleep, waking too early, or waking feeling unrefreshed that leads to daytime consequences. These daytime consequences may include daytime sleepiness, fatigue, irritability, feelings of depression or anxiety, difficulty concentrating, or impaired memory. According to the *Diagnostic and Statistical Manual of Mental Disorders (DSM-5),* these symptoms are typically present for 30 minutes or more for at least 3 days per week for 3 months or longer. An episode of insomnia may be provoked by an obvious trigger, such as a drastic change in personal or professional environment including marriage, divorce, death, change in career, or new child, medical illnesses, or certain types of medication. However, there may also be no identifiable trigger. Treatment for insomnia can take many forms, including medication sleep aids, or psychological therapies such as cognitive-behavioral therapy for insomnia, an evidence-based treatment that has shown very high efficacy and effectiveness in treating symptoms of insomnia.

SLEEP-DISORDERED BREATHING

Sleep-disordered breathing is a term for a collection of disorders that disrupt sleep as a result of multiple, brief periods of cessation of breathing. Obstructive sleep apnea, one of the more common forms of sleep-disordered breathing, occurs when the soft palette in the throat relaxes and blocks the airway during sleep. When this happens, breathing becomes difficult and sometimes impossible. When breathing is prevented, it triggers the individual to awaken in order to gasp for breath. These awakenings are often so brief that the individual is not even aware that breathing has stopped, or that they have been awake. Once breathing has resumed, the individual typically falls back asleep immediately, and the cycle begins again. According to the American Academy of Sleep Medicine, while mild sleep apnea is defined as 5-15 apneas, or cessations of breath, per hour, the most severe cases of sleep apnea can result in the individual waking more than 30 times per hour. This fragmentation of sleep can lead to both physiological and psychological consequences, including increased blood pressure and incidence of cardiovascular disease, chronic daytime sleepiness, fatigue, difficulty with attention, concentration, memory, and depression.

Although the exact causes of obstructive sleep apnea are not completely understood, rates of sleep apnea increase with increased age and weight. Additionally, because the relaxation of the muscles in the throat has been implicated in the manifestation of the disorder, an overall decrease in muscle tone within the body can result in the onset of sleep apnea. Physicians have established a brief measure used to determine the likelihood of having sleep apnea. The STOP-BANG includes questions with regard to snoring, tiredness, observations of cessation of breath during sleep, increased blood pressure, BMI score, age, neck circumference and gender. Although measures like the STOP-BANG are useful in identifying potential sleep apnea patients, formal diagnosis can only be made following an overnight sleep study including polysomnography.

Various treatments, including oral appliances, surgery and continuous positive airway pressure, have been developed for sleep apnea, and can be selected according to the comfort of the patient. Oral appliances are fitted by dentists and help re-align the jaw in order to keep the airway more open during sleep. Oral surgery can also be performed to reduce the size of the soft palette including the uvula, although the long term effectiveness of the treatment has been debated. To date, the most common and effective treatment for sleep apnea is the use of continuous positive airway pressure, or CPAP. CPAP is a device worn typically over the nose and mouth that utilizes pressurized air to keep the soft palette in place in order to keep the airway open. In order to be effective, however, the patient must continue to use CPAP throughout the course of the disorder.

NARCOLEPSY

Narcolepsy is a disorder that affects the regulation of the sleep/wake cycle producing excessive daytime sleepiness. Symptoms can, but do not always, include cataplexy, hypnogogic hallucinations and sleep paralysis. Cataplexy, one of the diagnostic symptoms of narcolepsy, is defined as a sudden loss of muscle tone prompted by strong emotion such as laughter or sadness. The loss of muscle tone can range from mild to severe weakness in limbs, with potentially complete loss of tone resulting in collapse. Hypnogogic hallucinations are visual or auditory perceptions in the absence of real stimuli which typically occur while the individual is falling asleep or waking up. Sleep paralysis, the last of the "tetrad of narcolepsy" is the phenomenon whereby the individual experiences the inability to move upon waking.

The cause of narcolepsy is now considered to be mainly genetic. Although the cause is genetic, diagnosis of narcolepsy does not rely on genetic testing. Instead, a combination of sleep measures is utilized including overnight polysomnography and the Multiple Sleep Latency Test (MSLT). The MSLT consists of an individual coming to a sleep laboratory during the day. Individuals are then given the opportunity to nap, every two hours, after having had a full night of sleep, the night before. Technicians monitor polysomnography to look for the signs and symptoms of narcolepsy, sleep onset latency, or how fast the individual falls asleep, and REM latency, or how fast the individual takes to begin REM sleep. Because of the excessive daytime sleepiness associated with the disorder, individuals with narcolepsy will typically show very fast sleep onset latency, and will enter REM faster than healthy individuals.

Treatment for narcolepsy involves treating each of the presenting symptoms separately. One can manage excessive sleepiness by utilizing stimulants, stimulant-like medications or napping regimens. Additionally, symptoms of cataplexy can be treated with two classes of antidepressant medications, tricyclics or selective serotonin reuptake inhibitors (SSRI's). Although there is no known cure for narcolepsy, successfully managing daytime sleepiness and cataplexy can allow an individual to lead a relatively asymptomatic life.

RESTLESS LEGS SYNDROME
Restless legs syndrome (RLS) is a disorder affecting the muscles in the legs during rest or at night, in the period just prior to sleep. According to the American Academy of Sleep Medicine, RLS results in an irresistible urge to move one's legs in order to reduce or eliminate painful or uncomfortable sensations in the legs. During the night, many individuals with RLS will experience periodic limb movements (PLM), where one will move their legs during sleep causing sleep fragmentation and disruption. The occurrence of PLM can be detected objectively using overnight polysomnography, but is not necessary for diagnosis. Although there are genetic factors that contribute to RLS, many cases have been found to be associated with iron deficiency. Certain types of medications may also lead to increased incidence or worsening of RLS.

Treatment of RLS can vary according to the severity of the disorder. In cases where iron deficiency is noted, iron supplements may alleviate or prevent symptoms. For more severe cases, or those that may not respond to treatment with iron, medications such as dopaminergic agents may improve both daytime symptoms and sleep quality. However, there are significant side effects associated with these types of medications, and they should not be used for the long-term management of RLS.

CIRCADIAN RHYTHM DISORDERS
Two of the most researched and common circadian rhythm disorders are advanced sleep phase syndrome (ASPS) and delayed sleep phase syndrome (DSPS). These two disorders, although manifesting at different times of day, are conceptually similar, in that they are disorders that prevent individuals from going to sleep or waking up at their preferred time. Individuals with ASPS feel excessively sleepy early in the evening, and as a result fall asleep and wake up earlier than they prefer. In contrast, individuals with DSPS, do not feel sleepy at their desired bedtime, and instead go to bed and wake up much later than preferred.

Treatment of circadian rhythm disorders, ASPS and DSPS, utilizes a variety of methods including chronotherapy, light therapy, or the use of melatonin supplements. Chronotherapy is the use of scheduled sleep/wake times in order to alter natural body rhythms. Chronotherapy can be used to treat ASPS and DSPS by moving scheduled bedtimes and wake times later, by an hour or more every day, until the preferred bed time can be achieved. As treatment for DSPS, chronotherapy involves moving the bedtime completely around the clock, eventually allowing one to achieve an "earlier" bedtime. This form of chronotherapy, however, may not be appropriate for all individuals since it can be very disruptive to a work or school schedule. Light therapy consists of the utilization of a light box which emits bright light. Bright light suppresses melatonin onset, which causes sleepiness and prompts sleep onset. With regard to ASPS, if melatonin is suppressed at night, sleep onset may occur later, at a more preferred time. In contrast, when light therapy is used in the morning, sleepiness may be decreased, allowing the individual to wake earlier, at a more preferred wake time. Lastly, as treatment for DSPS, melatonin supplements can be taken in the evening to mimic the naturally occurring process by which melatonin entrains the sleep/wake cycle, allowing sleep to occur earlier.

FURTHER READING

Allen, R. P., Picchietti, D., Hening, W. A., Trenkwalder, C., Walters, A. S., & Montplaisi, J. (2003). "Restless Legs Syndrome: Diagnostic Criteria, Special Considerations, and Epidemiology: A Report From the Restless Legs Syndrome Diagnosis and Epidemiology workshop at the National Institutes of Health". *Sleep Medicine*, 4(2), 101-119. The seminal paper describing the causes, treatments, and significance of restless legs syndrome.

Dauvilliers, Y., Arnulf, I., & Mignot, E. (2007). "Narcolepsy with Cataplexy". *The Lancet*, 369(9560), 499-511. A scientific article thoroughly describing narcolepsy with cataplexy.

Hening, W., Allen, R., Earley, C., Kushida, C., Picchietti, D., & Silber, M. (1999). "The Treatment of Restless Legs Syndrome and Periodic Limb Movement Disorder". An American Academy of Sleep Medicine Review. *Sleep*, 22(7), 970-999.

Mellinger, G. D., Balter, M. B., & Uhlenhuth, E. H. (1985). "Insomnia and Its Treatment: Prevalence and Correlates". *Archives of general psychiatry*, 42(3), 225-232. A scientific report describing an epidemiological sample of insomnia patients and selected treatments.

Sack, R. L., Auckley, D., Auger, R. R., Carskadon, M. A., Wright Jr, K. P., Vitiello, M. V., & Zhdanova, I. V. (2007). "Circadian Rhythm Sleep Disorders: Part I, Basic Principles, Shift Work and Jet Lag Disorders An American Academy of Sleep Medicine Review": An American Academy of Sleep Medicine Review. *Sleep*, 30(11), 1460.

Sack, R. L., Auckley, D., Auger, R. R., Carskadon, M. A., Wright Jr, K. P., Vitiello, M. V., & Zhdanova, I. V. (2007). "Circadian Rhythm Sleep Disorders: Part II, Advanced Sleep Phase Disorder, Delayed Sleep Phase Disorder, Free-Running Disorder, and Irregular Sleep-Wake Rhythm: An American Academy of Sleep Medicine review. *Sleep*, 30(11), 1484. This two-part review describes circadian rhythm disorders in detail.

Young, T., Peppard, P. E., & Gottlieb, D. J. (2002). "Epidemiology of Obstructive Sleep Apnea: A Population Health Perspective". *American journal of respiratory and critical care medicine*, 165(9), 1217-1239. A highly-cited study examining the incidence, health consequences and treatment of obstructive sleep apnea.

Jennifer R. Goldschmied and Patricia J. Deldin

SEE ALSO: Dreams; Insomnia; Sleeping Sickness; Sleepwalking

Spina bifida

A birth defect that results from a mistake early in the development of the spinal cord.

CAUSES AND SYMPTOMS

The development of the fetal nervous system is the most complicated process during pregnancy. It starts a few weeks after conception and continues until well after birth. The earliest steps are the most crucial, because the basic plan of the nervous system must be established accurately if it is to work properly later.

The central nervous system begins with the formation of a thickened layer of tissue, called the neural plate, along the back of the embryo. The edges of this plate curl up to form ridges, and the whole plate rolls up into a slender tube running from the head to the rump. This cylinder is then covered over by tissues that will form the surface of the back. The front end of this tube will soon expand to become the brain, and the rest of the tube will form the spinal cord. In order for these processes to proceed properly, the tube must seal itself along its entire length. If there are any gaps where the tube does not close, it will leak and will not be able to expand and develop properly. Without such expansion, all the later stages of nervous system development will also be prevented from occurring properly.

If the neural tube fails to seal, a small opening called a neuropore will remain at some point along its length. Depending on where the opening is, a variety of abnormalities can result. When the posterior region of the neural tube fails to close, the result is spina bifida. This flaw in the neural tube in turn affects the assembly of the muscle, bone, and skin in this region. In spina bifida, which means "divided spine," the vertebrae of the backbone do not join together properly.

The severity of spina bifida depends on how much damage has been done to the lower spinal cord region. In its mildest form, the only evidence of a problem may be that two of the bones in the spine fail to form quite right. If several vertebrae are involved, the membranes that protect the surface of the spinal cord can bulge outward, forming a ball-like mass in this region. The problems that result depend on how much of the spinal membrane is involved in this bulge. In the most severe cases, the vertebrae fail to protect the spinal cord, so that the nervous tissue itself is also involved and an opening to the outside remains at the base of the spinal cord. Additional problems with nervous system development may result, including improper fluid balances in the brain (hydrocephalus).

Because the brain and spinal column fail to develop properly in spina bifida, a variety of mental, behavioral, and physical symptoms can result. The nerve connections at the base of the spine are likely to be affected, resulting in paralysis in the lower back and legs, problems with bladder and bowel function, and loss of sensation. Because the development of the brain can also be affected, mental abilities may be impaired.

TREATMENT AND THERAPY

Effective measures have been developed to minimize the effects of spina bifida. Often, surgery is performed within twenty-four to forty-eight hours of birth to close any opening in the child's lower back and to reconstruct the spine and other tissues in this area. Problems with feet and legs may also be dealt with surgically. If the child has symptoms of hydrocephalus, the excess fluid will be drained. Bladder and bowel function will be regulated, such as by catheterization. Eventually, prosthetic devices may be fitted to assist the child's movement. Mental health and physical therapy experts will also be involved to assist in overcoming learning hurdles, monitoring physical development and training, and making emotional adjustments.

PERSPECTIVE AND PROSPECTS

Spina bifida has been known since ancient times, but little could be done then to ease the mental and physical damage that it causes. By the 1960s, surgical procedures were being developed that could repair the damage to the spinal cord and other parts of the lower back. Improvements in physical therapy methods, as well as improved prosthetic devices, also began to make physical activity a realistic prospect for these children.

Late in the twentieth century, new insights were gained into the causes of spina bifida. The mutated genes involved were identified, and it was learned why they do not work properly. Studies of neural tube defects in mice revealed how these defects occur and how best to prevent them.

It is now known that the diet of a pregnant woman can influence neural tube development. One of the most effective measures for preventing spina bifida has been shown to be the daily intake of folic acid. Recommended doses vary from 0.4 to 4.0 mg per day based on risk status, such as prior delivery of a baby with neural tube defects. Preconceptual counseling includes recommendations for prenatal vitamins (which contain significantly more folic acid than other multivitamins) to be taken even before pregnancy. In 2000, it was reported that a folic acid supplement program for pregnant women that took place over a six-year period in South Carolina cut in half the rate of neural tube defects, including spina bifida. Doctors now know that folic acid supplements starting at the point of conception can decrease the risk of spina bifida by as much as 75 percent.

For fetuses that develop spina bifida, fetal surgery, which occurs while the fetus is in the womb, has become an option for parents. Fetal surgery can improve brain malformations, making it unnecessary for many babies to need lifelong shunts-devices that allow drainage of fluid that has accumulated around the brain. Even with the demonstrated benefits of the surgery, however, there is no guarantee that the surgery can correct all neurological functions or that it will be successful for all babies. In fact, it has been shown that fetal surgery increases the risk of a baby being born prematurely, which poses a whole new set of problems.

Support organizations for families can help them cope with the challenges of caring for children with spina bifida. Physical therapy, counseling, and various group activities are available. Thanks to improved treatment and support, it is now possible for children with this condition to lead long and healthy lives.

INFORMATION ON SPINA BIFIDA

Causes: Birth defect
Symptoms: Bulging spinal cord, hydrocephalus, paralysis in lower back and legs, bladder and bowel malfunction, loss of sensation, mental impairment
Duration: Chronic
Treatments: Surgery, catheterization, prostheses, physical therapy, sometimes fetal surgery

---

FURTHER READING

Bloom, Beth-Ann, and Edward L. Seljeskog. *A Parent's Guide to Spina Bifida.* Minneapolis: University of Minnesota Press, 1988. Designed to assist the parents of children with spina bifida. The book includes chapters on the nature of the disorder and how it is treated, the medical problems associated with spina bifida, and how to help the afflicted child while he or she is growing up.

Kimball, Chad T. *Childhood Diseases and Disorders Sourcebook: Basic Consumer Health Information About Medical Problems Often Encountered in Pre-adolescent Children.* Detroit, Mich.:Omnigraphics, 2003. Offers basic facts about cancer, sickle cell disease, diabetes, and other chronic conditions in children and discusses frequently used diagnostic tests, surgeries, and medications. Long-term care for seriously ill children is also presented.

McLone, David. *An Introduction to Spina Bifida.* Reprint.Washington, D.C.: Spina Bifida Association of America, 1998. Aconcise report on spinal dysraphism and related disorders. Illustrations illuminate the text.

Martin, Richard J., Avroy A. Fanaroff, and Michele C. Walsh, eds. *Fanaroff and Martin's Neonatal-Perinatal Medicine: Diseases of the Fetus and Infant.* 2 vols. 8th ed. Philadelphia: Mosby/Elsevier, 2006. This classic reference work is one of the most comprehensive to date and features discussions on the diverse practice of neonatal-perinatal medicine, pregnancy disorders and their impact on the fetus, delivery room care, provisions for neonatal care, and the development and disorder of organ systems.

Moore, Keith L., and T. V. N. Persaud. *The Developing Human.* 8th ed. Philadelphia: Saunders/Elsevier, 2008. An outstanding textbook on human embryonic development, with specific information about the causes of congenital malformations and common defects occurring in each of the body's systems.

Nightingale, Elena O., and Melissa Goodman. *Before Birth: Prenatal Testing for Genetic Disease.* Cambridge, Mass.: Harvard University Press, 1990. Offering practical guidance to prospective parents, this volume addresses the question of whether or not to undergo testing, and if elected, how best to use the results.

Spina Bifida Association. http://www.sbaa.org. Promotes the prevention of spina bifida and strives to enhance the lives of all affected. Offers newsletter, physician

Howard L. Hosick

SEE ALSO: Spine, Vertebrae, and Disks

Stuttering

Stuttering is the most common speech disorder among adolescents and adults, and it has profound consequences for self-esteem. It usually begins in early childhood, as a result of both biological influences and learning processes. Modern therapy often focuses on treatments addressing behavioral aspects of stuttering.

INTRODUCTION

All people sometimes hesitate when they speak or repeat the starting sound or syllable of a word when they are nervous. These are examples of normal verbal disfluencies. Stutterers are different from normal speakers primarily because of the frequency of their problem, not because their speech problem is by itself unusual. Stuttering is a disorder involving the timing and rhythms of speech,Speech disorders not of articulation. Thus, it is quite different from other common speech defects. It is also the most common speech problem to affect teens or adults.

Stuttering is a universal phenomenon, impacting people of every society and language group on earth. It is approximately four times as common in boys as in girls. The disorder typically begins in the preschool years (almost always before age six) and, unless outgrown by adolescence, becomes progressively more pronounced. Some stutterers also exhibit cluttering, nonsensically vocalizing sounds. As the speaking problem worsens, the stutterer is likely to show other, related behavior problems such as nervous twitches or slapping oneself when trying to stop stuttering. Furthermore, a stutterer's self-esteem usually suffers; teens, especially, are self-conscious about this speech problem, which can lead to avoidance of speaking or to more pronounced social withdrawal.

POSSIBLE CAUSES

There are several possible causes of stuttering. Scientists do not seek to designate one as absolute; for different stutterers, different causes may apply. In addition, in any individual case, more than one cause may be relevant. For example, stuttering tends to run in families, suggesting a genetic contribution. This contribution may make an individual more likely to develop the stuttering problem, given the circumstances. About the only cause of stuttering that has been ruled out is imitation. No evidence exists that stuttering develops from a child's exposure to another stutterer.

A variety of physical differences between stutterers and nonstutterers have been investigated, with all aspects of the mouth and airways involved in speech production taken into account. When searching for a possible cause of stuttering, hearing problems should be considered, although stuttering is actually less common among the deaf. Nevertheless, partial hearing losses can influence confidence in learning to speak, and, in fact, the onset of the stuttering problem often corresponds with the earliest use of sentences. In the treatment of any speech defect, screening for hearing problems is an important preliminary step. Brain damage can also lead to neurogenic stuttering, although this trauma is not the usual cause of speech disfluencies.

While stress aggravates stuttering, it is not usually the cause of the speech disorder. Most stuttering problems develop gradually; parents of a stutterer typically cannot pinpoint when the problem began. Extremely stressful events have, however, been known to be direct causes of stuttering.

Most stuttering probably develops gradually during the time when children are beginning to speak in sentences and engage in conversation. Everyone shows verbal disfluencies; young children are even more likely to do so. Wendell Johnson argues that the difference between stuttering and nonstuttering preschoolers is not in the children, but in the perceptions of their parents. By overreacting to normal disfluencies, parents may impair a young child's self-confidence, instigating a vicious cycle: Low self-confidence creates more disfluency, which further lowers self-confidence. The cycle continues until the child is, in fact, a "stutterer."

The difficulty with this line of reasoning is that it imposes an unfair burden of guilt on the parents. In effect, concerned parents are accused of causing the problem by expressing their concern. While parental behavior may contribute to stuttering, most experts believe that the genetic evidence and the preponderance of boys among stutterers suggest a physical contribution as well. Moreover, treatment of speech disorders is most effective when begun early, and the social impact of stuttering makes early treatment even more critical; thus, parents of stutterers may not know whether they will do more harm by calling attention to the problem or by ignoring it.

TREATMENT APPROACHES

The best advice to parents is to be patient but watchful. First, parents should remember that all speakers show disfluencies, which are impacted by stress. The child learning to speak may require patience from the adult listener. Parents should not pressure a child who is attempting to express what, to the child, may be a complex idea. Parents should not finish a child's sentences. If a child's stuttering problem does not disappear with time, if it appears without obvious stressful circumstances, or if accompanying nervous behaviors develop, the parent should seek help. Patience and lack of pressure are extremely important with a diagnosed stutterer. The most helpful roles for the parent at this point are to provide unconditional emotional support and to cooperate with the therapist.

Many approaches to the treatment of stuttering emphasize controlling the problem rather than eliminating it. Stutterers are often advised to slow down their speaking and simply to stop and take a deep breath if stuttering begins. They may be advised to sigh before any speech attempt. Therapy is also concerned with self-esteem problems and with the social avoidance of stutterers, treating these as results, not causes, of stuttering.

DSM-IV-TR CRITERIA FOR STUTTERING (DSM CODE 307.0)

Disturbance, inappropriate for age, in the normal fluency and time patterning of speech

Characterized by frequent occurrences of one or more of the following:
- sound and syllable repetitions
- sound prolongations
- interjections
- broken words (such as pauses within a word)
- audible or silent blocking (filled or unfilled pauses in speech)
- circumlocutions (word substitutions to avoid problematic words)
- words produced with an excess of physical tension
- monosyllabic whole-word repetitions

Fluency disturbance interferes with academic or occupational achievement or with social communication

If speech-motor or sensory deficit is present, speech difficulties exceed those usually associated with these problems

---

Stutterers often develop their own control techniques. Some find, for example, that singing is easier than talking and take advantage of this to modify the pitch of their speech when a problem occurs. The best advice may be to do whatever works for any individual.

The decision whether or not to treat stuttering is complicated by the similarity of speech between early stutterers and nonstutterers and by the resulting difficulty in pinpointing the origin of the problem. Edward G. Conture has pointed out that therapists deal both with parents who are overconcerned about normal disfluency and with parents who are underconcerned about a real problem. Moreover, Conture has noted, the nature of treatment depends considerably on the age of the stutterer.

Young stutterers offer the best hope for treatment, before the complications created by social stigma occur or worsen. On the other hand, young stutterers present greater problems in diagnosis, as well as a need to counsel parents who are themselves experiencing stress related to the stuttering. For example, parents of stutterers frequently have great difficulty looking at their child when the child stutters. They feel their child's pain, but their own pained response may not be helpful. Additionally, young children may not understand instructions for speech exercises or may lack the patience to practice techniques. Teens are better able to cooperate with the activities of speech therapy, which involve following directions and practice. On the other hand, they may be uncooperative for a number of reasons: past negative therapy experience, fear of peer reactions to speech therapy, and normal adolescent resistance to adults.

Adult stutterers have the least likelihood of overcoming the problem but are highly motivated (although they also may have had bad experiences with past therapy efforts) and have the freedom to structure their own environments. The adult's freedom from parent and peer pressure can make psychotherapy for self-esteem problems more successful than it is for children and adolescents. On the other hand, the adult continues to face a tremendous social stigma, which can even take the form of job discrimination. Moreover, by this time in a stutterer's life, stuttering has become part of the person's identity, making change difficult.

SPEECH THERAPY

Specific speech therapy techniques are varied. Distraction techniques aim to divert the stutterer from the speech problem. The theoretical basis for this technique is that self-consciousness about speech aggravates stuttering. In one example of this type of therapy the stutterer crawls on the floor while speaking. These techniques often provide only temporary success because the general use of such methods in real-life situations is unlikely.

Desensitization techniques focus on training the stutterer to deal with situations that provoke stuttering. This requires analyzing all situations that produce stuttering. After a stress-free therapy environment is created, the "speech disrupters" are reintroduced one at a time, with the aim of strengthening the individual's tolerance for disruption.

Therapy is most effective for children when parents are involved, especially in terms of promoting self-esteem. Parents may require counseling also, both to deal with their own frustrations and to understand the impact of their and others' reactions on the stuttering child. In addition, parents are the most important members of the child's communication environment. The parents' roles, not only in their responses to the child's speech but also in their own manner of speaking with the child, largely structure that environment. For example, studies show that a child's stuttering diminishes when parents slow down their speech to a stuttering child.

An individual's self-esteem is central to effective therapy. Psychotherapy frequently deals with the psychological damage created by the stigma of stuttering. There are also numerous books on stuttering, many with a focus on self-help. Several authors advise stutterers of the needs, first, to increase their self-confidence and, second, to refrain from avoiding social interaction. For example, Johnson specifically emphasizes concentrating on one's "normal" speech instead of on one's stuttering. The idea is that the stutterer's preoccupation with stuttering has served to maintain and worsen the problem.

A common tactic in the self-help literature is to cite notable stutterers, including Moses, Aristotle, Thomas Jefferson, Winston Churchill, Charles Darwin, Annie Glenn, John Stossel, and Marilyn Monroe. Many significant stutterers have been known for their writing, and some have sufficiently coped to become public speakers, news reporters, or actors. This success may inspire a stutterer, enhancing a stutterer's self-esteem. Self-confidence is the common thread among all treatments, whether self-help, speech therapy, psychotherapy, or unconditional parental support.

CONTEMPORARY THEORIES

Descriptions of stuttering treatments can be found throughout history. Charles Van Riper listed several of the prescientific approaches, some dating to ancient Greece and Rome, including speaking with pebbles in the mouth (an ancient use of a distraction technique), exorcism, hot substances applied to the tongue, and bloodletting. At the beginning of the modern era, techniques included tongue exercises and surgery that deformed the tongue.

In the late nineteenth century, stuttering was described as a neurosis, or disorder caused by anxiety. Twentieth century psychoanalysts expanded on this theme in their treatment of stutterers. Through the first half of the twentieth century, the psychoanalytic view dominated theories and treatments of stuttering. According to this view, stuttering results from an unconscious conflict between the desire to speak and a preference to remain silent. The obvious tension experienced by stutterers, as well as their avoidance of speaking, supported this interpretation. The *Diagnostic and Statistical Manual of Mental Disorders* has included stuttering as a communications disorder.

Although some therapists remain influenced by psychoanalytic views, most contemporary therapists view the tension between wanting to speak and wanting to remain silent to be a result, not a cause, of stuttering. These therapists were more influenced by learning theory than psychoanalysis. For them, stuttering is considered the result of a process of learned reactions to specific environmental influences. Johnson's research on the similarities between preschool stutterers and nonstutterers, along with the differences among the perceptions of those same children's parents, strongly supports this interpretation. Most theorists and therapists also accept the role of genetic disposition in determining those likely to develop a stuttering disorder. In this view, therapy focuses on a stutterer's relearning and on control of the communication environment, especially the speech and reactions of the parents. Psychotherapy remains important not because psychological problems are seen as the cause of stuttering but because they appear to result from stuttering—from social stigma and frustrations in communicating with others.

The shift in professional views of stuttering may be attributed to the growing role in research of people who themselves have or have had a stuttering problem. Van Riper was such an individual, and he devoted his entire career to research and treatment of stuttering. The value

of his personal experience is found in his own solution: He became fluent when he stopped trying to hide his problem. Stuttering is a learned speech problem, with tremendous emotional consequences; stutterers are simply normal people coping with this problem.

SCIENTIFIC AND TECHNOLOGICAL ADVANCES

In the early twenty-first century, researchers used advanced imaging technologies such as magnetic resonance imaging (MRI) to achieve greater comprehension of brain anatomy and activity associated with stuttering. Investigators discussed their findings in professional journals and public media; those examining neurophysiological aspects detected that brain areas stutterers used to process their speech differed from the speech locations in brains of normal speakers. Scientists assessed gray-matter volume, left inferior frontal gyrus, and bilateral temporal regions associated with speech functions and white matter tracts linked to facial and larynx motor functions. Mark Onslow and his Australian Stuttering Research Centre colleagues noted stutterers' brains often contained more gyri and matter volume in speech parts of their brains than nonstutters. Other studies revealed that neuron connection flaws occurred in stutterers, and researchers hypothesized about whether the poor connections caused or were the result of stuttering. Aware that brain functioning affected speech, some therapists enhanced treatments to focus on physiological not psychological, intellectual, or social factors.

This knowledge of stutterers' brain functioning aided comprehension of other physical difficulties which many stutterers experienced, such as the inability to move their fingers quickly in rhythmic sequences needed to play some instruments. Scientists aware of brain activity in stutterers determined that the areas in brains associated with muscle control functions in tongues and other speech-related anatomy were adjacent to brain sites tied to finger movement.

Speech professionals considered that stuttering could be connected to mental stresses and traumas, emphasizing that more research would enhance comprehension of psychogenic stuttering. Researchers began studying the roles of anxiety and other psychological issues in stutterers' lives. Onslow and his colleagues determined that 60 percent of stutterers who were clinical trial participants admitted they had social phobia. Ross G. Menzies led a study of thirty-two adults who stuttered to evaluate how receiving speech restructuring treatment only or experiencing both cognitive-based therapy to address social phobia and speech restructuring treatment impacted the subjects' psychological health and stuttering. Some researchers evaluated groups of stutterers with psychological tests, such as the Minnesota Multiphasic Personality Inventory. Studies also considered how emotions in children influenced their speaking abilities and how stuttering provoked emotional abuse from peers.

Because of advances in communication technology, people who stuttered gained access to new therapeutic tools and methods. In 2008, the Hollins Communication Research Institute (HCRI) in Roanoke, Virginia, introduced its Hollins Fluency Program (HFP): Advanced Speech Reconstruction for Stuttering, which used computing and electronics technology to evaluate, readjust, and monitor a stutterer's speaking behavior to attain fluency. Ronald L. Webster, who founded HCRI, emphasized that HFP assisted people with varying forms and intensities of stuttering. During twelve days of therapy, HFP teaches stutterers how to stop muscle movements in their mouths, throats, and lungs associated with stuttering and practice alternative muscle behavior for fluent speaking. Clients interact with a computer program to study how to achieve specific movements of muscles for desired speech. A biofeedback component immediately assesses if clients have attained correct muscle motion while speaking. Approximately 93 percent of stutterers undergoing HFP achieved their desired results.

In January, 2009, the HCRI extended its therapy possibilities by developing an iPhone application to assess people's speaking behavior, in which stutterers carry iPhones while talking to family, friends, and people they encounter in public places. The iPhone application performs evaluations and presents feedback which had been restricted previously to the HCRI clinic computers. The mobility of the iPhone provides clients consistent assistance in environments where they most frequently speak instead of in artificial clinical surroundings.

FURTHER READING

Chang, Soo-Eun, et al. "Brain Anatomy Differences in Childhood Stuttering." *NeuroImage* 39 (2008): 1333-1344. Reports how imaging techniques assessed brain areas associated with speech and facial motor functions in three groups of children—fluent speakers, stutterers, and recovered stutterers—comparing data with imaging results in adults and emphasizing the importance of neuroplasticity in brain development.

Conture, Edward G. *Stuttering: Its Nature, Diagnosis, and Treatment.* Boston: Allyn & Bacon, 2001. A basic text aimed at speech therapy students. Emphasis on evaluation and treatment, highlighting important treatment differences related to the age of the stutterer. Includes numerous clinical examples and a complete case study in an appendix.

Davis, Stephen, Peter Howell, and Frances Cooke. "Sociodynamic Relationships Between Children Who Stutter and Their Non-Stuttering Classmates." *Journal of Child Psychology and Psychiatry* 43, no. 7 (2002): 939-947. Studied group of 403 children, ages eight through fourteen, of whom 16 stuttered, to observe how nonstutterers interact with stutterers. Discusses behavioral categories that the children used to describe their peers.

Guitar, Barry. *Stuttering: An Integrated Approach to Its Nature and Treatment.* 3d ed. Philadelphia: Lippincott Williams & Wilkins, 2006. Discusses basic stuttering information and addresses neurological diseases, emotional and psychological issues, trauma, brain imaging, neurogenic and psychogenic stuttering, and cluttering. Each chapter concludes with study questions and suggested projects. Tables, figures, bibliography.

Karrass, Jan, et al. "Relation of Emotional Reactivity and Regulation to Childhood Stuttering." *Journal of Communication Disorders* 39, no. 6 (November/December, 2006): 402-423. Researchers tested preschoolers who stuttered and a group who did not to assess how emotional issues might interfere with speech development. In addition to two laboratory-based speech tests of preschoolers, parents of the children tested responded to a survey about their children's emotional reactions and control.

Menzies, Ross G., et al. "An Experimental Clinical Trial of a Cognitive-Behavior Therapy Package for Chronic Stuttering." *Journal of Speech, Language, and Hearing Research* 51, no. 6 (December, 2008): 1451-1464. Evaluated the effect of singular and combined forms of cognitive behavior and speech restructuring therapies to aid stutterers with speaking problems and social anxieties twelve months after assistance from those therapies concluded.

Packman, Ann, Chris Code, and Mark Onslow. "On the Cause of Stuttering: Integrating Theory with Brain and Behavioral Research." *Journal of Neurolinguistics* 20, no. 5 (September, 2007): 353-362. Explains development of authors' syllable initiation theory to hypothesize about possible causation of stuttering, noting precedents investigating both healthy and damaged brain activity associated with speech.

Treon, Martin, Karen Blaesing, and Lloyd Dempster. "MMPI-2/A Assessed Personality Differences in People Who Do, and Do Not, Stutter." *Social Behavior and Personality: An International Journal* 34, no. 3 (April, 2006): 271-294. Study of sixty stutterers and sixty nonstutterers who were tested with the Minnesota Multiphasic Personality Inventory MMPI-2 and MMPI-A to detect any tendencies for psychological conditions sometimes associated with stuttering.

Nancy E. Macdonald; updated by Elizabeth D. Schafer

SEE ALSO: Anxiety

Thrombocytopenia

A bleeding disorder in which the blood contains an abnormally low count of functional platelets (thrombocytes).

CAUSES AND SYMPTOMS

Thrombocytopenia occurs when platelets are lost from the circulation faster than they can be replaced by the bone marrow where they are produced. It may result from either a deficiency in platelet production or an increased clearance rate from the blood. Clinically, thrombocytopenia is defined as a platelet count less than the normal levels of 150,000 to 350,000 per microliter of blood.

There are several specific causes of thrombocytopenia. In artefactual thrombocytopenia, antibodies in a person's blood cause platelets to stick together and cause a falsely low platelet count. In congenital thrombocytopenia, one of several rare genetic diseases causes low platelet counts. Another cause of thrombocytopenia is impaired platelet production, such as in leukemia or lymphoma, where the number of some other cell type in the bone marrow is increased, leaving fewer megakaryocytes for platelet production. Alternatively, the rate of platelet destruction can be increased as in disseminated intravascular coagulation (DIC), in which the blood clotting process is inappropriately activated. Antibodies in the blood, produced because of infections such as human immunodeficiency virus (HIV) or rheumatoid arthritis, can cause platelet removal. Idiopathic or immunologic thrombocytopenic purpura (ITP) causes thrombocytopenia through destruction of platelets by the patient's immune system.

Thrombocytopenia can also be attributable to an abnormal distribution of platelets, as when platelets are sequestered in a patient's enlarged spleen. Thrombotic thrombocytopenic purpura (TTP) is a disease resulting in thrombocytopenia. Platelets clump together in areas of clots to the extent that there are fewer platelets in other parts of the body. Finally, a massive transfusion of red blood cells can dilute platelets to thrombocytopenic levels. Thrombocytopenia ca cause excess bleeding and thus has several notable symptoms. Petechiae, rashes, and frequent bruising can appear on the skin, provoked by minor injury or pressure. Bleeding from wounds or body cavities may occur. At extremely low platelet counts, those below 20,000 per microliter, spontaneous bleeding occurs. The spleen and liver may be enlarged and sensitive to the touch if the thrombocytopenia is caused by splenic activity. Impaired clotting may cause blood to appear in the stool, urine, vomit, or sputum. Thrombocytopenic patients may also experience anemia, feel fatigued, or exhibit an elevated heart rate.

Low platelet counts increase the risk of bleeding, which becomes particularly dangerous when the count falls below 10,000 per microliter. Bleeding from the nose and gums is quite common. Serious hemorrhage can occur at the retina in the back of the eye, threatening vision. The most critical bleeding complication posing a risk to life is spontaneous bleeding in the head or in the lining of the gut.

TREATMENT AND THERAPY

The primary treatment for thrombocytopenia is to address the underlying cause of the deficiency. This is not always possible. If significant blood loss has occurred, then red blood cell or platelet transfusion may be necessary. However, in the condition of thrombotic thrombocytopenia purpura, the use of platelet concentrates is quite hazardous. Platelet growth factor can be used to stimulate increased platelet production in the bone marrow. Additionally, certain drugs such as aspirin and ibuprofen are to be avoided since they are known to cause antiplatelet activity.

If an infection is suspected as the cause of thrombocytopenia, then treatment such as antibiotics for the specific infection is often initiated. Some viral infections such as glandular fever caused by Epstein-Barr virus have no specific treatment, and only close monitoring is applied. If the thrombocytopenia is caused by the presence of cancer cells in the bone marrow, then treatment such as chemotherapy or radiotherapy is directed

---

INFORMATION ON THROMBOCYTOPENIA

Causes: Platelet deficiency or increased clearance from blood; may result from autoimmune response, genetic defect, infection, diseases such as leukemia, lymphoma, disseminated intravascular coagulation

Symptoms: Petechiae; rashes; frequent bruising; bleeding from wounds or body cavities; spontaneous bleeding; spleen and liver enlargement; blood in stool, urine, vomit, or sputum; anemia, fatigue; elevated heart rate

Duration: Chronic

Treatments: Depends on cause; may include red blood cell or platelet transfusion, platelet growth factor

---

at the abnormal cells. In such cases, the bone marrow may become damaged and blood platelet counts further lowered. Platelet transfusions are then given to prevent bleeding, until either the platelet count reaches acceptable levels or the bone marrow recovers its ability to produce sufficient numbers of platelets.

PERSPECTIVE AND PROSPECTS

Prior to the development of plasma exchange as an effective treatment in the 1970s, the mortality from thrombotic thrombocytopenic purpura–hemolytic uremic syndrome (TTP-HUS) was 90 percent. During those times, diagnosis was made using five clinical observations, including thrombocytopenia and fever. The availability of effective plasma exchange treatment has lowered the mortality rate to 20 percent. Early diagnosis is important, with thrombocytopenia and one other criterion the only requirements for initiation of treatment since 1991.

At the start of the twenty-first century, the treatment of children with idiopathic or immunologic thrombocytopenic purpura remained controversial. Platelet counts can be increased by treatment with corticosteroids, but clinical outcomes may not improve. Because most children spontaneously recover from severe thrombocytopenia in several days to weeks, only supportive care is sometimes recommended in this case.

FURTHER READING

Cattaneo, M. "Inherited Platelet-Based Bleeding Disorders." *Journal of Thrombosis and Haemostasis* 1, no. 7 (July, 2003): 1628–1636.

Chong, B. H. "Heparin-Induced Thrombocytopenia." *Journal of Thrombosis and Haemostasis* 1, no. 7 (July, 2003): 1471–1478.

Dugdale, David C. "Thrombocytopenia." *MedlinePlus*, March 14, 2012.

George, J. N. "Platelets." *The Lancet* 355, no. 9214 (April 29, 2000): 1531–1539.

Goldstein, K. H., et al. "Efficient Diagnosis of Thrombocytopenia." *American Family Physician* 53, no. 3 (February 15, 1996): 915–920.

McCrae, Keith R., ed. *Thrombocytopenia.* NewYork: Taylor&Francis, 2006.

MedlinePlus. "Platelet Disorders." *MedlinePlus*, May 22, 2013.

National Heart, Lung, and Blood Institute. "What Is Thrombocytopenia?" *NIH: National Heart, Lung, and Blood Institute*, September 25, 2012.

Reid, T. J., et al. "Platelet Substitutes in the Management of Thrombocytopenia." *Current Hematology Reports* 2, no. 2 (March, 2003): 165–170.

Warkentin, Theodore E., and Andreas Greinacher, eds. *Heparin-Induced Thrombocytopenia.* 4th rev. ed. New York: Marcel Dekker, 2007.

Michael R. King

SEE ALSO: Circulation

Thyroid disorders

Underactivity (hypothyroidism) or overactivity (hyperthyroidism) of the thyroid gland.

CAUSES AND SYMPTOMS

The thyroid gland normally weighs about twenty to thirty-five grams and is located in the neck just below the larynx, or voice box. The gland is named for the shield-shaped "thyroid" cartilage that forms the front of the larynx. The thyroid has two lateral lobes that are connected by an isthmus that crosses in front of the trachea. By placing a finger on the trachea below the larynx it is possible to feel the ridge-like isthmus pass under the finger after swallowing. The bilobed (two-lobed) shape of the rest of the gland can be felt just under the skin of the neck on either side of the midline, although its boundaries are normally indistinct except to a trained examiner.

The thyroid produces two major hormones. Thyroxine, a product of the follicular cells, is the major hormone produced by the thyroid that helps regulate metabolism. Within the thyroid are also parafollicular cells that produce calcitonin, an essential hormone involved in calcium metabolism. In the tissue of the thyroid are also embedded two pairs of parathyroid glands. The parathyroid glands produce parathyroid hormone, which is required to maintain normal levels of blood calcium. In the case of thyroid surgery, it is important that the parathyroid glands are not damaged or removed; otherwise, there may be life-threatening tetanus—the sustained contraction of muscles, including those needed for breathing.

The normal functioning of the thyroid results from an elaborate physiological control system involving the hypothalamus of the brain, the anterior lobe of the pituitary gland, and the thyroid gland. The hypothalamus produces thyrotropicreleasing hormone (TRH), which is passed by special blood vessels to the anterior lobe of the pituitary, the adenohypophysis. The TRH-stimulated cells in the adenohypophysis produce thyroid-stimulating hormone (TSH), which is released into the general circulation. When it reaches the thyroid gland, it stimulates the gland to produce thyroxine. Normally, thyroxine has a negative feedback effect on its own production; that is, thyroxine can inhibit the activity of the hypothalamus and the pituitary to maintain its concentration in the blood. Various thyroid disorders, which are more common in women than in men, can develop from tumors that either increase or decrease the hormones produced in these three interdependent structures.

The normal thyroid (or euthyroid state) produces mainly thyroxine, which is converted into triiodothyronine in the tissues of the body before it has its effects, which are generally to increase the metabolic rate of the body. Some triiodothyronine is directly produced by the thyroid. The thyroxine molecule contains iodide, the negative ion of iodine; iodine is therefore an essential component of one's diet. If iodine is not available in the diet—as in the case of vegetables grown in geographical areas glaciated in the past, such as mountainous terrain and the American Midwest—then the body cannot produce thyroxine. Industrialized countries have iodine added to table salt to ensure an adequate supply of this element in the diet. A lack of iodine, and therefore a lack of thyroxine, prevents the functioning of the negative feedback effect of thyroxine on the hypothalamus and pituitary, resulting in very low thyroxine levels and high TSH levels in the blood. High levels of TSH cause substantial growth of the thyroid, which will bulge from the neck as a goiter. A person with such a condition would be hypothyroid (that is, have lower-than-normal thyroxine levels in the blood) and may be affected by cretinism (mental impairment and stunted physical growth) if this condition occurs early in childhood.

Hypothyroidism can arise in other ways as well. Hashimoto's thyroiditis is a common type of hypothyroidism that is caused by an autoimmune reaction whereby white blood cells known as lymphocytes infiltrate the thyroid and gradually destroy its tissue. The presence of antibodies against normal thyroid proteins can be detected with this condition. The usual signs of hypothyroidism are an intolerance of cold, a low body temperature, a lower rate of metabolism, a tendency to sleep longer, a general lack of energy, infrequent bowel movements, constipation, possible weight gain, a puffy face and hands, a slow heart rate, cold and scaly skin, a lack of perspiration, and possible emotional withdrawal and depression.

Graves' disease, the most common type of hyperthyroidism, is an autoimmune disorder in which antibodies mimic the action of TSH and therefore stimulate the thyroid to produce excessive thyroxine. Sometimes, nodules develop in the thyroid that may produce the excessive thyroxine. Although the presence of a nodule in the thyroid may cause a person to suspect cancer, the nodules are usually benign. Hyperthyroidism may be associated with bulging eyes, but this orbitopathy does not always occur. Generally, there is an intolerance of heat, a loss of body weight, a high degree of nervousness, increased or decreased skin pigmentation, more frequent bowel movements, loss of hair, and a very rapid heart rate.

INFORMATION ON THYROID DISORDERS

Causes: Tumors, iodine deficiency, autoimmune disorders

Symptoms: In hypothyroidism, intolerance of cold, low body temperature, tendency to sleep longer, lack of energy, infrequent bowel movements, constipation, possible weight gain, puffy face and hands; in hyperthyroidism, bulging eyes, intolerance of heat, weight loss, nervousness, increased or decreased skin pigmentation, more frequent bowel movements, hair loss, rapid heart rate

Duration: Several months to chronic

Treatments: Thyroxine, antithyroid drugs (propylthiouracil, methimazole), radioactive iodine, surgery

TREATMENT AND THERAPY

Patients suspected of having hypothyroidism or hyperthyroidism will have their blood tested for levels of TSH and thyroxine. Ultrasonography can be used to detect tumors and serve as an anatomical guide for potential surgery. Hypothyroidism patients are prescribed a small oral dose (less than 1 milligram per day) of thyroxine, which is adjusted until a euthyroid state is obtained within a few months. Then the patient is maintained on thyroxine, with perhaps yearly checkups by a physician. For hyperthyroidism patients, several modes of treatment are possible. Antithyroid drugs, such as propylthiouracil (PTU) or methimazole, can be given to inhibit thyroxine synthesis. Radioactive iodine is commonly given to destroy part of the thyroid gland and thus reduce its thyroxine output. Second or even third doses of radioactive iodine may be given if the blood thyroxine levels remain high. Radioactive iodine is not used during pregnancy because damage to the fetal thyroid is likely. Additionally, surgery can be performed to remove enough thyroid tissue to restore normal thyroxine levels. Following any of the treatments, a hypothyroidism may be induced that will require that the patient receive thyroxine supplements. Finally, surgery can be used to reduce the bulging of the eyes caused by hyperthyroidism.

FURTHER READING

Bar, Robert S. *Early Diagnosis and Treatment of Endocrine Disorders.* Totowa, N.J.: Humana Press, 2003.

Braverman, Lewis E., ed. *Diseases of the Thyroid.* 2d ed. Totowa, N.J.: Humana Press, 2003.

Health Library. "Hyperthyroidism." *Health Library,* November 26, 2012.

Health Library. "Hypothyroidism." *Health Library,* March 15, 2013.

Hershman, Jerome M., ed. *Endocrine Pathophysiology: A Patient-Oriented Approach.* 3d ed. Philadelphia: Lea & Febiger, 1988.

Kovacs, William J.., and Sergio R. Ojeda, eds. *Textbook of Endocrine Physiology.* 6th ed. New York: Oxford University Press, 2012.

MedlinePlus. "Thyroid Diseases." *MedlinePlus,* May 30, 2013.

Melmed, Shlomo, and Robert Hardin Williams, eds. *Williams Textbook of Endocrinology.* 12th ed. Philadelphia: Elsevier/Saunders, 2011.

Ruggieri, Paul, and Scott Isaacs. *A Simple Guide to Thyroid Disorders: From Diagnosis to Treatment.* Omaha, Nebr.: Addicus Books, 2010.

Surks, Martin I. *The Thyroid Book.* Rev. ed. Yonkers, N.Y.: Consumer Reports Books, 1999.

John T. Burns, updated by Matthew Berria

SEE ALSO: Thyroid Cancer; Thyroid Gland, The

Tic disorders

A tic is defined as a sudden involuntary movement or twitch, usually in the face but sometimes in the neck or in other parts of the body, that occurs without any obvious external cause and that may also manifest itself in the victim's speech or breathing.

INTRODUCTION

The tics that occur with some frequency in young children and in adolescents are often confined to the face, particularly the eyes and lips, although these muscle contractions can also affect other parts of the body, notably the shoulders, the neck, the arms, the hands, and the trunk. They can also affect breathing and may be vocal.

Most people have had some experience with tics, but as people mature, the frequency of such tics usually diminishes. In cases of this sort, the condition is identified as transient tic disorder and does little to interfere with people's normal activities.

Some victims of the disorder, however, experience tics so frequently that it significantly affects their normal functioning. These people have chronic tic disorder, which, especially in its vocal manifestations, called coprolalia, makes it difficult for them to interact with people and to be involved in social and learning situations. Such people may erupt unexpectedly and quite frequently into loud streams of profanity directed to those around them. There usually is not any identifiable trigger for these eruptions, which often leave those who hear and see them bewildered and frightened.

Although coprolalia may be a transient condition, its manifestations require immediate attention, because those who have the condition are usually disruptive in social situations and in school settings. In some situations, this disruptiveness may cause victims of coprolalia to be isolated, because their presence in classroom settings can make it impossible for teachers to deal with them in average-sized classes.

CAUSES

The presence of tics in young people may be hereditary, although a genetic link has not been firmly established. Environmental causes appear to be present in some cases in which tics develop. It is also thought that stress may contribute to the occurrence of tics, and it has been observed that sometimes people who develop tics experience a reduction in their symptoms if their stress level is reduced.

Among adults, the overuse of caffeine, defined as more than the equivalent of five cups of coffee a day, can result in tics, twitches, or tremors that can be virtually eliminated if caffeine consumption is drastically reduced. The regular use of alcoholic beverages may also result in the tics, twitches, and tremors associated with the overuse of caffeine and can be controlled by eliminating alcoholic beverages from the patient's diet.

In some people, tics coexist with mental disorders and emotional instability, in which case they may be treated by psychologists or psychiatrists. Where a psychological basis exists for the condition, the reduction of stress is imperative.

TYPES AND FREQUENCY

Tics may be motor or verbal. Although they may disappear almost as quickly as they appeared, they are irresistible. Will power and distractions may mitigate them temporarily, but once the distraction disappears, the tic reappears. Researchers have found that tics do a great deal to relieve stress in those experiencing them, so they question the advisability of doing anything to prevent or discourage them.

Although tics are often associated with Tourette syndrome, they may also occur in people with Asperger syndrome, bipolar disorders, learning disabilities, and attention-deficit hyperactivity disorder (ADHD). Some neurologists have associated them with such conditions as chronic nail biting, nose picking, and air swallowing.

Tics often are closely associated with obsessive-compulsive disorders (OCDs). Those who experience transient tic disorders, defined as those that last for at least four weeks but for no longer than a year, generally exhibit behaviors associated with both motor and verbal (also called phonic) tics, sometimes simultaneously.

The American Psychiatric Associations' *Diagnostic and Statistical Manual of Mental Disorders: DSM-5* (2013) classifies three types of tic disorders: Tourette syndrome, persistent (or chronic) motor or vocal tic disorder, and provisional (formerly transient) tic disorder.

Transient tic disorders disappear as their victims mature. They are rarely found in people over eighteen years old. In some cases, however, the disorder follows its victims into adulthood, which usually complicates their lives considerably. However, as neurologist Oliver Sacks has shown in seven case studies involving those with Tourette syndrome, the most difficult type of tic disorder, some of those with the disorder have learned to live with it and lead productive lives in spite of it. Sacks cites case studies he has made of seven physicians who suffer from Tourette syndrome and practice actively in such fields as surgery, ophthalmology, and internal medicine.

A 2012 study conducted by the Centers for Disease Control indicates that 1 in 360 children between the ages of six and seventeen have Tourette syndrome. School-age boys develop Tourette syndrome (and tics in general) at a rate as high as five to one over their female counterparts.

The condition has been reported throughout recorded medical history. At one time, tics were considered to be evidence that those who had them, at least in their more extreme manifestations, were possessed. A degree of shame was associated with them. Tics were considered to stem from psychological causes well into the twentieth century, even though Tourette syndrome was identified in the last half of the nineteenth century.

In the United States, Tourette syndrome affects more whites than African Americans or Latinos. Young children suffer more frequently from Tourette than older children do. Children between twelve and seventeen are twice as likely to be diagnosed with Tourette syndrome than younger children.

Many tic disorders go unobserved and unreported. Therefore, some researchers have speculated that the actual occurrence of some kind of tic disorder may be as high as one in every hundred people between five and eighteen years old.

Young people who suffer from Tourette syndrome, even if they attend school, are often shunned by their classmates and may be dreaded by their teachers who view them as disruptive. Most school districts have some special education programs for those who need them, but a person with Tourette can seriously obstruct the learning processes of other students. Teachers on an intellectual level can understand the problems that face the person with Tourette, but this understanding does little to remedy the disruptions that such a student may create.

Students coping with Tourette syndrome have legal protection under Section 504 of the American with

Disabilities Act (ADA). This law protects the rights of all Americans with disabilities and is particularly relevant in educational and vocational training programs. Protection is granted under ADA to anyone whose physical or mental impairment places a limitation on them in one of several areas, including walking, seeing, hearing, speaking, breathing, and several other areas that are commonly found in those with Tourette. People with Tourette often have badly damaged self-images caused by their inability to fit into the social and educational settings in which most young people participate. Discussions of what Tourette syndrome is and of how it affects people often increase the understanding of the teenage tormentors of those with the syndrome.

TREATMENT

Most tic disorders are sufficiently mild and transient that they do not require treatment. Given time, the symptoms will probably diminish and finally disappear entirely. Those dealing with young people who have tic disorders are usually advised not to encourage them to suppress their tics because they often are essential in helping them release their stress and deal with their emotions.

For cases in which patients experience such severe tics that treatment is indicated, benzodiazepines and antipsychotic medications are sometimes employed. Such treatment is considered extreme and usually is resorted to only in cases in which there are such severe involuntary contractions of the muscles between the chest and the abdomen that the patient makes loud grunting noises and exhibits distinct symptoms of Tourette syndrome. In such cases, some instances of relief have been reported following acupuncture, acupressure, yoga, and massage.

Tourette syndrome usually involves two or more kinds of motor tics simultaneously as well as a phonic tic, generally coprolalia. Such extreme manifestations of this obsessive-compulsive disorder are infrequent and are usually dealt with both psychologically and medicinally. When it is considered necessary, however, limited doses of dopamine agonists, notably bromocriptine and pramipexole, may be administered.

Mild tics often respond to small quantities of a blood pressure medication, clonidine, or to an antiseizure medication, clonazepam. Multiple tics can be controlled by small doses of such antipsychotic drugs as haloperidol, pimozide, and fluphenazine, but each of these medications has significant side effects that cause most physicians to limit their use to the most extreme cases.

FURTHER READING

Bruun, Ruth Dowling, and Bertel Bruun. *A Mind of Its Own: Tourette's Syndrome—A Story and a Guide.* New York: Oxford UP, 1994. Print.

Burn, David, and Christopher Kennard. *Movement Disorders.* New York: Oxford UP, 2013. Print.

Cohen, Donald J., Ruth Dowling Bruun, and James F. Leckman, eds. *Tic and Tic Disorders: Clinical Understanding and Treatment.* New York: Wiley, 1999. Print.

Kushner, Howard I. *A Cursing Brain? The Histories of Tourette Syndrome.* Cambridge: Harvard UP, 1999. Print.

Kutscher, Martin L. *Kids in the Syndrome Mix of ADHD, LD, Asperger's, Tourette's, Bipolar, and More! The One Stop Guide for Parents, Teachers, and Other Professionals.* Philadelphia: Kingsley, 2005. Print.

Leicester, Mal. *Can I Tell You about Tourette Syndrome? A Guide for Friends, Family, and Professionals.* Philadelphia: Kingsley, 2014. Print.

Robertson, Mary M., and Simon Baron-Cohen. *Tourette Syndrome: The Facts.* 2nd ed. New York: Oxford UP, 1998. Print.

Sacks, Oliver. *An Anthropologist on Mars: Seven Paradoxical Tales.* New York: Knopf, 1995. Print.

Shimberg, Elaine. *Living with Tourette Syndrome.* New York: Simon, 1995. Print.

"Tourette Syndrome: Data and Statistics." *Centers for Disease Control and Prevention.* CDC, 9 June 2014. Web. 10 July 2014.

Williams, Mary E. *Tourette Syndrome.* Detroit: Gale, 2013. Print.

Woods, Douglas W., John C. Piacentini, and John T. Walkup, eds. *Treating Tourette Syndrome and Tic Disorders: A Guide for Practitioners.* New York: Guilford, 2007. Print.

R. Baird Shuman

SEE ALSO: Tourette Syndrome

Tourette syndrome

Tourette's syndrome is classified as a neuropsychiatric disorder because of its roots in neurological functioning, but its prominent features relate to a person's behavior and psychological/psychiatric functioning. The disorder is characterized by motor tics of the face, head, and other extremities that persist for more than one year. There are typically behavioral and cognitive symptoms linked to attention-deficit hyperactivity disorder and obsessive-compulsive disorder.

INTRODUCTION

Tourette's syndrome is named for Georges Gilles de la Tourette, the French physician who described the syndrome extensively in 1885. Tourette was the first to describe and publish a case study of a noblewoman who had the disorder. He later identified many of the symptoms that remain associated with the syndrome, including multiple tics, echolalia (the repetition of what is said by other people as if the patient was producing an echo of the other person's speech), and coprolalia (the use of obscene and vulgar language, often in a sexual context). The syndrome is considered to be rare, although estimates suggest it may occur in as many as one in two hundred individuals. Accurate estimates are difficult because of the variability of expression of the condition and the occurrence of multiple tics due to other causes. The incidence of Tourette's syndrome is much higher in children than in adults, and in many cases, motor and vocal tics disappear in adulthood. The incidence of Tourette's syndrome is greater in men than in women, as the generally accepted ratio of male to female patients is 4:1.

The onset of Tourette's syndrome usually occurs in childhood, with the average age of onset being seven years, although cases can occur earlier or later. Typically, the symptoms initially are simple motor tics and progress to more complex motor and vocal tics, although there is considerable variability among patients. The tics often go through periods of waxing and waning, and reach their peak around age ten, after which point they decrease and often disappear in later adolescence.

When Tourette first characterized the syndrome in 1885, he described symptoms in multiple members of a single family. The genetic basis of Tourette's syndrome is still not completely understood, but family studies have indicated that biological relatives of patients appear to have significantly greater risk of developing the syndrome than do relatives of unaffected persons.

Although there is no cure for Tourette's syndrome, medications have been found to be useful in reducing tics and some of the associated abnormal behaviors. However, many medical practitioners hesitate to prescribe these medications unless symptoms significantly interfere with an individual's day-to-day functioning.

Haloperidol is the most well-known medication used to treat Tourette's syndrome.

A surgical procedure called deep brain stimulation (DBS) has yielded promising results by substantially reducing or eliminating tics in affecting individuals. However, this procedure is still experimental and not yet an available or recommended form of treatment.

CLINICAL FEATURES

The presence of motor and vocal tics in young children is not uncommon, occurring in up to 19 percent of children. The type, frequency, and duration of tics are important in classifying the type of disorder that may be affecting a child. The American Psychiatric Association's *Diagnostic and Statistic Manual of Mental Disorders: DSM-IV-TR* (rev. 4th ed., 2000) lists four disorders that involve the presence of motor or vocal tics. Tourette's syndrome is considered as a diagnosis when both motor and vocal tics persist for more than one year. The diagnostic criteria for Tourette's syndrome include multiple motor and one or more vocal tics that have been present at some time during the illness, although not necessarily concurrently. The tics occur many times during a day (usually in bouts), nearly every day or intermittently throughout a period of more than a year. The anatomic location, number, frequency, complexity, and severity of the tics may change over time. There is usually a rostral to caudal movement (from the head to the trunk of the body) of tics that will repeat itself. Onset occurs before the age of eighteen. Occurrence is not exclusively during psychoactive substance intoxication or due to known central nervous system disease, such as Huntington chorea and postviral encephalitis.

The tics that are associated with Tourette's syndrome may be motor tics if movements are involved, or they may be vocal tics if sound is produced. The syndrome commonly begins with facial tics such as blinking, grimacing, and nose twitching. Other involuntary movements may involve head shaking, arm flapping, shoulder shrugging, and foot movements. Head banging and other forms of self-abuse may occur, although these are quite rare. Tics may be simple, as is the case with eye blinking. They may be complex and involve a number of muscle groups, such as jumping up and down or imitating movements of another person. Simple tics tend to be replaced by complex tics, and the severity and frequency of tics tends to wax and wane over time. This can be the most puzzling aspect of the disorder, and research has suggested it is very difficult to predict the course of the tics over time. In

DSM-IV-TR CRITERIA FOR TOURETTE'S SYNDROME

TOURETTE'S DISORDER (DSM CODE 307.23)

Both multiple motor and one or more vocal tics (sudden, rapid, recurrent, nonrhythmic, stereotyped motor movements or vocalizations) at some time during the disorder, although not necessarily concurrently

Tics occur many times a day (usually in bouts) nearly every day or intermittently throughout a period of more than one year; during this period, no tic-free periods of more than three consecutive months

Onset before age eighteen

Disturbance not due to direct physiological effects of a substance (such as stimulants) or a general medical condition (such as Huntington's disease or postviral encephalitis)

some situations, tics are initially mild but become more severe, and in other situations, they may remit for undetermined periods of time. Tics tend to worsen under conditions of stress and tend to subside when the patient is concentrating on some task or activity. Rarely are they present during sleep. As individuals age, it becomes possible to suppress the tics with voluntary effort. A burst of tics generally follows the period of conscious suppression to relieve the mounting inner urge. Some people with Tourette's syndrome have been able to have successful careers as actors, professional athletes, and surgeons.

The most severe aspects of Tourette's syndrome, from a social point of view, are coprolalia and copropraxia (an involuntary use of obscene gestures).Copropraxia Although it is a common belief, it is not correct to think that coprolalia and copropraxia are found in nearly all people with Tourette's syndrome. In fact, coprolalia is found in less than one-third of the cases, and copropraxia is far less common.

Most individuals with Tourette's syndrome have other mental health concerns, although the severity of these issues varies considerably. The two most common comorbid conditions include attention-deficit hyperactivity disorder (ADHD) and obsessive-compulsive disorder (OCD). Studies have suggested that ADHD occurs in 50 to 60 percent of individuals with Tourette's syndrome and typically develops before the onset of tics. The incidence of OCD and Tourette's syndrome occurs in 30 to 70 percent of cases. OCD symptoms become more

evident as the child matures and in many cases become the primary clinical issue in late adolescence and adulthood. The OCD symptoms in individuals with Tourette's syndrome are more often described as sensorimotor compared with individuals with just OCD. That is, individuals with Tourette's syndrome report physical sensations before tics or repetitive behaviors, whereas individuals with OCD describe specific thoughts and anxiety before compulsive behaviors. Although Tourette's syndrome is a chronic disorder, symptoms are usually much more severe in childhood, with the severity of tics peaking by about ten years of age. The tics tend to improve or disappear entirely in more than half of affected adults.

ETIOLOGY

The cause of Tourette's syndrome is not known. It represents a unique diagnosis that involves both neurology and psychiatry. For much of its history, Tourette's syndrome was considered primarily a psychiatric disorder because of the presence of motor and vocal tics and other atpyical behaviors often associated with the syndrome. Psychiatric comorbidity does appear to be a primary feature of Tourette's syndrome, but it is often a secondary consequence of the emotionally disabling physical features. As effective treatment with medications came into use, it became apparent that there was an underlying biochemical basis for the syndrome. The drug haloperidol, which is a dopamine receptor blocker, gave good results in controlling tics, indicating that somehow there was an increased sensitivity of the dopamine system in patients with Tourette's syndrome. Some research suggests that serotonin also plays a role in Tourette's syndrome, but the primary neurotransmitter of interest is dopamine. Other studies have found some evidence of subtle abnormalities in the basal ganglia of the brain. Recent experimental procedures have successfully used deep brain stimulation (DBS) on medial regions of the thalamus, a region with connections to the basal ganglia and brain cortex. The preliminary success of this procedure underscores the basal ganglia as an important brain structure involved in Tourette's syndrome. There have been surprisingly few autopsies to study Tourette's syndrome patients. Both gross and fine anatomical studies have not yielded conclusive findings, but results indicate that multiple structures of the brain may be involved in the syndrome.

Although a familial association of Tourette's syndrome has long been known, two problems have contributed to the difficulty of genetic studies: the problem of variable expressivity and the problem of incomplete penetrance. With variable expressivity, there is a range of phenotypes resulting from a given genotype, and this is very characteristic of Tourette's syndrome, where clinical features range from very mild to very severe. In incomplete penetrance, a genotype that should give rise to a certain expression or phenotype is not expressed at all, and this also seems to be true of Tourette's syndrome. In addition, there is no universal agreement as to what the Tourette syndrome phenotype is. In spite of the limitations, considerable progress has been made in the understanding of the inheritance of Tourette's syndrome.

The agreement between Tourette's syndrome exhibited by both members of monozygotic twins is about 50 percent, compared to 10 percent for dizygotic twins. Since the value for monozygotic twins is less than 100 percent, this indicates that nongenetic and environmental factors play a role in etiology.

Most family studies indicate that Tourette's syndrome is probably due to an autosomal dominant gene with incomplete penetrance. Although simple tics do not seem to have a familial relationship, severe tics do show such a relationship, with relatives of a patient being at an increased risk for tics, if not necessarily severe tics. Relatives of patients also are at increased risks for ADHD and OCD, indicating a possible genetic relationship of the disorders. Although the human genome has been scanned, no single gene has been found that is associated with Tourette's syndrome.

TREATMENT

No medication has been found to eliminate the symptoms of Tourette's syndrome completely. Good progress has been made in using medications in controlling and improving motor and vocal tics and some of the behavioral symptoms. Haloperidol acts as a depressant of the central nervous system and is successful in helping suppress symptoms in many patients. Side effects of haloperidol include drowsiness and alterations in mood, and may be severe enough to limit its use. Also, the effectiveness of haloperidol tends to diminish over time in many patients. Other drugs in use may have fewer side effects than haloperidol, but all drugs may have side effects. If behavioral disorders such as OCD and ADHD present problems, other medications such as risperidone (Risperdal) may need to be prescribed. In general, physicians are reluctant to prescribe medications unless the tics are severe and significantly affecting an individual's daily functioning. The combination of cognitive behavior therapy and medication yields the most significant improvements in children. Other nondrug treatments, such as adaptations to diet, have been recommended.

Since the symptoms of Tourette's syndrome may change over time, it is critical to monitor the levels of medications employed. Since Tourette's syndrome can be a chronic and potentially a socially debilitating disorder, supportive psychotherapy should be available for not only patients but also their families. Until the inheritance of Tourette's syndrome is understood more fully, genetic counseling will continue to be difficult. General information about recurrence risks and gender differences in the incidence of Tourette's syndrome may be transmitted. It also is essential to inform family members and patients of the variability of expression of the disorder in patients and how symptoms may change over time in the same individual.

FURTHER READING

Brill, Marlene Targ. *Tourette Syndrome*. Brookfield, Conn.: Twenty-first Century Books, 2002. An excellent overview of Tourette's syndrome through the eyes of someone with the disorder. It is well researched and written for a broad audience.

Hayden, Michael R., and Berry Kremer. "Basal Ganglia Disorders." *In Emery and Rimoin's Principles and Practice of Medical Genetics*, edited by David L. Rimoin, J. Michael Connor, and Reed E. Pyeritz. 3d ed. New York: Churchill Livingstone Press, 1996. Reviews basal ganglia disorders that involve involuntary movement syndromes, including Tourette's syndrome.

Hyde, Thomas M., and Daniel R. Weinberger. "Tourette's Syndrome: A Model Neuropsychiatric Disorder." *The Journal of the American Medical Association* 273, no. 6 (1995): 498-501. An overview of Tourette's syndrome with useful information on a case report, genetics, environmental-genetic interactions, and treatment.

Kurlan, Roger, ed. *Handbook of Tourette's Syndrome and Related Tic and Behavioral Disorders*. 2d ed. New York: Marcel Dekker, 2005. An extensive examination of the syndrome that covers its history, associated diagnoses, neurobiology, diagnosis, genetics, and clinical cases.

Kushner, Howard I. *A Cursing Brain? The Histories of Tourette Syndrome*. Cambridge, Mass.: Harvard University Press, 1999. The book examines the history of Tourette's syndrome with exceptionally interesting historical details. There is information concerning the etiology, progression, and treatment of the disorder from the nineteenth century up to the 1980's.

Leckman, James F., and Donald J. Cohen, eds. *Tourette's Syndrome: Tics, Compulsions—Developmental Psychopathology and Clinical Care*. New York: John Wiley & Sons, 1999. A useful book for doctors, students, and families of people with Tourette's syndrome. The book combines basic information and clinical care from neurobiological, developmental, and psychodynamic perspectives.

Shimberg, Elaine. *Living with Tourette's Syndrome*. New York: Simon & Schuster, 1995. A personal account of living with Tourette's syndrome that serves as a good resource for family and individuals with the syndrome.

Donald J. Nash; updated by Martin Mrazik

SEE ALSO: Tic Disorders

Vision disorders

Poor vision caused by diseases or abnormalities of the eyes.

CAUSES AND SYMPTOMS

The most common defects in human vision are nearsightedness (myopia), farsightedness (hyperopia), and astigmatism. All three of these conditions are called refractive errors because the cornea-lens focusing system of the eye bends light rays either too much or too little, so that the image formed on the retina is blurred. Fortunately, refractive errors can be corrected by means of eyeglasses or contact lenses. Millions of people use some form of vision correction.

Myopia and hyperopia are caused by a mismatch between the focusing power of the cornea-lens combination and the length of the eyeball. For a nearsighted person, the incoming light comes to a focus in front of the retina; a diverging lens is needed to move the image farther back. For a farsighted person, the situation is reversed; a converging lens is prescribed to provide extra focusing power.

The problem of astigmatism is attributable to a difference in the focal length of the eye for two perpendicular directions, which can occur if the eyeball is slightly deformed (like a grape being squeezed between two fingers). The curvature of the corneal surface would be different in two perpendicular planes. An optometrist can correct for astigmatism by prescribing glasses with different focal lengths in the two planes. The prescription

---

INFORMATION ON VISION DISORDERS

Causes: Infection, disease, allergies, injury, cataracts, glaucoma, refractive errors (nearsightedness, farsightedness, astigmatism)

Symptoms: Vary; may include eye redness, itchiness, or inflammation; blurred or disrupted vision; bleeding or hemorrhaging from eyes

Duration: Acute to chronic

Treatments: Depend on cause; may include medicated eye drops, corrective lenses, laser surgery, antibiotics, corneal transplantation

---

must specify the angle at which the deformation of the eyeball is maximized.

A vision problem that is common among older adults is the formation of cataracts, in which the lens of the eye becomes cloudy. Cataracts are a normal part of the aging process, like wrinkled skin or gray hair. In rare cases, however, children have them at birth or after an eye injury. Cataracts form on the inside of the lens capsule, not on the surface of the eye. Once started, their growth is irreversible. While vision can often helped through the use of eyeglasses and stronger lighting, the only entirely effective treatment is surgical removal of the defective eye lens, followed by implantation of an artificial (plastic) replacement. With developments in ophthalmology, such microsurgery has a success rate of better than 95 percent. What causes eye cataracts in the elderly is not yet well understood. One suggested explanation is the Maillard reaction, in which glucose and protein molecules combine when heated to form a brown product. This chemical reaction is responsible for the browning of bread or cookies during baking. The same process is thought to occur even at body temperature, but very slowly over a period of years. It has been suggested that the onset of cataract formation can be delayed by a good diet, regular exercise, and a generally healthy lifestyle.

Glaucoma is a vision problem that afflicts about 2 percent of the adult population, normally after the age of forty. Excessive fluid pressure develops inside the eye, causing damage to the optic nerve. Peripheral vision gradually decreases—a decrease that the patient may not even notice until it is detected by an optometrist during an eye examination. The usual treatments are medicated eyedrops to reduce pressure and laser surgery to improve fluid drainage. Glaucoma has nothing to do with red or watery eyes because these symptoms occur on the exterior of the eyeball.

The retina is a paper-thin membrane at the back of the eye, nourished by a network of tiny blood vessels. A frequent problem encountered by diabetics is the enlargement and possible hemorrhaging of these blood vessels. For older adults, macular degeneration is a condition associated with arteriosclerosis, sometimes leading to retinal bleeding. The most sensitive, central region of the retina deteriorates, causing an irreversible loss in reading ability that cannot be corrected with glasses.

Another retinal problem is its detachment from the back wall of the eye. This is an emergency situation requiring immediate medical attention. A detached retina can be caused by an accumulation of fluid behind the retina resulting from leakage through a small tear in the membrane. It can also come from a blow to the eye, as with a sports injury. Laser surgery has become an effective treatment for the various types of retinal damage.

TREATMENT AND THERAPY

During an eye examination, the optometrist tries to detect any deviations from normal vision. If the patient is nearsighted or farsighted or has astigmatism, appropriate corrective lenses can be prescribed. If cataracts, glaucoma, or a retinal problem exists, the patient will be referred to an ophthalmologist, who has received specialized medical training in eye surgery.

The history of eyeglasses has been traced back to the thirteenth century, when Roger Bacon, a Catholic scholar, wrote about using convex glass to make writing appear larger. Some medieval paintings show elderly noblemen wearing eyeglasses. No significant innovations were made until Benjamin Franklin invented bifocals in 1780, to aid people whose eyes did not focus properly at either near or far distances. Until the late 1940s, prescription eyeglasses were always made out of glass. Then plastic lenses were introduced; they had the advantages of lighter weight and greater resistance to breakage. The main problem with plastic is that it scratches more easily, but coatings have been developed to overcome this drawback.

An alternative to eyeglasses came in the 1950s with the development of contact lenses. They were made out of a hard plastic and covered the front of the cornea, floating on a thin layer of tears. They provided good vision but were uncomfortable to insert. Also, hard contacts cannot transmit oxygen and carbon dioxide to nourish the surface of the cornea, causing dryness and irritation

for the wearer. Such lenses are now virtually obsolete. Daily-wear soft contact lenses became available in the 1970s. They were much more comfortable than the hard plastic material and were gas-permeable. The soft lenses had an affinity for infection-causing bacteria, however, requiring a tedious, nightly sterilizing procedure with heat or chemicals. The technology of contact lenses continues to evolve. More recent developments are soft contacts for extended wear (up to two weeks without removal), bifocal gas-permeable contacts, and inexpensive, disposable contacts (to be discarded after two or three weeks). Contact lens wearers are cautioned to have regular eye checkups to make sure that the cornea is not being damaged.

Starting in the 1970s, eye specialists began to investigate the possibility of reshaping the eyeball to do away with eyeglasses completely. The first attempt utilized a hard lens pressing directly against the cornea to flatten it, in much the same way that orthodontic braces are used to straighten teeth. The change induced in the shape of the eye generally was only temporary, so lenses still were needed afterward.

A Soviet physician, Svyatoslav Fyodorov, developed Radial Keratotomy (RK), a surgical procedure to flatten the cornea permanently. A series of shallow incisions is made in the outer part of the cornea in a radial pattern, like the spokes of a wheel. The center of the cornea is not touched. As the incisions heal, the cornea bulges slightly near the edges, thus reducing its curvature in the middle. In this way, a permanent cure for nearsightedness can be accomplished. While thousands of patients underwent RK surgery between 1980 and 1993, the procedure remained controversial. The main problem was that the number of incisions and their depth could overcorrect or undercorrect the original refractive error. Also, some ophthalmologists were concerned about possible long-term aftereffects of scars on the cornea. RK soon decreased in popularity.

Another technique to alter the shape of the cornea is called keratomileusis. The outer half of the patient's cornea is removed and frozen, and then reshaped with a computer-controlled lathe to a predetermined curvature. After thawing, the cornea is sewn back into place, where it acts as a permanent contact lens. Keratomileusis can correct both myopia and hyperopia.

The laser, invented by physicists in the 1960s, is a very intense beam of light that can be adapted particularly well for surgery on the retina of the eye. The light beam passes successively through the transparent cornea, aqueous fluid, and lens without being absorbed. Its energy is then concentrated into a tiny spot on the retina, causing localized vaporization, or "welding," to occur. Laser-assisted in situ keratomileusis (LASIK) became quite popular at the end of the twentieth century. In LASIK surgery, the cornea is reshaped to help patients overcome myopia, hyperopia, or astigmatism. The procedure is done with a cool beam laser that removes thin layers of tissue from selected sites on the cornea to change its curvature. Success rates are high: 90 to 95 percent of the patients get 20/40 vision, and 65 to 75 percent of the patients get 20/20 vision or better. Lasers can also be used to excise leaking blood vessels and to repair or reattach a damaged retina.

Another surgical technique is to use a corneal transplant from an organ donor. The new cornea is shaped to the proper curvature with a lathe and is sewn on top of the patient's own cornea. The standard treatment for cataracts is surgical removal of the defective lens, followed by implantation of an artificial, plastic lens. Ophthalmologists routinely perform cataract surgery using only local anesthetic, so that the patient can go home without an overnight hospital stay.

Glaucoma, a condition of excess pressure in the eye, affects millions of people and has caused thousands of cases of blindness. The first line of treatment is the use of daily medication in the form of eyedrops to reduce the fluid pressure. Eventually, surgery may be necessary. The procedure used enlarges an opening at the edge of the iris to allow for better drainage of the aqueous fluid between the lens and cornea. The incision can be made with either a miniature scalpel or a laser. Glaucoma damage to the optic nerve cannot be repaired, but prompt treatment can prevent further deterioration of vision.

PERSPECTIVE AND PROSPECTS

The human eye is the most important sense organ for individuals to gather information about their environment. An amazingly high 40 percent of all nerve fibers going to the brain come from the retina of the eye. Any defect or deterioration from normal vision is a serious limitation. During the Middle Ages, few people learned to read and write, so the need for seeing at close range was not important. In modern society, however, people with poor eyesight are greatly handicapped. For example, students, computer operators, airplane pilots, and athletes cannot function without good vision.

Society is gradually becoming more sympathetic to people with handicaps, including blindness. Braille printing, guide dogs, and books recorded on audiotape are helpful developments for the blind. The U.S. Congress in 1992 passed the Americans with Disabilities Act, which mandates improved access for the visually impaired in facilities that serve the general public. Nevertheless, retaining good vision and preventing further deterioration will continue to be a vital part of overall health care.

FURTHER READING

Anshel, Jeffrey. *Healthy Eyes, Better Vision: Everyday Eye Care for the Whole Family.* Los Angeles: Body Press, 1990.

Berns, Michael W. "Laser Surgery." *Scientific American* 264 (June, 1991): 84–90.

Buettner, Helmut, ed. *Mayo Clinic on Vision and Eye Health: Practical Answers on Glaucoma, Cataracts, Macular Degeneration, and Other Conditions.* Rochester, Minn.: Mayo Foundation for Medical Education and Research, 2002.

Cassel, Gary H., Michael D. Billig, and Harry G. Randall. *The Eye Book: A Complete Guide to Eye Disorders and Health.* Baltimore: Johns Hopkins University Press, 2001.

"Eye Health and Safety." *Prevent Blindness America,* 2011.

"Healthy Eyes." *National Eye Institute,* 2013.

Parker, James N., and Philip M. Parker, eds. *The Official Patient's Sourcebook on Myopia.* San Diego, Calif.: Icon Health, 2004.

"Refractive Errors." *MedlinePlus,* May 20, 2013.

Sardegna, Jill, et al. *The Encyclopedia of Blindness and Vision Impairment.* 2d ed. New York: Facts On File, 2002.

Sutton, Amy L. *Ophthalmic Disorders Sourcebook.* 3d ed. Detroit, Mich.: Omnigraphics, 2008.

Sutton, Amy L., ed. *Eye Care Sourcebook: Basic Consumer Health Information About Eye Care and Eye Disorders.* 3d ed. Detroit, Mich.: Omnigraphics, 2008.

"Vision Impairment and Blindness." *MedlinePlus,* May 28, 2013.

"What Is Low Vision?" *EyeSmart.* American Academy of Ophthalmology, 2013.

Hans G. Graetzer

SEE ALSO: Eyes

Diversity

Biracial heritage

The United States has always contained many racial and ethnic groups, but during the twenty-first century the country has become more diverse than ever. Many individuals' heritages are not only bi-racial, but also multi-racial. Acknowledging this, the United States Census is now designed to allow an individual to designate more than one racial or ethnic heritage. The Census Bureau collects race data according to U.S. Office of Management and Budget guidelines, and all data are self-identified. That is, people choose their own race or ethnicity. The Census definitions are popular constructs that generally reflect a social definition of race as recognized in the United States, not a scientific, biological, or genetic definition.

INTRODUCTION

According to the U.S. Census, as of 2010, "white" Americans (those with their predominant heritage from one or more of many European countries) are the racial majority, with 63 per cent of the population. Hispanic and Latino Americans (roots in Spain or Latin America) made up about 18 per cen, the largest ands fastest growing minority. African-Americans were 13 per cent, and Asians about 5 per cent. Native Americans constituted about 1 per cent.

Vine Deloria, Jr., the renowned Native American author, educator, and activist, was fond of saying that race does not exist (as a valid concept in biology or anthropology), but racism does, in politics and history. While ethnicity does influence culture, race, per se, is not regarded as a valid biological concept in the scholarly world. That has not kept it from being influential as a device to aggravate social tension.

RACE, RACISM AND THE U.S. CENSUS

The U.S. Census has attempted to describe the country's multi-racial character since its beginning, with categories reflecting assumptions that have been dominant at any particular time. Given the shifting nature of racial and ethnic categories in the Census, any attempt to use its information to compare how the country's proportion of different groups has changed over time should be undertaken with care. The changing nature of Census categories also indicates just how little racial categories have to do with science. They are socially constructed, and change swiftly with popular attitudes.

The treatment of race and ethnicity in the Census has changed a great deal over the years. In 1790, the main questions involved "slave" and "free" individuals. In 1820, the term "colored" (mixed white and black) was introduced, along with a question that counted "foreigners not naturalized." This question was refined in 1830 as "The number of White persons who were foreigners not naturalized." In 1850, a form was added to indicate whether a person was "W" (white), "B" (black), or "M" (mulatto, or mixed).

By 1870, a "C" (Chinese, indicating anyone of East Asian heritage) was added, along with "AI" (American Indian). In 1890, Japanese and Chinese were counted separately. In 1900, American Indians were asked to indicate whether they lived on or off reservations, and what proportion of their heritage was "white." The 1910 Census asked for information about a respondent's "mother tongue." By 1920, "Hindu" (South Asian), Filipino, and Korean categories had appeared. These were removed after 1940, but re-introduced in 1970, with "East Indians" (formerly called Hindus) being classified as "white."

In the 1930 Census, the "mulatto" category was removed. A person with any African-American heritage at all was to be listed as Negro under the "one drop" rule (one drop of Negro blood made the person African-American for Census purposes). This included some respondents whose heritages were partially American Indian, who were recorded under that category only if they were predominantly racially and culturally Native American, and recognized as such within their communities (a standard that was much more restrictive than having one drop of blood). The Census at that time also asked whether American Indians of mixed European ancestry were accepted as "white" or "Indian" in a community context, to gauge assimilation.

Census forms were openly patriarchal in 1930 – that is, anyone with interracial ancestry was recorded as the father's race. Also, in 1930, for the first (and only) time, the term "Mexican" appeared on Census forms, to include persons born there, or whose parents were Mexican. The Census had no such category for anyone else of Latin American ancestry, and Mexican-Americans were to be counted as "white."

The same confusion was reflected in court decisions. In 1935, for example, a federal judge ruled that three Mexican immigrants could not obtain U.S. citizenship because they were not "white," as U.S. law of the time required. Responding to diplomatic pressure, President

Franklin D. Roosevelt intervened and instructed all agencies of the federal government, including the Census Bureau, to classify persons of Mexican descent as "white," thus beginning decades of categorical confusion on Census forms regarding how to classify persons of Latino heritage. The category "Mexican" thus vanished from Census forms after 1940.

Late in the twentieth century, the U.S. Census increased its list of specific racial categories (such as East Indian, Guamanian, Vietnamese, Samoan, and others). The list was still woefully incomplete given the number of different peoples actually present in the United States, so some groups were being counted and others left out. In 1990, the Census allowed bi- or multiple heritages as a write-in option, but did not include them in its tallies. The first race listed was assigned to a person (a listing of black-white was listed as black, for example).

In 2000 a list of several racial categories was offered and respondents were invited to choose more than one and, for the first time, these choices were also reported. That year, nearly 9 million people checked more than one category. The largest category was mixed "white" and Native American or Alaska Native. It is probable that many other people of mixed heritage did not report it. At about the same time the American Anthropological Association requested that the Census remove the word "race" from its forms in favor of "ethnicity" on grounds that "race" has no precise meaning in human biology or studies of societies. The Census did not adopt this recommendation on its forms for 2010.

ETHNIC UNDERSTANDING: SEATTLE'S "FOUR AMIGOS"

Multi-ethnicity continues to increase in the United States even as the Census wrestles with ways to measure it. For example, the Seattle area has rapidly become much more multi-ethnic as leaders of different minorities have learned to cooperate in pursuit of common goals, providing a national laboratory for Martin Luther King, Jr.'s concept of a multi-racial nation. Starting in the 1960s, leaders of Asian, Black, Latino, and Native American communities planned common strategies.

Native leader Bernie Whitebear led an initial sit-in that turned a piece of surplus Army land into the Daybreak Star, an enduring urban Indian service and cultural center. The creation of Daybreak Star occurred within the context of fishing-rights assertions in the face of state power at about the same time. Roberto F. Maestas led another occupation that founded El Centro

de la Raza, which also evolved into a service, educational, and cultural center. Larry Gossett, a one-time black student militant, and later a King County Council member, spearheaded a multicultural movement to change the name of King County (which includes Seattle) from honoring nineteenth-century slaveholder William Rufus DeVane King to honor Dr. King's legacy. Filipino Bob Santos led a movement to preserve Seattle's best-known Asian neighborhood in the face of outside development.

Each member of this group openly acknowledged his bi- or multi-racial heritage, and explored ways of celebrating his own heritage while upholding the validity of others. Maestas, who died in 2010, was fond of saying that he was partially European (Hispanic, from Spain), partially Native American (Pueblo, from New Mexico), and partially black, and that he loved all the parts. Santos was Filipino, with its mix of Hispanic and multiple Asian roots. He also, through his wife, is married into an "Indiopino" (American Indian and Filipino) family. Whitebear, who died in 2000, was Native American and European, and Gossett is African and European-American.

These four leaders became close friends, later known as "The Four Amigos" or, in jest, "The Gang of Four." Each developed a constituency that supported the others in fishing-rights assertions, demonstrations by minority construction workers, and building occupations, putting bodies on the line, even risking arrest. As a result communities formed as their goals were reached.

All four leaders shared a dream that Martin Luther King would have recognized. Although each of them would deny that social change is the work of a few individuals, or that decades of complex social and political change could be summarized in a few short words (in any language), the Four Amigos shared ideas about how people should co-operate, as well as the passion and organizing skills required to rally many hundreds of people who took part in confrontations during which they often risked arrest. Many in Seattle who initially resisted these ideas and tactics came to respect, and even to embrace them over the years.

FURTHER READING

Deloria, V. Jr. (1988). *Custer died for your sins: An Indian manifesto*. Norman, OK: University of Oklahoma Press. This book is a scathing indictment of attitudes toward race and racism.

Santos, B. and Iwamoto, G. (2015). *The Gang of Four: Four, four communities, one friendship.* Seattle, WA: Chin Music Press Inc. This account traces the unity of Latino, Black, Asian, and American Indian communities in Seattle.

Prewitt, K. (2013) *What is your race? The Census and our flawed efforts to classify Americans.* Princeton, NJ: Princeton University Press. This book argues that racial and ethnic categories should be dropped from the U.S. Census.

U.S. Census Bureau. (2015). "Race." http://www.census.gov/topics/population/race.html. This is the official U.S. Census web page on race and ethnicity.

Bruce E. Johansen

SEE ALSO: Racism

Hate crimes

Hate crimes are criminal offenses, such as murder, assault, arson, or vandalism, that are motivated by the offenders' bias against the race, nationality, religion, ethnicity, disability, or sexual orientation of the targeted person. The motives for these crimes are rooted in learned behaviors and discrimination that may have been present for generations.

INTRODUCTION

The term "hate crime" is a relatively new term, though bias-motivated crime has a much longer history. Advocates who were addressing violent crime in the United States that targeted African Americans, Asian Americans, and Jewish Americans in the 1980s are believed to have coined the term. Since the coining of the term, federal and state governments, as well as social scientists, have made efforts to formally define hate crimes for the purposes of collecting statistics and improving law-enforcement and prevention efforts.

The Federal Bureau of Investigation (FBI) defines a hate crime as a "a criminal offense against a person, property or property motivated in whole or in part by the offender's bias against a race, religion, disability, sexual orientation, or ethnicity/national origin." However, complete agreement on what constitutes a hate crime has not been reached.

In the past, although these criminal acts could be prosecuted, the punishment did not include a consideration of the bias motivating the crime. Thus, painting a swastika on the door of a Jewish person's home was considered a crime because the graffiti defaced property and a law existed against vandalism, but not because the act was done to intimidate the resident. Hate crime laws allow the psychological harm done to a victim to be factored into the determination of whether any special sanctions should occur. Research has suggested that the victim of a hate crime experiences more harm than does the victim of a similar crime not motivated by bias or hate. In 2009, the United States Congress passed the Matthew Shepard and James Byrd Jr. Hate Crimes Prevention Act, which provides federal funding and assistance to state, local, and tribal jurisdictions to assist in the investigation and prosecution of hate crimes. The law also created a new federal criminal law that criminalizes causing bodily injury when the crime was committed because of the actual or perceived race, color, religion, or national origin of any person, or when the crime was committed because of the actual or perceived religion, national origin, gender, sexual orientation, gender identity, or disability of any person and the crime affected interstate or foreign commerce or occurred with federal special maritime and territorial jurisdictions. The law removed the requirement that the victim be engaged in a federally protected activity, such as voting or attending a public school, at the time of the crime.

The law is named after Matthew Shepard and James Byrd Jr., who were both victims of violent hate crimes in 1998 in US states that had no existing hate crime laws at the time.

CAUSES

The central cause of these crimes is hate, which most often is the result of fear, anger, and ignorance. Hate crimes are acts of bias, bigotry, and intolerance toward an identified group. Though individuals and small groups may be the actual victims, the ultimate target of the perpetrators is the group to which the victims belong. For example, a hate crime offender may target and beat a black man in order to intimidate all African Americans in the community. Perpetrators of hate crimes seek to terrorize the larger group by criminal acts against its members.

The beliefs and prejudices held by hate crime offenders are learned and can go back for generations. Perpetrators develop an "us-versus-them" outlook, in which they hold that their own group is superior and correct in its view and that the other group is inferior.

The other group's members may be seen as interlopers. In addition, they may be made the scapegoats for what is perceived to be wrong in a society. In this way, the other group is made responsible for economic problems, crime, and the other ills of society. Often when an identifiable group migrates into an area (community, state, or country), the resident group sees the immigrants as a drain on—or competitor for—the available resources and views their removal as the only solution. Research indicates that some of the most extreme biased responses are sparked by a perceived threat to the cultural integrity of the perpetrators' ingroup by members of an outgroup. Typically, a hate group or hate crime perpetrator does not know much about the identified group. In fact, the less people know about an identified outgroup, the stronger their prejudices will be. Social psychology research has identified a phenomenon known as the "outgroup homogeneity effect," by which people tend to see members of groups that they are not apart of as more homogenous than members of their own group, empowering stereotypes and leading to deindividuation of outgroup members.

Researchers Jack McDevitt, Jack Levin, and Susan Bennett, in a 2002 study published in the *Journal of Social Issues,* classified hate time offenders into four categories based on the psychological and situational factors that led to hate crimes: thrill-seeking perpetrators are motivated by a desire for excitement and power; defensive perpetrators are motivated by protecting their community from perceived outsiders; retaliatory perpetrators commit violence in response to a real or perceived hate crime against their own group by members of the target group; and missionary perpetrators are typically members of hate groups who are deeply motivated by bigotry and see it as their "mission" to intimidate or eliminate the other group. These categories are widely used by law enforcement officers in the investigation and identification of hate crimes. Thrill-seeking is thought to be the most common motivation for hate crime offenders.

VICTIMS AND OFFENDERS

Potential hate crime victims are those who are or are thought to be members of an identifiable group. These victims differ from victims of random crimes in that hate crime victims are specifically selected as a crime target due to their race, ethnicity, nationality, religion, sexual orientation, gender identity, or disability. They were not victimized for what they were doing or what they had in their possession, but for what and who they are. Con-

sequently, these victims cannot alter their behaviors to protect themselves from possible future ttacks.

While all violent crime puts victims at risk for psychological distress, victims of violent hate crimes are even more likely to suffer from depression, anxiety, anger, and posttraumatic stress disorder than victims of comparable violent crimes that are not motivated by bias and hate. Furthermore, hate crimes send a message to all members of a given group that their neighborhood, school, workplace, or community is hostile and dangerous to them. Hate crimes victimize not only the targeted individuals but members of their group at large. Members of the targeted group may experience psychological distress, heightened anxiety, and lowered self-esteem.

In the United States, the most frequent profile of a hate crime offender is a young white man, usually one who has low self-esteem and is socially isolated. Research demonstrates that the perpetrators of hate crimes also demonstrate above-average levels of aggression and antisocial behavior. However, most offenders do not have a diagnosable psychopathology. Alcohol and drug use can contribute to their behavior. Other characteristics of offenders include a history of abuse and of witnessing violence used as a coping method.

These hate crime offenders hold stereotypical beliefs that cause them to view the entire identified group as a threat. Out of their need for belonging, they may be attracted to hate groups, where people share their beliefs. Though less than 10 percent of the reported hate crimes are committed by members of organized hate groups, these groups can produce splinter groups or influence individuals who come in contact with them. Areas where there are high levels of hate-group activity and membership typically report higher numbers of hate crimes.

Offenders may plan their crimes over a period of time or act spontaneously on finding a target. However, there is a strong premeditated component to hate crimes compared to other criminal offenses. People who commit hate crimes are more likely to deliberate on and plan their attacks than the perpetrators of nonbias-related crimes, and some may even travel long distances to seek out members of their targeted group. Though their crimes may appear irrational to most people, the perpetrators see them as logical and defensible, the natural result of the cultural climate that fostered the hate ideology.

HATE CRIME STATISTICS

According to FBI statistics, there were 5,796 reported hate crime incidents involving 6,718 criminal offenses in the United States in 2012. Approximately 49 percent of these hate crimes were racially motivated, with 66 percent of racially motivated hate crimes involving anti-black bias, 22 percent involving anti-white bias, 4 percent involving anti-Asian/Pacific Islander bias, and 3 percent involving anti–American Indian bias. The next most common types of hate crimes, in descending order, were motivated by bias against sexual orientation (19 percent), religion (19 percent), ethnicity or nationality (12 percent), and disability (1.5 percent). Nearly 60 percent of all hate crimes motivated by ethnicity or nationality bias targeted Hispanic and Latino individuals. Of the 6,718 hate crime offenses reported in 2012, nearly 60 percent involved crimes against persons and 38 percent involved crimes against property.

Approximately 28 percent of all reported hate crime offenses in 2012 involved property damages and vandalism, 23 percent involved simple assault, 22 percent involved intimidation, and 12 percent involved aggravated assault.

Of the 5,331 hate crime offenders whose race was reported in 2012, approximately 55 percent were white, 23 percent were black, 9 percent were groups made up of individuals of various races, 0.9 percent were Asian or Pacific Islander, and 0.9 percent were American Indian.

The majority of victims of antireligious hate crimes were Jewish (62 percent), followed by Muslims (12 percent), Catholics (6 percent), Protestants (3 percent), and atheists or agnostics (0.9 percent). Of the individuals targeted due the offender's bias against disability, approximately 80 percent were targeted due to mental disability and 20 percent were targeted due to physical disability.

HATE CRIME VERSUS TERRORISM

When compared, hate crimes and terrorist acts share many of the same characteristics. They are acts of intimidation, acts against an identifiable group, and attempts to send a message of hostility and induce fear. However, terrorism tends to be national or international in scope and to be better organized and planned than most hate crimes. Terrorists tend to seek large gatherings with many potential victims, partly because of the greater expected media coverage. Terrorists also tend to have political motives and often seek the removal of the targeted group, particularly if it is a government group or occupying force. Some theorists have argued that terrorism is an "upward crime," in which a perpetrator of lower social standing targets members of the majority or the dominant group in society, whereas hate crimes are largely committed by members of the dominant group against members of minority groups.

FURTHER READING

Cheng, Wen, William Ickes, and Jared B. Kenworthy. "The Phenomenon of Hate Crimes in the United States." *Journal of Applied Social Psychology* 43.4 (2013): 761–94. Print.

Deloughery, Kathleen, Ryan D. King, and Victor Asal. "Close Cousins or Distant Relatives: The Relationship between Terrorism and Hate Crime." *Crime and Delinquency* 58.5 (2012): 663–88. Print.

Gerstenfeld, Phyllis B. *Hate Crimes: Causes, Controls, and Controversies*. 3rd ed. Los Angeles: Sage, 2013. Print.

King, Ryan D., and Gretchen M. Sutton. "High Times for Hate Crimes: Explaining the Temporal Clustering of Hate-Motivated Offending." *Criminology* 51.4 (2013): 871–94. Print.

Mason-Bish, Hannah, and Alan Roulstone. *Disability, Heat Crime and Violence*. London: Routledge, 2013. Print.

McDevitt, J., J. Levin, and S. Bennett. "Hate Crime Offenders: An Expanded Typology." *Journal of Social Issues* 58.2 (2002): 303–17. Print.

Merino, Noël, ed. *Hate Crimes*. Detroit: Greenhaven, 2009. Print.

Paulson, Lawrence N. *Hate Crimes: Legal Issues and Legislation*. New York: Nova Science, 2008. Print.

Post, Jerrold M., Cody McGinnis, and Kristen Moody. "The Changing Face of Terrorism in the 21st Century: The Communications Revolution and the Virtual Community of Hatred." *Behavioral Sciences and the Law* 32.3 (2014): 306–34. Print.

Schafer, J., and J. Navarro. "The Seven-Stage Hate Model: The Psychopathology of Hate Groups." *FBI Law Enforcement Bulletin* 72.3 (2003): 1–8. Print.

Shively, Michael, and Carrie F. Mulford. "Hate Crime in America: The Debate Continues." *National Institute of Justice Journal* 257 (2007): 8–13. Print.

Richard L. McWhorter

SEE ALSO: Racism; Sexism; Stereotyping

LGBT teens and parental acceptance

Adolescence is fraught with challenges so numerous that they may seem never ending. Experiencing romantic relationships can be one of the most exciting and one of the most difficult aspects of growing into adulthood. One's sexual orientation is often brutally scrutinized by peers and more often by family. An adolescent self – identified as lesbian, gay, bisexual, or transgender not only has to deal with the common "growing pains" of an everyday teenager but also has the very sensitive task of disclosing their sexual identity to their parents and family members. This is often a turning point in one's family accompanied by depression, rejection, and questioning of one's self-worth. By bringing awareness to this highly sensitive area of adolescent development, more can be done to educate young adults and their families navigating these waters as to where they can turn for help and support.

INTRODUCTION

Defining commonly used and interchangeably used terms when exploring adolescent sexuality can help shed light on what can be a very confusing part of normal human development. Genetic, hormonal, and anatomic characteristics determine whether a person is a biologic female or male. Biologic sex typically is defined by medical assessment of genitalia during infancy. Anatomic sex usually is viewed as a binary concept, male or female. Children are typically raised according to their biologically or anatomically assigned sex, with little additional thought given to the individual's psychological or behavioral self-identification.

The term "questioning" is used when an individual is within the process of exploring one's own sexual orientation, investigating influences that may come from their family, religious upbringing, and internal motivations.

Gender identity is an individual's innate sense of being male, female, or somewhere in between. Gender role is society's expectations of attitudes, behaviors, and personality traits typically based on biologic sex. Masculinity and femininity are main concepts conveying these cultural associations. Gender expression is how gender is presented to the outside world but does not necessarily correlate with gender identity.

Sexual orientation is defined as the type of sexual, romantic, physical, and/or spiritual attraction one feels for others. An individual is often labeled based on the gender relationship between him or her and the people he or she is attracted to. Sexual orientation is not synonymous with sexual activity. Many adolescents may identify themselves as lesbian, gay or bisexual without having had any sexual experience with someone of the same sex. Others have sexual experiences with a person of the same sex but do not consider themselves lesbian, gay or bisexual. This is particularly relevant during adolescence because experimentation and discovery are normal and common during this developmental period.

Current models of gender theory move beyond two dimensions and include variations of self-identification and terminology such as: gender variance, gender queer, gender fluid, two-spirit, or transgender. In general, transgender refers to individuals whose gender role or gender identity is not congruent with their biologic or anatomically assigned sex. An individual is commonly referred to as "transitioning" if he or she is undergoing the process of moving from one sex/gender to another. Sometimes, this is done by hormone or surgical treatments. Gay is a term used to describe a man who is attracted to men, but often used and embraced by women to describe their same-sex relationships as well. The term lesbian is traditionally used to describe a woman who's emotional, romantic, and/or sexual desires are geared towards other women. The term heterosexual or straight is used to describe someone who is sexually attracted to another person of the opposite sex. People that define themselves as bisexual are intimately involved, romantically, emotionally, and/or sexually, with both men and women. The acronym "LGBT" is used to refer to individuals part of the lesbian, gay, bisexual, or transgender community.

SOCIAL AND CULTURAL INFLUENCES

Influences on adolescent sexual development may include factors such as involvement of family, peers, and social networks, traditions related to race, ethnicity, culture, or religion which may have codes of conduct regarding sexual behavior, and one's immediate environment such as their neighborhood or school. Because there are so many different influences, sexual development can and usually does look very different from person to person.

A great amount of time and emotional energy is devoted to the development of sexual identity in adolescence. In the early teenage years, there is a preoccupation with romantic issues. During this time, mixed gender social groups naturally begin to form. In late teenage years, romantic relationships become central to social life. A vast majority of teens report having at least one relationship during this time that is defined as "serious". Individuals may spend more time with their chosen partner than they do with their family.

Although very normal, this time in adolescent development can be overwhelming with new feelings, desires, and changing social dynamics. It's no wonder that family, in particular parental involvement is a crucial source of support when going through this process.

PARENTAL INVOLVEMENT

Parental communication has been positively related to the delaying of the initiation to sexual intercourse among teens. Higher family cohesion promotes more vigilant and competent decision making. Open family communication stressing responsibility, education about sexually transmitted infections, sexuality, and contraception positively influences adolescent decision making. Teens who talked with parents about sexual behavior are more likely to use contraception than their peers who do not have this type of relationship with their parents. This being said, it can be very difficult to initiate these lines of communication, especially if one is questioning their sexual identify. According to an article written by Kathleen A. Commendador in 2010 reviewing the studies of the past 25 years in the area of parental involvement in sexual development, most adolescents perceive their parents as the most important factor in influencing their long-term decisions and parental views have the highest influence on sexual opinions, beliefs, and attitudes. In other words, teen sexual development begins in the home with parental figures. Parental disapproval, particularly maternal disapproval, throughout the period of sexual development can greatly impact one's sense of self as they progress to adulthood.

COMING OUT AND PARENTAL ACCEPTANCE

The term "coming out" can be defined as recognizing one's sexual orientation, gender identity, or sexual identity, and to be open about it with oneself and with others. This process does not end with informing close friends or family members of one's sexuality. This process does not have to happen all at once. It can be lifelong depending on how one chooses to do it. Many individuals deem this as pivotal or life changing. What can be a very freeing experience for some can be a traumatic event for others if support from family and community members is not present. It can be very difficult to predict how someone will react, especially when coming out to parents.

It is realistic to think that parental reaction to coming out may not be positive. Being mentally prepared for any reaction, positive or negative, is important. Some parents may react as if they had already known of their child's sexual orientation and were just waiting for their child to say it. Others may be open and accepting from the very beginning while others may initially go into a period of grieving. This period has been described as parental grieving for the loss of what they imagined to be in their child's future. The "white picket fence" idealistic dream of a perfect adult life may seem to dissolve in some parent's minds when their children identify as not heterosexual. A parent can be said to be grieving the life that they thought their child would have. Parents may even feel guilty as if they have somehow caused this to happen to their child or that a wrong decision has lead to their child identifying as LGBT.

Studies have been conducted examining the impact of parental acceptance on the behaviors of teens in the LGBT community. A study done by researchers Ryan, Huebner, Diaz, and Sanchez in 2009 suggested associations between parental rejecting behavior during adolescence and use of illegal drugs, depression, attempted suicide, and sexual health risk by LGBT young adults. It has been said that although parents may go through an initial grieving period, many eventually move towards acceptance. Accepting and rejecting behaviors can co-occur as families adjust to learning about their child's LGBT identity. Acceptance and affirmation parental behaviors have been linked to mental health and behavior risks in young adulthood such as high self-esteem, increased social support, and better health status including decreased depression, substance abuse, sexual risk behavior, and suicidal ideation.

The Family Acceptance Project (FAP) is an initiative that works to prevent health and mental health risks for lesbian, gay, bisexual and transgender (LGBT) children and youth, including suicide, homelessness and HIV, in the context of diverse familial, cultural, and faith communities. This project not only combats the negative outcomes of parental rejection, it also stresses the need for focus to be placed on the positive outcomes of parental openness and acceptance. According to research conducted as part of this act, family acceptance did not vary based on gender, sexual identity, or transgender identity. In other words, it did not appear that families and parents are more accepting of females than males who identify as LGBT. It appears that ethnicity and religious or cultural affiliation change the rates of acceptance among families. For example, the FAP found that Latino families, religious families regardless of religion, immigrant families, and families of low socioeconomic status appear to be less accepting of LGBT adolescents.

SUPPORT

It's important to be prepared when coming out. Know where to go for support in case things get tough at home or school. Family members, parents, and friends are going through this process along with the adolescent coming out. Education can be one of the best ways to raise awareness of the importance of parental acceptance and support. The organization Parents, Families and Friends of Lesbians and Gays (PFLAG), a support group for parents of gays, lesbians, bisexual, and transgender persons, is an excellent resource for ways to support LGBT teens. Again, parental acceptance may not happen right away or at all. It's important to be aware of this and know that sexual discovery and determination of sexual identity is a natural, normal part of growing up. LGBT teens are not alone. Having the courage to come out to the world as one's true self is one of the most difficult things teens for to do. Know there is hope and support out there, even if it's not at home.

FURTHER READING

LaSala, M. (2011, March, 12). Should you come out to your parents? *Psychology Today*. Retrieved from: https://www.psychologytoday.com/blog/gay-and-les-bian-well-being/201103/should-you-come-out-your-parents. This article provides tips for deciding when to come out to family and parents. The author also provides suggestions as to when not to come out to parents, such as when physical or emotional violence may be an issue.

The Family Acceptance Project (FAP). http://family-project.sfsu.edu/. This website offers resources for families with LGBT teens. It focuses on new research about the impact that families and parents have on the life of teens. It also provides educational materials for families wanting to know more about how to support their teens.

It Gets Better Project. http://www.itgetsbetter.org/. This website offers support to LGBT teens facing challenges because of their sexuality. It also offers teens opportunities to join support groups and meet others that share their struggle.

Neece, R. (2011, November 12). The parent crap: 10 tips for coming out. *Huffington Post*. Retrieved from: http://www.huffingtonpost.com/randy-neece/the-parent-crap-10-tips-for-coming-out_b_2104164.html. This article also provides tips when deciding how and when to come out to family members. It stresses the importance of mental preparation when going into this situation.

Parents, Families and Friends of Lesbians and Gays (PFLAG). https://community.pflag.org/. This is the nation's largest organization for parents, families, friends, and allies united with people who are lesbian, gay, bisexual, or transgender. It has many chapters throughout the U.S. and this website has information on how to get involved in a local chapter.

The Trevor Project. http://www.thetrevorproject.org/. This organization is dedicated to providing crisis intervention and suicide prevention for LGBT teens.

Ryan, C., Russell, S., Huebner, D., Diaz, R., & Sanchez, J (2010). Family acceptance in adolescence and the health of LGBT young adults. *Journal of Child and Adolescent Psychiatric Nursing*, 23, 205- 213. This article explores the relationships between various families and LGBT teens and how a positive reaction with parental acceptance can be a protective factor for LGBT teens against issues such as drug use and suicide.

Theresa Mastronardi

SEE ALSO: Depression; Gender Roles and Conflicts; LGBT Teens and Peer Acceptance; Self-Esteem; Teenage Suicide

LGBT teens and peer acceptance

The centuries-old childhood saying "Sticks and stones will break my bones, but names/words will never hurt me," suggesting that negative words or verbal bullying will not hurt a person, and, therefore, should be ignored or at least downplayed, may be long past its time. For many adolescents, especially for LGBT teens, words are usually quite hurtful and often have lasting emotional, psychological, and at times physical effects.

INTRODUCTION

There is no other time in life when peer acknowledgement and acceptance is more sought after and needed than in adolescence, and no other group needs the acknowledgement and acceptance of their peers more than LGBTs. While adolescence and all its difficulties present problems for all teens, LGBT teens have a unique set of circumstances that present additional burdens. Studies show conclusively that LGBT teens are routinely bullied, both verbally and physically, harassed, and marginalized by their peers. Such treatment and negative experiences often results in higher rates of depression, suicidal thoughts, suicide attempts, and substance abuse for LGBT teens; in addition, LGBT teens' education may be compromised as they often miss school or drop out altogether as they do not feel school offers them a safe environment.

LGBT-UNIQUE PROBLEMS

Adolescence, a difficult time of transition from childhood to adulthood, is an especially vulnerable time for many. It's a time when self-awareness and awareness of place in one's social structure is forming and often solidifying. The need to have a sense of belonging and "fitting in" the need for the all-important peer acknowledgement and acceptance, are at a lifetime high. With a "heightened awareness" and, as Toomey, et al. refer to as the "sense of an imaginary audience," or a heightened self-consciousness or sense of being constantly watched and judged, teens are at one of the most vulnerable points of their lives. Bullying of any kind, and any words or actions that place teens in the position of being an "outsider" are difficult, and studies show that this is heightened for LGBT teens.

School, for better or worse, is the center of most young people's universe, so experiences there are all the more important. Society has generally viewed schools as safe, somewhat benign places where children, adolescents, and teens directly and indirectly learn vitally important socialization skills needed for lifetime growth and success. In addition, students, as they mature, learn not only by their peers' words and actions, but also by their subconscious ability to pick up on "cues," that teach them where they as individuals "fit" into the larger picture. It could be stated that there is no other time in a person's life that the need to "fit in" is more keenly felt, the need, as Anderman calls it, of a sense of "school belonging." And the sense of "school belonging" can be especially important for LGBT teens as "coming out" to family is often a difficult experience, so peer acceptance may be their only avenue of support.

Studies, including the biennial "National School Climate Survey," of the Gay, Lesbian & Straight Education Network (GLSEN) point to higher rates of depression, suicidal thoughts, and suicidal attempts by LGBT students than their straight peers. LGBT teens are also more prone to substance-abuse. And physical bullying and assaults can result in teens missing school or dropping out as they do not feel safe at school. As Russell states "For too many LGBT and gender variant students, school victimization has resulted in school failure, poorer grades, and restricted life chances that limit vocational and career development and undermine their human potential."

All students that suffer from verbal or physical abuse, bullying, harassment and marginalization are negatively affected, but as Martin-Storey and Crosnoe point out, studies show there is a "unique role of harassment due to sexual minority status." In fact, according to a study by Swearer and colleagues, "boys who were bullied because they were called gay experienced great psychological distress, greater verbal and physical bullying, and more negative perceptions of their school experiences than boys who were bullied for other reasons." And in addition, LGBT boys often experience more harassment than LGBT girls. As Toomey points out "biological sex may be a moderator in the backlash toward gender nonconformity."

SOLUTIONS

School boards, school administrators, and teachers, in fact, all adults that interact with teens must approach the problems uniquely faced by LGBT teens in a similar way that they would tackle any biased or prejudiced behavior. Policies should be formed and implemented. Actions must be taken, as inaction or non-action on the part of teachers can be interpreted as tacit approval of harassment and bullying. In addition, teachers should be offered sensitivity training to ensure that they are not implicitly harassing LGBT teens, for example, using or allowing insidious, casual remarks such as "that's so gay."

Gay-Straight Alliances (GSAs), started by the Gay Straight Alliance Network in 1998, are student-run clubs that offer a safe place or environment for students to meet to discuss sexual orientation and identity to work toward elimination of LGBT harassment and bullying. The Gay Straight Alliance Network offers a directory of nationwide GSAs and information and resources on how to establish a GSA. GSAs have proven to be effective in promoting better understanding and fostering a safe and non-judgmental environment.

Schools are the center of the universe for most teens, and the place where the vast majority of their socialization occurs. Society at large dictates what is considered "normal," and teens, in their need for a sense of peer acceptance and school belonging, want to conform to the norm. Negative experiences, especially bulling, leave scars for all that suffer, but LGBT teens are a particularly vulnerable minority group and, as studies show, suffer more than most of their peers.

FURTHER READING

Anderman, EM (2002) School effects on psychological outcomes during adolescence. *Journal of Educational Psychology* 94(4): 795-809

Centers for Disease Control and Prevention (CDC) "LGBT Youth," http://www.cdc.gov/lgbthealth/youth. htm Includes "LGBT Youth Resources," "Resources for Educators and School Administrators," and "Resources for Parents and Family Members."

Diaz, EM, Kosciw, JG, & Greytak, EA (2010) School connectedness for lesbian, gay, bisexual, and transgender youth: In-school victimization and institutional supports. *The Prevention Researcher* 17(3): 15-17

Gay, Lesbian & Straight Education Network, http://www. glsen.org, includes link to *The 2013 National School Climate Survey: The experiences of lesbian, gay, bisexual and transgender youth in our nation's schools*

Gay-Straight Alliance Network, https://www.gsanet-work.org

Heck, NC, Livingston, NA, Flentje, A, Oost, K, Stewart, BT, and Cochran, BN (2014) Reducing risk for illicit drug use and prescription drug misuse: High school Gay-Straight Alliances and lesbian, gay, bisexual, and transgender youth. *Addictive Behaviors* 39(4): 824-828

Martin-Storey, A & Crosnoe, R (2012) Sexual minority status, peer harassment, and adolescent depression. *Journal of Adolescence* 35(4): 1001-1011

Roe, SL (2015) Examining the role of peer relationships in the lives of gay and bisexual adolescents *Children & Schools* 37(2): 117-124

Russell, ST, Ryan, C, Toomey, RB, Diaz, RM, & Sanchez, J. (2011) Lesbian, gay, bisexual, and transgender adolescent school victimization: Implications for young adult health and adjustment. *Journal of School Health* 81: 223-230

Schuster, MA & Bogart, LM (2015) A longitudinal study of bullying of sexual-minority youth *New England Journal of Medicine* 372(19): 1872-1874

Swearer, SM, Turner, RK, & Givens, JE (2008) "You're so gay!": Do different forms of bullying matter for adolescent males? *School Psychology Review* 37(2): 160-173

Toomey, RB, Ryan, C, Diaz, RM, & Russell, ST. (2011) High school Gay-Straight Alliances (GSAs) and young adult well-being: An examination of GSA presence, participation, and perceived effectiveness. *Applied Developmental Science* 15(4): 175-185

Toomey, RB, Ryan, C, & Diaz, RM (2010) Gender-nonconforming lesbian, gay, bisexual, and transgender youth: School victimization and young adult psychosocial adjustment. *Developmental Psychology* 46(6): 1580-1589 (scholarly)

Watson, S & Miller, T. (2012) LGBT oppression *Multicultural Education*, Summer 2012: 2-7

Claire B. Joseph

SEE ALSO: Bullying; Dealing with Bullying; Dealing with Peer Pressure; Depression; Teens and Alcohol Abuse; Teens and Drug Abuse; Teenage Suicide

Racism

Those studying racism examine the phenomenon of negative attitudes and behavior by members of the majority toward those who belong to racial and ethnic minorities. The topic of racism, which straddles the boundaries between social psychology and sociology, is connected with the study of intergroup relations, cognition, and attitudes in general..

INTRODUCTION

The social and psychological study of prejudice and discrimination, including prejudice and discrimination against African Americans, has a long history; the term "racism," however, did not enter the language of social psychology until the publication of the Kerner Commission Report of 1968, which blamed all-pervasive "white racism" for widespread black rioting in American cities. While usually applied to black-white relations in the United States, the term is also sometimes used with regard to white Americans' relations with other minority groups, such as Asians or Latinos, or to black-white relations outside the United States, for example, in Britain, Canada, or South Africa. Most of the studies and research on racism have focused on white racism against blacks in the United States.

Racism is seen by many social psychologists not as mere hatred but as a deep-rooted habit that is hard to change; hence, subvarieties of racism are distinguished.

Psychoanalyst Joel Kovel, in his book *White Racism: A Psychohistory* (1970), distinguishes between dominative racism, the desire to oppress blacks, and aversive racism, the desire to avoid contact with blacks. Aversive racism, Samuel L. Gaertner and John Dovidio find, exists among those whites who pride themselves on being unprejudiced. David O. Sears, looking at whites' voting behavior and their political opinions as expressed in survey responses, finds what he calls symbolic racism: a resentment of African Americans for making demands in the political realm that supposedly violate traditional American values. Social psychologist James M. Jones distinguishes three types of racism: individual racism, the prejudice and antiblack behavior deliberately manifested by individual whites; institutional racism, the social, economic, and political patterns that impersonally oppress blacks regardless of the prejudice or lack thereof of individuals; and cultural racism, the tendency of whites to ignore or to denigrate the special characteristics of black culture.

Where Dovidio and Gaertner find aversive racism, Irwin Katz finds ambivalence. Many whites, he argues, simultaneously see African Americans as disadvantaged (which creates sympathy) and as deviating from mainstream social norms (which creates antipathy). Such ambivalence, Katz contends, leads to exaggeratedly negative reactions to negative behaviors by an African American, but also to exaggeratedly positive reactions to positive behaviors by an African American. He calls this phenomenon ambivalence-induced behavior amplification.

The reasons suggested for individual racism are many. John Dollard, Neal E. Miller, and others, in *Frustration and Aggression* (1939), see prejudice as the scapegoating of minorities to provide a release for aggression in the face of frustration; in this view, outbursts of bigotry are a natural response to hard economic times. Muzafer and Carolyn Sherif, in *Groups in Harmony and Tension* (1953) and later works, see prejudice of all sorts as the result of competition between groups. Theodor Adorno and others, in *The Authoritarian Personality* (1950), view prejudice, whether directed against blacks or against Jews, as reflective of a supposedly fascist type of personality produced by authoritarian child-rearing practices. *In Racially Separate or Together?* (1971), Thomas F. Pettigrew shows that discriminatory behavior toward blacks, and the verbal expression of prejudices against them, can sometimes flow simply from a white's desire to fit in with his or her social group. Finally, both prejudice and discrimination, many psychologists argue, are rooted

in those human cognitive processes involved in the formation of stereotypes.

RACISM AND STEREOTYPES

Stereotypes are ideas, often rigidly held, concerning members of a group to which one does not belong. Social psychologists who follow the cognitive approach to the study of racism, such as David L. Hamilton, Walter G. Stephan, and Myron Rothbart, argue that racial stereotyping (the tendency of whites to see blacks in some roles and not in others) arises, like any other kind of stereotyping, from the need of every human being to create some sort of order out of his or her perceptions of the world. Although stereotypes are not entirely impervious to revision or even to shattering in the face of disconfirming instances, information related to a stereotype is more efficiently retained than information unrelated to it. Whites, it has been found, tend to judge blacks to be more homogeneous than they really are, while being more aware of differences within their own group: This is called the out-group homogeneity hypothesis. Whites who are guided by stereotypes may act in such a way as to bring out worse behavior in blacks than would otherwise occur, thus creating a self-fulfilling prophecy.

Why is stereotypical thinking on the part of whites about African Americans so hard to eliminate? The history of race relations in the United States deserves some of the blame. Some mistakes in reasoning common to the tolerant and the intolerant alike—such as the tendency to remember spectacular events and to think of them as occurring more frequently than is really the case (the availability heuristic)—also occur in whites' judgments about members of minority groups. In addition, the social and occupational roles one fills may reinforce stereotypical thinking.

Pettigrew contends that attribution errors —mistakes in explaining the behavior of others—may have an important role to play in reinforcing racial stereotypes. The same behavioral act, Pettigrew argues, is interpreted differently by whites depending on the race of the actor. A positive act by a black might be ascribed to situational characteristics (for example, luck, affirmative action programs, or other circumstances beyond one's control) and thus discounted; a positive act by a white might be ascribed to personality characteristics. Similarly, a negative act might be ascribed to situational characteristics in the case of a white, but to personality characteristics in the case of a black. The tendency of whites to view the greater extent of poverty among blacks as solely the result of lack of motivation can be seen as a form of attribution error.

POLICY GUIDES

Institutional racism occurs when policies that are nonracial on their face have differential results for the two races. For example, a stiff educational requirement for a relatively unskilled job may effectively exclude blacks, whose educational preparation may be weaker, at least in part because of past racial discrimination. The policy of hiring friends and relatives of existing employees may also exclude blacks, if blacks have not historically worked in a particular business. In both cases, the effect is discriminatory even if the intent is not.

Somewhat connected with the concept of institutional racism is Pettigrew's notion of conformity-induced prejudice and discrimination. A classic example is that of the precivil-rights-era southern United States, where urban restaurant owners, regardless of their personal feelings about blacks, refused them service out of deference to local norms. Another example is the case of the white factory worker who cooperates with black fellow workers on the job and in union activities but strenuously opposes blacks moving into his neighborhood; norms of tolerance are followed in one context, norms of discrimination in the other.

The concept of symbolic (sometimes called "modern") racism, a form of covert prejudice said to be characteristic of political conservatives, arose from a series of questions designed to predict whether white Californians would vote against black political candidates. It has been used to explain opposition to school busing to achieve integration and support for the 1978 California referendum proposition for limiting taxes. John B. McConahay shows that white experimental subjects who score high on the modern racism scale, when faced with hypothetical black and white job candidates with identical credentials, are more likely than low scorers to give a much poorer rating to the black candidate's résumé.

Aversive racism cannot be detected by surveys. Since aversive racists wish to maintain a nonprejudiced self-image, they neither admit to being prejudiced nor discriminate against blacks when social norms clearly forbid it; when the norms are ambiguous, however, they do discriminate. In a New York City experiment, professed liberals and professed conservatives both got telephone calls from individuals identifiable from their speech patterns as either black or white. At first, the caller said he had the wrong number; if the recipient of the call did not

hang up, the caller then asked for help regarding a disabled car. Conservatives were less likely to offer help to the black, but liberals were more likely to hang up when they were told by the black that a wrong number had been called. In another experiment, white college students proved just as willing to accept help from a black partner as from a white one when the help was offered. When the subjects had to take the initiative, however, discomfort with the reversal of traditional roles showed up: More asked for help from the white partner than from the black one.

Both symbolic and aversive, but not dominative, racists manifest ambivalence in their attitudes toward blacks. Katz's concept of ambivalence-induced behavior amplification has been tested in several experiments. In one experiment, white college student subjects were told to insult two individuals, one black and one white. After they had done so, they proved, when asked for assistance in a task later on, more willing to help the black they had insulted than the white person.

The effect of the availability heuristic in reinforcing stereotypes is seen in the case of a white who is mugged by a black criminal. If the victim knows no other blacks, he or she may well remember this one spectacular incident and forget the many blacks who are law-abiding. The effect of occupational roles in reinforcing stereotypes can be seen in the example of a white police officer who patrols a black slum neighborhood and jumps to the conclusion that all blacks are criminals.

Experiments on stereotyping indicate that white subjects remember the words or actions of a solo black in an otherwise all-white group better than they do the words or actions of one black in a group of several blacks. With a mixed group of speakers, some white and some black, white experimental subjects proved later to be more likely to confuse the identities of the black speakers than those of the white speakers, while remembering the race of the former. The self-fulfilling prophecy concept has been tested in experiments with white subjects interviewing supposed job candidates. The white subjects were more ill at ease and inarticulate interviewing a black candidate than in interviewing a white one; in turn, the black candidate was more ill at ease than the white one and made more errors.

Since most such experiments use college students as subjects, there is inevitably some doubt about their generalizability to the outside world. Nevertheless, it seems likely that the evidence from social psychology experiments of just how deeply rooted racial bias is among white Americans has played at least some role in leading governments to adopt affirmative action policies to secure fairer treatment of blacks and other minorities in hiring procedures.

HISTORY AND DEVELOPMENTS

Although the study of racism per se began with the racial crisis of the 1960s, the study of prejudice in general goes back much further; as early as the 1920s, Emory Bogardus constructed a social distance scale measuring the degree of intimacy members of different racial and ethnic groups were willing to tolerate with one another. At first, psychologists tended to seek the roots of prejudice in the emotional makeup of the prejudiced individual rather than in the structure of society or in the general patterns of human cognition. For many years, the study of antiblack prejudice was subsumed under the study of prejudice in general; those biased against blacks were thought to be biased against other groups, such as Jews, as well.

In the years immediately following World War II, American social psychologists were optimistic about the possibilities for reducing or even eliminating racial and ethnic prejudices. Adorno's *The Authoritarian Personality,* and *The Nature of Prejudice* (1954), by Gordon Allport, reflect the climate of opinion of the time. Allport, whose view of prejudice represented a mixture of the psychoanalytic and cognitive approaches, used the term "racism" to signify the doctrines preached by negrophobe political demagogues; he did not see it as a deeply ingrained bad habit pervading the entire society. Pettigrew, who wrote about antiblack prejudice from the late 1950s on, cast doubt on the notion that there was a specific type of personality or pattern of child rearing associated with prejudice. Nevertheless, he long remained in the optimistic tradition, arguing that changing white people's discriminatory behavior through the enactment of civil rights laws would ultimately change their prejudiced attitudes.

The more frequent use by social psychologists of the term "racism" from the late 1960s onward indicates a growing awareness that bias against blacks, a visible minority, might be harder to uproot than that directed against religious and ethnic minorities. Social psychologists studying racial prejudice shifted their research interest from the open and noisy bigotry most often found among political extremists (for example, the Ku Klux Klan) to the quiet, everyday prejudices of the average apolitical individual. Racial bias against blacks came to

be seen as a central, rather than a peripheral, feature of American life.

Responses to surveys taken from the 1940s to the end of the 1970s indicated a steady decline in the percentage of white Americans willing to admit holding racist views. Yet in the 1970s, the sometimes violent white hostility to school busing for integration, and the continuing social and economic gap between black and white America, gave social psychologists reason to temper their earlier optimism. The contact hypothesis, the notion that contact between different racial groups would reduce prejudice, was subjected to greater skepticism and ever more careful qualification. Janet Schofield, in her field study of a desegregated junior high school, detected a persistence of racial divisions among the pupils; reviewing a number of such studies, Stephan similarly discerned a tendency toward increased interracial tension in schools following desegregation. The pessimism suggested by field studies among younger teenagers was confirmed by experiments conducted in the 1970s and 1980s on college students and adults; such studies demonstrated the existence, even among supposedly nonprejudiced people, of subtle racism and racial stereotyping.

Yet while social psychological experiments contribute to an understanding of the reasons for negative attitudes toward blacks by whites, and for discriminatory behavior toward blacks even by those whites who believe themselves to be tolerant, they do not by any means provide the complete answer to the riddle of racial prejudice and discrimination. Unlike many other topics in social psychology, racism has also been investigated by journalists, historians, economists, sociologists, political scientists, legal scholars, and even literary critics. The techniques of social psychology—surveys, controlled experiments, and field studies—provide only one window on this phenomenon.

FURTHER READING

Allport, Gordon W. *The Nature of Prejudice.* 1954. Reprint. Cambridge: Addison, 1990. Print.

Augoustinos, Martha. "Psychological Perspectives on Racism." *InPsych.* Australian Psychological Society, Aug. 2013. Web. 25 June 2014.

Barndt, Joseph. *Understanding and Dismantling Racism: The Twenty-First Century Challenge to White America.* Minneapolis: Fortress, 2007. Print.

Bell, Derrick. *Faces at the Bottom of the Well: The Permanence of Racism.* New York: Basic, 1992. Print.

Campbell, Duane. *Choosing Democracy: A Practical Guide to Multicultural Education.* 4th ed. Boston: Allyn, 2009. Print.

Dovidio, John F., and Samuel L. Gaertner, eds. *Prejudice, Discrimination, and Racism.* 1986. Rpt. San Diego: Academic, 1992. Print.

Gilroy, Paul. *Against Race: Imaging Political Culture beyond the Color Line.* Cambridge: Belknap, 2001. Print.

Katz, Irwin. *Stigma: A Social Psychological Analysis.* Hillsdale: Lawrence Erlbaum, 1981. Print.

\Katz, Phyllis A., and Dalmas A. Taylor, eds. *Eliminating Racism: Profiles in Controversy.* New York: Plenum, 1988. Print.

Marsh, Jason, Rodolfo Mendoza-Denton, and Jeremy Adam Smith. *Are We Born Racist? New Insights from Neuroscience and Positive Psychology.* Boston: Beacon, 2010. Print.

Oshodi, John Egbeazien. *History of Psychology in the Black Experience: Perspectives Then and Now—A Psychology in the Perspective of the History of the Africans and People of African Descent.* Lanham: UP of America, 2012. Print.

Pettigrew, Thomas F., et al. *Prejudice.* Cambridge: Belknap, 1982. Print.

Steele, Shelby. *The Content of Our Character: A New Vision of Race in America.* New York: HarperPerennial, 1998. Print.

Stephan, Walter G., and David Rosenfield. "Racial and Ethnic Stereotypes." *In the Eye of the Beholder: Contemporary Issues in Stereotyping.* Ed. Arthur G. Miller. New York: Praeger, 1982. Print.

Sue, Derald Wing, and David Sue. *Counseling the Culturally Diverse: Theory and Practice.* Hoboken: Wiley, 2013. Print.

Trepagnier, Barbara. *Silent Racism: How Well-Meaning White People Perpetuate the Racial Divide.* Boulder: Paradigm, 2007. Print.

West, Cornell. *Race Matters.* 2d ed. Boston: Beacon, 2001. Print.

Paul D. Mageli; updated by Frank A. Salamone

SEE ALSO: Biracial Heritage; Hate Crimes; Stereotyping

Religion and spirituality

Teens and young adults have a variety of religious and spiritual beliefs and experiences, similar to adults. Adolescence is a unique time in an individual's faith development because individuals are often exposed to information and experiences that broaden one's perspective, including one's faith. Adolescence and young adulthood can also be a time of questioning and exploring one's religious and spiritual beliefs.

INTRODUCTION

Religion can be a sensitive and a divisive topic for some. When people hear the words religion and spirituality many people have some kind of automatic response. Religion is often a topic that people do not want to discuss at parties or at the family dinner table because it can create heated discussions. Religion and spirituality can be hard for people to discuss because it is often a highly individual experience and people frequently form differing, strong, opinions about religion.

Religion can have different roles in an individual's life. Religious and spiritual beliefs can be a highly personal thing. To some individuals it is very important and influences their worldviews, morals, and political views. To others, religion has less salience in their daily lives and has little impact on how they interact with the world. At some point in life, almost everyone thinks critically about what he or she believes about religion. Faith is considered one's trust in a set of beliefs and can even refer to the practice of one's religious beliefs. Everyone has some kind of belief system that governs the way in which he or she sees the world. This perspective may or may not include a religious or spiritual outlook.

Similarly to adults, teens and young adults have a wide variety of beliefs including monotheism (belief in one god or deity), duo-theism (belief in at least two gods or deities), polytheism (belief in multiple gods or deities), non-theism (does not depend on a god or deity), spiritualism (belief that humans can communicate with spirits of the deceased), agnosticism (belief that whether or not there is a supreme deity or deities is unknowable), atheism (belief that there is no supreme deity or deities) and many others. There are all types of religions practiced among teens with varying degrees of religious commitment.

RELIGION VS. SPIRITUALITY

Religion consists of beliefs and traditions that influence an individual's worldview and sometimes involves a deity or deities. The word spirituality is frequently used, although there are multiple interpretations of the word. In general, spirituality is often used to discuss a personal transformation or an individual's subjective experience. A common phrase is "spiritual but not religious" which refers to individuals who do not participate in organized religion but who considers themselves spiritually connected to the world. Other people might consider themselves both religious and spiritual. These terms are labels people often use to identify themselves to others.

BY THE NUMBERS

According the National Study of Youth and Religion (NSYR) around 80% of teenagers say they believe in God. A little more than 70% said they felt very close or somewhat close to God and 65% reported praying at least once each week. Over half indicated that they attend services two to three times each month. These statistics reflect the fact that many teens are thinking about religion and describe themselves as faithful. Despite the evidence of student involvement, the NSYR found that adolescents often had a difficult time articulating their beliefs and often described religious beliefs that are somewhat distant from the stated beliefs of the religious tradition to which they belonged.

FAITH DEVELOPMENT

During childhood, family life often has a large influence on one's religious beliefs. Children are usually most exposed to the faith of their parents or family. It is normal for children to be curious about religion and to accept the stories and traditions they are typically exposed to. During adolescence many youth begin to learn more about faith from sources outside the family such as friends, teachers, and the media. During the teenage years, faith can sometimes help teens shape their identity. Adolescence can be a time of experimentation and religious beliefs are no exception. Some students may become deeply involved in religious activities while others might experiment with other than mainstream religions simply to learn about them.

For the majority of teenagers, attendance at religious events declines during high school. However, researchers at UCLA found that teens often still retain their religious identity despite a decline in organized religious participation. In the late teen years and into early adulthood, a number of students are able to critically reflect upon their faith or their beliefs. Often this process occurs when young adults begin to transition into adulthood. This process if often sparked by events such as moving away from home, working in new environments, and forming serious romantic relationships. This is a time when people might begin to question things they have always believed or thought to be true. It is normal for people to express doubt in their faith tradition of origin and to go through a phase of determining whether or not they want to remain in that faith. For some, this can be a difficult and lengthy process, while for others it is an easy transition. During this time many young adults seek out peers to learn of other's experiences. Some might turn to religious or spiritual leaders, parents, media, and books to explore the emotions tied to their experience.

Photo: iStock

179

BENEFITS

Some research has shown that religion has positive benefits for people, including teens. Interestingly, more religious youth tend to perform better in school, be more involved in extracurricular activities, and are even more likely than non-religious peers to wear seatbelts. Other benefits include less delinquent behavior, less tobacco and drug use, and a higher likelihood of staying in high school. There is also a higher rate of volunteerism among religious teens compared to non-religious teens.

FUTURE DIRECTIONS

While several major studies have been conducted on youth and religion, these seem to have primarily focused on mainstream religions that reflect the majority population and less on the religious experiences of minority individuals. Additionally, there could be more research conducted on the lived religious experiences of young adults as opposed to just research on the religious practices of young adults.

FURTHER READING

Associated Press. (2005, February 23). "Study: Most U.S. Teens Serious About Religion". *NBC News*. Retrieved from: http://www.nbcnews.com/id/7019023/ns/us_news/t/study-most-us-teens-serious-about-religion/#.VXnqaEuv0pE. This article reviews findings from the National Study of Youth and Religion. They discuss general trends among teenagers relating to religion and specifically talk about teens' knowledge of their faith traditions.

Barooha, J. (2014, September 12). "Religion In College: How Has Your Faith Changed. *Huffington Post*. Retrieved from: http://www.huffingtonpost.com/2012/09/04/religion-in-college-how-has-your-faith-changed-in-college_n_1853154.html. This article references a study conducted by the Social Science Research Council as part of the National Longitudinal Study of Adolescent Health. The study researched adolescents who disaffiliate with religion and who stop attending religious services.

Briggs, D. (2014, October 29). "The No. 1 Reason Teens Keep the Faith As Young Adults". *Huffington Post*. Retrieved from: http://www.huffingtonpost.com/david-briggs/the-no-1-reason-teens-kee_b_6067838.html. This article discusses results from the National Study of Youth and Religion that suggest that religious beliefs are best predicted by the religious involvement of parents.

Dorfman, J. (2003, December 22). "Religion is Good For All of Us, Even Those Who Don't Follow One". *Forbes*. Retrieved from: http://www.forbes.com/sites/jeffreydorfman/2013/12/22/religion-is-good-for-all-of-us-even-those-who-dont-follow-one/. This article reviews some of the research on benefits people receive from practicing religion as well as benefits society as a whole receives from having religious citizens. The author examines possible benefits for kids, adolescents, and adults.

Wheeler, M. (2011, June 17). "Teens Maintain Their Religion as Part of Their Identity During Turbulent High School Years". *UCLA Newsroom*. Retrieved from: http://newsroom.ucla.edu/releases/teens-maintain-their-religion-208066. This article focuses on a study that investigates how a teen's ethnic identity influences their religious identity and participation.

Alyssa Tedder-King

SEE ALSO: Decision Making; Meditation

Sexism

Sexism is prejudice against persons on the basis of their gender. Sexism may exist at the interpersonal level, where it is expressed in individual beliefs and behaviors; alternatively, it may become institutionalized when social institutions and practices encourage gender bias.

INTRODUCTION

The psychological basis for sexism, as for other forms of prejudice, is the human tendency to form stereotypes about persons who are members of certain social groups. Stereotypes may be either positive or negative; they consist of sets of interrelated beliefs and expectations that a person holds about a particular social group. When these stereotypes affect people's interpersonal behavior, sexism can result, leading to prejudice—a negative attitude toward a social group—and discrimination.

Gender stereotypes are reflected in beliefs and attitudes about the general nature of men and women as members of distinct social groups. In addition, gender stereotypes are related to the development of expectations about men's and women's psychological characteristics, interests, aptitudes, and behaviors. For example, if a person believes that women are more nurturant than men, then he or she might expect that women are more likely than men to be employed as child-care workers. In turn, these expectations may affect how people behave in social situations. The presence of different expectations for male and female performance may lead to differential treatment on the basis of gender. For example, if the director of a child-care center expects women to be superior nursery school teachers, then he or she may be likely to discriminate against males who apply for an available teaching position.

AMERICAN GENDER STEREOTYPES

Psychological research has established that gender stereotypes are quite pervasive in American culture. Considerable attention has been directed toward identifying the content of gender stereotypes. Psychologists are interested in the particular nature of beliefs that individuals hold about men and women in American culture. In a classic study, Paul Rosenkrantz, Inge Broverman, and their colleagues asked Americans to describe characteristics of the typical American man and woman. Their findings, which were first reported in the late 1960s, have been supported by subsequent research. Thus, their research appears to provide an accurate portrayal of the gender stereotypes commonly held by American adults.

These researchers found that subjects tended to describe men and women in terms of two different clusters of psychological traits, or personality characteristics. Women were more likely to be characterized by a group of traits that could be summarized as representing an expressiveness cluster. That is, men and women agreed that, as a group, women were caring, warm, and emotionally expressive. In contrast, men were characterized by a group of traits that could be described as an instrumentality cluster. In this instance, the typical man was perceived to be assertive, dominant, and competent. Thus, perceptions of men and women, as members of social groups, were conceived in terms of opposing psychological characteristics.

In the early 1980s, Kay Deaux and Laurie Lewis conducted a series of studies that elaborated on this pioneering research. They hypothesized that instrumentality and expressiveness are only two possible distinctions between men and women. Deaux and Lewis believed that additional factors were likely to play an important role in gender stereotyping. In their research program, male and female subjects were given a list of gender-relevant characteristics. Subjects then were asked to estimate the likelihood that a man or woman possessed each

characteristic. The results of these studies indicated that gender stereotypes do in fact consist of a number of related components. Subjects reliably associated certain psychological traits, role behaviors, occupations, and physical characteristics with gender.

The male stereotype consisted of the instrumentality cluster coupled with masculine psychological and physical characteristics. Subjects perceived the typical male to be strong, masculine, likely to hide his feelings, sexy, and muscular. Men typically were described as breadwinners and as being likely to take the initiative in encounters with the opposite sex. The typical male roles included blue-collar worker, businessman, athlete, and "macho man." In contrast, the female stereotype consisted of the expressiveness personality cluster coupled with feminine psychological and physical characteristics. Subjects described the typical woman as being smart and attractive, but also feminine, sensitive, and emotional. Women often were stereotyped as housewives and were perceived to be likely to be engaged in domestic chores such as child rearing and cooking. On the other hand, female stereotypes were not simply relegated to the domestic role. Subjects also held stereotypes that were representative of female athletes, businesswomen, and "sexy women."

Although there appears to be some overlap between male and female categories, it is clear that gender stereotypes do parallel the common roles that men and women typically assume in society. In addition, men and women are perceived to be members of distinctly different social groups. For the most part, people expect men and women to display opposing psychological characteristics and role behaviors. Finally, it should be noted that psychologists have found remarkable cross-cultural similarity in the content of gender stereotypes.

THE CONSTRAINTS OF STEREOTYPES

A large body of psychological research has investigated the effects of sexism. Some psychologists have investigated how gender stereotypes may influence people's perceptions of women in certain social roles (for example, as leaders). Others have studied how the use of sexist language might be related to the formation and maintenance of gender stereotypes.

The effects of gender stereotypes are particularly pronounced when people must form first impressions and make social judgments about others on the basis of little information. Natalie Porter and her colleagues have studied the factors that persons consider when they are asked to identify the leader of a small group. They asked subjects to view a photograph of an all-male group, an all-female group, or a mixed-sex group. Subjects were then asked to guess which person in the photograph held the position of group leader.

First, Porter and her colleagues found that subjects were likely to rely on spatial configuration as an important cue in determining which person was the leader of the group. In the cases of all-male and all-female groups, the majority of subjects identified the person at the head of the table as the group leader. When the group consisted of both male and female members and a male was seated at the head of the table, this person also was designated as leader by a majority of subjects. When a female occupied the head position in a mixed-sex group, however, her position at the table was disregarded. In this situation, any of the other males in the group was selected. It is clear from these results that women are less likely than men to be seen as leaders of mixed-sex groups. The results of this study are consistent with the content of gender stereotypes described by Deaux and Lewis.

SEXISM AND LANGUAGE

Gender stereotypes are also apparent in the everyday use of language. For example, many linguists have pointed out that the English language traditionally has regarded the male linguistic forms as normative. The male-as-normative principle refers to the tendency for "man" to be used to refer to all human beings. Thus, the male is considered to be the representative, or prototype, of the human species. An example of the male-as-normative principle is the use of the pronoun "he" as a generic pronoun that is intended to refer to both males and females. An example is, "While stress is a normal concomitant of our daily lives, man's ever-increasing pace of life may in fact shorten his life span."

The use of the male-as-normative principle has been subjected to two primary criticisms. First, the use of a male-gendered pronoun is often ambiguous. When a writer asserts that "man's ever-increasing pace of life may in fact shorten his life span," the reader may assume that men are more susceptible to the negative effects of stress than women. An alternative interpretation is that humans, regardless of sex, are negatively affected by stress. The second criticism focuses on issues of gender equality. The use of the male-as-normative principle implies that women are exceptions to the general rule. Critics argue that the use of the male generic encourages people to think exclusively of males rather than including

females. Further, they claim that language and thought are closely related and that sexist language may foster gender stereotypes.

In the early 1980s, psychologist Janet Shibley Hyde investigated the effects of sexist language on children's thought processes. She was particularly interested in discovering whether children understood the male-as-normative principle. She asked elementary school children to complete a story about another child. Each of the children was given a sentence with which to begin his or her story (for example, "When a kid goes to school, _____often feels excited on the first day."). One-third of the sentences provided "he" in place of the blank, one-third included "they," and one-third included "he or she." Hyde found that children's stories indeed were influenced by the use of gender pronouns. When "he" or "they" was provided to the child, fewer than 20 percent of the stories were about females. This effect was especially pronounced when boys were tested. Not one boy who was provided with the pronoun "he" wrote a story about a girl. In contrast, when the pronouns "he or she" were supplied, 42 percent of the stories were about females. Hyde concluded that when children hear the word "he," even when used as a generic pronoun, they tend to think of males.

A number of practical suggestions have been made to avoid the use of sexist language. One simple change is to use the pronoun "they" in place of "he." The results of Hyde's study, however, would suggest that the use of "he or she" would be a better alternative. Others have argued that the single pronouns "he" and "she" might be used with equal frequency throughout written text. Such suggestions are not trivial. Since the 1970s, many textbook publishers have issued guidelines that forbid the use of sexist language. The American Psychological Association (APA) has provided similar guidelines for manuscripts that are submitted for publication in journals published by the APA.

DIFFERENTIAL PSYCHOLOGY

Psychological research investigating the causes and effects of sexism is rooted in the specialized field of differential psychology, which investigated ethnic and gender differences in psychological variables such as intelligence and mental abilities. As early as 1879, Gustave Le Bon provided a description of gender differences in which he noted women's innate inferiority to men, an observation echoed by many other differential psychologists of that period. Hence, the tendency to observe differences between social groups was reflected in both the attitudes and the research efforts of early psychological researchers and continues today.

Historically, social psychologists have studied people's beliefs about differences between social groups and their attitudes toward members of other social groups. The first study of stereotypes was conducted in 1922 by Walter Lippmann, a public opinion researcher. His identification of the stereotype concept provided a means for the scientific study of ethnocentrism. The rise of fascism and its thesis of group superiority and inferiority in pre-World War II Europe concerned many social scientists and provided an impetus for the development of systematic studies of intergroup relations. While perceptions of different ethnic groups were the focus of social psychological studies of stereotypes conducted before the 1940's, the study of gender stereotypes was initiated by the publication of a study conducted by Samuel Fernberger in 1948.

Social psychologists continued to study stereotypes and their relation to prejudice in the post-World War II era. Gordon Allport's *The Nature of Prejudice* (1954) provided a theoretical model that explained the process of stereotyping and the development and maintenance of prejudice. In Allport's view, stereotypes are negative attitudes toward the members of other groups that are accompanied by rigid, inflexible thought processes. His conceptualization of stereotypes and prejudice remained unchallenged until the late 1960s, when social psychological research demonstrated that categorization and stereotyping were normal consequences of human thought processes.

The political unrest that characterized American society during the Vietnam War era was reflected in an explosion of social psychological studies of racism and sexism. In addition, the prevailing societal concerns about political and social inequality coincided with demands among feminist scholars for the conduct of nonsexist psychological research. This resulted in the emergence of a new field in the early 1970s, the psychology of women. Nonsexist, gender-fair psychological research has been promoted as a legitimate field of study by the establishment of a specialized section within the APA (Division 35) that is dedicated to the psychology of women. Scholarship in this field is dedicated to the study of sexism, gender differences and similarities, and other aspects of gender role socialization.

FURTHER READING

Bem, Sandra Lipsitz. *The Lenses of Gender: Transforming the Debate on Sexual Inequality.* New Haven, Conn.: Yale University Press, 1994. Print.

Calogero, Rachel M., and John T. Jost. "Self-Subjugation Among Women: Exposure to Sexist Ideology, Self-Objectification, and the Protective Function of the Need to Avoid Closure." *Journal of Personality and Social Psychology* 100.2 (2011): 211–28. Print.

Keonig, Anne M., et al. "Are Leader Stereotypes Masculine? A Meta-Analysis of Three Research Paradigms." *Psychological Bulletin* 137.4 (2011): 616–42. Print.

McClean, Vernon, and Cornelia Wells, eds. *Racism and Sexism: A Collaborative Study.* 2d ed. Dubuque, Iowa: Kendall/Hunt, 2006. Print.

Mills, Sara. *Language and Sexism.* New York: Cambridge University Press, 2008. Print.

Sleeter, Christine E., and Carl A. Grant. "Race, Class, Gender, and Disability in Current Textbooks." *The Textbook as Discourse: Sociocultural Dimensions of American Schoolbooks.* Eds. Eugene F. Provenzo, et al. New York: Routledge, 2011. 183–215. Print.

Swann, William B., Judith H. Langlois, and Lucie Albino Gilbert, eds. *Sexism and Stereotypes in Modern Society.* Washington, D.C.: American Psychological Association, 1998. Print.

Tavris, Carol, and Carole Wade. *The Longest War: Sex Differences in Perspective.* 2d ed. New York: Harcourt Brace Jovanovich, 1984. Print.

Thorne, Barrie, Cheris Kramarae, and Nancy Henley. *Language, Gender, and Society.* Rowley, Mass.: Newbury House, 1983. Print.

Walsh, Mary Roth, ed. *The Psychology of Women: Ongoing Debates.* New Haven, Conn.: Yale University Press, 1987. Print.

Williams, John E., and Deborah L. Best. *Sex and Psyche: Gender and Self Viewed Cross-culturally.* Newbury Park, Calif.: Sage Publications, 1990. Print.

Cheryl A. Rickabaugh

SEE ALSO: Gender Roles and Conflicts; LGBT Teens and Parental Acceptance; LGBT Teens and Peer Acceptance; Rape and Sexual Assault; Sexual Consent; Sexual Harassment; Stereotyping

Stereotyping

A stereotype is a negative label stuck on people or groups based on a widely held, fixed, oversimplified standard, conventional image or idea. They can be based on many factors, including age, race, ethnicity, gender, sexual identity, profession, and physical appearance. Stereotyping is a form of prejudice or bias. Stereotypes are generally harmful and dangerous as they affect how people view and treat others, and how people view themselves and formulate their identities and self-worth. Adolescents, who are at an especially vulnerable age, need to become aware of stereotypes and how they affect their assumptions and actions. With education and understanding comes empowerment to counteract or combat stereotypes.

INTRODUCTION

It's a frustrating fact of life that everyone makes judgments about people based on their characteristics and appearance and how their first impressions relate to deep-seated societal assumptions or stereotypes about these characteristics and appearances. Where do stereotypes come from, how did they get started, and how are they perpetuated? There might be a tiny kernel of truth in the basis of stereotypes, but the ideas have been magnified and oversimplified and over time have insidiously become a part of the social fabric, societal assumptions, and mindsets.

Adolescence is a difficult time of transition from childhood to adulthood. It's a time of great changes, physically, psychologically, and emotionally. It's a time to push boundaries, when adolescents are trying to "find themselves" and their place in an oftentimes complex and confusing world. Dealing with stereotypes makes this whole process much more difficult and stressful and can affect every aspect of their lives, including their relationships with parents, family, teachers, and peers. Stereotypes can affect adolescents' self-esteem and behavior, often resulting in self-fulfilling prophecies. For example, if a person is convinced that they're "bad at math," they will fail a math test regardless of how much they've studied for it.

Society is bombarded by media, including the internet and social media, movies, TV, music, and video games, with explicit and implicit stereotypes and explicit and implicit messages on how people should behave and dress and which body images are preferred or rejected. In

addition, advertisers perpetuate stereotypical thinking in their messages and images, promoting products in a way that feeds into cultural assumptions and mindsets. And much of this is geared towards adolescents because they have enormous buying power. In fact, in its 2006 Policy Statement "Children, Adolescents, and Advertising," the American Academy of Pediatrics reported that "children and adolescents are attractive consumers: teenagers spend $155 billion/year, children younger than 12 years spend another $25 billion, and both groups influence perhaps another $200 billion of their parents' spending per year."

STEREOTYPING ABOUT ADOLESCENTS

Adolescents are often described in many negative ways. They're often assumed to be rebellious, moody, difficult, withdrawn, isolated, risk-takers, and abusers of drugs and alcohol. Now the physical, psychological and emotional upheavals of adolescence may very well result in some rebelliousness and moodiness. However, there is no "one size fits all" experience for adolescents, and it is detrimental to all to assume that turning 13 will automatically change an adolescent into a "monster."

In fact, it's interesting to note that a study by Buchanan & Hughes shows that when parents' expectations and assumptions that their children, regardless of past behavior or past parent-child relationships, will conform to negative stereotypes when they become teenagers, may very well backfire and result in just such bad behavior. In other words, teens whose parents expect bad behavior are more likely to exhibit bad behavior. For example, teens whose parents expect them to do drugs or drink excessively may be less likely to resist temptation, impulse, and self-control, and feel that if their parents already think they're doing it, why not just do it?

STEREOTYPING BY ADOLESCENTS

It's ironic that while adolescents suffer the ill effects of negative stereotyping, they are not immune to stereotyping others; in fact adolescents have a rigid set of peer stereotypes and peer "classifications." They judge their peers based on race, ethnicity, gender, sexual identity, looks, style of dress and hair style, jewelry, body art, social positions, and interests. Adolescents are categorized as nerds, geeks, dweebs, dorks, jocks, popular or unpopular, and often associated with cliques, not to mention gangs. Adolescents also categorize their peers by scholastic assumptions, e.g., boys are better at math, or girls are better at English. And racial stereotyping often mirrors society's prejudices.

EXTRA STRESSES OF STEREOTYPING

Steele & Aronson's classic 1995 article describes the concept of "stereotype threat," which Inzlicht & King define as "a situational predicament in which individuals suspect their behaviors could be judged on the basis of negative stereotypes about their group instead of personal merit."

Yong quotes scientist and TV personality Dr. Neil Degrasse Tyson who, when working towards his Ph.D. in astrophysics, was one of seven African-Americans in a nationwide field of 4,000. Tyson stated that "In the perception of society my academic failures are expected and my academic successes are attributed to others," calling such stereotyping an "emotional tax."

Even more stressful is what Inzlicht & King describe as "stereotype threat spillover," where stereotype threats have "lingering effects that continue to influence people after they leave threatening environments, such that it has residual effects on behavior even in areas unrelated to the impugning stereotype." For example, the residual stress of dealing with stereotypes in the past could lead to future bad behavior including aggressive behavior and overeating.

COPING WITH STEREOTYPING

Like any type of prejudice or bias, stereotyping is, unfortunately, a deeply ingrained part of our society; however, this does not mean that it must be accepted. To overcome or combat stereotyping, adolescents and their parents, families, and teachers must become aware of their insidiousness and detrimental effects, and, through education, become empowered to counter them and alleviate them. Adolescents and their families and teachers need to examine their communities and how stereotyping affects their general health and well-being, especially their sense of identity and self-worth. Parents and teachers can implement strategies and programs that shift the focus from negative stereotyping of adolescents to promoting their positive actions. Sensitivity training that includes acceptance of each individual's worth can have a positive effect on all involved.

FURTHER READING

American Academy of Pediatrics Committee on Communications (2006) Children, adolescents, and advertising. *Pediatrics 2006* 118(6): 2563-2569

Buchanan, CM & Hughes, JL. (2009) Construction of social reality during early adolescence: can expecting storm and stress increase real or perceived storm and stress? *Journal of Research on Adolescence* 19(2): 261-285

Centers for Disease Control and Prevention (CDC) Adolescent Health Publications & Resources http:www.cdc.gov/healthyouth/adolescenthealth/publications.htm

Fox, MG & Sokol, L. (2011) *A cognitive therapy guide to overcoming self-doubt and creating unshakable self-esteem: think confident, be confident for teens.* Oakland, CA: New Harbinger Publications, Inc.

Inzlicht, M & King, SK. (2010) Stereotype threat spillover: how coping with threats to social identity affects aggression, eating, decision making, and attention. *Journal of Personality and Social Psychology* 99(3): 467-481

National Library of Medicine's MedlinePlus "Teen Health" http://www.nlm.nih.gov/medlineplus.teenhealth.html

Steele, CM & Aronson, J. (1995) Stereotype threat and the intellectual test performance of African-Americans. *Journal of Personality and Social Psychology* 69(5): 797-811

Steele, CM. (1997) A threat in the air: How stereotypes shape intellectual identity and performance. *American Psychologist* 52(6): 613-629

Yong, E. (2013) Armor against prejudice. *Scientific American* 308(6):77-80

Claire B. Joseph

SEE ALSO: Racism; Sexism

Drugs, Alcohol, and Addictions

Addictive personality and behaviors

There are many types of personalities and personality features associated with problems related to addictive behavior. No single personality type or disorder exists alone in this relationship. Furthermore, personality and addictive behavior may influence each other: Personality may cause some addictive behavior, and some addictive behavior may encourage the development of certain personality features or even personality disorders.

INTRODUCTION

Addiction is a condition in which individuals engage in habitual behaviors or use of substances in a way that is maladaptive and causes them harm or distress. Fascination with the idea of an addictive personality and related behavior dates to 950 BCE, to the works of Homer, the Greek poet, and perhaps before that to the writings of Laozi, a Chinese philosopher and imperial adviser. These men studied human nature and wrote about the uncontrollable allure of certain desires, which led to behaviors that were likely to cause personal and cultural destruction. Thus, these two writers were exploring the realm of personality: the intellectual, emotional, interpersonal, and intrapersonal structure of an individual that is exhibited through consistent patterns of thinking, worldview, self-view, and behavior.

Some researchers have asked whether a single psychological predisposition or a multilevel series of complications is involved in the addictive personality or whether virtually any personality is vulnerable to addiction. Researchers administering personality tests to individuals with addictive behavior problems have found a variety of notable personality traits. Sometimes these traits precede the addiction, and sometimes they seem to be caused by or exacerbated by the addiction. These findings are highly controversial and have fueled many heated discussions.

Symptoms, or indications of a problem, with personality are varied. For some individuals with addictive behavior problems, aggressive energy and antiauthority issues seem to be at the core of their personality. Indulgence in the addictive behavior is accompanied by the release of aggressive impulses, resulting in a feeling of euphoria. This feeling of relief is then associated with the outlet used, and it seduces the user to attempt a duplication of the original process, thus reexperiencing the euphoria.

Inadequate self-esteem is a psychological predisposition thought to be a common source of imperceptible pain, and the inability to handle the pain can lead to a desire to find an outlet to reduce the pain. In fact, according to research by Zhanshen Chen, socially based pain can last longer than physical pain and, in effect, do more damage. Thus, as a risk factor to addiction, pain suffered because of self-esteem issues is a substantial consideration. Some individuals with addictive behavior problems want to control the pain but lack the necessary social, psychological, and biological tools to do so. Other symptoms that may be identified early enough to allow preventive measures to be taken include poor impulse control; intolerance and low frustration level, leading to a need for control; and rigidity and extremes in action and thoughts.

Behavior with addictive characteristics may involve alcohol and other drugs, food, work, sex, gambling, exercise, video-game playing, television watching, and even Internet-related behavior. Online gaming, role-playing, and sexual interactions based on the Internet have addictive features. However, these behaviors must receive much greater study before they can be recognized as actual addictions. The notion of an addictive personality developed in the twentieth century partially because some individuals displayed more than one behavior with addictive characteristics or, when one addictive behavior was given up, one quickly replaced it. Some have seen this process of substitution as a form of generalization in which behaviors form an addictive behavior pattern. Problems such as manipulation, denial of responsibility, displacement of emotions, and general dishonesty in lifestyle may provoke this process. In general, however, the addictive process can be periodic, cyclic, sporadic, or continuous, depending on a person's life patterns, resources, and basic personality. In fact, research indicates that any personality can become addicted.

PERSONALITY THEORIES

Different personality theories present conflicting ideas about addiction, adding to the controversy surrounding this topic. Psychoanalysts believe that addiction is a result of unconscious conflicts and of fixation on the pleasure principle, which states that one's energy in life is directed toward reducing pain and that one's innate drives control one's actions. Although some neo-Freudians disagree with the cause of pain, most agree with the basic concept. Social learning and behavioral psychologists believe that an addictive personality is molded through shaping—the slow and continual development of a behavior—with continuous reinforcement along the way, based on the mores prevalent in an individual's society. The need to be accepted becomes a person's driving force.

Cognitive psychologists hold that an addictive personality is formulated by the way a person receives, processes, stores, and retrieves sensory information. Also important is the nature of the attributes the person ascribes to the addictive substances or behaviors; those ascribing more power, whether it is there or not, may be at higher risk. An individual may develop very positive expectancies for what the behavior can do for them, whether or not their attributions and beliefs are true. If the substance or behavior produces a positive effect, then the person is likely to repeat the process so that the effect can be duplicated. In essence, people become addicted to the pleasurable results of the substance before they become addicted to the particular path taken to achieve them.

Humanistic psychologists concentrate on the present, focusing on the fact that people have choices, yet many people do not know how to make proper ones because of trauma experienced during youth. To the humanist, the idea of the family is important, particularly how love was expressed and experienced, because through love, people can believe in themselves enough to be able to make positive choices.

The proponents of trait theory contend that people are born with certain tendencies and preferences of action, which may or may not be genetic; the evidence is inconclusive. Trait theorists seem to agree, however, that society and the family have a strong influence on people and that some people are predisposed toward compulsive behavior from an early age.

Biological studies have been conducted to explore the suspected link between addictive behavior and genes, substance use disorders suggesting that, at least in part, a tendency toward addiction may be inherited. Studies suggest that certain people may inherit impaired neurological homeostasis, which is partly corrected by their addiction. The sons of fathers with alcohol dependence have a higher "body sway" (the degree to which a person sways when standing upright with the eyes closed) than do sons of men without alcohol dependence; "body sway" decreases when the sons are intoxicated. Sons of men with alcohol dependence have a higher rate of addiction than daughters do, no matter which parent reared the children.

People with "familial essential tremor," an inherited disorder, have less tremor when drinking and have a higher rate of alcohol dependence. Also, while alcohol-dependent people do not have higher levels of arousal at rest, they become more aroused when stressed, as measured by heart rate, and are slower to return to rest.

The majority of controlled scientific studies on genetics have been conducted on the alcoholic population. Consequently, the studies are inconclusive when discussing addiction and any related personality problems overall. However, the studies do add evidence to the possible link between biology and behavior.

SELF-REGULATION

Research seems to indicate that addiction is a multilevel problem with complex roots in psychology, sociology, biology, and genetics. Among the symptoms of addictive behavior are tendencies toward excessiveness, compulsion, and obsessions. Compulsions are impulses that are difficult to resist, while obsessions are compelling ideas or feelings that are usually somewhat irrational. These tendencies have prompted many to wonder about the existence of an addictive personality.

For some, this tendency can be traced back to childhood and used as a warning sign. If the tendency is identified in advance, efforts can be made to alter the child's first impulse and slowly, over time and with much positive reinforcement, show the child alternative, acceptable behavior. When the child can be taught to achieve self-regulation in a positive way, within acceptable social limits, there is a better chance for positive achievement as an outcome. Self-regulation is a process whereby individuals manage their feelings, reactions, and thoughts in response to internal and external events. In a culture where excessiveness is common, however, teaching balance and self-regulation can be difficult. This is because immediate gratification may be promoted and reinforced in such a culture.

Whether addictive behavior is learned for survival, passed on genetically, or is an intricate combination of both, apparently, a set of personal features can predispose a person toward addiction, or, at the least, can place a person in a high-risk group. If these symptoms can be identified early enough, the chance to teach potential addicts the path toward balance increases, and the compulsive lifestyle can be decreased or channeled in a healthy way.

ADDICTION TREATMENTS

Addictions and the victims of addictions have been studied and described at least since the beginning of written language, and probably since humanity first communicated by storytelling. As such, many treatments and related self-help efforts have developed over the years. In 1935, in Ohio, Robert Smith and William Wilson organized Alcoholics Anonymous (AA). AA is not a formal program of treatment but instead a self-help resource consisting of a group of people with alcohol problems who are in various stages of recovery, from those desiring to quit to those who have achieved very long-term abstinence from alcohol. It is a program in which most individuals work through a series of steps as they make progress in their recovery.

The value of AA is world renowned. The organization is considered by most professionals and nonprofessionals who have contact with it to be one of the more far-reaching recovery resources in the world, in terms of the many ways in which it may help its attendees. The twelve-step program, an idea that AA started, transcends the boundaries of alcohol problems and has been applied to many addictions. AA is run by people recovering from alcohol problems who desire to remain abstinent. They are primarily nonprofessionals who simply seek to help other individuals who desire to quit. However, not until the early 1970s did addiction gain national and international attention through significant progress based on research funded by the US government.

In 1971, the National Institute on Alcohol Abuse and Alcoholism conducted research that showed addiction to be threatening American society. Afterward, a concentrated effort was made to study individuals addicted to alcohol and other drugs, with an attempt to find symptoms that could predict individuals at high risk for developing such problems. The federally funded studies would ostensibly find ways to help prevent and reduce the tremendous health, social, and economic consequences of addiction in the United States. Assessing dependence potential and discovering vulnerability or high-risk factors through demographic characteristics, psychological status, and individual drug history became the focus of studies. The funding of these studies became a critical component in the fight to better understand addiction. As a result, many promising treatments became available for individuals and families seeking help for problems with addiction and behaviors with addictive features. Treatment goals also expanded to address not only those with a desire to quit but also those who want to cut down

on their use or prevent use altogether. Such approaches include cognitive behavioral treatments focusing on relapse prevention, readiness-to-change treatments such as motivational interviewing, programs for adolescents such as multisystemic family therapy, harm-reduction strategies focused on reducing the risks and problems associated with substance use while also potentially reducing use, and a wide variety of pharmacological approaches involving the use of prescription medications to stave off addictions.

Internationally, studies indicate that technologically advanced societies seem to give rise to more kinds of dependency than do more slowly developing countries, a fact which could help researchers focus on some societal misconceptions of overall health. For example, in the United States and some other similarly advanced societies, there exists a tendency toward instant gratification. People who are tense are advised to take a pill. People who are lonely can call a certain number for conversation. People who are bored might have an alcoholic drink. People who are unhappy might eat. Ideally, societies, governments, and researchers will unite to unveil all possible symptoms of addiction, to identify those at high risk for addiction, and to employ successful recovery methods.

FURTHER READING

Anderson, Robert E., Gordon E. Barnes, and Robert P. Murray. "Psychometric Properties and Long-Term Predictive Validity of the Addiction-Prone Personality (APP) Scale." *Personality and Individual Differences* 50.5 (2011): 651–56. Academic Search Complete. Web. 13 Feb. 2014.

Khantzian, Edward J. *Treating Addiction as a Human Process*. Northvale, NJ: Aronson, 1999. Print.

McNeece, C. A., and D. M. DiNitto. *Chemical Dependency: A Systems Approach*. 4th ed. Needham Heights, MA: Allyn, 2012. Print.

Mulé, S. Joseph, ed. *Behavior in Excess: An Examination of the Volitional Disorders*. New York: Free, 1981. Print.

Orford, Jim. *Excessive Appetites: A Psychological View of Addictions*. 2nd ed. New York: Wiley, 2001. Print.

Thombs, Dennis L., and Cynthia J. Osborn. *Introduction to Addictive Behaviors*. New York: Guilford, 2013. Print.

Twerski, Abraham J. *Addictive Thinking: Understanding Self-Deception*. 2nd ed. Center City, MN: Hazelden, 1997. Print.Wilson, Bill. Alcoholics Anonymous. 3rd ed. New York: Alcoholics Anonymous, 1999. Print.

Frederic Wynn; Updated by Nancy Piotrowski

SEE ALSO: Codependency; Families and Substance Abuse; Intervention; Media and Substance Abuse; Recognizing the Symptoms; Recovery

ADHD medications

Attention-deficit/hyperactivity disorder (ADHD) is a condition in which people have trouble focusing and paying attention. As a result, those with ADHD may be hyperactive, act without thinking, or have trouble following through with tasks. According to the Centers for Disease Control and Prevention, ADHD is the most common neurodevelopmental disorder of childhood and, although usually diagnosed in childhood, it may last into adulthood. The ideal treatment for ADHD is usually a combination of medication and behavioral therapy, but there is no single best treatment. Any good treatment plan, however, should include close monitoring and adjustments in medication treatment regimens as needed.

INTRODUCTION

Attention deficit/hyperactivity disorder has been described in historic literature for the last 200 years, predominantly showing children with characteristic behaviors of hyperactivity, impulsivity, and inattention which continue to be seen in those with the diagnosis today. Charles Bradley, in 1937, was the first to depict the positive effect of stimulant medications in children with symptoms of ADHD. It took another twenty five years for any further research to be pursued in the area. According to Consumer Reports, ADHD is a common neurobiological disorder which affects between 5-8% of school-aged children today, 60% of which continue with symptoms into adulthood. Although it has been thought that ADHD affects three times the number of boys than girls, recent research is finding that the number of females affected with ADHD is nearly equal to that of boys. The sales of ADHD medications have been quite profitable, with an estimated $12.9 billion in sales in 2014. The National Resource Center on ADHD notes that ADHD medications, such as stimulants, have been shown to be effective, with 70-80% of children responding positively to the medications. Not all who receive treatment have similar effects, with some showing great benefits while others experience moderate effectiveness and some only manage to see modest results. While stimulants have overall good results, the risk for abuse does exist. It has been noted that teenagers and college students without an ADHD diagnosis take ADHD medication to pull all-nighters or focus for exams. Stimulants also have the potential to decrease appetite, thus the allure to abuse medication for weight loss.

OVERVIEW OF ADHD MEDICATION TREATMENT

Those individuals diagnosed with Attention Deficit/ Hyperactivity disorder can be treated with a stimulant or nonstimulant medication, both of which have been shown to be safe and effective when used under the supervision of a physician and as they are intended. In the short term, 60-80% of children and adolescents on stimulants and/or non-stimulants see improvements in attention, hyperactivity, and concentration. Medication for ADHD is usually a daily medicine and due to the forgetfulness among child and adolescent patients, and stigma that may be associated with the medication and diagnosis, compliance is at times an issue. There are several different forms of medication, including short-acting, long acting, liquid, and patches which may help patients have an easier time with medication compliance. Stimulant medication has been in use since 1937 and currently includes methylphenidate (Ritalin, Concerta), mixed salts of single entity amphetamine product (Adderall, Adderall XR), and dextroamphetamine (Dexedrine, Dextrostat). Non-stimulant medications include atomoxetine (Strattera), antidepressants such as tricyclics and bupropion, and antihypertensives such as clonidine.

STIMULANT MEDICATIONS

Psychostimulant medications are the most widely used medication to help treat patients with ADHD. Although stimulants help between 70-80% of patients manage their symptoms, they are not a cure for the disorder. The American Medical Association (AMA) reported that "pharmacotherapy, particularly stimulants, has been extensively studied. Medication alone generally provides significant short-term symptomatic and academic improvement" and "the risk-benefit ratio of stimulant treatment in ADHD must be evaluated and monitored on an ongoing basis in each case, but in general is highly favorable." Stimulant medications include methylphenidate (Ritalin, Concerta), mixed salts of single entity amphetamine product (Adderall, Adderall XR), and dextroamphetamine (Dexedrine, Dextrostat), all of which work on the neurotransmitter dopamine. Dopamine works in the brain centers which control pleasure, movement, and attention. When taken in the manner that is prescribed, stimulants help patients with attention and ADHD. However, when taken in ways other than prescribed, dopamine levels in the brain can be increased and can lead to addiction.

Methylphenidate (Ritalin, Concerta) is a short-acting medication which begins to work in 15-20 minutes. This medication is taken by mouth and the effects usually wear off by nighttime. Most physicians see improvement when the patient takes the medicine three times a day. Methylphenidate is available in both brand name and generic which allows for patients to have lower cost options. Concerta is the extended release version of methylphenidate, which was approved by the FDA in 2000 It has three different compartments that release the medication at different times of the day to provide longer acting effect of the medicine. Price of Concerta is more expensive as it is longer acting and generic is not yet available. Common side effects with methylphenidate include appetite suppression, mild sleep disturbance, and irritability. Some patients on high doses can see motor tics but these normally resolve by lowering the dose.

Mixed salts of single entity amphetamine products (Adderall, Adderall XR) have a variable length of action which ranges from 3.5-8 hours, depending on the dose. These medications are taken orally and have similar side effects to those seen with methylphenidate and include decreased appetite, mild sleep disturbance, and irritability. Amphetamines are available in both brand name and generic options thus allowing for cheaper medication options for patients.

Dextroamphetamine (Dexedrine, Dextrostat) is a short acting medication that begins to have effect in 20-30 minutes and lasts 4-5 hours. Dexedrine is a sustained release capsule, which releases part of the dose in the capsule in the first hour and the rest of the dose in the next 3.5 hours. Side effects are similar to the other stimulant medications and include mild sleep disturbance, decreased appetite, and irritability. These medications are available in both brand name and generic which helps keep costs under control for patients.

NON-STIMULANT MEDICATION

Some children, adolescents, and adults respond equally, if not better to non-stimulant medication than to the traditional stimulant medication used in the treatment of ADHD. Non-stimulants can be used when there is a contraindication to the use of stimulants, the patient has experienced a side effect to stimulants or the patient/patient family prefers not to use a stimulant for personal reasons. Atomoxetine (Strattera) was approved by the FDA in 2002 for use in ADHD. It is not a stimulant or an antidepressant. It works on a different neurotransmitter in the brain, called norepinephrine and helps to alleviate symptoms of inattention, hyperactivity, and impulsivity. Unlike stimulants which are controlled substances, atomoxetine is not and, therefore, doctors can provide refills and samples of the medications. However, atomoxetine is not as fast acting as stimulants and usually takes 3-4 weeks for patients to start seeing results with symptoms. The most common side effects with Strattera include dizziness, decreased appetite, fatigue, upset stomach, nausea, and mood swings. Strattera is not available in generic form thus the cost is high and it may be difficult for some patients to continue on the medication for financial reasons.

ANTIDEPRESSANTS

Antidepressants such as bupropion and tricyclics have been used with less frequency to treat ADHD symptoms. Not many studies have been done on the effects of antidepressants on ADHD symptoms thus these medications should be used with caution. Tricyclics and bupropion work on dopamine and norepinephrine; the neurotransmitters in the brain that have been linked with ADHD and these seem to be more effective than other antidepressants that work on serotonin, another neurotransmitter in the brain. Antidepressants are not FDA approved for the treatment of ADHD and side effects can include an increased risk in suicidal thoughts in children and adolescents.

ANTIHYPERTENSIVES

Clonidine is an antihypertensive medication which has been used to treat high blood pressure but has shown to be helpful in treating the symptoms of ADHD in some patients. When used in combination with a stimulant medication, the benefits are moderate. Clonidine has been shown to help ease tics in children with both tics and ADHD. Common side effects of clonidine include dry mouth, drowsiness, low blood pressure, and low heart rate. Clonidine is generic so more affordable than some other treatment options.

RISK OF ABUSE WITH ADHD MEDICATIONS

Although stimulant medication has a low risk of leading to addiction, there is potential for abuse especially among teenagers and college students. As mentioned earlier, students without a diagnosis of ADHD have used stimulant medication in order to pull all-nighters to study for exams and work on school projects. With the common side effect of decreased appetite, it has been noted that teenagers may also turn to ADHD medication as a form of weight loss. In children and teenagers, the rate of misuse has been reported between 5-8% whereas college students have a larger abuse rate of 5-35%. Out of those students who have reported using ADHD medication without a diagnosis, 26-63% state they used the medication to help boost academic performance. Out of the three most commonly prescribed stimulants, dextroamphetamine and amphetamines have a higher risk for abuse as opposed to methylphenidate. Some users have reported crushing the medication to snort it or dissolve in water and inject. This use poses great risk and can lead to severe complications and even death. According to a study by Setlink, Bond, and Ho; "Calls related to teenaged victims of prescription ADHD medication abuse rose 76%, which is faster than calls for victims of substance abuse generally and teen substance abuse." Almost one-third of teenagers have reported knowing a friend who abuses ADHD medications.

FUTURE DIRECTIONS

Although research continues on the cause of ADHD in children, adolescents, and adults, it is still unknown as to what exactly leads to a patient developing ADHD. Research is continuing to look at brain imaging and animal models to help unravel the missing pieces of ADHD and studies are being conducted in the long term effects and outcomes of children with ADHD. This is a fairly new field of study that still has many unanswered questions with room for further research and development of treatment.

FURTHER READING

Kastrenakes, J. (2015, May 14). Uninsured and minority kids are less likely to be diagnosed with ADHD. Retrieved from: http://www.theverge.com/2015/5/14/8603483/adhd-diagnosis-statistics-nchs This article reviews the disparities in ADHD diagnosis amongst children and discusses how minority race and insurance standing play a role in either over diagnosis or under diagnosis of children with ADHD.

Rettner, R. (2013, April 2). ADHD medications: 5 vital questions and answers. Retrieved from: http://www.livescience.com/28370-adhd-medication-side-effects.html This article reviews 5 common questions patients and families have in regards to ADHD medications. They cover such questions as what are the short term and long term effects of medications, when a child should start medication, once started how long do you need to continue, if symptoms are mild do medications need to be started, and what steps can be taken to minimize overuse of ADHD medications.

Rodriguez, D. Medications to treat ADHD. Retrieved from: http://www.everydayhealth.com/adhd/adhd-drugs.aspx Accessed June 9, 2015. This article reviews the most common medications prescribed in the treatment of ADHD. It looks at not only the medications discussed in this article but a few other common medications that were not highlighted in this publication.

Whelan, L. (2015, February 24). Sales of ADHD meds are skyrocketing. Here's why. Retrieved from: http://www.motherjones.com/environment/2015/02/hyperactive-growth-adhd-medication-sales. This article reviews the reasons as to why we are seeing an increase in the sales of ADHD medication. It looks into the growing number of diagnoses in the developed world and delves into how the Affordable Care Act will increase mental health coverage and may increase the number of children diagnosed with ADHD.

Brittany Casey and Christine D. McFarlin

SEE ALSO: Antidepressants; Attention-Deficit Hyperactivity Disorder (ADHD); Ritalin

Alcohol and its effects

Ethanol, the type of alcohol found in alcoholic beverages, is a colorless, flammable substance with psychoactive (mind-altering) properties. The amount of alcohol in the body is usually measured as the blood alcohol content (BAC), expressed as the percentage of alcohol per liter of blood. Moderate intake of alcohol can have some health benefits; however, excessive or prolonged use has many detrimental effects on the body.

MIXING DIFFERENT TYPES OF ALCOHOL

Is there any truth to the saying, "beer before liquor, never been sicker; liquor before beer, you're in the clear"? Beliefs about the sequence of drinking may stem from the rate at which the body processes alcohol. The liver can efficiently process one standard-sized alcoholic drink per hour only, although men can process more alcohol per hour than can women. What constitutes one drink? Twelve ounces of beer, five ounces of wine, and one shot (1.5 ounces) of hard liquor are generally equivalent in their alcohol content.

The amount of alcohol in the blood rises more quickly after drinking liquor than after drinking beer. If a person drinks liquor before beer, he or she is likely to feel the effects of the alcohol sooner. This may encourage one not to consume as much, decreasing the chances of getting sick from overdoing it. Drinking beer before liquor, on the other hand, may make one feel ill because, having had little or no immediate effect from the beer, a person may be motivated to consume higher concentrations of alcohol by drinking shots or drinking stronger mixed drinks.

A more scientific explanation for the common belief is that different types of alcohol contain different amounts of compounds called congeners. Drinks that contain high quantities of congeners may increase hangover symptoms. Clear beverages like vodka, gin, and white wine contain less congeners than darker drinks like brandy, whisky, rum, and red wine. Mixing the congeners may increase stomach irritation.

SHORT-TERM EFFECTS

Alcohol is absorbed into the bloodstream through the lining of the stomach, so measurable amounts can be present within five minutes of ingestion. If alcohol is consumed after eating a heavy meal, its absorption is slowed. Alcohol is metabolized (broken down) in the liver. One to two hours are required to metabolize one drink.

Alcohol is a central nervous systemcentral nervous system depressantsalcohol (CNS) depressant; small amounts can produce euphoria and relaxation while large amounts can result in coma or death. Furthermore, moderate alcohol intake (a maximum of one or two drinks per day) may have some health benefits; excessive and regular consumption can be severely detrimental to one's health.

Different degrees of BACblood alcohol content produce different effects, including euphoria, lethargy,

mental confusion, stupor, vomiting, and coma. These effects are outlined here.

Euphoria (BAC of 0.03 to 0.12 percent). Symptoms include improved mood, increased sociability, increased self-confidence, increased appetite, inhibited judgment, impaired fine-muscle coordination, and flushed appearance. At this level, the person may laugh more readily, be friendlier, become more socially aggressive, or do things he or she would not normally do. Of note, a BAC of 0.08 percent, the threshold for driving under the influence, is set for every US state.

Lethargy (BAC of 0.09 to 0.25 percent). Symptoms include impaired comprehension and memory, sedation, slowed reflexes, blurred vision, and ataxia (lack of coordination), which is manifested by difficulties in balancing and walking. At this level, the person may forget phone numbers, addresses, or where he or she has parked a car. Driving or operating machinery could result in serious injuries or fatalities. If walking, the person could trip or fall.

Mental confusion (BAC of 0.18 to 0.30 percent). Symptoms include pronounced confusion, labile emotions (abrupt mood changes, laughing or crying readily), increased ataxia, decreased pain sensation, slurred speech, staggering, sensory impairment (sight, hearing, and touch), vomiting, and dizziness, which is often associated with nausea. This level is sometimes referred to as falling-down-drunkenness, and the person at this level of intoxication is severely impaired.

Stupor (BAC of 0.25 to 0.40 percent). Symptoms include severe ataxia, vomiting, unconsciousness (may be intermittent), slowed heart rate, slowed respirations, and urinary incontinence. At this level, death can occur from respiratory depression or from vomiting (if while unconscious, the person aspirates vomit into his or her lungs).

Coma (BAC of 0.35 to 0.50 percent). Symptoms include unconsciousness, markedly depressed reflexes (for example, pupils do not respond to light), severe respiratory depression, and severely slowed heart rate. At this level the drinker has alcohol poisoning, and death at this point is not uncommon.

Aftereffects from an acute drinking episode persist for up to twenty-four hours. Consumption of alcohol within several hours before going to sleep results in the drinker falling asleep more promptly. Consumption of one alcoholic beverage may increase total hours of sleep and may decrease awakening during the night. Higher consumption, however, results in the disruption of sleep patterns and prevents a restful night's sleep. The person falls asleep promptly; however, once most of the alcohol has been metabolized, the person experiences (because of a rebound effect) episodes of wakefulness and light, unproductive sleep. The following morning, the person who consumed two or more alcoholic beverages awakens fatigued and may experience a hangover, which can include headache, nausea, thirst, sensitivity to light and noise, diarrhea, and dysphoria (depression, anxiety, and irritability). Some of these symptoms are caused by dehydration, which can occur even with moderate alcohol consumption.

A single episode of drinking at the euphoric level (BAC of 0.03 to 0.12 percent) can have long-term consequences. Inappropriate comments or behavior while under the influence can result in the breakup of a relationship or the loss of a job. Driving under the influence—even if below the legal limit of 0.08 percent—can result in a traffic accident, which might cause serious injuries.

The presence of 30-50 milligrams of alcohol per every 100 milliliters of blood represents one average drink (a glass of beer or wine or an ounce of hard liquor). People who abuse alcohol may not stop drinking unitl much higher levels result in confusion, unconsciousness, coma, or even death.

LONG-TERM EFFECTS
In general, regular abusers of alcohol fall into two categories of use: alcoholism and alcohol abuse. Alcoholism is a chronic condition in which a person depends on regular ingestion of alcoholic beverages. Alcoholics are unable to control their drinking and continue to drink even when doing so interferes with their health, interpersonal relationships, and work.

Alcohol abuse is excessive drinking—enough to cause problems in daily life—without the person having complete dependence on alcohol. The long-term effects of regularly consuming more than one or two alcoholic beverages are profound and include medical, neuropsychiatric, and social problems. Both alcoholics and alcohol abusers are more susceptible to the long-term effects of alcohol abuse. These are caused by the direct effects of alcohol on the body and by resultant poor nutrition. Heavy drinkers may have a poor diet because much of their caloric intake often comes from alcoholic beverages.

Long-term alcohol abuse has medical, neuropsychiatric, and social consequences. Medical effects include diabetes, an impaired immune system, kidney infections and kidney failure, pneumonia, gastritis (inflammation of the stomach) and esophagitis (inflammation of the esophagus), and the following, all of which are common in alcoholics:

Cancer. Includes many forms of cancer, such as throat, esophagus, stomach, colon, rectum, liver, and kidney cancers. The combination of tobacco and alcohol markedly increases the risk of cancer, particularly cancers of the mouth and throat.

Cardiovascular disease. Hypertension (high blood pressure), heart failure, cardiomyopathy (damage to the heart muscle), and stroke.

Pancreatitis (inflammation of the pancreas). Acute pancreatitis is the sudden onset of inflammation, which may result in death. Chronic pancreatitis can continue for many years and can ultimately lead to death.

Ulcers of the stomach or duodenum (upper portion of the stomach). A perforated ulcer is a life-threatening situation.

Cirrhosis of the liver. This condition can lead to liver failure and death. Cirrhosis can produce portal hypertension (increased blood pressure in the venous system within the liver). Portal hypertension can produce esophageal varices (dilated blood vessels in the esophagus). Esophageal varices are prone to rupture and can result in a fatal hemorrhage.

Vitamin deficiencies. Vitamin deficiencies, which are usually caused by a poor diet, can result in a number of severe health problems.

Obesity. The appetite-stimulating effect of alcohol coupled with the calories in alcohol can result in obesity in some alcohol abusers.

Long-term neuropsychiatric effects of alcohol abuse include confusion; impaired memory; dementia; antegrade amnesia (also known as blackouts, the loss of memory following an episode of heavy drinking); tremors; peripheral neuropathy (numbness of the feet and hands); hallucinations (auditory and visual); fear, anxiety, and a sense of impending doom; an obsession with drinking; sexual dysfunction, including decreased libido and erectile dysfunction (inability for a male to get an erection); and delirium tremens, or DTs (tremors or convulsions). DTs occur during an episode of withdrawal from alcohol.

Long-term social effects of alcohol abuse include traffic fatalities or injuries to self or others, dysfunctional home life, spousal battery, child abuse, disruption of interpersonal relationships outside the home, injury or accidents at work, loss of a job or promotion, and codependency (a condition in which an alcoholic manipulates or controls others, such as his or her spouse, children, friends, and coworkers).

FETAL ALCOHOL SPECTRUM DISORDER

Fetal alcohol spectrum disorderfetal alcohol spectrum disorder (FASD) is a general category for the long-term effect of alcohol consumption on the fetus of a pregnant woman who also is an alcoholic. FASD involves varying degrees of physical and mental abnormalities. The best known and most thoroughly researched form of FASD is fetal alcohol syndrome (FAS).

Children with FAS are often born with a low birth weight and have varying degrees of facial abnormalities, mental retardation, CNS disorders, skeletal abnormalities, and heart defects. The facial abnormalities include microcephaly (small head and brain), small eyes, thin upper lip, and a small, upturned nose. The CNS disorders include vision and hearing problems, poor coordination, learning disabilities, and sleep problems. The skeletal abnormalities include deformities of the limbs, joints, and fingers. The heart defects include atrial septal defects (defects in the wall separating the upper heart chambers) and ventricular septal defects (defects in the wall separating the lower heart chambers).

Two other forms of FASD are alcohol-related neurodevelopmental disorder (ARND) and alcohol-related birth defects (ARBD). Persons with ARND may have intellectual, behavioral, and learning disabilities. During childhood, they tend to perform poorly in school and have difficulties with mathematics, attention, judgment, memory, and impulse control. Persons with ARBD have abnormalities that include hearing problems and problems of the heart, skeletal system, and kidneys.

Affected children cannot be cured; however, the following factors can improve a child's quality of life: early recognition of the disorder (before the age of six years); enrollment in special education programs; and a nurturing, stable, home environment. FASD is preventable if a woman stops drinking when she learns that she is pregnant.

A February 2011 study found that counseling about alcohol use during pregnancy is often inadequate. A study of 12,611 women who delivered infants from 2001 through 2008 found that, despite the substantial number of women who continue to consume alcohol during pregnancy, health care providers do not routinely assess alcohol consumption or counsel all women about alcohol's harmful effects. As with other alcohol-related disorders, nutrition and other factors (such as abuse of prescription drugs or illegal substances) play a role in the development of FASD.

A safe level of alcohol consumption, which will prevent FASD, is not known; however, no cases of FASD have been reported in which the pregnant woman consumed an occasional alcoholic beverage or even consumed a larger amount on a few occasions. A large study (11,513 children) published by researchers at University College London in October 2010 found that children at age five years who were born to women who drank one or two alcoholic beverages per week during pregnancy were not at increased risk for any behavioral or cognitive problems.

ALCOHOL COMBINED WITH OTHER SUBSTANCES

Many abusers of alcohol also abuse other substances. Sometimes, the combination has a synergistic effect—the combined effect is significantly more harmful than either substance alone. These harmful effects can occur with both short- and long-term use of alcohol plus another substance or substances. These substances include tobacco, marijuana, CNS depressants, CNS stimulants, prescription drugs, and over-the-counter (OTC) medications.

Tobacco. The combination of alcohol and tobacco greatly increases the risk of many types of cancers. The risk of oral (mouth and tongue) cancer is extremely high in smokers (or tobacco chewers) who also drink alcohol in excess. Smoking is a particularly difficult habit to quit. For example, studies have found that heroin addicts who had given up the drug for more than one year found it more difficult to quit smoking than breaking a heroin habit. Other studies have found that it is more difficult to quit smoking than to quit using cocaine.

Marijuana. Marijuana is a commonly used recreational drug and is frequently used with alcohol. The combination of the two can be particularly lethal. When a marijuana smoker also has overindulged in alcohol, vomiting is not uncommon. This reaction removes some of the alcohol from the stomach, but this reflex is suppressed with marijuana. As a result, more alcohol remains in one's system, increasing the result of alcohol poisoning. Even small amounts of alcohol and marijuana increase the risk of a traffic accident. Alcohol slows reaction time and alertness, and marijuana further impairs the driver. For example, marijuana reduces the frequency of a driver's visual searches (that is, of looking right and left before entering an intersection or before changing lanes).

CNS depressants. Alcohol is a CNS depressant. Co-ingestion (mixing) of alcohol and other CNS depressants, such as heroin, barbiturates, tranquilizers, analgesics (pain relievers), and sedatives, is particularly harmful. Reports have shown that more than 70 percent of fatal heroin overdoses are caused by the co-ingestion of heroin and another depressant, such as alcohol. The drug interaction can lead to depressed breathing and slowed heart rate, resulting in unconsciousness. The unconscious state can progress to coma and death. While unconscious, the person may vomit and aspirate the vomitus into his or her lungs, which frequently causes death. A 2010 study found that alcohol is more detrimental to one's health than is heroin.

CNS stimulants. CNS stimulants, such as cocaine, methamphetamine, and caffeine, interact with alcohol. Researchers have found that cocaine and alcohol combine in the liver to produce cocaethylene, which intensifies the euphoric effect of cocaine. Cocaine by itself has been associated with sudden death; however, cocaethylene is associated with a greater risk of sudden death than cocaine alone.

Methamphetamine is a potent stimulant. Studies have suggested that when combined with alcohol, it increases the risk of alcohol poisoning. Caffeine is a mild stimulant, compared with cocaine and methamphetamine. However, the combination of alcohol and caffeine has added risks. Not uncommonly, a person who has overindulged is offered a cup of coffee to "sober up." However, the caffeine in the coffee does not improve sobriety—it merely produces a state of wide-awake drunkenness. The increased alertness coupled with the augmented self-confidence from alcohol increases the risk of unsafe activity, such as driving an automobile.

Prescription or nonprescription medication. Many prescription drugs, such as antipsychotics and antidepressants, interact with alcohol. In addition, some OTC products, such as sleep aids and cold remedies, also may have an interaction. It is prudent for one taking any medication to read the label of the medication before consuming alcohol.

MODERATE ALCOHOL INTAKE

Moderate drinking (up to three drinks per occasion or seven drinks per week) may have some health benefits. This level of drinking might reduce the risk of heart disease, of dying from a heart attack, and of developing gall-

stones, and it might possibly reduce the risk of stroke and diabetes. Drinking red wine might be particularly beneficial. The so-called French paradox observes that the French have a relatively low incidence of coronary artery disease, despite high rates of smoking, low rates of exercise, and high rates of diets that are relatively high in saturated fat. The answer to this paradox might lie in the consumption of red wine by the French.

Red wine contains resveratrolresveratrol, which is an antioxidant. Experimental evidence shows that resveratrol may have anti-inflammatory, anticancer, and blood-sugar-lowering properties, all of which promote cardiovascular health. Despite the positive evidence, the health benefits of resveratrol are subject to controversy. The appetite-stimulating properties of alcohol have been found to benefit the elderly, whose health can suffer from a lack of appetite. A variety of tonics containing alcohol are on the market, and they often improve appetite. They also often improve sleep patterns.

FURTHER READING

Fisher, Gary, and Thomas Harrison. *Substance Abuse: Information for School Counselors*, Social Workers, Therapists, and Counselors. 4th ed. Boston: Allyn & Bacon, 2008. Incorporating actual clinical examples with solid research, this text provides counselors and social workers with a detailed overview of alcohol and other drug addictions.

Ketcham, Katherine, and William F. Asbury. *Beyond the Influence: Understanding and Defeating Alcoholism*. New York: Bantam, 2000. The authors define alcoholism as "a genetically transmitted neurological disease," and not the result of a character defect or moral weakness. They explain in exhaustive detail the effects of "the drug alcohol" on the human body and brain in both alcoholics and nonalcoholics.

Ludwig, Arnold. *Understanding the Alcoholic's Mind: The Nature of Craving and How to Control It*. New York: Oxford UP, 1989. Informative text for those who treat alcoholics, live with alcoholics, or who are alcoholics.

Miller, William R. *Rethinking Substance Abuse: What the Science Shows, and What We Should Do about It*. New York: Guilford, 2010. Reviews what is known about substance abuse and offers overviews of biological, psychological, and social factors in the treatment of substance abuse. Anticipates future developments and evaluates them for their possible impact on prevention and treatment.

WEBSITES OF INTEREST
Al-Anon and Alateen
http://www.al-anon.alateen.org
Alcoholics Anonymous
http://www.aa.org
National Institute on Alcohol Abuse and Alcoholism
http://www.niaaa.nih.gov

Robin L. Wulffson

SEE ALSO: Alcohol Poisoning; Binge Drinking; Fetal Alcohol Syndrome; Hepatitis; Liver Cancer; Pregnancy and Alcohol; Teens and Alcohol Abuse

Alcohol poisoning

Alcohol poisoning is an illness caused by consuming a large amount of alcohol in a short time. It usually occurs after binge drinking, in which a person rapidly ingests five or more drinks in sequence. Alcohol poisoning also can result in coma and death. The amount of alcohol in the body is usually measured as blood alcohol content (BAC) and is expressed as the percentage of alcohol per liter of blood. Alcohol consumption is also measured by the number of drinks a person consumes.

HANGOVER

A hangover is the body's way of indicating that overindulging in alcoholic beverages is unhealthy. An effective treatment for hangovers would undermine the body's own defense system against drinking too heavily. It is important to understand how alcohol consumption and hangovers are related.

After a person stops drinking, his or her blood alcohol concentration (BAC) begins to drop. Hangover symptoms peak around the time the BAC is 0.0. Alcohol acts as a diuretic (increases urine output), leading to dehydration and the loss of electrolytes. Although alcohol initially acts as a sedative, drinking actually disrupts the sleep cycle, causing a person to wake up fatigued. Finally, acetaldehyde, a toxic by-product of the body's breaking down of alcohol, causes many hangover symptoms.

There is no scientific evidence to support any method to rid the body of hangover symptoms. However, hangover remedies remain well known and often used, despite the evidence. Strong black coffee, for example, is a favorite among persons with a hangover, who reason that a jolt of caffeine will restore energy to their body. However,

caffeinated beverages, like alcohol, are diuretics and only worsen dehydration.

Additionally, the modest benefits of acetaminophen (Tylenol) may not be worth the increased risk of liver toxicity that can occur in the presence of alcohol. Ibuprofen and aspirin are safer for the liver, but they may worsen any stomach irritation caused by drinking excesses. One should not expect to recover by drinking more alcohol. The additional alcohol will be metabolized, and the unavoidable hangover will return as the person's BAC drops.

CAUSES

Most alcohol poisoning cases are caused by ethanol poisoning (C_2H_5OH), which is a component of alcoholic beverages, namely beer, wine, and hard liquor. Ethanol has been produced by the fermentation of sugar since antiquity. Other alcohol poisoning cases are caused by methanol poisoning (CH_3OH) or isopropyl alcoholIsopropyl alcoholalcohol poisoning (C_3H_8O). Methanol is primarily used in the production of other chemicals; it is sometimes used as an automotive fuel. Isopropyl alcohol is a component of rubbing alcohol and is widely used as a solvent and a cleaning fluid.

All forms of alcohol are flammable and colorless, and all are readily available in the marketplace. Although the purchase of alcoholic beverages in the United States is generally restricted to adults age twenty-one years and older, minors often obtain the product through a third party, sometimes even their parents, without difficulty.

RISK FACTORS

A number of factors increase the risk of becoming ill through alcohol poisoning. They include the following:

- Rate of drinking. The more rapidly a person consumes a given amount of alcohol, the more likely the risk of alcohol poisoning. One to two hours are required to metabolize one drink.
- Gender. Young men age eighteen through twenty-five years are the most likely to experience alcohol poisoning; however, women are more susceptible to alcohol poisoning than men because they produce less of an enzyme that slows the release of alcohol from the stomach.
- Age. Teenagers and college-age youth are more likely to engage in binge drinking; however, the majority of these drinking-related deaths occur in persons age thirty-five to fifty-four years. This older age group often does not metabolize alcohol

as readily as younger persons and is more likely to have an underlying health problem that increases the risk.

- Body mass. A heavier person can drink more alcohol than a lighter person and still register the same BAC. For example, a 240-pound man who drinks two cocktails will have the same BAC as a 120-pound woman who consumes one cocktail.
- Overall health. Persons with kidney disease, liver disease, heart disease, or other health problems may metabolize alcohol more slowly. A person with diabetes, for example, who binge drinks might experience a dangerous drop in blood sugar level.
- Food consumption. A full stomach slows the absorption of alcohol, so drinking on an empty stomach increases the risk.
- Drug use. Prescription and over-the-counter drugs might increase the risk of alcohol poisoning. Ingestion of illegal substances, such as cocaine, methamphetamine, heroin, and marijuana, also increases the risk.

SYMPTOMS

Alcohol poisoning symptoms include confusion, stupor, or unconsciousness; respiratory depression (slow breathing rate); irregular breathing (a gap of more than ten seconds between breaths); slow heart rate; low blood pressure; low body temperature (hypothermia); vomiting; seizures; and pale or blue skin.

SCREENING AND DIAGNOSIS

The BAC is a definitive test for alcohol poisoning. Persons with alcohol poisoning often have a BAC of 0.35 to 0.5 percent. By way of comparison, a person is considered to be driving under the influence in all US states if his or her BAC is 0.08 percent or higher. Other blood tests include those that check a person's complete blood count (CBC) and those that check levels of glucose, urea, arterial pH (acid), and electrolytes.

TREATMENT AND THERAPY

Treatment consists of supportive measures until the body metabolizes the alcohol. This includes insertion of an airway (endotracheal tube) to prevent vomiting and aspiration of stomach contents into the lungs; close monitoring of vital signs (temperature, heart rate, and blood pressure); provisions of oxygen; medication to increase blood pressure and heart rate, if necessary; respiratory

support, if necessary; maintenance of body temperature (blankets or warming devices); and administration of intravenous fluids to prevent dehydration. In such cases, glucose should be added if the person is hypoglycemic, that is, if the person has low blood sugar (also, thiamine is often added to reduce the risk of a seizure). Another form of treatment is hemodialysis (blood cleansing), which might be needed for a dangerously high BAC (of more than 0.4 percent). Hemodialysis also is necessary if methanol or isopropyl alcohol has been ingested.

PREVENTION

The best prevention against binge drinking is education, especially of persons who participate in at-risk activities. Young men make up the group with the highest risk of alcohol poisoning. Often, young men have a sense of invincibility and they may disregard helpful advice from any source. Peer pressure is probably the best deterrent; however, it also is a factor that can encourage binge drinking. Furthermore, children with a good parental relationship are less likely to drink to excess.

FURTHER READING

Fisher, Gary, and Thomas Harrison. *Substance Abuse: Information for School Counselors, Social Workers, Therapists, and Counselors.* 5th ed. Upper Saddle River, NJ: Merrill, 2012. Incorporating clinical examples with solid research, this text provides counselors and social workers with a detailed overview of alcohol and other drug addictions.

Ketcham, Katherine, and William F. Asbury. *Beyond the Influence: Understanding and Defeating Alcoholism.* New York: Bantam, 2000. The authors define alcoholism as "a genetically transmitted neurological disease," and not something that results from a character defect or from moral weakness. Explains in detail the effects of "the drug alcohol" on the human body and brain in both alcoholics and nonalcoholics.

Miller, William R., and Kathleen M. Carroll, eds. *Rethinking Substance Abuse: What the Science Shows, and What We Should Do about It.* New York: Guilford, 2010. Reviews what is known about substance abuse and offers overviews of biological, psychological, and social factors involved in the treatment of substance abuse. It also anticipates developments and evaluates them for their potential impacts on prevention and treatment.

Olson, Kent R., et al., eds. *Poisoning and Drug Overdose.* 6th ed. New York: McGraw-Hill, 2012. A resource for poison control centers, toxicologists, and health care practitioners for the diagnosis, treatment, and management of poisonings caused by exposure to industrial, therapeutic, illicit, and environmental chemicals.

WEBSITES OF INTEREST
Al-Anon and Alateen
http://www.al-anon.alateen.org
Alcoholics Anonymous
http://www.aa.org
National Institute on Alcohol Abuse and Alcoholism
http://www.niaaa.nih.gov
National Institute on Drug Abuse
http://www.nida.nih.gov

Robin L. Wulffson

SEE ALSO: Alcohol and Its Effects; Binge Drinking; Teens and Alcohol Abuse

Amphetamine abuse

Amphetamine abuse is the repeated, high-dose, nonmedical use of amphetamines, which are potent, highly addictive central nervous system stimulants. Abuse continues despite the user's inability to function normally at home, school, and work.

CAUSES
Amphetamines are rapidly absorbed once ingested. When they reach the brain, they cause a buildup of the neurotransmitter dopamine. This leads to a heightened sense of energy, alertness, and well-being that abusers find to be pleasurable and productive for repetitive tasks. Tolerance develops rapidly, leading to the need for higher doses.

Amphetamines are easy to obtain, often through diversion from legal use, and they are relatively inexpensive. Using them does not carry the social stigma or legal consequences associated with the use of other stimulants, such as methamphetamine and cocaine.

RISK FACTORS
Amphetamine abuse is widespread and has been present almost since their introduction for medical use in the 1930s. Amphetamines were widely abused by soldiers during World War II to maintain alertness during long hours on duty. They are still used by some military personnel in combat settings.

After the war, amphetamines became popular among civilians, especially students who used them to keep awake for studying and as appetite suppressants and recreational drugs. By the 1960s, about one-half of all legally manufactured amphetamines were diverted for illegal use. With greater control over distribution of commercially manufactured amphetamines, manufacture by clandestine laboratories increased dramatically. In addition, the Internet has become a popular source for nonprescription amphetamines.

Abuse now occurs primarily among young adults (age eighteen to thirty years). A common venue for their abuse is the rave, an all-night music and dance concert or party. Use among males and females is evenly divided, except for intravenous use; in this case, males are three to four times more likely to use the drug intravenously. Abusers can rapidly become both physically and psychologically dependent on amphetamines, with a compulsive need for the drug.

SYMPTOMS
Physical symptoms of amphetamine abuse include euphoria, increased blood pressure, decreased or irregular heart rate, narrowing of blood vessels, dilation of bronchioles (the breathing tubes of the lungs), heavy sweating or chills, nausea and vomiting, and increases in blood sugar. High doses can cause fever, seizures, and cardiac arrest.

Frequent, high-dose abuse can lead to aggressive or violent behavior, ending in a psychotic state indistinguishable from paranoid schizophrenia. Features of this state include hallucinations, delusions, hyperactivity, hypersexuality, confusion, and incoherence. One such delusion is formication, the sensation of insects, such as ants, crawling on the skin. Long-term use can result in permanent memory loss.

SCREENING AND DIAGNOSIS
Routine blood and urine testing do not detect amphetamines in the body. Abusers who use pills or who snort amphetamine leave no outward signs of the abuse. Smokers may use paraphernalia to use the drug. Abusers who inject the drug will have needle marks on their skin.

A change in behavior is the primary clue to amphetamine abuse. The abuser develops mood swings and withdraws from usual activities and family and friends. Basic responsibilities and commitments are ignored or carried out erratically. The abuser becomes hostile and argumentative. Any change in a person's appearance, such as sudden weight loss, or in behavior, such as agitation or change in sleep patterns, should be addressed. Such changes may indicate amphetamine abuse. Experts recommend that parents focus their concern with the youth's well-being, and not on the act of abuse.

TREATMENT AND THERAPY
Symptoms of amphetamine withdrawal can develop within a few hours after stopping use. Withdrawal symptoms include nightmares, insomnia or hypersomnia (too much sleep), severe fatigue or agitation, depression, anxiety, and increased appetite. Severe depression can produce suicidal thoughts. Withdrawal symptoms usually peak within two to four days and resolve within one week.

No specific medications are available for directly treating amphetamine abuse. However, antidepressants can be helpful in the immediate and post-withdrawal phases. Some research suggests that serotonergic uptake inhibitors, such as fluoxetine, might be helpful in treating amphetamine abuse.

The National Institute on Drug Abuse recommends psychotherapeutic intervention utilizing a cognitive behavioral approach. Such an approach helps the abuser learn to identify counterproductive thought patterns and beliefs and to change them so that his or her emotions and actions become more manageable. The abuser is also taught how to improve coping skills to address life's challenges and stresses. Narcotics Anonymous and amphetamine-specific recovery groups are also helpful.

PREVENTION
As there are medical indications for amphetamines, experts recommend that prescription formulations be kept from potential abusers. Pill counts should be taken regularly. Young people should be taught the differences between medical use and illegal abuse. Parents should ensure that their children are not attracted to social settings or activities where amphetamine abuse is or might be encouraged or tolerated.

FURTHER READING
Abadinsky, Howard. *Drug Use and Abuse: A Comprehensive Introduction.* 7th ed. Belmont, CA: Wadsworth, 2011. Focuses on what drugs are abused, how they are abused, and how abuse is treated or prevented. Amphetamine abuse is covered in chapter 12.

Julien, Robert M. *A Primer of Drug Actions.* 11th ed. New York: Worth, 2008, A concise, nontechnical guide to the mechanisms of action, side effects, uses, and abuses of psychoactive drugs. A section in chapter 7 discusses amphetamines.

Kuhn, Cynthia, Scott Swartwelder, and Wilkie Wilson. *Buzzed: The Straight Facts about the Most Used and Abused Drugs from Alcohol to Ecstasy.* 3rd ed. New York: Norton, 2008. Contains an informative, easy-to-read section on hallucinogens and their effects.

Lowinson, Joyce W., et al., eds. *Substance Abuse: A Comprehensive Textbook.* 4th ed. Philadelphia: Lippincott, 2005. A comprehensive textbook. Chapter 16 covers amphetamines.

WEBSITES OF INTEREST
"Amphetamines and Related Disorders." Encyclopedia of Mental Disorders
http://www.minddisorders.com/A-Br/Amphetamines-and-related-disorders
Narcotics Anonymous
http://www.na.org
National Institute on Drug Abuse
http://www.nida.nih.gov

Ernest Kohlmetz

SEE ALSO: Methamphetamine; Teens and Drug Abuse

Antidepressants

Patients with depression were routinely treated with psychotherapy until the 1950s, when the first antidepressants were developed. Many medications have been developed to treat depression, with varying degrees of effectiveness and various side effects.

INTRODUCTION
In the early 1950s, psychotherapy was being used to treat people with major depression, but researchers were looking for more effective means of treatment, including pharmaceuticals. The first antidepressant, iproniazid, was discovered accidentally while it was being used to treat tuberculosis. This monoamine oxidase inhibitor (MAOI) was found to improve the mood of the patients it was used to treat, and this suggested that depression could be treated through pharmacological means. When this first antidepressant was found to cause damage to

the liver, it was replaced by imipramine, the first tricyclic antidepressant. Although imipramine was effective in treating nearly two-thirds of the cases of major depression, it was accompanied by a number of side effects, including sleepiness, palpitations, dry mouth, and constipation.

SECOND-GENERATION ANTIDEPRESSANTS

Over the next quarter century, there were many attempts to synthesize antidepressants that were not fraught prowith side effects. It became apparent that both MAOIs and tricyclics affected multiple neurotransmitters and thus had numerous side effects. Therefore, researchers directed their attention to the development of a medication that would affect a single neurotransmitter only. In 1971, the first antidepressant medication to block the uptake of only one neurotransmitter was released in the form of fluoxetine (Prozac). This medication, still widely used, was the first selective serotonin reuptake inhibitor (SSRI). Since the 1970s, the second-generation antidepressants Prozac, paroxetine (Paxil), and sertraline (Zoloft) have been the most commonly used antidepressants.

ADDITIONAL ANTIDEPRESSANTS

The pharmaceutical industry has improved technology to the point where drug makers are capable of producing antidepressant medications that act on more than one neurotransmitter without causing large numbers of side effects. This category of drugs is commonly referred to as the dual reuptake inhibitors. The most common of these dual reuptake inhibitors are the serotonin-norepinephrine reuptake inhibitors (SNRIs). SNRIs include venlafaxine (Effexor) and duloxetine (Cymbalta). These SNRIs increase the levels of both serotonin and norepinephrine (noradrenaline) in the brain by inhibiting the reabsorption of these neurotransmitters by brain cells. Although the mode of action by which these dual reuptake inhibitors function is uncertain, it is believed that the increased levels of serotonin and norepinephrine in the brain enhance the transmission of nerve impulses, thereby improving and elevating affect. These and other modern antidepressants fall into the category of atypical antidepressants. Medications that are considered atypical antidepressants do not easily fit in any other category of drugs while inhibiting the uptake of several neurotransmitters within the brain. Another commonly used drug in this category is buproprion (Wellbutrin). These medications are typically taken orally and in pill form.

NATURAL ANTIDEPRESSANTS

There are dozens of over-the-counter remedies and supplements that are marketed as antidepressants. For many of these substances, there is little, if any evidence of their safeness or effectiveness. One herbal supplement, St. John's wort, is quite commonly used to counter depression and has been shown to be highly effective in some studies. This herbal remedy comes from a plant with yellow flowers. Derivatives of this plant were first used medicinally in ancient Greece. Although St. John's wort was initially used to treat pain or for sedation, it has come to be used mainly as an over-the-counter antidepressant. Studies are ongoing to determine if St. John's wort really has antidepressant effects or if people are merely responding to their own expectations (creating a placebo effect).

FURTHER READING

Baumel, S. *Natural Antidepressants: Tried and True Remedies from Nature's Pharmacy.* New York: McGraw-Hill, 1998. Print.

Breggin, Peter R. *The Anti-Depressant Fact Book: What Your Doctor Won't Tell You About Prozac, Zoloft, Paxil, Celexa, and Luvox.* Cambridge: Perseus, 2001. Print.

Glenmullen, J. *The Antidepressant Solution: A Step-by-Step Guide to Safely Overcoming Antidepressant Withdrawal, Dependence, and "Addiction."* New York: Simon & Schuster, 2006. Print.

Hansen, R. A., et al. "Efficacy and Safety of Second-Generation Antidepressants in the Treatment of Major Depressive Disorder." *Annals of Internal Medicine* 143 (2005): 415–26. Print.

Kee, Joyce LeFever, Evelyn R. Hayes, and Linda E, McCuistion. *Pharmacology: A Patient-Centered Nursing Process Approach.* 8th ed. St. Louis: Elsevier, 2014. Print.

Kirsch, Irving. *The Emperor's New Drugs: Exploding the Antidepressant Myth.* New York: Basic, 2011. Print.

Hart, Carl L., and Charles Ksir. *Drugs, Society, and Human Behavior.* New York: McGraw-Hill, 2011. Print.

Muir, Alice Jane. *Overcoming Depression.* New York: McGraw-Hill, 2013. Print.

Sharp, Katherine. *Coming of Age on Zoloft: How Antidepressants Cheered Us Up, Let Us Down, and Changed Who We Are.* New York: Harper Perennial, 2012. Print.

Robin Kamienny Montvilo

SEE ALSO: Anxiety; Bipolar Disorder; Depression

Barbiturates

Barbiturates are a family of central nervous system depressant drugs with considerable abuse potential. Historically, they have played important roles in the treatment of sleep disorders, anxiety, seizures, and muscle spasms. Largely replaced by benzodiazepines, they retain clinical usefulness mainly as anticonvulsants and anesthetics.

MEDICINES CLASSIFIED AS BARBITURATES
- Amytal sodium
- Butisol sodium
- Luminal
- Nembutal sodium
- Phenobarbital
- Seconal sodium

HISTORY OF USE
In 1864, German scientist Adolf Von Baeyer synthesized barbituric acid by condensing urea and malonic acid. The name reportedly came from a friend of the discoverer, or from the day of Saint Barbara. The acid itself did not induce any effect on the central nervous system. Subsequently, more than twenty-five hundred barbiturate compounds with pharmacological properties have been obtained.

In 1903, Emil Fischer and Joseph von Mering discovered an effective sedative, diethylbarbituric acid or barbital, which entered medicine under the trade name Veronal. Another barbiturate, phenobarbitalphenobarbital (Luminal), was introduced in 1912.

By the mid-twentieth century, barbiturates became the most widely used sedativesedatives-hypnotic medication and the most popular substances of abuse. Their lipid solubility rendered them quick to act and increased their hypnotic properties, but it decreased the duration of action. Collectively referred to as downers, barbiturates were taken alone or with ethanol to produce a feeling of relaxation and euphoria. In the United States, barbiturate abuse and addiction markedly increased in the 1950s and 1960s. The drugs became especially popular with actors and entertainers, as a way to cope with stress and uncertainty. (Elvis Presley chronically overused barbiturates, and an empty bottle of pentobarbitalpentobarbital [Nembutal] was found on Marilyn Monroe's nightstand after her death.) As safer drugs for people with sleep disorders became available, the use of barbiturates for this purpose declined.

The beginning of the twenty-first century, however, saw a modest increase in the popularity of barbiturates as substances of abuse. According to a national survey on drug use and health by the US Substance Abuse and Mental Health Services Administration, in the first years of this century an estimated 3.1 million people age twelve years and older had misused barbiturates. Deaths caused by overdose and suicide attempts using barbiturates still occur.

Barbiturates today are used clinically for anesthesia, pediatric sedation, status epilepticus treatment, and seizure prevention, and, in certain instances, for cases of traumatic brain injury. Some barbiturates are used to treat insomnia. Lesser known uses for barbiturates include treatment of essential hand tremor, cyclic vomiting, and hyperbilirubinemia in neonates. Among advocates of euthanasiaeuthanasiaand barbiturates and among those who commit suicide, barbiturates remain one of the most commonly employed drugs. Pentobarbital is the drug of choice for veterinary anesthesia and euthanasia.

EFFECTS AND POTENTIAL RISKS
Barbiturates are classified according to their duration of action. The effects of ultra-short-acting drugs, such as Pentothal (used in surgical settings), last less than one hour. Short-acting barbiturates (such as Nembutal and Seconal) act for three to four hours and are more likely to be abused. The effects of intermediate-acting barbiturates (such as Amytal) last for six to eight hours, and those of long-acting barbiturates (such as Veronal and Luminal) last approximately twelve hours.

Like other sedative-hypnotic drugs, barbiturates produce relaxation or sleep. The mechanism underlying their effect is thought to be an enhancement of the neural inhibition induced by the neurotransmitter gamma-aminobutyric acid.

At regular doses, the effects of barbiturates vary depending on the user's previous experience with the drug, the setting of use, and the mode of administration. A particular dose taken in the evening, for example, may induce sleep, whereas it may produce relaxed contentment, euphoria, and diminished motor skills during the day. Some users report sedation, fatigue, unpleasant drowsiness, nausea, vomiting, and diarrhea. A paradoxical state of excitement or rage also can occur. Users may experience a "hangover" phenomenon the day after drug administration. Hypersensitivity reactions, sensitivity to sunlight (photosensitivity), decreased sexual function, and impaired memory also have been reported. Tolerance to sedative and hypnotic effects develops after regular use.

Above-regular dosage of barbiturates induces a state of intoxication similar to that caused by ethanol. This resemblance, and tolerance development, may prompt some users to increase their drug intake. Mild intoxication is characterized by drunk-like behavior with slurred speech, unsteady gait, lack of coordination, abnormal eye movements, and an absence of alcohol odor.

The therapeutic dosage of any barbiturate is close to the lethal dose. Because of this narrow therapeutic window, severe intoxication or drug-induced death can easily occur. Intentional or accidental overdose results in extreme drowsiness, respiratory depression (with slow breathing), hypotension, hypothermia, renal failure, decreased reflexes, and, ultimately, coma and death. A person with suspected barbiturate overdose should be seen by a physician without delay.

Barbiturate use can cause both psychological and physical dependency and severe, even life-threatening, withdrawal symptoms (such as anxiety, insomnia, tremors, increased heart rate, delirium, and seizures). Persons who want to stop taking this medication should do so under medical supervision only. Concomitant use of other sedative hypnotics, such as alcohol and benzodiazepines, leads to potentially dangerous synergistic effects.

FURTHER READING

Doweiko, Harold E. *Concepts of Chemical Dependency.* 7th ed. Belmont, CA: Brooks, 2009. An accessible textbook that includes a discussion of barbiturate effects and abuse.

Goldberg, Raymond. *Drugs across the Spectrum.* 6th ed. Belmont, CA: Wadsworth, 2010. A popular drug textbook with a subchapter discussing the effects of barbiturates and the health implications of their use.

Lynton, Richard. "Barbiturates." *Haddad and Winchester's Clinical Management of Poisoning and Drug Overdose.* Eds. Michael W. Shannon, Stephen W. Borron, and Michael Burns. 4th ed. New York: Saunders, 2007. A well-written, authoritative chapter on barbiturates and their pharmacology, uses, and overdose potential.

Shannon, Joyce Brennfleck, ed. *Drug Abuse Sourcebook.* 3rd ed. Detroit: Omnigraphics, 2010. A comprehensive resource for information on the abuse of depressants, including barbiturates.

WEBSITES OF INTEREST

"CNS Depressants." National Institute on Drug Abuse http://www.drugabuse.gov/publications/research-reports/prescription-drugs/cns-depressants
US Drug Enforcement Administration. Drug Information: Barbiturates
http://www.justice.gov/dea/concern/b.html

Mihaela Avramut

SEE ALSO: Depressants Abuse; Prescription Drug Abuse

Below the bulimia threshold

Bulimia, also called bulimia nervosa, is a psychological disorder that involves repeated binge eating accompanied by inappropriate actions to prevent weight gain. The binge involves eating a very large amount of food in a limited time, and feeling out of control during the eating. The inappropriate actions most typically are self-induced vomiting, but also may include misuse of laxatives or other medication, extreme fasting, or excessive exercise. The binge-purge cycle occurs at least once a week for three months or longer. People with bulimia are overly concerned about their body shape and weight.

INTRODUCTION

Approximately 1-2% of adolescent and young adult women have bulimia, most commonly middle or upper-middle-class older adolescent and young adult women in countries that highly value thinness. The binge eating/purging episodes frequently begin during or immediately after dieting, but many stressful life events may also precipitate onset.

Bulimia is classified as mild (purging 1-3 times/week), moderate (purging 4-7 times/week), severe (purging 8-13 times/week), or extreme (purging more than 14 times/week). The pattern of purging may be chronic or episodic, and without treatment typically lasts for several years. People with bulimia have increased risk of death from all causes and from suicide.

Risk factors for bulimia include weight concerns, low self-esteem, depression, and anxiety. Also, risk increases for people who internalize a thin body ideal or who experienced childhood sexual or physical abuse.

Even though bulimia is classified as a psychological disorder, biology as well as culture has an influence. On the biological side, the disorder seems to run in families.

Relatives of patients with eating disorders are 4 to 5 times more likely than the general population to develop eating disorders. On the culture side, bulimia occurs in about equal rates in most industrialized countries, but at least until recently was not typically found in developing countries, where access to food is often a daily concern. In the United States, most people with bulimia are white, but bulimia has been noted in other ethnic groups as well.

The food eaten during a binge typically is junk rather than fruits and vegetables. The amount of food is more than most people would eat under similar circumstances, but varies from person to person. Most people with bulimia readily understand that they binge eat and that this is an unhealthy thing to do. Continual snacking throughout the day would not be considered binge eating. Because bulimia has biological, psychological, and cultural components, ideal treatment addresses all three.

BIOLOGY

Bulimia has a number of potentially serious medical consequences. Self-induced vomiting is very harmful to the mouth, and typically leads to excessive cavities, loss of dental enamel, and other tooth and gum problems. Repeated vomiting also leads to enlarged salivary glands, which give the face a chubby appearance. Other harmful effects of repeated vomiting are tears in the esophagus, calluses or scars on the back of the hands, and changes in the body's chemicals. Chemical changes, called electrolyte imbalance, can lead to heart complications, seizures, and kidney failure, all of which can be fatal. Overuse of laxatives can lead to excessive constipation or permanent colon damage. Another potential problem is amenorrhea (absence of menstrual periods).

Ironically, people with bulimia typically develop more body fat than their non-bulimic peers. Further, people with bulimia are usually of normal weight or slightly overweight. Vomiting is not particularly effective at reducing caloric intake. It typically eliminates approximately 50% of the calories recently consumed, less if there is a delay.

PSYCHOLOGY

Bulimia often occurs with other psychological problems. Most people with bulimia report having an anxiety disorder at some point during their lives. Many people with bulimia report mood disorders, particularly depression, at some point in their lives. Also, people with bulimia are at higher risk than their non-bulimic peers for problems with substance abuse.

Most people with bulimia feel that their popularity and self-esteem are largely determined by their weight, no matter what are their other accomplishments. They are intensely preoccupied with how others view them. If they are successful, they consider themselves frauds, because if others really knew them, they would not seem adequate, self-sufficient, or worthwhile. Many young women with bulimia have a diminished sense of personal control, such that fear of losing control pervades their awareness. They have no confidence in their own abilities and strikingly low self-esteem. They also display more perfectionistic attitudes than most people. Like people with anorexia, an eating disorder that involves excessive fasting, they have a distorted body image.

Shame and secrecy surrounding eating are common in people with bulimia. They typically skip regular meals and social eating occasions, preferring to eat alone. Rather minor incidents related to eating, such as having a candy bar, may activate their fear of gaining weight, and set off a round of purging.

For some people, dieting leads to increased chances of developing bulimia. However, many people go on strict diets, but only a few of them develop bulimia or any other eating disorder. The underlying psychological factors may be emotional instability, poor impulse control, and excessive perfectionism.

A competitive environment seems to increase the chances of developing bulimia. Also, people with bulimia report a desire to have an empty stomach. At risk groups include athletes, dancers, models, and sorority women. In one 2-year research project that followed 11- to 14-year-old girls in ballet school, at least one quarter of them developed an eating disorder.

Young people with bulimia often seek out one another on websites where they find support and even sometimes inspiration or detailed information about how to get rid of the extra calories they consumed during a binge. Famous people who have reported being bulimic include: Paula Abdul, Justine Bateman, the Barbi twins, Melanie C (Sporty Spice), Princess Diana, Sally Field, Jane Fonda, Cheryl James (Salt of Salt-n-Pepa), Elton John, Lindsay Lohan, Joan Rivers, and Britney Spears.

CULTURE

The vastly different rates of bulimia in different groups supports the idea that there is a cultural component. In developed countries, such as the United States, there are strong media messages, particularly from television and fashion magazines, that thin is beautiful and the only way to be successful. Some young people find it very hard to resist these messages.

The ideals of beauty have changed, and thinness was not always considered attractive. Until the 1950's, in the United States, curvy and plump bodies were the accepted body type. Marilyn Monroe, for example, was a size 14.

No one factor seems to cause bulimia. Rather, people with bulimia seem to have some of the same biological vulnerabilities (such as being highly responsive to stressful events) as people with anxiety and/or mood disorders. Add to this biological vulnerability severe psychological and social pressure to be thin, and some people will develop bulimia.

TREATMENT

Drugs and psychological treatments with proven effectiveness for anxiety disorders are also the treatments of choice for bulimia. There are also prevention programs designed to overcome cultural ideals of extreme thinness.

The body's hypothalamus gland influences eating as well as the levels of various chemicals, one of which is serotonin. Low serotine is associated with impulsivity and binge eating. Thus, drugs that are used to treat bulimia influence the production of serotonin. In particular, anti-depressants that influence serotonin are the drugs of choice. Prozac is specifically approved for treatment of bulimia, and may help even if the person is not depressed. Other antidepressants that target serotonin and may be used for bulimia are Zoloft, Paxil, and Luvox. It is not clear whether the low serotonin causes the development of bulimia, or whether the bulimia causes the low serotonin.

There are several types of psychological approaches to treating bulimia. Cognitive-behavioral therapy starts with teaching the physical consequences of binge eating and purging, and the fact that vomiting and laxative abuse does not control weight but does have many harmful consequences. Also, the treatment includes scheduling 5-6 meals per day that include small, manageable amounts of food, and no more than a 3-hour interval between planned meals and snacks, so that there are no long periods without some food. Next, cognitive treatment focuses on altering dysfunctional thoughts and attitudes about body shape, weight, and eating. The treatment teaches coping strategies for resisting the impulse to binge and purge, including arranging activities so that the person will not be alone after eating.

Cognitive-behavioral treatment is effective, more effective than drugs alone, and seems to last, though it does not work for all people with bulimia.

Another psychological approach is family therapy, which helps parents intervene when their teenage child has bulimia. Also, interpersonal therapy addresses difficulties in close relationships, and improves communication and problem-solving. Both family therapy and interpersonal therapy can help people with bulimia. Combining drugs and psychological treatments boosts chances of success.

Prevention applied to at-risk young people can reduce chances of ever developing bulimia. Prevention programs teach that weight gain after puberty is normal, and that excessively controlling calories can cause more weight gain rather than less. One program targeted sorority women and included a health education program delivered through the internet. Interactive software included text, audio, and video components and online self-monitoring journals and behavior change assignments. The 8-week program had weekly assignments, including posting a message to a discussion group. Also, someone contacted participants via email if they missed assignments. This program helped a lot.

Bulimia can be treated outside the hospital. The National Eating Disorders Association is a large nonprofit organization in the United States dedicated to preventing eating disorders.

FURTHER READING

Hay P.P.J., Bacaltchuk, J., Stefano, S., & Kashyap, P. (2009). Psychological treatments for bulimia nervosa and binging. Cochrane Database of Systematic Reviews. Summarizes in lay language a scientific study in in which researchers reviewed 48 studies involving over 3000 people with bulimia. Findings were that cognitive behavior therapy is helpful in treating bulimia.

National Eating Disorder Association website: https://www.nationaleatingdisorders.org/bulimia-nervosa. An overview page contains symptoms, warning signs, health consequences, and links to more detailed information. Also, there are links to talk to someone in person or chat online with a counselor (mostly during business hours), or take an eating survey.

Mayo Clinic website: http://www.mayoclinic.org/diseases-conditions/bulimia/basics/definition/con-20033050. Contains information about symptoms, risk factors, consequences, and how to prepare for as well as what to expect when seeing a physician about bulimia.

WebMD website: http://www.webmd.com/mental-health/eating-disorders/bulimia-nervosa/bulimia-nervosa-credits. Includes symptoms, health consequences, and good guidelines for managing stress in healthy ways.

Lillian M. Range

SEE ALSO: Anorexia Nervosa and Bulimia Nervosa; Antidepressants; Anxiety; Body Image and Girls; Compulsive Overeating; Depression; Eating Disorders; Exercising Addiction; Mood Disorders; Staying in a Healthy Weight Range

Binge drinking

Binge drinking is the rapid consumption of five or more alcoholic beverages in succession. Binge drinking often occurs in group settings and can lead to coma and death. The amount of alcohol in the body is usually measured as the blood alcohol content, which is expressed as the percentage of alcohol per liter of blood. Alcohol consumption is also measured by the number of drinks ingested.

COLLEGE BINGE DRINKING

Binge drinking, or heavy episodic drinking, is one of the most serious problems on college campuses. According to the Centers for Disease Control and Prevention, binge drinking is defined as consuming five or more drinks in about two hours for males and consuming four or more drinks in about two hours for females.

Binge drinking not only leads to alcohol overdose (poisoning) but also leads to drunk driving, accidents, poor school performance, risky sexual activity, property damage, illicit drug use, and death. Furthermore, studies suggest that heavy drinking in adolescence is strongly associated with heavy drinking in young adult life. Rather than "growing out" of binge drinking behavior, many young persons "grow into" a pattern of alcohol dependence or abuse.

CAUSES

Ethanol (C_2H_5OH) is the psychoactive (mind-altering) component of alcoholic beverages, namely beer, wine, and hard liquor. Since antiquity, ethanol has been produced by the fermentation of sugar.

Alcohol is a flammable and colorless liquid and is readily available on the marketplace. Although the sale of alcoholic beverages in the United States and many other developed nations is generally restricted to adults over the age of twenty-one years, minors can often obtain the product through a third party, sometimes even their parents, without difficulty.

Peer pressure is a major factor in binge drinking. Teenagers and young adults who have never consumed alcohol, or who have consumed only an occasional alcoholic beverage, may succumb to peer pressure in a party environment and engage in binge drinking through drinking games. Party attendees are sometimes encouraged to partake in drinking with a beer "bong," which facilitates binge drinking. (A beer bong is a funnel attached to a hose. The drinker lies on his or her back, and one or more bottles of beer are funneled into his or her mouth.)

Significant evidence exists that genetic factors are involved in the development of alcoholism. The interaction of genes and environment is complex and, for most people with alcohol dependence, many factors are involved. Since 1989, the US government-funded Collaborative Study on the Genetics of Alcoholism (COGA) has been tracking alcoholism in families. COGA researchers have interviewed more than fourteen thousand people and sampled the DNA (deoxyribonucleic acid) of hundreds of families. Researchers have found evidence for the existence of several alcohol-related genes. COGA researchers are increasingly convinced that certain types of alcoholics are representative of a number of genetic variations.

RISK FACTORS

The following factors increase risk of binge drinking:

- Rate of drinking. Rapid consumption of a given amount of alcohol increases the risk of alcohol poisoning. One to two hours are required to metabolize one drink.
- Gender. Young men from age eighteen through twenty-five years are the most likely group to engage in binge drinking; thus, they are at the highest risk for alcohol poisoning. However, young women also engage in binge drinking and are more susceptible to alcohol poisoning because women produce less of an enzyme that slows the release of alcohol from the stomach than men.
- Age. Teenagers and college-age youth are more likely to engage in binge drinking; however, the

majority of deaths from binge drinking occur in persons age thirty-five to fifty-four years. The persons in this age group often do not metabolize alcohol as readily as younger persons and are more likely to have underlying health problems that increase the risk.

- Body mass. A heavier person can drink more alcohol than a lighter person and still register the same blood alcohol content (BAC). For example, a 240-pound man who drinks two cocktails will have the same BAC as a 120-pound woman who consumes one cocktail.
- Overall health. Persons with kidney, liver, or heart disease, or with other health problems, may metabolize alcohol more slowly. Persons with diabetes who binge drink might experience a dangerous drop in blood sugar level.
- Food consumption. A full stomach slows the absorption of alcohol; thus, drinking on an empty stomach increases the risk.
- Drug use. Prescription and over-the-counter drugs might increase the risk of alcohol poisoning. Ingestion of illegal substances, such as cocaine, methamphetamine, heroin, and marijuana, also increase the risk.

SYMPTOMS

Symptoms of alcohol poisoning include respiratory depression (slow breathing rate); confusion, stupor, or unconsciousness; slow heart rate; low blood pressure; low body temperature (hypothermia); vomiting; seizures; irregular breathing (a gap of more than ten seconds between breaths); and blue-tinged skin or pale skin.

SCREENING AND DIAGNOSIS

The BAC test is a definitive measure of alcohol in the blood and, hence, of blood poisoning. Persons with alcohol poisoning often have a BAC of 0.35 to 0.5 percent. By comparison, the BAC level that marks driving under the influence is 0.08 percent in all US states. Other screening tests include complete blood count and other tests that check levels of glucose, urea, arterial pH, and electrolytes in the blood.

TREATMENT AND THERAPY

Acute treatment consists of supportive measures until the body metabolizes the alcohol; acute treatment includes insertion of an airway (endotracheal tube) to prevent vomiting and aspiration of stomach contents into the lungs; close monitoring of vital signs (temperature, heart rate, and blood pressure); oxygen administration; medication to increase blood pressure and heart rate, if needed; respiratory support, if needed; and maintenance of body temperature (blankets or warming devices). Acute treatment also includes the administration of intravenous fluids to prevent dehydration (glucose should be added if the person is hypoglycemic, and thiamine is often added to reduce the risk of a seizure). Further treatment includes hemodialysis (blood cleansing), which might be needed for dangerously high BAC levels (more than 0.4 percent). Hemodialysis also is necessary if methanol or isopropyl alcohol has been ingested.

Follow-up treatment for binge drinking requires the aid of a health care professional skilled in alcohol abuse treatment. A treatment plan includes behavior-modification techniques, counseling, goal setting, and use of self-help manuals or online resources. Counseling on an individual or group basis is an essential treatment component. Group therapy, which is particularly valuable because it allows interaction with others who abuse alcohol, helps a person become aware that his or her problems are not unique. Family support is a significant component of the recovery process, so therapy may include a spouse or other family member.

Binge drinking may be a component of other mental health disorders. Counseling or psychotherapy may be recommended. Treatment for depression or anxiety also may be a part of follow-up care. Beyond counseling and medication, other modalities may be helpful. For example, in September 2010, researchers at the University of California, Los Angeles released the results of a clinical trial on a unique therapy that applies electrical stimulation to a major nerve that emanates from the brain. The technique, trigeminal nerve stimulationtrigeminal nerve stimulation, reduced participants' depression an average of 70 percent in an eight-week period.

Care also may include long-term pharmaceutical treatment, including the oral medications disulfiram, acamprosate, and naltrexone. Disulfiramdisulfiram (Antabuse), which is taken orally, produces unpleasant physical reactions to alcohol ingestion; these reactions include flushing, headaches, nausea, and vomiting. Disulfiram, however, does not reduce the craving for alcohol. One drug that can reduce craving is acamprosateacamprosate (Campral). Another drug, naltrexonenaltrexone (ReVia), may reduce the urge to drink, and it blocks the pleasant sensations associated with alcohol consumption. Oral medications are not foolproof, however; if a person wants to return to drinking, he or she can simply stop taking the medication.

To avoid (or manage) relapses and to help deal with the necessary lifestyle changes to maintain sobriety, aftercare programs and support groups are essential for the recovering alcoholic. Regular attendance at a support group, such as Alcoholics Anonymous, is often a component of follow-up care.

Although death can occur from binge drinking, most alcohol-related fatalities occur in automobile accidents caused by driving under the influence. Also, women who binge drink are vulnerable to sexual assault while in an alcohol-induced stupor. Repeated episodes of binge drinking can result in permanent physical injury and in reduced quality of health. Brain and liver damage is common in repetitive binge drinkers. A young adult who binge drinks often progresses to alcoholism in adulthood.

PREVENTION

The best way to prevent binge drinking is to educate persons who partake in at-risk behaviors. The highest risk for binge drinking occurs among young men, who often have a sense of invincibility and who often disregard advice from any source. Peer pressure is probably the best deterrent; it also is a factor that can encourage binge drinking. Finally, children with a good parental relationship are less likely to drink to excess.

FURTHER READING

Fisher, Gary L., and Thomas C. Harrison. *Substance Abuse: Information for School Counselors, Social Workers, Therapists, and Counselors.* 5th ed. Upper Saddle River, NJ: Merrill, 2012. Incorporating clinical examples with solid research, this text provides counselors and social workers with a detailed overview of alcohol and other drug addictions.

Ketcham, Katherine, and William F. Asbury. *Beyond the Influence: Understanding and Defeating Alcoholism.* New York: Bantam, 2000. The authors define alcoholism as "a genetically transmitted neurological disease" and not the result of a character defect or moral weakness. They explain the effects of "the drug alcohol" on the human body and brain in both alcoholics and nonalcoholics.

Miller, William R., and Kathleen M. Carroll, eds. *Rethinking Substance Abuse: What the Science Shows, and What We Should Do about It.* New York: Guilford, 2010. Reviews what is known about substance abuse and offers overviews of biological, psychological, and social factors involved in the treatment of substance abuse. Also anticipates prevention and treatment developments and evaluates them for their overall possible effects.

Olson, Kent R., et al., eds. *Poisoning and Drug Overdose.* 6th ed. New York: McGraw-Hill, 2012. A resource for poison control centers, toxicologists, and health care practitioners for the diagnosis, treatment, and management of poisonings from exposure to industrial, therapeutic, illicit, and environmental chemicals.

WEBSITES OF INTEREST

Al-Anon and Alateen
http://www.al-anon.alateen.org
Alcoholics Anonymous
http://www.aa.org
National Institute on Alcohol Abuse and Alcoholism
http://www.niaaa.nih.gov
National Institute on Drug Abuse
http://www.drugabuse.gov

Robin L. Wulffson

SEE ALSO: Alcohol Poisoning; Peer Pressure; Teens and Alcohol Abuse

Body modification addiction

Body modification is the intentional physical altering of one's body, often for aesthetic reasons, by means of piercing and tattooing, for example. Personal modification is mediated by numerous psychological and social constructs (such as religion, culture, self-esteem, and identity development). Dealing with body modification addiction is focuses on how to understand, balance, and differentiate issues of self-mutilation versus issues of self-empowerment and identity formation, in the context of a person's unique cultural background.

BACKGROUND

Body modification's long history is rooted in the practice of more clearly marking or imposing meaning upon a particular person by physically changing their appearance. The practice of body piercing and tattooing, for example, has enabled cultures to more closely monitor religious affiliation, social groups, and social status for thousands of years.

Modern understandings of body modification have evolved in nuanced ways. While some cultures continue to use modification rituals in the ways of predecessors, other cultures have seen body modification practices take a more provocative turn, away from tenets of group affiliation or rite-of-passage and toward self-expression and identity formation.

The latter part of the twentieth century and the beginning of the twenty-first century have seen a steep increase in body modification (in both the volume of people choosing to modify their body and in the larger cross-section of society engaging in the practice). Body modification has become so popular that it has become difficult to assign a person to a particular subgroup (or subculture) based solely on the chosen modification. Historically, this was the principal reason why people chose to modify their body.

The most common motivators behind the practice of body modification include art and fashion, individuality (control), group affiliation, and personal transformation. As such, the tenor of body modification research has shifted slightly over the years, away from issues of self-mutilation and toward a greater appreciation for and understanding of how such practices align with one's self-structures and ongoing personal narrative.

Finally, a powerful undercurrent to these motivators is that of addiction. A question that remains is this: What exactly is a person becoming addicted to when his or her body modification rituals intersect with obvious patterns of addictive behavior?

TRANSITIONAL RESEARCH

Sociological research on issues related to body modification has been largely replaced with research aimed at identifying existing personality structures that make body modification more likely. This transition has been made, in part, because issues of body modification have become so prevalent in society. Body modification is now a mainstream practice, so drawing lines between specific social groups and exploring their derivations has become something of an antiquated notion.

Psychological research has instead taken up the issue of underlying motivational factors and existing personality structures that make it more likely for someone to pursue specific body modification (body piercing, tattooing, and plastic surgery, in particular). Additionally, while there is a dearth of research focused exclusively on body modification addiction, valuable research is available to help one better understand the mechanisms that lead to addictive behavior. Of particular importance is research that values pluralism and examines body modification addiction through several, competing theoretical modalities.

Modern research is far more collaborative and inclusive when it comes to understanding body modification and treating body modification addiction. Research now considers traditional, well-accepted medical underpinnings of addiction, longstanding sociological precedents inherent to all body modification, and the complex self-processes and personality structures that may predispose people to body modification, all of which has helped advance research in this area. As such, what may have once fallen into the realm of psychopathology is now considered more broadly and more carefully.

MOTIVATORS AND ADDICTIVE BEHAVIOR

An addiction, by definition, is a behavior that persists despite negative consequences. In the case of body modification addiction, the negative consequences can include infections (sometimes severe), the perpetuation of unhealthy coping mechanisms, and potential pathological stigma (among others). Underlying these consequences are complex representations and expressions of the self, including prevalent cultural dynamics and experiences in one's early history that led to a specific self-identity.

Considerable research has looked at the most prevalent motivators and personality traits common to people who engage in body modification. This research has helped advance the discussion about how to best identify and treat body modification addiction. It considers, for example, external and internal triggers, conflicts that arise, and factors that interfere with goal-setting and necessary support systems.

Perhaps most important to any treatment of addiction is identifying the motivation in place to help reduce (and ultimately stop) the negative behavior. A preliminary, vital step would be considering why it is that someone is engaged in the behavior in the first place (before even considering why it is that they want to change). Taken together, evaluating motivational factors and personality constructs that contribute to a specific behavior is a crucial first step for any treatment.

With respect to body modification, considerable overlap exists between motivators and personality traits common to those who engage in this behavior. Typically, the average body modifier is one who seeks sensation and control and one who is (often) driven by art and fashion, individuality, group affiliation, and personal transformation. Those addicted to body modification typically strive to hold on to specific memories, experiences, and values (positive and negative).

CURRENT UNDERSTANDINGS

How might one answer a person who asks why he or she cannot stop a child from piercing his or her body? Before answering this question, one may want to consider how body modification addiction differs from other substance-based addictions.

Whereas tracing the derivation of one's substance-based addiction is more "paint-by-numbers" (linear), tracing the derivation of one's body modification addiction is more comparable to a fresco painting, with layers upon layers of factors contributing to the overall portrait. It can be difficult to navigate to a particular place in time, or event, that led to a specific body modification addiction. Instead, it is better to consider the range of factors that can make body modification addiction so complex. This is precisely what modern research is aiming to do.

Discriminative overtones have been largely replaced with questioning and curious inquiry about how (and why) people choose to modify their body, about what is driving their proclivity to do so, and about possible patterns or character traits common to those who modify often. The body has been an artistic canvas for thousands of years. It also has become more than an object. The body has become the vehicle through which people assert control in their lives, transform and heal in the face of trauma, and tell the world how they would like to be identified.

Much has been written about the ways in which people use their body to reclaim some aspect of their life, empower themselves, and express themselves in a therapeutic way. As such, a twenty-first-century understanding of body modification has been elevated by research examining theories of the self and embracing pluralism. What is known about body modification addiction has been greatly enhanced by research into motivational factors and personality constructs common to those who engage in this behavior. Future research should continue this trend, examining the powerful representations of the self and cultural factors that shape human identity.

FURTHER READING

Nathanson, Craig, Delroy L. Paulhus, and Kevin M. Williams. "Personality and Misconduct Correlates of Body Modification and Other Cultural Deviance Markers." *Journal of Research in Personality* 40 (2006): 779–802. Print. Examines cultural factors and unique personality constructs inherent to body modification practices. Methods used are predominantly self-report. The use of the word deviance separates this research from others that look specifically at issues of personality.

Pitts, V. *In The Flesh: The Cultural Politics of Body Modification*. New York: Palgrave, 2003. Examines the societal and psychological evolution of understandings of body modification.

Suchet, Melanie. "The 21st Century Body: Introduction." *Studies in Gender and Sexuality* 10.3 (2009): 113–18. Print. Outlines competing theoretical formulations common in body modification research, looking specifically at self-structures and incorporating psychoanalytic tenets into body modification research.

Winchel, Ronald M., and Michael Stanley. "Self-Injurious Behavior: A Review of the Behavior and Biology of Self-Mutilation." *American Journal of Psychiatry* 148 (1991): 306–17. Print. Outdated but fascinating analysis of body modification practices and research evolutions. While this article is quite good, it is compelling to consider how the scope of current research has changed since its publication.

Wohlrab, Silke, et al. "Differences in Personality Characteristics Between Body-Modified and Non-Modified Individuals: Associations with Individual Personality Traits and Their Possible Evolutionary Implications." *European Journal of Personality* 21.7 (2007): 931–51. Print. A seminal work comparing personality traits between persons with and without body modifications. Work on gender-related issues is particularly revealing.

Wohlrab, Silke, Jutta Stahl, and Peter M. Kappeler. "Modifying the Body: Motivations for Getting Tattooed and Pierced." *Body Image* 4.1 (2007): 87–95. Print. Discusses the volume of research that looks at the various motivators for body modification and describes in detail the history of research in this area.

Joseph C. Viola

SEE ALSO: Attention-Seeking Behavior; Body Image and Girls; Body Image and Guys; Piercings and Infections

Caffeine and mental health

Caffeine is a mild stimulant drug found in common foods, beverages, and over-the-counter medications. While its use is generally nonproblematic and part of many people's daily routines, overuse or misuse can lead to physical and mental health problems.

INTRODUCTION

Caffeine is a legal drug that in its natural form has a bitter taste. Chemically, it is a xanthine-type drug, which is alkaloid in nature, meaning that it is nitrogen based. It is a mild diuretic, or substance that encourages urination, and a mild stimulant. Stimulants are a broad group of substances that can excite the body's central and peripheral nervous system and the cardiovascular system. Because of these properties, stimulants can have therapeutic and otherwise desirable effects. In fact, stimulants and their derivatives have been used to treat conditions such as drowsiness, narcolepsy, asthma, attention-deficit hyperactivity disorder (ADHD), autism, and obesity.

Caffeine is commonly found in coffee, tea, and other beverages, such as soft drinks and energy drinks. It is also present in chocolate, cocoa, over-the-counter medications for avoiding drowsiness, and even some headache remedies. The general effect of caffeine is mild relative to other stimulants; nonetheless, caffeine is considered a psychoactive substance. Its most basic effect is to trigger increased alertness; other, positive effects such as enhanced cognitive performance and increased selective attention remain the subject of debate. The most common form of administration of the drug is oral ingestion. Because caffeine products are mild stimulants, legal, and available worldwide, they are part of daily rituals in many countries. People gather to drink caffeinated beverages, enjoying them as part of social rituals. Therefore, as with other drugs, some psychosocial benefits are associated with caffeine.

DISORDERS RELATED TO CAFFEINE USE

As with any drug, pros and cons of usage exist; potential problems can occur if caffeine is not used properly. In fact, from a physical health perspective, regular overuse of caffeine can result in mild to serious gastrointestinal problems such as gastroesophageal reflex disease (GERD). Untreated, such conditions can result in ulcers and erosion of the esophageal tract. Problems such as GERD have been associated with cancer. Therefore, in terms of the link between caffeine and GERD, caffeine intake may be a controllable factor relevant to cancer prevention. Regular use of caffeine can also lead to tolerance, the need to use more of a drug to achieve a previous effect or the use of the same amount resulting in a lessened effect. Frequently when this happens, individuals may also be subject to caffeine withdrawal symptoms, such as headaches, if they stop using the drug. Such effects contrast markedly to the more severe withdrawal syndromes—confusion, depression, and fatigue—experienced by individuals dependent on stimulants such as amphetamine.

In addition to physical problems, caffeine is associated with at least three types of mental health problems in which it is a causative factor. These conditions are known as "caffeine-related disorders." One of these problems is caffeine intoxication, which is characterized by a pattern of symptoms: When individuals consume more than two or three cups of coffee, they may show symptoms such as a flushed face, physical agitation, muscle twitches, excitement, restlessness, nervousness, insomnia, diuresis, gastrointestinal problems, and a feeling of inexhaustibility. When an individual shows many of these symptoms, experiences distress or impairment, and the problems are not because of other problems, clinicians diagnose caffeine intoxication. Again, review of these symptoms underscores that caffeine is mild relative to other stimulants, such as amphetamines, which can cause paranoia, panic, psychosis, rapid pulse rates, hallucinations, aggression, violence, suicidal or homicidal tendencies, bruxism (teeth grinding), arrhythmias, heart damage, and even seizures.

A few other disorders are known as "caffeine-induced disorders," a subset of substance-induced disorders, which are problems caused by taking a drug. Caffeine-induced sleep disorder occurs when the use of caffeine significantly disturbs an individual's sleep. Caffeine-induced anxiety disorder occurs when caffeine use causes a person to experience distressing anxiety, a mood state characterized by extreme fear, worry, and uneasiness that may be cognitive, emotional, or physical. In a few case studies, extremely high doses of caffeine has reportedly induced psychosis, with the affected person exhibiting symptoms such as paranoid delusions and bizarre behavior. With caffeine-induced disorders, clinicians must rule out other causes, such as a primary sleep disorder, anxiety disorder, or other existing psychiatric condition. One method of doing this is to observe if the person continues to have symptoms after they have abstained from caffeine. If symptoms persist, a caffeine-related diagnosis is dismissed. If the symptoms do not persist, the problem is deemed related to the use of caffeine.

FURTHER READING

Bourne, Edmund, and Lorna Garano. *Coping with Anxiety: Ten Simple Ways to Relieve Anxiety, Fear, and Worry.* Oakland: New Harbinger, 2003.

Chu, Yi-Fang. *Coffee: Emerging Health Effects and Disease Prevention.* Ames: Wiley-Blackwell, 2012. Print.

Epstein, Lawrence, and Steven Mardon. *The Harvard Medical School Guide to a Good Night's Sleep.* New York: McGraw-Hill, 2006.

Goiney, Christopher, Devin Gillaspie, and Clara Alvarez Villalba. "Addressing Caffeine-Induced Psychosis: A Clinical Perspective." *Addictive Disorders & Their Treatment* 11.3 (2012): 146–49. Print.

Hale, Jamie. "Caffeine's Effect on Your Thinking." PsychCentral.com. *Psych Central,* 15 Apr. 2012. Web. 24 Feb. 2014.

Inaba, Darryl S., and William E. Cohen. *Uppers, Downers, and All-Arounders: Physical and Mental Effects of Psychoactive Drugs.* 7th ed. Ashland: CNS, 2011. Print.

Kassel, Karen Schroeder. "Decreasing Your Caffeine Intake." *Health Library.* EBSCO Information Services, 2 June 2012. Web. 20 Feb. 2014.

Rosen, Winifred, and Andrew T. Weil. *From Chocolate to Morphine: Everything You Need to Know about Mind-Altering Drugs.* Rev ed. Boston: Houghton-Mifflin, 2004. Print.

Weinberg, Bennette Alan, and Bonnie K. Bealer. *The World of Caffeine: The Science and Culture of the World's Most Popular Drug.* New York: Routledge, 2002. Print.

Nancy A. Piotrowski

Cocaine and its effects

Cocaine use disorder is when the use of cocaine harms a person's health or social functioning, or when a person becomes dependent on cocaine. The powdered form of cocaine can be snorted or dissolved in water and injected. Crack is cocaine in a rock crystal form. It can be heated so its vapors can be smoked. Cocaine use disorder is treat-

able. But, it takes hard work. Talk to your doctor if you think you have this condition.

CAUSES

Cocaine stimulates the brain to release large amounts of the hormone dopamine. Dopamine results in the euphoria commonly reported by cocaine abusers. As a person continues to use cocaine, a tolerance is developed. This means that higher doses and more frequent use are needed to maintain the euphoria.

RELEASE OF DOPAMINE IN THE BRAIN

The dopamine connecting to the receptors causes a euphoric feeling. This occurs naturally, but cocaine causes an exaggerated response that can lead to addiction. When a cocaine user stops using abruptly, a crash or withdrawal occurs. This results in an extremely strong craving for more cocaine. It also results in fatigue, loss of pleasure in life, depression, anxiety, irritability, suicidal thoughts, and sometimes paranoia. These withdrawal symptoms often prompt the user to seek more cocaine.

RISK FACTORS

Cocaine use disorder is more common in young men and in those aged 18-25 years old. However, cocaine use disorder can occur in anyone at any age.

SYMPTOMS

Symptoms associated with cocaine use disorder include:

* **Short-term effects include:**
- Euphoria
- Increase in energy
- Excessive talking
- Being mentally alert
- Decreased need for food and sleep
- Dilated pupils
- Increased temperature
- Increased heart rate
- Increased blood pressure
- Bizarre, erratic, or violent behavior
- Vertigo
- Muscle twitches
- Paranoia
- Restlessness, irritability, and anxiety
- Heart attack
- Seizures
- Sudden death

* Long-term effects include:
- Cravings that can't be controlled or predicted
- Increased tolerance
- Increased dosing
- Use of cocaine in a binge
- Increased irritability, restlessness, and paranoia
- Paranoid psychosis
- Hearing sounds that aren't there

* Medical complications include:
- Heart rhythm abnormalities
- Heart attack
- Chest pain
- Respiratory failure
- Stroke
- Seizure
- Headache
- Abdominal pain
- Nausea
- Chronic runny nose or septal perforation

DIAGNOSIS

Your doctor will ask about your symptoms and medical history. A physical exam will be done. The doctor will ask specific questions about your cocaine use, including how long you have been using the drug and how often.

TREATMENT

Talk with your doctor about the best treatment plan for you. Treatment programs may be inpatient or outpatient and may:

- Require that you have already stopped using cocaine
- Involve a detoxification program

MEDICATIONS

There are currently no medications to specifically treat cocaine use disorder. Treatment with medication focuses on the symptoms of euphoria and craving. Medications that have shown some promise include:

- Modafinil—wakefulness promoting agent
- N-acetylcysteine
- Topiramate—seizure medication
- Disulfiram
- Agonist replacement therapy
- Baclofen
- Antidepressants—may be helpful for people in the early stages of stopping cocaine use

BEHAVIORAL THERAPY

Behavioral therapies to help people quit using cocaine are often the only available, effective treatment for cocaine use disorder. Therapies include contingency management. With this program, people receive positive rewards for staying in treatment and remaining cocaine-free. Also, cognitive behavioral therapy helps people to learn how to abstain and remain abstinent from cocaine.

REHABILITATION PROGRAMS

In rehab programs, people with cocaine use disorder stay in a controlled environment for 6-12 months. During this time, they may receive vocational rehab and other support to prepare them to return to society.

PREVENTION

The best way to prevent cocaine use disorder is to never use cocaine. It is highly addictive and illegal.

FURTHER READING

Amato L, et al. "Dopamine agonists for the treatment of cocaine dependence". *Cochrane Database Syst Rev.* 2011;(12):CD003352..

Carson-DeWitt R, ed. *Encyclopedia of Drugs, Alcohol, and Addictive Behavior.* 2nd ed. New York, NY: MacMillan Reference Books; 2000.

Cocaine abuse. *EBSCO DynaMed website.* Updated February 15, 2013. Accessed February 20, 2013.

Degenhardt L, Hall W. "Extent of illicit drug use and dependence, and their contribution to the global burden of disease". *Lancet.* 2012;379:55-70

DrugFacts: Cocaine. *National Institute on Drug Abuse* website. Accessed. Updated March 2010. Accessed February 20, 2013.

Karila L, Reynaud M. *Therapeutic approaches to cocaine addiction.* [article in French] Rev Prat. 2009;59(6):830-834.

Research report series: Cocaine. *National Institute on Drug Abuse* website. Updated September 2010. Accessed February 20, 2013.

WEBSITES

Cocaine Anonymous
http://www.ca.org/
National Institute on Drug Abuse
http://www.nida.nih.gov
Cocaine Anonymous of Southern Ontario
http://www.ca-on.org/

Native Alcohol and Drug Abuse Counseling Association of Nova Scotia
http://nadaca.ca/

Krisha McCoy, updated by Michael Woods

SEE ALSO: Teens and Drug Abuse

Codependency

Codependency is a set of behaviors that people living with alcoholics, drug addicts, or troubled persons tend to develop. Codependents engage in excessive caretaking of the alcoholic, drug addict, or troubled person, and little or no caretaking of themselves. Although the caretaking is intended to control the behavior of the alcoholic, drug addict, or troubled person, it actually enables the person to stay addicted and to remain blameless for the addiction.

INTRODUCTION

Codependency is a behavioral pattern that has been identified as existing in pathological relationships. These behaviors can develop in childhood and are a response to living in a dysfunctional family or relationship. Typically these families have "rules" that prohibit dealing with family issues and feelings in a direct way. These families usually have an alcoholic, drug-addicted, mentally ill, or chronically ill member. Family members focus their attention on this troubled member to the exclusion of other family members. Family members are taught to care for the "ill" member and to do what is necessary to keep this person content. They learn to repress their feelings, to try to be perfect, and to ignore their own needs. The family attempts to keep the problems of the "ill" member a secret.

Codependent people tend to be caretakers of others and typically ignore their own needs and feelings. They have difficulty trusting other people and attempt to control others by their behavior, often by trying to be perfect or by taking over the care of the other person. Codependents are attracted to people who cannot be counted on to meet their needs and who are inconsistent and unreliable. Typically, codependent people are unable to nurture and care for their own emotional needs. Codependency tends to be passed on from one generation to the next.

Codependent behavior is based on a need to control others and to change their behavior. Codependents attempt to control others by being perfect and loving all the time; always responding to requests for assistance even when they do not want to help; trying to be in control of things all the time; and trying to do what the other person wants them to do, not what they actually want to do. Because they make little attempt to meet their own needs and are often abused by another or simply overwhelmed with all that they have to do, codependents tend to be anxious and depressed. Often, this is why they seek treatment. Initially, they are usually treated for depression.

Although codependent people appear to be taking responsibility for another person, they are actually wishing that the other person would take care of them. They are unable to ask for what they want, but they expect the other person to make them feel cared for and happy. Because the other person is incapable of making them feel cared for and happy, codependents never have their wants met.

Codependents become attached to other people to the point that they are willing to suppress their own feelings to maintain the relationship. Some codependent behavior is considered to enable people who are alcoholic, drug addicted, or sick to avoid taking responsibility for their behavior and for changing this behavior. It is thought that most alcoholics and drug addicts have an enabler to make excuses for their addiction or alcoholism. The lives of the codependent and the alcoholic or drug addict become pathologically intertwined. Codependents tend to be attracted to people who are alcoholic, drug addicted, or troubled, so they tend to have relationship after relationship with such people.

Some groups feel that what is deemed codependent behavior is actually normal spousal or relationship behavior, in which one person cares for the other. Certainly wives and mothers engage in much caretaking. However, it is the degree of caretaking and attachment that differentiates the codependent from the normal wife or mother. Healthy spousal and parental relationships do not enable cared-for persons to avoid responsibility for their behaviors, nor do they force the family members to deny their own needs.

POSSIBLE CAUSES

Codependency behaviors were initially identified in the families of alcoholics and drug addicts. These same behaviors have more recently been identified in pathological family situations, including families in which spousal or child abuse is occurring, families with poor

---

CHARACTERISTICS OF CODEPENDENT PEOPLE

According to the National Mental Health Association, the following are characteristics of codependent individuals:

- an exaggerated sense of responsibility for the actions of others
- a tendency to confuse love and pity, with the tendency to "love" people they can pity and rescue
- a tendency to do more than their share, all of the time
- a tendency to become hurt when people do not recognize their efforts
- an unhealthy dependence on relationships; the codependent will do anything to hold on to a relationship, to avoid a feeling of abandonment
- an extreme need for approval and recognition
- a sense of guilt when asserting themselves
- a compelling need to control others
- lack of trust in self and/or others
- fear of being abandoned or alone
- difficulty identifying feelings
- rigidity/difficulty adjusting to change
- problems with intimacy/boundaries
- chronic anger
- lying/dishonesty
- poor communication
- difficulty making decisions

---

communication patterns, and families with a mentally or chronically ill member. Codependency does not develop in all families with mentally or chronically ill members; rather it will develop only in those families in which the sick person is controlling the family and in which the parents exhibit codependent behaviors. It is possible for families to function normally in this situation. However, in homes with alcoholics, drug addicts, or abusers, it is much harder to avoid codependency.

DIAGNOSING

Codependent behavior is diagnosed by the identification of codependent behavior patterns. Codependent people often experience anxiety, depression, or both. The symptoms that are seen in the codependent person are controlling behavior, distrust of others, perfectionism, repression of feelings, problems with intimacy, caretaking, hypervigilance, stress-related illnesses, insomnia, low self-esteem, dependency, denial, weak boundaries, anger, sexual problems, and poor communication skills. Once people learn codependent patterns, they are likely to apply these behaviors to other relationships, even though the new relationships are unlike the one that spawned these behaviors. They may establish codependent relationships with their counselor, physicians, friends, bosses, and other authority figures. Codependency becomes the only way they know to establish relationships with other people.

People of all ages can demonstrate symptoms of codependency, although typically the symptoms appear in childhood. This behavioral pattern usually continues for the rest of people's lives unless they have long-term counseling to identify their behaviors and assist them in changing these behaviors.

TREATMENT OPTIONS

The treatments for codependency include long-term counseling and support groups. In counseling, codependent people are taught to identify their own needs, to deal with their feelings, to be assertive, to refuse when they do not want to do something, to communicate their needs to others, and to care for and nurture themselves. Sometimes during treatment, a person forms a codependent relationship with his or her counselor and tries to appear perfect to this person. At this point, counseling ceases to be effective because the patient has stopped working on problem behaviors. This negates the purpose of counseling, which is to learn to change codependent behavior patterns. Consequently, it may be helpful for codependents to periodically change counselors.

Codependency support groups such as Co-Dependents Anonymous, based on the twelve-step program of Alcoholics Anonymous, have developed. The twelve steps involve accepting that one's life is out of control and asking a higher power for assistance, but some people are repelled by references to a higher power. Some codependency groups are geared toward specific codependency issues, such as living with an alcoholic or in a dysfunctional family. Usually they deal with general issues of codependency without consideration of the attractive behavior. Groups vary in their effectiveness, so codependents may have to try several groups before they find one that is helpful to them.

THE HISTORY OF TREATMENT

Codependency was first discussed in the late 1970's. At this time, it was noticed that people addicted to drugs or alcohol tended to have relationships with people with a particular set of behaviors. However, as early as the 1940's, spouses, particularly wives, of alcoholics met and formed support groups to deal with the behavior of their spouses. At first, these groups were called Al-Anon, in reference to the Alcoholics Anonymous groups for alcoholics. As mental health professionals became more familiar with these behavior patterns, they realized that the behaviors occurred not only in people in relationships with alcoholics and drug addicts but also in people in relationships with people with other compulsive behaviors such as gambling, overeating, and some sexual behaviors. These same behavior patterns were discovered in adult children of alcoholics, people in relationships with emotionally disturbed or chronically ill people, and in professionals in helping professions, such as nurses and social workers.

FURTHER READING

Babcock, Marguerite, and Christine McKay, eds. *Challenging Codependency: A Feminist Critique.* Toronto, Ont.: University of Toronto Press, 1995. This collection of essays criticizes the label of codependency as damaging to women and challenges some of codependency's tenets.

Beattie, Melody. *Beyond Codependency: And Getting Better All the Time.* New York: Harper & Row, 1989. Beattie focuses on recovery from codependency in this book. She uses frequent examples of codependents to demonstrate her points.

_____. *Codependent No More: How to Stop Controlling Others and Start Caring for Yourself.* Center City, Minn.: Hazelton, 1992. This classic work defines codependent behavior and gives examples of codependents and their lives. The main focus of the book is to assist readers in identifying their codependent behaviors and changing their lives.

_____. *The New Codependency: Help and Guidance for Today's Generation.* New York: Simon & Schuster, 2009. In this self-help book, Beattie clears up misconceptions about codependency and provides self-assessments regarding various codependent behaviors.

Lewis, Rebekah. *Doormats and Control Freaks: How to Recognize, Heal, or End Codependent Relationships.* Far Hills, N.J.: New Horizon, 2005. Lewis provides a twelve-step plan for increasing self-esteem and creating healthy relationships.

Weinhold, Barry K., and Janae B. Weinhold. *Breaking Free of the Codependency Trap.* Rev. ed. Novato, Calif.: New World Library, 2008. Two clinicians provide step-by-step tools that people can follow to end codependent behavior.

Christine M. Carroll

SEE ALSO: Addictive Personality and Behaviors

Compulsive overeating

A pattern of behavior in which a person routinely ingests large quantities of food beyond the feeling of fullness without the ability to stop

SIGNS

It is estimated that 4 million American adults are compulsive overeaters.

The behavior is nearly twice as common in women as in men, and it typically begins before the age of twenty years. The primary sign of compulsuve overeating is regularly eating large quantities of food uncontrollably without physical hunger. Other food related behaviors include eating rapidly, eating to the point of physical discomfort, eating alone and secretly, hiding food to eat later, hiding the evidence of eating, and eating food that has been discarded or is about to be discarded.

Compulsive overeaters have a preoccupation with food, spending an inordinate amount of time on meal planning, food shopping, and cooking and eating. They make furtive trips to convenience stores, fast food restaurants, and late night grocery stores. They recognize that their eating habits are not normal and feel powerless to stop eating voluntarily. They turn to food for comfort and yet use it as a reward. Their rapid weight gain brings them feelings of guilt, shame, disgust, and self-loathing. They cannot separate their identity from their weight; in weighing themselves, for example, how they feel about themselves is dictated by the number on the scale. They believe that they will be better persons once they are thin, so they try various diets with a sense of desperation.

Although weight may be lost initially, it is often regained, plus more.

UNDERLYING CAUSES

Researchers have not conclusively determined the underlying causes of compulsive overeating. Studdies have investigated genetic predispositions to food addiction, in which a person's metabolism of foods, such as sugar, wheat, and fats, affects the same area of the brain affected by other addictive substances, such as cocaine. Other brain studies have examined compulsive overeating as a biochemically based impulse disorder somewhat similar to kleptomania, hypersexuality, compulsive shopping, and gambling addiction. A connection to dopamine in the brain has been shown, as well as hypersensitivity to the pleasurable properties of food.

Some medical professionals consider compulsive overeating to be a means of self- medicating for clinical depression. In some cases, the resulting rapid weight gain may be a protective mechanism to cope with physical or sexual abuse. The behavior also may serve to numb painful emotions of rejection, abandonment, and low self-esteem. One study showed that compulsive overeaters produce more cortisol in response to stress than do normal eaters; cortisol is known to stimulate the drive to eat, leading to obesity. Chronic stress has an apparent connection to the preference for high-energy foods that contain large amounts of sugar and fat.

NEGATIVE EFFECTS

The unbalanced diet of the compulsive overeater who typically chooses sweets and starches, has adverse health consequences, such as high serum cholesterol level, high blood pressure, and increased risks for heart attack, stroke, kidney failure, and diabetes. This diet may also result in lethargy, moodiness, irritability, and depression

In some cases, self-harming may be used to dissociate from emotional pain by substituting physical pain that releases endorphins. Compulsive overeaters who self-harm usually hold themselves to unreasonably high standards, have difficulty expressing their emotions, and are repulsed by their own bodies. The extreme and rapid weight gain contributes to varicose veins, blood clots in the legs, sciatica, arthritis, and bone deterioration. It may also cause shortness of breath and sleep apnea.

TREATMENT

Like alcoholism, compulsive overeating is considered to be a disease in that it involves treatment and recovery

and cannot be overcome by willpower alone. However, it is also a behavior that may be managed by behavior modification therapy. A typical initial exercise is to keep a food diary, a written record of the kind and quantity of food eaten,the time and place of eating, and the emotional context. This diary is then analyzed to identify habits, underlying emotions, and foods that trigger uncontrollable eating. The next step usually is to consult a nutritionist to devise a healthy food plan with adequate calories for energy, necessary nutrients, and fiber for improved digestion. A third step is to identify and practice healthy activities—emotional coping mechanisms—that substitute for food; these activities may include exercise, meditation, and spending time with friends.

Persons can seek support from professional counseling or from a twelve-step program such as Overeaters Anonymous. In some cases, drug therapy with antidepressants may be appropriate.

FURTHER READING

Academy for Eating Disorders. http://www.aedweb.org.

National Eating Disorders Association. http://www.nationaleatingdisorders.org.

Ross, Carolyn Coker. *The Binge Eating and Compulsive Overeating Workbook: An Integrated Approach to Overcoming Disordered Eating.* Oakland, Calif: New Harbinger, 2009. With distinct sections on healing the body, mind, and spirit, this book offers a whole-body plan for regaining physical and emotional health.

Sheppard, Kay. *Food Addictions: The Body Knows.* Rev. ed. Deerfield Beach, Fla.: Health Communications, 1993. Written by a certified eating-disorder specialist, this book addresses the addictive influences of the metabolism of flour and sugar, as well as the psychological need for support and self-healing.

Bethany Thivierge

SEE ALSO: Food Addiction; Obesity; Overeaters Anonymous

Cough and cold medications

Dextromethorphan (DXM) is a highly effective and safe cough medicine that has been available over the counter since 1958. It is found in many cold, flu and sinus medications in combination with other medications and therefore often found in the family medicine cabinet. When used as recommended it is highly effective but when used in excess it has many side effects that have become susceptible to drug abuse. Because of its ready availability and inexpensive cost it is abused particularly by adolescents

The abuse of DXM is a problem not only in itself but also because, as with many over-the-counter preparations, it also contains other substances that, in high doses, can be dangerous or addictive. This problem is compounded by the fact that DXM is also available online in tablet, capsule and powder forms allowing purchasers to increase the dose with fewer negative side effects and to mix it with any combination of other substances of their choice. DXM can also be purchased illegally premixed with other drugs such as ecstasy or methamphetamine.

INTRODUCTION

Teen abuse of over-the-counter medications (OTC's) is common because the cost is not prohibitive, they are easily attainable, and there is a mistaken impression they are not as dangerous as other types of drugs. In most US states there are few legal barriers to prevent teens from buying them. Cough medicine containing DXM has been a popular way to get high in this age group. Research indicates that there has been a slow shift downward in the number of users since 2008 but that in 2014, 2.5% of 8th graders and 4.2% of 12th graders had used DXM in the previous year to get high. There has been much discussion about how addictive it is but some users admit it they had cravings for DXM after use.

HEALTH EFFECTS

The recommended dosage as a cough medicine for adults is 15 to 30 milligrams (mg) every 6 to 8 hours. As abusers increase dosage from 100 to 400mg, the following stages are observed: mild stimulation at 100mg approximately or about 3oz of cough syrup. As the dose is increased there is euphoria, hallucinations and distorted visual perceptions. A sense of being separated from one's body occurs between 500mg-1500mg. A dose of 500mg would be about 16oz of a typical cough or cold remedy. The high dose effects are similar to phenycyclidine (PCP) and ketamine. The greatest risks in individuals are injuries or accidents resulting from the moderate to high dosage effects. However even the OTC drugs are combined with other active ingredients or medications that can dramatically increase the risk of negative side effects. Overdoses have occurred that can be serious or life threatening. As with other drugs, response at a given dosage will not be the same for everyone. Researchers have found that as many as 10% of Caucasians are more vulnerable to overdose since they metabolize the drug more slowly than the average person putting them at greater risk. Continued use can lead to insomnia, distress or discomfort. In more extreme cases there can be a loss of contact with reality along with a confused state.

In the cough syrup form, users are advised by other abusers to take the drug in quickly so the DXM can be rapidly absorbed before the consumption of the large

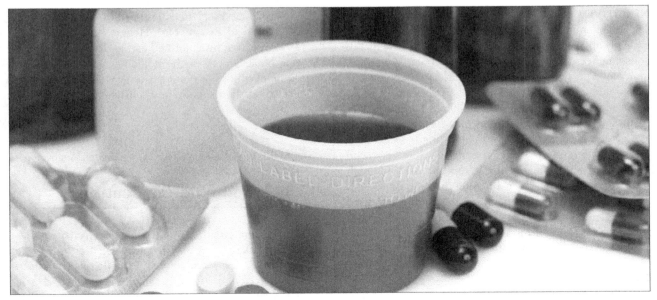

Photo: iStock

quantities of syrup causes vomiting: one of the classic negative effects of the use of this drug. This makes the online supply of this substance more appealing since users can determine how they want to ingest it, liquid, capsule etc. There are also web sites available describing the most expeditious ways to use the substance for enhanced effects. As with other illicit purchases the user has little information about the purity or drug combinations they are purchasing.

In cold remedies the DXM is not found alone but in combination with other medications such as acetaminophen, pseudoephedrine and antihistamines. High doses in combination with alcohol have resulted in death. It is well documented that acetaminophen in high doses can cause liver damage, however this type of injury takes some time to be detected while the individual many continue to use the drug, enhancing the seriousness of the liver injury. Mixtures of DXM and pseudoephedrine can cause significant increases in blood pressure and mixtures of high doses of DXM and antihistamines can lead to central nervous system and cardiovascular toxicity. DXM in combination with antidepressants can cause agitation, hallucinations, rapid heart rate and blood pressure changes. High doses in combination with promethazine-codeine have resulted in dimished respiration and death. This can be exacerbated by concurrent alcohol consumption. The greatest short-term risk of DXM is derived from distorted visual perception resulting in injuries or accidents.

IDENTIFYING USERS

Parents may have difficulty identifying teens who use cough medicine as a recreational drug since they have many characteristics similar to other drug abusers in their age group: including withdrawl from family, changes in appearance, poor performance in school, loss of friends or development of new friendships with whom they have drug use in common, mood shifts, inability to focus, changes in appetite or depression. Several slang terms are used that may be a signal to parents that their teens are abusing this drug such as: Skittles, Triple C, Poor Man's Ecstasy, Red Devils etc. The injectable form of DXM is referred to as Romilar or K.

Teens believe that in addition to its availability DXM is a safe drug to use and that it will not be detected with drug testing. It is a fallacy however, as DXM is a part of the panel of drugs routinely measured in post-accident or pre-employment testing.

STATE AND FEDERAL REGULATION

Since 2012, eight states have passed laws that limit or prohibit the sale of cough medicines to minors. Purchasers must provide proof of age or a prescription before they can buy the formula, but then only in small quantities. Highly addictive drugs such as morphine, oxycodone or codeine are classified as controlled substances by the federal government but DXM has not been included at this time. There has been consideration at the federal level by the Drug Enforcement Administration and Food and Drug Administration to make DXM- containing medications available only by prescription.

FURTHER READING

Consumer Healthcare Products Association. Dextromethorphan: Preventing teen cough medicine abuse. Retrieved from: www.chpa.org/dex.aspx. An in-depth, but not too complex, look at the value of over-the-counter- medications as well as the legislation affecting DXM and the possible directions of future legislation.

Logan BK, Goldfogel G, Hamilton R, Kuhlman J (2009). Five deaths resulting from abuse of dextromethorphan sold over the internet. *J Anal Toxicol* 33(2): 99-103. A report of 3 separate incidences where 5 male teens were killed following DXM over doses.

National Institutes of Health. U.S. National Library of Medicine. Dextromethorphan. Retrieved from: http://www.nlm.nih.gov/medlineplus/druginfo/meds/a682492.html. The article from the US National Medical Library describes in simple format the correct use of DXM, side effects and overdose and provides other valuable information about the abuse of this compound.

Annette O'Connor

SEE ALSO: Cross-Addiction; Over-the-Counter (OTC) Drugs

Crack

Crack is a solid form of cocaine made by dissolving powdered cocaine in a mixture of baking soda or ammonia with water. The mixture is boiled into a solid form and then broken into chunks. Crack is a powerful stimulant that reaches the brain in about eight seconds and pro-

duces an intense high that lasts between five and ten minutes.

HISTORY OF USE

Crack first appeared in the US cities of Los Angeles, San Diego, and Houston in the early 1980s, reportedly as a means of moving a large amount of cocaine that was available in the United States in the 1970s. The major crack epidemic, as it came to be called, took place between 1984 and 1990, mostly in poor, urban areas in the United States. By 2002, the United Kingdom reported a crack epidemic, and today, crack is used worldwide.

Since about 2000, the use of crack has decreased substantially, though it has not disappeared. Young adults (at levels as high as 65 percent) report having tried crack at least once; however, repeat-usage percentages are significantly lower. Arrest rates for crack possession are also dramatically lower than those of the 1980s and 1990s, with some cities showing crack-arrest percentages in the single digits.

There are several explanations for these lowered rates, including higher prices for cocaine and also changes in how the law handles charges for crack possession. However, the most significant cause for the decrease in the use of crack is the dramatic rise in methamphetamine use. Methamphetamine's low cost, easy availability, and extremely addictive nature make it popular among drug abusers.

EFFECTS OF USE

Crack is a stimulant that artificially increases the levels of dopamine released from the brain. Also, crack prevents dopamine from being "recycled" by the body, leading to an excess of dopamine with repeated use. This excess causes an overamplification of the dopamine-receptor neurons and leads to a disruption of normal neural communications. For example, the brain loses the ability to properly respond to pleasurable stimuli, which causes the drug user to seek more drugs to feel any pleasure. While the initial response of the brain to this massive dopamine buildup is a drug-induced euphoria, an increase in self-confidence, and increased high energy, these effects become harder and harder to attain as the dopamine system becomes damaged, leading to addiction and tolerance.

RISKS OF USE

Crack affects not just the brain but also almost every system in the body. One of the most strongly affected is the pulmonary system. Because crack is inhaled using high temperatures (90 degrees Celsius, or 194 degrees Fahrenheit), users often suffer burned lips, tongue, and airways. Another common side effect of crack use is a cough with black sputum, which is caused by the butane torches used to heat the smoking pipes. Other crack-related respiratory illnesses include pulmonary edema (also known as crack lung), asthma, and adult respiratory distress syndrome.

Sudden death from cardiac arrest is another danger to crack users, especially those who drink alcoholic beverages while using crack. (Any polydrug use increases the risk of sudden cardiac arrest.) Psychiatric trauma also is common in crack users and may include severe paranoia, violent behavior, and hallucinations (including delusional parasitosis, or Ekbom's syndrome, the belief that one is infested with parasites; this can cause a person to violently scratch themselves).

Crack users are especially at risk for infections with the human immunodeficiency and hepatitis viruses. Shared needles are one source; the other source is the exchange of sex for drugs. This often places women at an especially high risk. Another danger is tuberculosis and other saliva-borne diseases, which are passed by sharing a common crack pipe.

The so-called crack-babies epidemic has been weighted by myth and misinformation, leading people to believe that a generation of children became an essentially lost generation. Studies show that the stereotype of the crack baby, born addicted to crack and facing insurmountable developmental issues and an inability to bond, is simply false. The reality is more complicated. Independent of other issues, such as alcohol and tobacco abuse and poor physical environment, many of these babies are living normal lives.

Further research shows that the area of the body most affected in these children is the dopamine system that develops early in the fetal cycle; the system may show long-term effects of crack and cocaine exposure. A child also may have a mild behavioral disorder or a subtler developmental phenotype that resembles attention deficit hyperactivity disorder. Cognitive and attention systems may be affected, and these children may require help from a special-needs program.

FURTHER READING

Laposata, Elizabeth A., and George L. Mayo. "A Review of Pulmonary Pathology and Mechanisms Associated with Inhalation of Freebase Cocaine ('Crack')."

American Journal of Forensic Medicine and Pathology 14 (1993): 1–9. Print. A review of the respiratory conditions that result from inhalation of crack, ranging from burned lips and airways from the crack pipe to pulmonary edema and hemorrhage.

Lejuez, C. W., et al. "Risk Factors in the Relationship between Gender and Crack/Cocaine." *Experimental and Clinical Psychopharmacology* 15 (2007): 165–75. Print. A study that examines the psychological and socioeconomic reasons why women are more at risk from using crack.

Thompson, Barbara L., Pat Levitt, and Gregg D. Stanwood. "Prenatal Exposure to Drugs: Effects on Brain Development and Implications for Policy and Education." *Nature* 10 (2009): 303–12. Print. A comprehensive look at the effects of several different types of prenatal drug use, including how crack use specifically affects the development of the dopamine system, which can have long-term effects on cognitive and attention systems.

S. M. Willis

SEE ALSO: Cocaine and Its Effects; Teens and Drug Abuse

Cross-addiction

Cross-addiction involves the transfer of an addiction from one harmful substance or behavior to another. It also involves the abuse of more than one mind-altering substance at a time. Scientists now understand that addiction is a physiological problem caused both by nature and by nurture. A person who becomes an addict often inherits a sensitive brain and develops behavioral habits that lead to chemical changes in the brain. These changes, in turn, lead the person to use toxic substances against his or her will.

DOPAMINE D2 RECEPTORS IN ADDICTION

The PET images show that repeated exposure to drugs depletes the brain's dopamine receptors, which are critical for one's ability to experience pleasure and reward. This can lead to the transfer of one drug addiction to another.

Research confirms that all drugs of abuse, including alcohol, marijuana, nicotine, amphetamines, barbiturates, opiates, and heroin, work on the same neurological pathways in key areas of the brain—in particular, dopamine receptors and the limbic system, a primitive area focused on meeting basic needs. Dopamine is a "feel-good" chemical that tricks the limbic system into equating drugs with pleasure or relief, and even with survival.

In people who are genetically predisposed to addiction, the release of dopamine is more intense, and it unleashes what is known as the phenomenon of craving. Such persons cannot limit their intake of an addictive drug because of this craving. People who do not come from a family of addicts or alcoholics can, through force of habit, still become addicted to toxic drugs and experience the same phenomenon.

Often when a person attempts to quit a drug of choice, he or she will use another drug to satisfy the craving and essentially keep the reward pathways of the brain in hypersensitive mode. Alternatively, cross addicts who have no desire to quit will mix a cocktail of drugs to get a desired effect.

RISK FACTORS

The dopamine hypothesis suggests that if a person is addicted to one drug, they are at higher risk of becoming addicted to another. For people who are trying to quit a particular drug, cross-addiction can lead to a relapse of the original drug-taking behavior because of the sustained craving and because of impaired decision-making abilities.

SYMPTOMS

The symptoms of addiction feature three characteristics: chemical dependency, drug-taking habits, and denial of dependency and habits. Chemical dependency involves four components: craving, or the compulsion to ingest a mood-altering substance; impaired control of the amount ingested on any given occasion; physical dependence, which produces a period of withdrawal when the drug is discontinued; and tolerance, or the need for more of the drug to feel its effects.

Cross addicts are often in extreme denial. They tend to be more secretive than alcoholics and will hide their behavior from friends and family members. Because most drugs are illegal, cross addicts often suffer from paranoia.

SCREENING AND DIAGNOSIS

Cross-addictions are far more dangerous than alcoholism alone, because mixing drugs and alcohol can lead to death sooner. As with alcoholism, cross-addiction requires a certain amount of self-diagnosis to be treatable.

Dependence can be diagnosed when the person admits to three or more of the following: taking substances in greater amounts than intended; a persistent desire to cut down or stop using fails to change the behavior; frequent intoxication or presence of withdrawal symptoms that interfere with functioning; spending significant amounts of time acquiring drugs or dealing with the consequences of use; giving up activities in order to use drugs; persistent use despite adverse consequences; marked tolerance; withdrawal symptoms; and the use of drugs to treat withdrawal symptoms.

TREATMENT AND THERAPY

Intensive therapy and treatment are required to break an addiction without transferring that addiction. The first step is building self-awareness and an understanding of the nature of addiction. Sobriety must be the first priority, and it should be affirmed and nurtured daily.

If a person transfers an addiction from one substance to another, the brain remains in addictive mode; the neural associations and pathways have no opportunity to become disabled and dormant. Thus, the cycle of cross-addiction can be broken only by stopping the drug-taking and by remaining totally abstinent from all mind-altering drugs.

Acute withdrawal symptoms, such as sweating and nausea, can last a couple of weeks. Postacute withdrawal symptoms can happen for two years. These bouts tend to last three or four days and produce irritability, mood swings, variable energy, low enthusiasm, disturbed sleep, and difficulty concentrating. The first two years are the most difficult; after five years of abstinence, relapse is uncommon.

PREVENTION

Recovery is a lifelong process that requires new coping skills. Relaxation is chief among them; rigorous honesty and avoiding high-risk situations also will help prevent a relapse.

People who have been addicted to one drug must be vigilant, because cross-addiction can occur by happenstance. A recovering alcoholic, for example, may go to the dentist and be prescribed pain medicine, to which he or she develops a chemical dependency. Without thinking about it, the patient begins to increase the dosage and frequency of the pain medication and may seek unnecessary refills. Not all doctors learn about the physiology of addiction, so to protect oneself, a recovering addict must be wary when taking prescription medications.

FURTHER READING

Christopher, James. *How to Stay Sober: Recovery without Religion.* New York: Prometheus, 1988. Approaching recovery from a secular point of view, this book counsels self-reliance and self-respect instead of reliance on a higher power. Suggests new coping skills and provides a weekly diary for the first year of sobriety.

Johnson, Marlys C., and Phyllis Alberici. *Cross-Addiction: The Hidden Risk of Multiple Addictions.* New York: Rosen, 1999. Discusses the nature of drug addiction, how addiction to one substance can be transferred to another, and how to recover from addiction.

Kipper, David, and Steven Whitney. "Cross-Addiction." *The Addiction Solution: Unraveling the Mysteries of Addiction through Cutting-Edge Brain Science.* Kipper, David, and Steven Whitney. New York: Rodale, 2010. Draws on composite case histories to illustrate how the innovative personal recovery program works by customizing treatment for a diverse group of addicts abusing a variety of substances, from the first day of treatment to successful resolution.

Ries, Richard, and Shannon C. Miller. *Principles of Addiction Medicine.* Philadelphia: Lippincott, 2009. A text for physicians and mental health professionals on all aspects of drug and alcohol addiction from the American Society of Addiction Medicine.

Laura B. Smith

SEE ALSO: Addictive Personality and Behaviors

Cutting and self-mutilation

Cutting and self-mutilation are behaviors in which a person injures his or her own body; these behaviors are not usually suicide attempts. Some examples of self-injury are cutting, burning, hair pulling, and head banging.

RISK FACTORS AND RELATED CONDITIONS

Although self-injury can occur at any age, it usually begins in adolescence. It was originally thought that women were more likely than men to engage in self-injury, but later research indicates that the incidence is equal among women and men. The research also indicates that about 1 percent of the US population engages in various types of self-injury.

Persons who self-injure commonly have a history of abuse, including sexual, physical, or emotional abuse.

Self-injury is often associated with other mental health problems, such as eating disorders, substance abuse, obsessive-compulsive disorders, schizophrenia, depression, bipolar disorder, borderline personality disorder, anxiety disorders, post-traumatic stress disorder, dissociative disorders, panic disorder, and phobias.

Persons who engage in self-injury often come from homes where expressing anger and other emotions is (or was) forbidden. They frequently have low self-esteem and exhibit perfectionism. Also, they are likely to be impulsive and to have poor problem-solving skills. However, self-injury does not indicate the severity of mental illness or the ability of the person to function and lead a relatively normal life.

WHY PERSONS SELF-INJURE

There are many reasons for self-injury. One is using the behavior to provide a way to deal with overwhelming feelings, such as anger, extreme sadness, anxiety, depression, stress, sense of failure, self-hatred, or the helplessness of a trauma. Persons who self-injure have difficulty coping with severe emotional pain.

Self-injury can serve as a distraction from emotional pain, a way to express feelings that the person is unable to describe, or a way to feel a sense of control over something that is uncontrollable. Persons who self-injure often describe a feeling of calmness and relief of their intense feelings after they have injured themselves. Other self-injurers describe feeling emotionally numb and empty. For these persons, the self-injury allows them to feel something. Some are communicating their distress and expressing a need for help through self-injury. Others are punishing themselves for some imagined wrong.

Other persons use self-injury to prevent something worse from happening to them. This is unrealistic thinking, in which the person feels that if something bad is happening to him or her now, nothing else bad can happen. Others use self-injury to separate themselves from their feelings, which fade in the face of the physical pain. Most likely self-injury leads to the release of endorphins in the brain. These substances are natural pain relievers and tranquilizers.

It is thought that some persons self-injure to seek attention and to manipulate others. This is unlikely because most self-injurers are ashamed of the injuries that they cause, and they will hide their self-inflicted injuries. It is common for self-injurers to wear shirts with long sleeves and full-length pants in all types of weather to hide their injuries. The exceptions to this are persons who are developmentally disabled and persons with organic brain disease. They are likely to engage in self-injury without also trying to hide the injury or the behavior. In these instances, the behavior is caused by their brain injury.

SYMPTOMS AND TREATMENT

No single therapy exists to treat persons who self-injure, and there is no consensus as to the most effective treatment. Typically, treatment must be developed based on the needs and other mental health conditions of the self-injurer. Possible helpful medications include antidepressants, antipsychotic drugs, and minor tranquilizers.

Often-used psychotherapeutic approaches include cognitive-behavioral therapy, dialectical-behavior therapy, and psychodynamic psychotherapy. The type of psychotherapy also depends on the other psychological illnesses of the client. In severe cases of self-injury, the person may be hospitalized to exert some control over the behavior.

Psychotherapy usually begins with an exploration of why the person self-injures. The therapist will teach alternative behaviors to use when the person feels like self-injuring. These alternatives include physical activities, journaling, and talking with friends or family members. Alternative actions also may be taught, such as snapping an elastic band that is wrapped around the self-injurer's wrist. While this action does cause some pain, it does not cause injury. Biofeedback may be used to help the person identify the feelings that lead to the urge to self-injure.

It is important that the person understands that treatment, especially self-treatment, takes time, hard work, and motivation. If the self-injurer is an adolescent or child, family therapy may be necessary to identify what triggers the self-injuring behavior. Group therapy also may be used to provide the person with supportive relationships with others who are dealing with similar issues. Self-injurers who are developmentally disabled can be taught how to accomplish goals without using self-harming behaviors.

BIBLIOGRAPHY

Hollander, Michael. *Helping Teens Who Cut: Understanding and Ending Self-Injury.* New York: Guilford, 2008. Explains self-injury and debunks the many myths surrounding self-mutilation and cutting behavior. Outlines advanced treatment principles.

Smith, Melinda, and Jeanne Segal. "Cutting and Self-Harm." Jan. 2012. Web. 17 Apr. 2012. http://www.

helpguide.org/mental/self_injury.htm. This article is aimed at helping the self-injurer understand why he or she self-injures. Includes information on obtaining support and assistance.

Strong, Marilee. *A Bright Red Scream: Self-Mutilation and the Language of Pain.* New York: Virago, 2005. First published in 1999, this work examines self-injury and the psychology of pain through case studies.

Sutton, Jan. *Healing the Hurt Within: Understanding Self-Injury and Self-Harm, and Heal the Emotional Wounds.* 3rd ed. Oxford, England: How to Books, 2007. The author, a psychotherapist, describes the reasons for self-injury with case studies and includes information on helping the self-injurer.

Christine M. Carroll

SEE ALSO: Anxiety; Depression; Teen Suicide

Date rape drugs

Date rape drugs are typically odorless, colorless, and taste-less substances that are often combined with alcohol and other drinks. The drugs sedate and incapacitate an unsuspecting person, leaving that person unable to resist a sexual assault.

COMMON DATE RAPE DRUGS

Rohypnol (flunitrazepam), gamma hydroxybutyrate (GH-BGHBand date rape), and ketamine are common date rape drugs. Alcohol and ecstasy are also used to commit sexual assaults. All of these drugs affect judgment and behavior and can put a person at risk for sexual assault or risky sexual activity.

Rohypnol use began to gain popularity in the United States in the early 1990s. It is a benzodiazepine (chemically similar to sedative-hypnotic drugs such as Valium or Xanax) and is illegal in the United States. It is legal in Europe and Mexico, where it is prescribed for sleep problems and used for anesthesia. It is exported to the United States illegally.

Rohypnol is a pill that dissolves in liquid. Some of these pills are small, round, and white. Newer pills are oval and green-gray in color. When placed into a drink, the pills' dye makes clear liquids turn bright blue and dark drinks turn cloudy. However, this color change is often difficult to see in a dark drink, such as cola or dark beer, or in a darkened room, such as a nightclub or bar.

Also, pills with no dye are still available. The pills also can be ground into a powder.

GHB (Xyrem) is a central nervous system depressant that was approved by the US Food and Drug Administration (FDA) in 2002 for use in the treatment of narcolepsy (a sleep disorder). This approval came with severe restrictions, including its use only for the treatment of narcolepsy, and with the requirement that it be monitored by the FDA through a patient registry.

GHB also is a metabolite of the inhibitory neurotransmitter gamma-aminobutyric acid. It exists naturally in the brain, but at much lower concentrations than those found when GHB is abused. GHB comes in a few forms: a liquid with no odor or color, a white powder, and a pill. It can make a drink taste slightly salty.

Ketamine is legal in the United States for use as an anesthetic for humans and animals. It is mostly used with animals. Veterinary clinics are sometimes burglarized for their ketamine supplies. Ketamine comes as a liquid and a white powder.

EFFECTS ON THE HUMAN BODY

The sedative-hypnotic effects of date rape drugs are powerful. The drugs can affect a person quickly and without that person's knowledge, which makes them especially appealing to potential perpetrators of assault. The length of time that the effects last varies and depends on how much of the drug is taken and if the drug is mixed with other drugs or alcohol. Alcohol makes the drugs even stronger and can cause serious health problems, even death.

The effects of Rohypnol occur within thirty minutes of ingestion and can last for several hours. A victim may look and act like someone who is drunk. He or she might have trouble standing, might have slurred speech, or might pass out. GHB takes effect in about fifteen minutes and can last three or four hours. A small amount of GHB can have a big effect. Ketamine is fast-acting. A victim might be aware of what is happening but unable to move. Ketamine also causes memory problems. Later, a victim might not remember what occurred while drugged.

It is often difficult for a person to know if he or she has been drugged and assaulted. Most victims do not remember details of the incident. The victim might not be aware of the attack until eight or twelve hours after it occurred, after the drug effects wear off.

Date rape drugs can leave the body quickly. By the time a victim receives help, the drug involved in the attack is likely out of the person's system. However, there are other signs that indicate a person might have been drugged, including the following, in which the person feels drunk and has not had any alcohol or feels like the effects of drinking alcohol are stronger than usual; wakes up feeling hung over and disoriented or having no memory of a period of time; remembers having a drink, but cannot recall anything after that; finds that his or her clothes are torn or are not fitting properly; or feels like he or she had sex but cannot remember having sex.

Persons who have ingested a date rape drug should get medical care immediately. As with any sexual assault, it is important that the victim not urinate, douche, bathe or shower, brush teeth, wash hands, change clothes, or eat or drink before seeing a medical professional. Doing so may destroy evidence of the assault. The hospital will use a rape kit to collect any evidence. The victim should ask the hospital to take a urine sample that can be used to test for date rape drugs. Rohypnol stays in the body for several hours and can be detected in the urine up to seventy-two hours after ingestion. GHB leaves the body within twelve hours.

FURTHER READING

Adams, Colleen. *Rohypnol: Roofies—"The Date Rape Drug."* New York: Rosen, 2007.

Albright, J. A., S. A. Stevens, and D. J. Beussman. "Detecting Ketamine in Beverage Residues: Application in Date Rape Detection." *Drug Testing and Analysis* 4.3–4 (2011). Print.

Németh, Z., B. Kun, and Z. Demetrovics. "The Involvement of Gamma-Hydroxybutyrate in Reported Sexual Assaults: A Systematic Review." *Journal of Psychopharmacology* 24.9 (2010): 1281–87. Print.

WEBSITES OF INTEREST

Center for Substance Abuse Research
http://www.cesar.umd.edu/cesar/drugs/rohypnol.asp
National Institute on Drug Abuse
http://www.drugabuse.gov/publications/infofacts/club-drugs-ghb-ketamine-rohypnol
Project GHB
http://www.projectghb.org
WomensHealth.gov
http://www.womenshealth.gov/publications/our-publications/fact-sheet/date-rape-drugs.pdf

Claudia Daileader Ruland

SEE ALSO: Rape and Sexual Assault; Sexual Assault and Drug Use

Depressants abuse

Depressants represent a broad category of substances, with or without clinical use, which reduce the activity of the central nervous system. Included in this category of substances are ethanol, sedative-hypnotics (barbiturates, benzodiazepines), barbiturate-like compounds (chloral hydrate, methaqualone, meprobamate), narcotics (opium, morphine, codeine), marijuana, antihistamines, and some inhalants. Frequently, the term depressants abuse is used in a restricted sense, to designate specifically the nonmedical use of sedative-hypnotic drugs.

CAUSES

Humans have always sought to alleviate the effects of stress and to reduce anxiety, depression, restlessness, and tension. Alcohol and kava kava are two of the oldest depressant agents. The nineteenth century brought synthetic substances such as bromide salts and chloral hydrate. These were followed by barbiturates and benzodiazepines, which were introduced in the twentieth century.

Depressant abuse is on the rise because of the wide availability of drugs by prescription or through the illicit marketplace. Examples of illegal depressants of abuse include the date rape drugs flunitrazepamflunitrazepam (RohypnolRohypnol) and gamma-hydroxybutyric acid-gamma-hydroxybutyric acid (GHB, a natural depressant).

Overall, short-acting agents are more likely to be used nonmedically than those with long-lasting effects. Because of their wider margin of safety, benzodiazepines have largely replaced barbiturates. They now constitute the most prescribed central nervous system (CNS) depressants—and the most frequently abused, usually to achieve a general feeling of relaxation. However, barbiturates and barbiturate-like drugs still pose clinical problems, as many young people underestimate the risks these drugs carry. Non-benzodiazepine sedatives, such as zolpidem (Ambien), also can generate misuse and dependence.

Most sedative-hypnotic drugs work by enhancing the inhibitory activity of the neurotransmitter gamma-aminobutyric acid, thus reducing CNS activity and promoting relaxation and sleep. They are usually prescribed to treat sleep disorders, anxiety, acute stress reactions, panic attacks, and seizures. In higher doses, some agents become general anesthetics. Chronic use results in tolerance and dependence (both psychological and physical).

RISK FACTORS

Barbiturate abuse occurs most commonly in mature adults with a long history of use, while benzodiazepines are favored by younger persons (those younger than forty years of age). Two main categories of people misuse depressant drugs. The first category comprises people who receive depressant prescriptions for psychiatric disorders or who obtain them illicitly to cope with stressful life situations. These persons have a high risk of becoming dependent, especially if they receive high doses, take the drug for longer than one month, and have a history of substance abuse or a family history of alcoholism. However, if dose escalation is not evident and drugs are not used to achieve a state of intoxication, chronic benzodiazepine users should not be considered abusers.

A second important category comprises people who use sedative drugs in the context of alcohol or multiple-drug abuse. These people may take benzodiazepines to alleviate insomnia and anxiety (sometimes induced by stimulants), to increase the euphoric effects of opioids, and to diminish cocaine (or alcohol) withdrawal symptoms.

SYMPTOMS

People who abuse depressants often engage in drug-seeking behaviors that include frequently requesting, borrowing, stealing, or forging prescriptions; ordering and purchasing medication online; and visiting several doctors to obtain prescriptions. These behaviors often accompany changes in sleep patterns and irritable mood and increased alcohol consumption. Recreational use and self-medication with depressants may lead to accidental overdoses and suicide attempts. Many persons use a "cocktail" of alcohol and depressant medications for enhanced relaxation and euphoria. This practice is dangerous, as it carries a high risk of overdose.

Sedative-hypnotic drug intoxication resembles alcohol, painkillers, and antihistamine intoxication. It presents with impaired judgment, confusion, drowsiness, dizziness, unsteady movements, slurred speech, and visual disturbances. Young adults attempting to get high may show excitement, loss of inhibition, and even aggressive behavior. Acute GHB intoxication leads to sleep and memory loss. These manifestations occur without alcohol odor on the breath, unless the abuser combined the drug with alcohol. In the case of barbiturates, the behavioral effects of intoxication can vary depending on the time of day, the surroundings, and even the user's expectations.

Tolerance to barbiturates is not accompanied by an increase in lethal dose, as it is with opiates. For this reason, an overdose can be fatal. Signs and symptoms of barbiturate overdose vary, and they include lethargy, decreased heart rate, diminished reflexes, respiratory depression, and cardiovascular collapse.

All sedative-hypnotics can induce physical dependence if taken in sufficient dosage over a long time. Withdrawal from depressant medication results in a "rebound" of nervous system activity. In a mild form, this leads to anxiety and insomnia. In cases of more severe dependence, withdrawal manifests with nausea, vomiting, tremors, seizures, delirium, and ultimately, death. Therefore, discontinuation of prescription drugs necessitates close medical supervision.

SCREENING AND DIAGNOSIS

To evaluate a person who might abuse depressant medication, a doctor will obtain a thorough medical history, ask questions about current and previous drug and alcohol use, and perform a physical examination. A psychiatric evaluation may also be required. The diagnosis of depressant drug abuse relies on evidence of dose escalation, on obtaining multiple prescriptions, and on taking the drug for purposes other than those stated in the prescription.

Multiple tests detect the presence of drugs and also potential medical complications. These include drug screening (urine and blood), electrolyte and liver profiles, an electrocardiogram, and X-ray and magnetic resonance imaging.

TREATMENT AND THERAPY

Therapeutic strategies for depressants abuse vary according to the drug used, the severity of the manifestations, and the duration of drug action. Common therapies include detoxification, which involves the use of agents that reverse the effects of the drug (for example, using Flumazenil for benzodiazepine abuse and using Naloxone for narcotics abuse). Other common therapies include the use of medications that mitigate withdrawal symptoms, counseling in inpatient or outpatient settings, support groups, and relaxation training. When a person receiving treatment has combined a CNS depressant with alcohol or other drugs, all aspects of this addiction have to be addressed and treated.

PREVENTION

Sedative-hypnotic medication should be used only as prescribed. Combinations of CNS depressants (such as alcohol/drug or over-the-counter drug/prescription medication) pose high risks and should be avoided.

People who are unsure of a drug's effects, or who suspect dependence, should consult a pharmacist or a doctor. Those people who are contemplating the discontinuation of a CNS depressant or who are experiencing withdrawal symptoms should seek medical care immediately.

A careful assessment is necessary before prescribing depressant medication in persons with a history of drug abuse. These individuals require close monitoring. Also, caregivers and health care providers should verify that there are no alternative sources for obtaining the drug of abuse.

FURTHER READING

Hanson, Glen R., Peter J. Venturelli, and Annette E. Fleckenstein. *Drugs and Society*. 9th ed. Sudbury, MA: Jones, 2006. An easy-to-read textbook that includes a comprehensive review of CNS depressants and their effects and patterns of abuse.

Parker, James N., and Philip M. Parker. *The Official Patient's Sourcebook on Prescription CNS Depressants Dependence*. San Diego, CA: Icon, 2002. Useful resource for patients and caregivers, covering all aspects of depressant dependence.

Sadock, Benjamin J., and Virginia A. Sadock. *Kaplan and Sadock's Synopsis of Psychiatry: Behavioral Sciences/ Clinical Psychiatry*. 10th ed. Philadelphia: Lippincott, 2007. Popular psychiatry textbook for students and health care practitioners that discusses depressants abuse.

Sue, David, Derald Wing Sue, and Stanley Sue. *Understanding Abnormal Behavior*. Boston: Wadsworth, 2010. Accessible textbook that includes a well-written discussion of depressants misuse.

WEBSITES OF INTEREST

National Institute on Drug Abuse
http://www.drugabuse.gov/publications/research-reports/prescription-drugs/cns-depressants
US Drug Enforcement Administration
http://www.justice.gov/dea/concern/depressants.html

Mihaela Avramut

SEE ALSO: Antidepressants; Depression

Designer drugs

Designer drugs are illegal synthetic analogs of controlled substances that possess similar pharmacological qualities. Designer drugs encompass a wide range of potent, unpredictable, and potentially deadly stimulants, depressants, hallucinogens, and opiates. Common designer drugs include methamphetamine, ecstasy, China white, lysergic acid diethylamide (LSD), phencyclidine (PCP), ketamine, and gamma hydroxybutyric acid (GHB).

FOXY

Foxy is a hallucinogenic drug in the tryptamine family, similar to psilocybin (mushrooms). It is used recreationally as a psychedelic.

Foxy most frequently appears in tablet or capsule form. The drug was first synthesized by Alexander Shulgin, and its chemical creation was reported by him in 1980. With the placement of MDMA (ecstasy) under legal control in the United States in 1985, foxy began to appear in the illicit-drug street trade.

Foxy, named in 1999, was first called Eve to contrast with Adam, a name used occasionally for ecstasy. Foxy soon became more widely known as a designer street drug and became popular in dance clubs and raves and other such venues, where the use of club drugs, particularly ecstasy, was well established.

HISTORY OF USE

Designer drugs became popular in the 1970s as a way to bypass existing regulations on controlled substances. After the Controlled Substances Act (1970) restricted the availability of illicit substances, clandestine chemists began modifying and manufacturing synthetic alternatives with similar pharmacological effects. Designer-drug production and trafficking became widespread, producing cheaper and stronger alternatives.

Some designer drugs were originally intended for medical use; others were created strictly for recreational use. The first designer drugs included hallucinogens and synthetic substitutes for heroin and amphetamine.

By the 1980s, many designer drugs became known as club drugs and gained popularity among young abusers at underground dance parties, bars, and nightclubs called raves. These raves became the place to sell and use club drugs, such as ecstasy, to enhance the club experience. The combining of designer drugs emerged as a common practice to enhance euphoric effects. Mixing ketamine, a hallucinogenic tranquillizer, with the stimulant methamphetamine became known as trail mix, while using ecstasy with LSD was called candy flipping.

Designer drugs remained legal until the 1980s, when their psychological and physical hazards became fully recognized. The drugs caused numerous overdose deaths worldwide. By 1986, the widespread manufacture and misuse of designer drugs prompted legislators in the United States to modify the Controlled Substances Act and add the Federal Analog ActFederal Analog Act to include all chemically similar substances and possible derivatives as controlled substances.

Designer drugs make up a substantial portion of the illegal drug market. Newer classes of designer drugs such as spice, K2, 2C-B, and bath salts are continually being developed, marketed, and sold by illegal chemists. Despite efforts to curb designer drug production, their abuse and popularity continues to be a concern.

COMMON DESIGNER DRUGS

Common designer drugs include hallucinogens and depressants as well as synthetic substitutes for heroin and amphetamine. The most popular amphetamine or speed analogs include methamphetamine and methylenedioxymethamphetamine (MDMA, or ecstasy).

Methamphetamine, known as meth, crystal, ice, speed, and crank, is one of the most addictive designer drugs available. It is commonly used at clubs for its intense rush of euphoria. By the 1960s, methamphetamine abuse reached epidemic proportions.

MDMA has both stimulant and hallucinogenic properties and is related to amphetamine and mescaline. Ecstasy is a party drug designed to produce a rush of euphoria followed by heightened sociability and hallucinations.

A popular synthetic heroin alternative is China white, which encompasses a variety of fentanyl derivatives (painkillers with opiate-like properties similar to but more potent than heroin). China white gained popularity as a recreational drug among heroin users as a cheaper alternative.

Hallucinogenic designer drugs include LSD and PCP. LSD, or acid, is the most widely known of the hallucinogenic drugs. It is an extremely potent semisynthetic psychedelic drug derived from lysergic acid. PCP, or angel dust, derivatives were popular in the 1970s. PCP, originally developed as a surgical anesthetic, is a dangerous and unpredictable hallucinogen; users typically experience horrifying and violent hallucinations.

Several designer drugs, such as ketamine and GHB, exhibit depressant and hallucinogenic qualities. Ketamine is a tranquilizer with powerful hallucinogenic properties that is known to induce out-of-body and dreamlike states. GHB, known as cherry meth and liquid ecstasy, initially was used as a bodybuilding agent to stimulate muscle growth. GHB is a popular recreational drug at nightclubs and is sometimes used as a "date rape" drug.

EFFECTS AND POTENTIAL RISKS

Designer drugs are often lethal substitutes; they are mixed with unknown impurities and are many times more potent than the original substance they mimic. Designer drugs can act as stimulants, depressants, hallucinogens, and painkillers (opiates).

Designer drugs exhibit different effects at varying doses. Stimulants, like methamphetamines, increase brain activity by increasing the neurotransmitter dopamine, producing euphoria, excitement, and increased energy. Depressants, such as GHB, slow the central nervous system through endorphin-like mechanisms, inducing relaxation, contentment, and sedation. Hallucinogens, such as LSD, bind to serotonin receptors in the brain, producing sensory distortions. Opiates, including China white, act through opioid receptors to alter pain responses. Although the effects of each designer drug are different, all can be lethal.

Designer drugs are abused for their intoxicating effects. The short-term effects of designer drugs include increased euphoria, excitement, and energy. Negative short-term effects include nausea, vomiting, anxiety, depression, confusion, irritability, amnesia, dilated pupils, impaired speech, visual disturbances, hallucinations, behavioral changes, disturbed sleep, muscle cramps, panic attacks, shaking, clenched teeth, drooling, chills, increased perspiration, increased heart rate, hypertension, and sudden death.

Long-term designer drug use can lead to anorexia, dehydration, social withdrawal, anhedonia (inability to experience pleasure), violent behavior, suicidal behavior, paranoia, psychosis, stroke, seizures, convulsions, paralysis, coma, lung disease, kidney, heart, and respiratory failure, blood vessel damage, permanent brain damage, and death.

Most designer drugs are highly addictive; physical and psychological tolerance and dependence develops quickly. Users crave larger doses of the drug to achieve the original high. Mixing designer drugs with other substances increases the risk of accidental overdose and death.

FURTHER READING

Clayton, Lawrence. *Designer Drugs.* New York: Rosen, 1998. Provides basic information about the various types of designer drugs, their effects, and causes for abuse and addiction.

Gahlinger, Paul M. *Illegal Drugs: A Complete Guide to Their History, Chemistry, Use, and Abuse.* New York: Plume, 2004. A comprehensive guide to the history, chemical properties, health effects, and medical uses of both legal and illegal drugs.

Goldberg, Raymond. *Drugs across the Spectrum.* 6th ed. Belmont, CA: Wadsworth, 2010. Discusses the history, health effects, treatment, prevention, and legal issues associated with drug addiction and its effects on society.

Hanson, Glen R., Peter J. Venturelli, and Annette E. Fleckenstein. *Drugs and Society.* 10th ed. Sudbury, MA: Jones, 2009. Examines the effects of drug use and abuse on individuals and society. Provides detailed information on drug laws, commonly abused drugs, and substance abuse treatment and prevention options.

Olive, M. Foster. *Designer Drugs.* Philadelphia: Chelsea House, 2004. Presents information on the history, health effects, production, distribution, and regulations associated with designer drugs.

WEBSITES OF INTEREST

eMedicineHealth.com
http://www.emedicinehealth.com/club_drugs/article_em.htm
National Institute on Drug Abuse
http://www.drugabuse.gov

Rose Ciulla-Bohling

SEE ALSO: Hallucinogens and Their Effects; LSD; Mushrooms/Psilocybin; PCP

Drug testing

Drug testing is done to ensure the safety of the general public, to maintain standards at schools and places of employment, and to make sure that athletes do not gain unfair advantage through the use of performance-enhancing drugs. The goal of these tests is detect whether a person has used drugs such as alcohol, marijuana, cocaine, amphetamines, barbiturates, benzodiazepines, lysergic acid diethylamide (LSD), opiates, phencyclidine (PCP), synthetic hormones, and steroids. Commonly used drug tests analyze a person's breath, urine, saliva, sweat, blood, or hair.

DEFINITION AND BASIC PRINCIPLES

Drug testing in the workplace and schools has become commonplace. A variety of tests are used to detect elevated levels of the most common drugs that can impair job performance or are illegal to use. The importance of drug testing has continued to increase since the Controlled Substances Act of 1970 placed all regulated drugs into five classifications based on their medicinal value, their potential to harm people, and their likelihood of being abused or causing addiction. Schedule I drugs have no known medical value and are most likely to be abused, while Schedule V drugs have little potential for abuse. These scheduled drugs are called controlled substances because their use, manufacture, sale, and distribution are subject to control by the federal government.

There are two general types of drug testing. Federally regulated drug testing, according to the National Institute on Drug Abuse (NIDA), requires testing for cannabinoids (THC, marijuana, hashish), cocaine, amphetamines, opiates (morphine, heroin, and codeine), and PCP. Nonfederally regulated drug testing is often used to test athletes in various sports for the use of creatine, hormones, steroids, and other performance-enhancing drugs. Additional tests are used to detect barbiturates and alcohol.

Urinalysis is typically used as a preliminary test because it is less expensive and more convenient than the other tests. Saliva tests and breathalyzers are commonly used. Blood tests, although less frequently employed because they are generally more expensive and invasive, are more dependable, as are hair strand tests. A preliminary positive test using urinalysis must be confirmed by diagnostic tests completed in an analytical laboratory setting, which can take several days to complete. These diagnostic tests include the analytical instruments of gas chromatography (GC), mass spectrometry (MS), ion scanning, high-pressure liquid chromatography (HPLC), immunoassay (IA), and inductively coupled plasma spectrometry (ICP-MS).

BACKGROUND AND HISTORY

The detection of ingested drugs in various body fluids first sparked the interest of the ancient alchemists. In 1936, Rolla N. Harger of Indiana University patented the Drunkometer, a breath test to measure a person's level of alcohol intoxication. In 1954, Robert F. Borkenstein of Indiana University invented the breathalyzer, which had the benefit of greater portability, to measure blood-alcohol content. However, it was not until the widespread use of recreational drugs in the 1960's that the National Institute of Drug Abuse was established to monitor drug use. With its creation, federal funding became available to researchers to develop drug testing methods, which led to rapid advances. In 1973, physician Robert L. DuPont was appointed director of the National Institute of Drug Abuse. As director, DuPont implemented the use of the urine test and further developed immunoassays to test for several controlled substances.

In 1981, an airplane crashed on the USS Nimitz, and the investigation into the incident revealed drug use to be a contributing factor. As a result, the United States Navy began random drug testing of all active-duty personnel in 1982. In the 1980's, the U.S. Department of Transportation began to test all of its employees. In September, 1986, President Ronald Reagan signed Executive Order 12564, making drug testing mandatory for federal employees and all employees in safety-sensitive positions, such as employees in the nuclear power industry. The National Institute of Drug Abuse extended this mandatory testing to include truck drivers working in the petroleum industry. This testing has come to be regulated by the Substance Abuse and Mental Health Services Administration (SAMHSA), which is part of the U.S. Department of Health and Human Services.

HOW IT WORKS

Because of the commercial availability of so many masking agents, the most effective drug testing occurs when the subject has had no previous notification. Thus, random drug testing is very effective and has become common in the workplace, schools, and for athletes. The National Collegiate Athletic Association and the National Football League provide only one to two days notice before drug testing, and the United States Olympic Committee has a no-notice policy for drug testing.

The first commonly available drug testing method was the breathalyzer, followed by urinalysis. The usage of saliva tests continues to increase, while sweat tests remain the least-used testing method. Blood tests require additional medical staff and are also the most invasive testing method; therefore, although they are very accurate, they are not as commonly used as urinalysis. Hair tests are very accurate but do not detect drug use in the last four to five days. In terms of validity for legal purposes, any of these preliminary, or screening, tests must be confirmed by an analytical technique, most often gas chromatography/mass spectrometry, performed by trained personnel within a diagnostic laboratory.

Breath. Borkenstein received a patent in 1958 for the breathalyzer, which determines an individual's blood-alcohol content (BAC) from a breath sample. The ethanol in the breath of an individual reacts with the dichromate ion, which has a yellow-orange color, in the presence of acid to form the green chromate ion. This color change from pale orange to green can easily be observed. All fifty states and the District of Columbia have laws that forbid a person to drive with a BAC of 0.08 percent or greater, a level at which the individual is judged to be legally impaired.

Urine. Urinalysis became a common method of detecting drugs in the 1980's and has continued to be widely used. The urine sample is collected and sealed to ensure that it remains tamper-free. It is generally subjected to an immunoassay test first because this test is very fast.

Saliva. Testing of oral fluids is becoming increasingly common because of its convenience for random testing, and it is more resistant to adulteration than urine samples. Saliva testing can detect cocaine, amphetamine, methamphetamine, marijuana, bezodiazepines, PCP, opiates, and alcohol if the substance was ingested between six hours and three days before the test was administered.

Sweat. Although traditionally not considered to be as useful as the other methods because of the dilute sample obtained, patches that can be worn on the skin and collect samples over several hours are increasingly popular. This method of drug testing is preferred by government agencies such as parole departments and child protective services in which urine testing is not the method of choice.

Blood. Because blood tests are the most invasive and expensive method, requiring additional medical personnel, they are not as widely used as the other tests as a screening method. However, blood testing is very accurate and reliable, so it is often used to confirm a positive result from another type of drug test.

Hair. Hair samples from any part of the body can be used and are extremely resistant to any type of tampering or adulteration. Special fatty esters are permanently formed in the hair as a result of alcohol and drug metabolism, and therefore, this method is very reliable.

Gas Chromatography/Mass Spectrometry (GC/MS). This tandem analytical instrumentation must be done by trained personnel within a laboratory setting and therefore is not as convenient as the other testing methods. However, it is much more accurate and is used to confirm more rapid, preliminary tests. The gas chromatograph is able to separate molecules based on their attractive interactions with the material that packs a column. Molecules take varying amounts of time to travel, or elute, from the column, resulting in different retention times, or amounts of time retained on the packing material of the column. These separated molecules are then ionized in the mass spectrometer, which is able to produce molecular weight information.

APPLICATIONS AND PRODUCTS

Drug Test Dips. Test strips known as drug test dips, dip strips, drug test cards, or drug panels use a single immunoassay panel to test for several common drugs at once. Specific reactions between antibodies and antigens allow marijuana, cocaine, amphetamine, opiates, and methamphetamine to be detected in urine samples. These assay strips are so easy to use that the staff of many schools, sports clubs, and offices can use them. However, they must be used only as a preliminary test. Positive results should be confirmed using gas chromatography/mass spectrometry conducted by an independent diagnostic laboratory.

The test strip is removed from its protective pouch and allowed to equilibrate to room temperature. Meanwhile, a urine sample is obtained in a small cup and also allowed to equilibrate to room temperature. The test strip is dipped vertically, with the arrow on the test strip pointing down into the sample, and remains immersed in the urine sample for ten to fifteen seconds. Then the test strip is removed from the urine sample and placed

on a flat, nonabsorbent surface. After five minutes, the test strip is checked for the appearance of any horizontal lines. The appearance of a colored line in the control region of the dip strip and a faded color line in the test region of the dip strip indicates a negative test and that the concentration of a drug is too low to be detected. If only one line appears in the control region, with no line visible in the test region, then the test is considered to be positive for the presence of drugs. The test is considered to be invalid if only one line appears in the test region or no line appears at all. An invalid test is usually the result of either not following the procedure correctly or not using a large enough urine sample.

The test strips for marijuana use a monoclonal antibody to detect levels of THC, the active ingredient in marijuana, in excess of 50 nanograms per milliliter (ng/ml), the level recommended by SAMHSA. Methamphetamine can be detected in urine samples for three to five days after usage by using a test strip equipped with a monoclonal antibody. A positive test indicates a level in excess of 1,000 ng/ml. A test strip detects the major metabolite of cocaine, benzoylecgonine, for up to twenty-four to forty-eight hours after use. Morphine in excess of 2,000 ng/ml can also be detected by using a test strip containing a specific antibody. Morphine is the primary metabolite product of heroin and codeine.

Kits. Drug tests used for fast, preliminary screening include easy-to-use kits that can test samples of urine, saliva, breath, hair, or sweat. Of these tests, the hair test for drugs is considered to be the most accurate but is still considered to be a preliminary test. To confirm preliminary results or to obtain results for legal purposes, a sample of saliva or urine must be sent to a laboratory when a more reliable test such as GC/MS must be performed. It can take three to seven days to obtain the results. Urine drug test kits are less expensive than other tests, provide instantaneous results, and are easy to store. However, because of variations in metabolism rate, there can be a three-day to one-month detection window, making these tests easier to adulterate than the saliva, hair, sweat, or blood tests.

Adulteration of Specimens. Adulteration generally refers to intentional tampering with a urine sample, and certain substances can be added to urine to create a false-negative test result. Adulteration of urine samples is a common problem because four urine samples is a common problem because four types of masking products—dilution substances, synthetic urine, cleaning substances, and adulterants—are readily available. More than four hundred readily available commercial products can mask urine samples. Dilution substances, including diuretics, lower the concentration of drug in a sample. An individual can either ingest one of these substances before submitting a urine sample or add the substance directly to the urine sample. Synthetic and dehydrated human urine can be bought and submitted for testing. An individual can also purchase a cleaning substance such as an herbal supplement for $30 to $70 and ingest the substance before submitting a sample. The herbal supplement reacts chemically with the drug to essentially nullify its active ingredient. Adulterants are chemicals that can actually react with the drugs, but these are actually added to the sample rather than ingested by the individual.

Methods to Detect Adulteration. Several methods can be used to detect the use of some type of adulterant. If the specific gravity of urine is outside the normal range of 1.003 and 1.030, then the sample may have been diluted. Another indication of adulteration via dilution is to test the level of creatine. If the level is too low (less than 5 milligrams, or mg, per deciliter) then dilution took place. Oxidants, such as pyridinium chlorochromate (PCC), bleach, or hydrogen peroxide, can react chemically with the drug to essentially nullify it. One commonly sold PCC adulterant is called Urine Luck. Tests can also detect the presence of any type of additional oxidant. If the pH (acidity-alkalinity) value of the urine is outside the normal range of 4.0 to 9.0, then an adulterant was added. Two common adulterants are sold under the names of Whizzies or Klear, and these react chemically with drugs in the urine by oxidizing the active ingredient in marijuana. Another chemical reaction occurs when an adulterant called Clear Choice or Urine Aid prevents enzyme activity in the test, which results in the presence of glutaraldehyde, which causes a false negative. Among the states that have passed laws to prevent the sale of masking agents are Florida, South Carolina, North Carolina, New Jersey, Maryland, Virginia, Kentucky, Oklahoma, Nebraska, Illinois, Pennsylvania, and Arkansas.

IMPACT ON INDUSTRY

Drug testing was initially developed for military use and then mandated for federal employees. However, the widespread use of recreational drugs beginning in the 1960's caused private sector employers and then academic institutions to routinely administer drug tests. As a result, a huge market has developed not only for rap-

id, on-site testing methods but also for at-home testing methods, which many parents use to monitor their children. This demand produced explosive growth by companies that manufacture on-site or at-home drug testing kits, and the kits are sold by mass merchandisers and in drugstores such as Target, Walmart, Walgreens, and CVS. In addition, many of these inexpensive kits can be purchased on the Internet.

CAREERS AND COURSE WORK

An interest and aptitude for biology, chemistry, and quantitative classes are important prerequisites to pursuing a career in drug testing. Additional required characteristics include the ability to solve problems, pay close attention to detail, work under pressure, have good manual dexterity, and have normal color vision. Depending on the requirements of the state of residence, a person needs a certificate or license or an associate's degree in biology, chemistry, or medical technology to be employed as a clinical laboratory technician, medical technician, or clinical laboratory technician. Specific information regarding certification can be obtained from the board of registry of the American Association of Bioanalysts and the National Accrediting Agency for Clinical Laboratory Sciences. Typical job duties involve drug sample collection and storage and operation of automated analyzers, often wearing protective gloves and safety glasses. In May, 2008, the median annual salary for a technician was about $35,000.

A bachelor's degree is required to work as a technologist or scientist and earn a higher salary of about $50,000. In addition to a higher salary, a bachelor's degree allows a person to take on more responsibility and possibly advance into supervisory and managerial positions. The ideal bachelor's degree is medical technology, which requires courses in chemistry, biology, microbiology, statistics, computers, and mathematics. To pursue research or become a laboratory director, a master's or doctoral degree is necessary. Employment in the drug testing field is projected to grow at the rate of 14 percent through 2016, which is faster than the average, according to the U.S. Department of Labor. Typical employers include forensic science laboratories, research and development laboratories, and quality assurance laboratories in industry, government, schools, or hospitals.

SOCIAL CONTEXT AND FUTURE PROSPECTS

Mandatory testing is regulated by SAMHSA, part of the U.S. Department of Health and Human Services. This mandatory testing does not yet test for semisynthetic opioids, such as oxycodone, oxymorphone, and hydrocodone, which are often used to relieve pain but have the potential to be abused. However, many employers, athletic organizations, and schools test for these drugs, and ongoing research is directed toward increasing the convenience and reliability of methods of detecting these drugs. Because so many masking agents are readily available, random testing without prior notification is the most effective method, although it is not without controversy. Schools are increasingly performing random drug testing, often leading to protests that the tests are an invasion of privacy and a violation of Fourth Amendment rights.

Organizations such as the International Olympic Committee, National Collegiate Athletic Association, National Basketball Association, and National Football League monitor athletes for the use of more than one hundred anabolic-androgenic steroids. Efforts are being made to eliminate the use of performance-enhancing drugs in all sports. The International Olympic Committee led a collective initiative in creating the World Anti-Doping Agency (WADA) in Switzerland in 1999. WADA created a code in an attempt to standardize regulation and procedures in all sporting countries and keeps a list of prohibited substances. Banned substances include anabolic steroids, hormones, masking agents, stimulants, narcotics, cannabinoids, glucocorticosteroids, and for some sports, alcohol and beta-blockers during competition. Also forbidden are methods of enhancing oxygen transfer (such as blood doping) and gene doping. The UNESCO International Convention Against Doping in Sport, which came into force in 2007, is a global treaty designed to help governments align their policies with the WADA code.

FURTHER READING

Jenkins, Amanda J., and Bruce A. Goldberger, eds. *On-Site Drug Testing.* Totowa, N.J.: Humana Press, 2002. Discusses on-site methods of testing for drugs in hospital, criminal, workplace, and school settings. Looks at many specific tests, discussing their efficacy and their underlying principles.

Karch, Stephen B., ed. *Workplace Drug Testing.* Boca Raton, Fla.: CRC Press, 2008. Examines regulations and mandatory guidelines for federal workplace drug testing and describes techniques. Provides sample protocols from the nuclear power and transportation industries.

Liska, Ken. *Drugs and the Human Body with Implications for Society.* Upper Saddle River, N.J.: Pearson/Prentice Hall, 2004. Simply describes the various classes of drugs and drug testing methods.

Mur, Cindy, ed. *Drug Testing.* Farmington Hills, Mich.:Greenhaven Press/Thomson Gale, 2006. A collection of essays on drug testing in schools and the workplace, discussing efficacy and ethical issues such as privacy.

Pascal, Kintz. *Analytical and Practical Aspects of Drug Testing in Hair.* Boca Raton, Fla.: CRC Press, 2006. Looks at advances in the use of strands of hair for drug testing in the workplace and in forensic crime laboratories and techniques for detecting specific drugs.

Thieme, Detlef, and Peter Hemmersbach. *Doping in Sports.* Berlin: Springer, 2010. Examines sports doping from its beginning, covering the use of anabolic steroids, erthyropoietin, human growth hormone, and gene doping in humans and the doping of race horses. Effects of the drugs, detection methods, and regulations are also discussed.

WEB SITES

Drug and Alcohol Testing Industry Association
http://www.datia.org
Substance Abuse and Mental Health Services Administration
http://www.samhsa.gov
Substance Abuse Program Administrators Association
http://www.sapaa.com
U.S. Department of Labor
Drug-Free Workplace Adviser
http://www.dol.gov/elaws/drugfree.htm
World Anti-Doping Agency
http://www.wada-ama.org

Jeanne L. Kuhler

SEE ALSO: Intervention; Teens and Drug Abuse

Drunk driving

By law, a driver is considered to be impaired by alcohol if his or her blood alcohol content is 0.08 percent (0.08 grams of alcohol per 100 milliliters of blood) or higher. A driver is any operator of a motor vehicle, which includes motorcycle, truck, and passenger vehicle.

SOBRIETY CHECKPOINTS

The sobriety checkpoint, or roadblock, is a law enforcement tool used to arrest drunk drivers and to deter driving while intoxicated. Specifically, sobriety checkpoints occur when law enforcement officers set up a roadblock and stop cars to determine if their drivers have been drinking alcohol. According to the US Centers for Disease Control and Prevention, accidents involving drunk drivers were reduced by 20 percent in US states that have sobriety checkpoints.

Sobriety checkpoints raise a number of concerns, however. One is racial profiling and another is the targeting of unlicensed drivers. If a driver is unlicensed, his or her car can be impounded, making money for the state but penalizing drivers stopped at checkpoints who were not drunk. A third issue is the constitutionality of a sobriety checkpoint. Opponents say it violates the constitutional (Fourth Amendment) right against unreasonable searches.

DRUNK DRIVING LAWS

Every US state has enacted a law making it illegal to drive with a blood alcohol contentblood alcohol contentand drunk driving (BAC) of 0.08 percent or higher. Also, each US state has set the minimum drinking age to twenty-one years and has established a zero-tolerance law that prohibits people less than twenty-one years of age from driving after drinking. The majority of zero-tolerance laws set the drinking limit to a BAC of 0.02 percent. Drivers convicted of alcohol-impaired driving face suspension or revocation of their license.

Drivers who refuse to undergo BAC testing or who fail the test can have their license taken away immediately under a process called administrative license suspension. This process is practiced in forty-one states and the District of Columbia, and the length of time a license is suspended ranges from seven days to one year, depending on the state. Many states will consider restoring driving privileges during a suspension if the person demonstrates a special hardship (such as needing to drive to work).

A mechanism that prevents suspended or probationary drivers from operating a vehicle while impaired by alcohol is the ignition interlock device. This device is attached to the vehicle's ignition and forces the driver, before being able to start the vehicle, to blow into the device for an analysis of the driver's blood alcohol level; a device that registers a BAC of 0.08 or above will lock the vehicle's ignition.

EFFECTS OF ALCOHOL

Alcohol is quickly absorbed into the bloodstream and travels throughout the body and to the brain within thirty to seventy minutes of having an alcoholic drink. A standard alcoholic beverage (such as a twelve-ounce beer, a five-ounce glass of wine, or one shot of liquor) contains about one-half ounce (exactly 0.54 ounces) of alcohol.

All of these types of alcohol will affect BAC in the same way. How quickly a person's BAC rises will depend on how quickly he or she drinks the beverage, on the amount he or she drinks, on the amount of food in the person's stomach, and on his or her weight and gender. Having food in the stomach helps slow the absorption of alcohol through the stomach walls into the bloodstream. Moreover, heavier people have more water in their body, and this water dilutes their BAC. Females typically have less water and more body fat than men, and alcohol is not easily absorbed into fat cells, so more alcohol is absorbed into the bloodstream.

The effects brought on by alcohol start to appear with a BAC of 0.02 percent. These effects include a loss of judgment and a decline in the driver's ability to quickly track moving objects or perform two tasks at a time. Once a person's BAC reaches 0.05, the risk of a fatal crash substantially increases. At this level, the person is less alert and coordinated, has trouble focusing, has trouble steering the vehicle, and is slower to respond to emergency driving situations. At a BAC of 0.08 percent, muscle coordination is poor and the driver will have problems concentrating and controlling the vehicle, will have short-term memory loss, will have problems processing information (for example, signal detection), and will show impaired reasoning and depth perception. With a BAC of 0.10 the driver's reaction time and control deteriorates, thinking slows further, and driving becomes even more difficult. By the time a driver's BAC reaches 0.15 percent, he or she shows a major loss of balance, impaired processing of information, inattention, and little control of the vehicle.

STATISTICS

The National Highway Traffic Safety Administration's National Center for Statistics and Analysis (NCSA) tracks statistics on alcohol-impaired driving and reports these results annually. The NCSA states that any fatal crash in which a driver has a BAC of 0.08 percent or higher is an alcohol-impaired-driving crash, and fatalities resulting from this crash are alcohol-impaired-driving fatalities. They further clarify that alcohol-impaired does not mean that the crash or the fatality was solely caused by alcohol impairment.

Another source that monitors and reports statistics annually is the Insurance Institute for Highway Safety (IIHS). This organization uses data from the US Department of Transportation's Fatality Analysis Reporting System to analyze and report statistics.

FATALITIES

Some progress has been made to reduce alcohol-impaired driving and related injuries and deaths since about 1980. Reports from the NCSA and the IIHS show that from 1982 to 1994, the United States had a 32 percent decline in deaths among drivers with a BAC at or above 0.08. This decline has leveled off in fatalities per year and has ranged from 22 to 25 percent since 1994 through 2009. Looking at overall alcohol-impaired traffic fatalities (drivers or nondrivers), the United States had a 7.4 percent decline between 2008 and 2009.

The year 2009 had 10,839 alcohol-impaired traffic fatalities (or one death every forty-eight minutes), accounting for 32 percent of the total motor vehicle traffic fatalities in the United States. Drunk drivers made up sixty-seven percent of persons killed; 16 percent were passengers in the drunk drivers' vehicles, 10 percent were occupants in other vehicles, and 6 percent were not in a motor vehicle.

Time of day and day of the week also were important indicators of an increased incidence of alcohol-related-deaths. Midnight to 3 a.m. was the deadliest time for intoxicated drivers involved in crashes: 72 percent of these drivers had a BAC at or above 0.08 and 46 percent had a BAC at or above 0.15. The incidence of alcohol-impaired drivers involved in fatal crashes was four times higher at night (37 percent) than at daytime (9 percent) and was two times higher on weekends (31 percent) than on weekdays (16 percent).

The NCSA defined nighttime as starting at 6 p.m. and ending at 5:59 a.m. (daytime began at 6 a.m. and ended at 5:59 p.m.) and defined weekend as starting Friday at 6 p.m. and as ending Monday at 5:50 a.m. (Weekday was defined as Monday from 5 a.m. to Friday at 5:59 p.m.). The IIHS narrowed the timeframe for what defined nighttime (9 p.m. to 6 a.m.) and found that 62 percent of drivers with a BAC at or above 0.08 had died and 46 percent of drivers with a BAC at or above 0.15 had died during that time.

Of 1,314 children age fourteen years and younger who were killed in motor vehicle crashes, 181 (or 14 percent) died in crashes involving alcohol-impaired drivers. Fifty-one percent of these 181 children were in the vehicle of the alcohol-impaired driver and 15 percent were struck by the alcohol-impaired driver's vehicle (data not reported on the remaining 34 percent).

DRIVER CHARACTERISTICS

Of the 12,012 drivers involved in a fatal crash with a recorded BAC of 0.01 percent or higher, 84 percent had a BAC of at least 0.08 and 56 percent had a BAC of 0.15 or higher. The most common BAC recorded for drunk drivers involved in fatal crashes was 0.17 percent.

Age was a significant predictor of a person driving drunk and being involved in a fatal crash. Youthand drunk driving statistics between twenty-one and twenty-four years of age with a BAC of 0.08 or higher topped the list of fatalities at 35 percent, followed by twenty-five to thirty-four year olds (32 percent), thirty-five to forty-four year olds (26 percent), forty-four to fifty-four year olds (22 percent), sixteen to twenty year olds (19 percent), fifty-five to sixty-four year olds (13 percent), sixty-five to seventy-four year olds (7 percent), and age seventy-five years or older (3 percent). There was a consistently higher percentage of male drivers with a BAC at or above 0.08 percent who were involved in fatal crashes in every age group. More than one-half of men age twenty-one to thirty years (58 percent) and age thirty-one to forty years (53 percent) with a BAC at or above 0.08 and involved in a crash were killed.

For overall deaths of drunk drivers with 0.08 or higher, 40 percent were male and 22 percent were female, 29 percent were motorcyclists, 23 percent were drivers of passenger vehicles, 23 percent were drivers of light trucks, and 2 percent were drivers of large trucks. Drivers involved in a fatal crash with a reported BAC level of 0.08 or higher were eight times more likely than nondrinking drivers to have a previous impaired-driving conviction.

FURTHER READING

"The ABCs of BAC: A Guide to Understanding Blood Alcohol Concentration and Alcohol Impairment." 17 Feb. 2012. Web. http://www.stopimpaireddriving.org/ABCsBACWeb. Clearly explains the effects of alcohol and how it affects a person's driving abilities at different BAC levels.

Dasgupta, Amitava. *The Science of Drinking: How Alcohol Affects Your Body and Mind.* Lanham, MD: Rowman & Littlefield, 2011. A comprehensive study of the science of alcohol impairment.

"Impaired Driving." 17 Feb. 2012. Web. http://www.nhtsa.gov/Impaired. Features manuals, brochures, and toolkits on impaired driving.

"Traffic Safety Facts 2009 Data: Alcohol-Impaired Driving." 17 Feb. 2012. Web. http://www-nrd.nhtsa.dot.gov/pubs/811385.pdf. Provides detailed descriptive data and summaries on alcohol-impaired driving fatality by role, type of vehicle, gender, age, BAC levels, and US state.

WEBSITES OF INTEREST

Insurance Institute for Highway Safety
http://www.iihs.org
Mothers Against Drunk Driving
http://www.madd.org
National Commission Against Drunk Driving
http://www.ncadd.com
National Highway Traffic Safety Administration
http://www.nhtsa.gov
National Institute on Alcohol Abuse and Alcoholism
http://www.niaaa.nih.gov

Christine G. Holzmueller

SEE ALSO: Teens and Alcohol Abuse

E-cigarettes and other alternatives

Many alternatives have emerged to conventional tobacco cigarattes, including e-cigarettes (vaping), chewing tobacco, and hookahs. All of them have one thing in common: they are delivery systems for nicotine, a highy addictive drug that binds with the same receptors in the brain as heroin. The addictive nature of nicotine intensifies as more of it is injested, no matter how it is delivered. Use of e-cigarettes has been growing rapidly among high-school students in the United States, from a very small percentage before 2010 to 15 to 20 per cent in 2015. Smokeless tobacco has a mortality risk lower than that of conventional cigarettes, but the American Cancer Society calls it only "less lethal".

INTRODUCTION

E-cigarettes involve the delivery of nicotine to the brain via a vapor solution, so use of them is sometimes called "vaping." Unlike traditional tobacco cigarettes, they do not involve burning and inhalation of tobacco, which contains numerous unhealthy chemical compounds in addition to nicotine, some of which can cause cancer. Because of this, "vaping" is sometimes advanced as a relatively healthty alternative to tobacco cigarettes. The vapor itself may contain harmful chemical compounds, however. Although e-cigarettes are a relatively new technology, a substantial number of articles have appeared in the medical literature examining them, a very small sample of which are listed below under "Further Reading."

"We need a national debate on nicotine," said Mitch Zeller, director of the Center for Tobacco Products, part of the federal government's Food and Drug Administration (Nocera, 2015). Many public-health officials believe that e-cigarettes should be regulated as strenuously as tobacco-based products, so that teenagers will be legally prohibited from using them. In 2015, Zeller said that the FDA was conducting more than 50 studies aimed at evaluating the health risks of e-cigarettes and where to place them on "the continuum of risk" (Nocera, 2015). "I am fond of quoting Michael Russell," Zeller said, referring to a tobacco scientist who, during the early 1970s, recognized that nicotine was the addictive device in tobacco, as he said: "People smoke for the nicotine but die from the tar" (Nocera, 2015).

E-cigarettes were invented by Hon Lik in China during 2003, the same year that his father, a heavy smoker of tobacco, died of lung cancer. Hon himself quit smoking after inventing e-cigarettes, and advanced them in China beginning in 2004 as a smoking cessation aid. These devices usually contain a heating element that atomizes a liquid form of nicotine that satisfies the same craving as cigarette smoke. They contain propylene glycol, glycerin, and one of thousands of flavorings, along with nicotine. Some do not contain nicotine, but these don't sell very well (in 2015, more than 95 per cent of e-cigarettes contained nicotine). Vaping aerosols also have been found to contain very small amounts of variuos toxicants as well as heavy metals, but at much lower levels than tobacco smoke.

USAGE AND EFFECTS OF E-CIGARETTES WORLDWIDE

As of 2015, several million people worldwide were using e-cigarettes, a number that was increasing rapidly. In some countries, among young people, e-cigarette use by 2014 had exceeded that of tobacco cigarettes. Tobacco companies were moving into the market. Most e-cigarette smokers use them every day, and a large proportion continued to use tobacco products as well. Many traditional cigarette smokers used e-cigarettes in places where smoking tobacco is illegal.

The United Kingdom's National Health Service has concluded that e-cigarettes may be somewhat safer than tobacco cigarettes, but long-term effects on the body are presently unknown, lacking adequate clinical trials. The United States Food and Drug Administration (FDA) largely agreed in 2014 that scientific evidence did not then exist to evaluate potential health risks of e-cigarettes, or their potential use as an aid to help smokers quit tobacco-based products.

A July 2014 World Health Organization (WHO) report said that "vaping" is not merely water vapor, and that it could pose health risks to adolescents and fetuses. The United States Centers for Disease Control warns that advertising of e-cigarettes as a "healthy" alternative to tobacco smoking may increase nicotine addiction among young people. In the meantime, fervent supporters of "vaping" have organized into groups and hosted "vape meets" in several U.S. cities to promote use of e-cigarettes. Some vapers (who call themselves "cloud-chasers") rig their e-cigarette devices to produce large amounts of vapor so they will be obvious in a provocative way. The Oxford dictionaries declared "vape" its "word of the year" in 2014.

As of 2015, about two-thirds of major countries had regulated "vaping" in some manner. Singapore, Brazil, and Uruguay had banned e-cigarette use. In Canada, sale of the devices remained legal, but without approval by Health Canada, the nicotine fluid used in these devices was technically illegal, a ban that was widely ignored.

HOOKAH

The hookah, a water pipe that vaporizes flavored tobacco through a basin of water has become popular in the United States, Europe, and elsewhere in the world, having arrived with immigrants from the Middle East. Its use stems from the early importation of tobacco to the Middle East from North America by the Dutch, perhaps as early as 1622. The name "hookah" came into English during British colonization of India during the nineteenth century. Its use spread so rapidly that some Britons were said to have preferred their hookah to their dinner.

In Arab lands, where alcohol is often forbidden by Islamic law, the hookah is usually shared in cafes, but in North America and Europe it has become established in some bars and taverns. Traditionally, the tobacco acquires its taste by being marinated in molasses. The tobacco is then placed above the water in the pipe's bowl with pierced foil and hot coals. The smoke is then drawn through water to filter and cool it. Unlike most foms of smoking, the hookah is shared as a social experience.

SMOKELESS TOBACCO

Tobacco without smoking　is available as "chew" in strands or twists (called chew, wads, or plugs) that are placed between the cheek and gums or teeth so thst nicotine is absorbed through the mouth. The interaction of the tobacco and saliva produces brown juice that users spit out. Another variation, snuff, is packaged in small pouches that also may be inserted between cheek and gum without producing spittle.

Dry snuff also may be inhaled as a powder. "Snus," another variation, also comes in small pouches that can be used like snuff. While these tobacco products have been marketed as safer than smoking tobacco, the Americsn Cancer Society asserts that they contain many of the same carcinogenic substances as any form of tobacco, although locations of cancers may change. For example, chewed tobacco raises the probability of tongue, throat, stomach, and pancreas cancers even as it may decrease incidence of lung and many other cancers that result from cigarette smoking. Smokeless tobacco is also just as addictive as any other form. Tobacco absorbed in the mouth also may accelerate tooth decay, and play a role in heart disease.

FURTHER READING

Cahn, Z., and Siege, M. (2011, February). Electronic cigarettes as a harm reduction strategy for tobacco control: a step forward or a repeat of past mistakes? *Journal of Public Health Policy* 32 (1): 16–31. http://www.palgrave-journals.com/jphp/journal/v32/n1/full/jphp201041a.html. This study argues that advocates of "vaping" who claim that it will reduce tobacco smoking may be blowing smoke.

Carroll-Chapman, S.L. and L.T Wu, L.T. (2014, March 18). E-cigarette prevalence and correlates of use among adolescents versus adults: A review and comparison. *Journal of Psychiatric Research* 54: 43–54. This academic treatment compares recent increases in e-cigarette use across age groups.

Nocera, J. "Smoking, vaping and nicotine." (2015, May 29). *New York Times*. http://www.nytimes.com/2015/05/26/opinion/joe-nocera-smoking-vaping-and-nicotine.html. Nocera asserts that nicotine addiction is a major issue, regardless of how it is delivered.

Orr, K.K. and Asal, N.J.. (2014, November). Efficacy of electronic cigarettes for smoking cessation. *Annals of Pharmacotherapy* 48 (11): 1502–1506. http://aop.sagepub.com/content/48/11/1502. Are e-cigarettes a suitable aid in smoking cessation? This is an early and rather indecisive study.

Rom, O.; Pecorelli, A., Valacchi, G. and Reznick, A.Z.. (2014). Are e-cigarettes a safe and good alternative to cigarette smoking? *Annals of the New York Academy of Sciences.* http://onlinelibrary.wiley.com/doi/10.1111/nyas.12609/abstract;jsessionid=9B9433762B3D9745FF3BB4E66E102071.f01t03. The authors conclude that further research is necessary to accurately compare the effects of "vaping" to those of tobacco smoking.

Osberg, M. (2014, February 25). "Vape life: welcome to the weird world of e-cig evangelists". *Verge.*

http://www.theverge.com/2014/2/25/5445662/vape-life-welcome-to-the-weird-world-of-e-cig-evangelists. This populor account delves into the world of vaping fanatics.

Suter, M.A., Mastrobattista, J., Sachs, M. and Aagaard, K. (2015). Is there evidence for potential harm of electronic cigarette use in pregnancy? *Birth Defects Research Part A: Clinical and Molecular Teratology* 103 (3): 186–195. The focus here is on the delivery of nicotine and birth defects. More research is advised.

Weaver, M., Breland, A., Spindle, T. and Eissenberg, T. (2014). Electronic cigarettes. *Journal of Addiction Medicine* 8 (4): 234–240. This treatment of e-cigarettes focuses on the fact that they are as addictive as any other form of nicotine.

Bruce E. Johansen

SEE ALSO: Smoking and Its Effects

Families and substance abuse

A family with a substance-abusing member often experiences long-lasting, deleterious consequences from that abuse. An individual member's substance abuse or addiction is also the family's substance abuse or addiction. Self-pity, hatred, resentment, guilt, and anger disrupt family life that, while never perfect, should ideally be health-promoting, protective, supportive, and positive. Powerful and dangerous emotions intoxicate and ruin the function- *al life of the family. Treatment, however, is available for family members and for the addict.*

CAUSES

Initial substance and chemical use is almost always voluntary, as the person decides to consume or not consume a substance; if they do consume, they decide how much. The person is in charge of the choices he or she makes.

Continued choices to use a drug produce chemical and structural changes in the brain that result in involuntary, compulsively driven needs to have the drug. This action compromises the functioning of the areas of the brain involved in the inhibition of drives. The urge is never more than temporarily satisfied, however. The substance, not the person, is in control.

What often starts as an experience of recreation, relaxation, excitement, experimentation, social bonding, or isolated escape from life's challenges becomes a need to satisfy and resupply. Users are now abusers, and abusers often become addicts of the substances they are using.

Substance abuse can involve any chemical, but more often they involve commonly used and legal substances such as tobacco (the nicotine in tobacco is addictive) and coffee or tea (the caffeine in coffee and tea is addictive) or illegal chemicals such as cocaine, heroin, and marijuana. Substances of abuse also include legal medications, such as anti-anxiety and pain medications, which require a physician prescription to obtain, and over-the-counter medications.

Although these substances are chemically quite varied, they all produce the same overt response in the abuser: an unrelenting need to achieve the next altered state of consciousness, be it a high, sleepiness or relaxation, or excitability. Satisfying the need becomes a priority over responsibilities with family, friends, or work. The addict becomes emotionally cut off from family, friends, and coworkers. Addiction and the quest to satiate the next urge control the addict's mental state.

Those struggling with addiction often have legal troubles and frequently use substances in dangerous situations (such as driving under the influence). The ability to resist the impulse to take the drug overtakes users' self-control, and they are left helpless and often beyond the help that their families and friends can typically provide.

RISK FACTORS

While vulnerability to substance addiction can come about for many reasons, the most common involve a prior history of substance abuse in one's family, which is dually suggestive of being exposed to and learning how to use substances (imitative, learned behavior), and a genetic predisposition to responding more strongly to drugs than might be true for the average person. The average person without an addiction is more likely to have been raised in a family free of substance and chemical abuse.

Geneticists are moving closer to identifying several genes and gene clusters that promote a much stronger pleasure response to certain substances than is typical in the average person. Neuroscientists, similarly, are increasing their focus on areas of the brain that become highly excitable in addicted persons exposed to drugs.

One in four families has one or more members who either abuses drugs or is addicted to drugs. This can be explained in part by research that shows that addiction and substance abuse occur more readily in persons with a family history in which a first-order relative is chemically addicted and in which there exists a genetic loading for an unusually pleasurable response to drugs and other substances. This extrapolates to one of every two families having to cope in a major way with a relation or close friend who abuses or is addicted to drugs.

Having a behavioral or mental problem or illness, even common ones like anxiety and depression, also increases the odds that one will develop an addiction. Also more likely to become addicted are persons who were neglected or physically or emotionally abused as children. Research also shows that even the delivery system employed, that is, how the drugs are ingested, puts someone on a faster track to addiction. Snorting and intravenous injection are the most dangerous methods that can lead to drug addiction.

IMPACT ON THE FAMILY

Persons do not intend to become addicts or substance abusers. People most often use substances to change an emotional state, to enhance a state of feeling good, or to combat a state of feeling bad.

Use easily becomes frequent use, frequent use increases the odds that use progresses to abuse; episodes of abuse, in turn, increase—and almost guarantee—the odds that addiction will overcome the person's state of mind and being. They live the life of addictive preoccupation; nothing else matters.

Having a substance-abusing member in a family has long-lasting, deleterious effects that take from the energy, bonds, and nurturance that characterize the traditional family group. The social dynamic in families is that each member reacts to all other members. Mothers react to spouses and their children. Fathers react to spouses and their children. Children react to each parent and their siblings. This mesh of reactions results in a long-term, developmentally progressive, complex social system that has its own lifecycle. A substance-abusing family member has an impact on this cycle, usually in one of three ways. Family members can respond to the substance abuse in a similar fashion.

The most prevalent of these three reactions is the desire to stay engaged with the substance abuser, and to advise, counsel, support, reason with, and show disappointment in the abuser while seeking the promise of abstinence and reform. This response by family members who love and are committed to each other is rarely effective, but nonetheless may last for decades. Engagement often produces depression and hopelessness in the family, which can then produce guilt and shame in the abuser. The pain of the guilt and shame is more than the abuser can withstand, and the negative emotions may drive him or her back to the substance of abuse.

The second most prevalent reaction, confrontation, usually arises some time after the addiction is accepted as a real problem, both for the family member and for the family. Confrontational responses generally have rapid onset with a short half-life. Most people cannot sustain high levels of intense anger and outrage. The addict often recoils in the face of such an emotional onslaught and will nervously try to avoid the drug or not get caught taking the drug. Inevitably, because the addiction or abuse is not being treated, its remission is brief; when it resurfaces, it will again be met by family outrage. The addict will then respond as before: recycling the pattern of abuse.

The third reaction, collaboration, can move family members from being contributors to and enablers of the problem to recognizing that, in the face of the disease, the family has become diseased itself; symptoms are often manifested in a long and varied series of unhelpful, maladaptive, dysfunctional responses that attempt the impossible: Remove the cause of the addiction, try to control the addiction, and find a cure for the addiction.

Engagement initially requires the emotional and psychological detachment from the addict and his or her disease. Genetic loading and family history notwithstanding, family members (often slowly) come to understand that they did not cause the disease, that they cannot (and have never been able to) control the disease, and that they cannot cure the disease.

TREATMENT FOR FAMILIES

Just as families have primary ways of reacting to their drug-abusing members, they also have fairly predictable developmental stages in reacting to these members. In the beginning, as an addict's behavior becomes harder to hide, family members begin to notice that something is wrong.

Family members will feel concerned and worried and will begin genuine attempts to look out for the troubled member's welfare. Families ask, remark, comment, suggest, and obtain promises of reduced or controlled use. Families will protect, make excuses, and try to carry on their normal lives. Slowly, as these efforts only prolong the addiction and delay treatment, families experience extreme emotional dissonance and self-doubt. Families become confused about whether they are tolerating addiction, enabling addiction, or just protecting themselves.

At this stage, families are immersed in the addiction, and treatment becomes necessary, even if the addict refuses. Often family members will employ a strategy of emotional or physical avoidance, a form of denial that parallels that of addicts.

For addicts and their families substance addictions are treatable diseases. As families accept the realities of the addiction, they can begin to make real changes. For most families, the treatment of choice will be a family-centered, twelve-step program such as Al-Anon or Nar-Anon. Individual family members may get their own treatment by meeting with a mental health specialist skilled at recognizing common dysfunctional family responses. As the family tends to its own health, it gets healthier. With the right kind of help comes healing, and the family can start to return to a normal way of life.

Family life involves intense emotions (good and bad), so it is almost impossible for families to have an engaged response without outside guidance, direction, and support. Help for families coping with addicted members is wide ranging. It comes in the form of twelve-step groups such as Al-Anon and Nar-Anon. Also available are licensed behavioral health care professionals who specialize in substance abuse treatment or specialized treatment centers or programs.

In addition to being an example of those invested in their own recovery, families can be huge catalysts for aiding the addicts' treatment and recovery processes. Ideally, the family should respond to the addiction with support and noninterference.

The role of the family is critical; its reactions will either promote health or enable disease. Though they may never have abused substances themselves, family members should accept that they are coping with more than the substance abuse habits of an individual member. They are facing a family disease, and they should seek help accordingly.

FURTHER READING

American Academy of Child and Adolescent Psychiatry. "Facts for Families." Washington, DC: AACAP, 2011. An informational guide series for parents and families facing a variety of real-world issues, including substance abuse and chemical addictions.

Barnard, Marina. *Drug Addiction and Families*. Philadelphia: Jessica Kingsley, 2007. The author, a senior research fellow at the Centre for Drug Misuse Research at the University of Glasgow, Scotland, has written extensively on the contributory role family environments can play in the development of substance misuse and abuse and how families can respond effectively.

Bradshaw, John. *On the Family: A New Way of Creating Solid Self-Esteem*. Deerfield Beach, FL: Health Communications, 1996. One of the best introductions to understanding families as systems with dynamic, reactive energies. Explains in clear, insightful language the family's role in supporting ongoing problematic and addictive behaviors in an individual family member.

Congers, Beverly. *Addict in the Family: Stories of Loss, Hope, and Recovery*. Deerfield Beach, FL: Health Communications, 2003. Generally regarded as a realistic yet inspirational read, this work includes real-life perspectives from family members coping with a loved one's addiction. Discusses the need for self-care.

Friel, John C., and Linda D. Friel. *Adult Children Secrets of Dysfunctional Families: Secrets of Dysfunctional Families*. Deerfield Beach, FL: Health Communications, 1988. Based in large measure on their extensive clinical experience with families coping with substance abuse, the authors discuss how family dynamics promote conditions that foster substance abuse.

Hayes, Steven, and Michael Levin. *Mindfulness and Acceptance for Addictive Behaviors: Applying Contextual CBT to Substance Abuse and Behavioral Addictions*. Oakland, CA: New Harbinger, 2010. Hayes is a pioneer in the application of mindfulness in treatment of substance abuse and addictions in general. A readable work focused on helping the reader apply this approach to many types of substance addictions.

WEBSITES OF INTEREST

Families Anonymous
http://www.familiesanonymous.org
National Institute on Drug Abuse
http://www.drugabuse.gov
Substance Abuse and Mental Health Services Administration
http://www.samhsa.gov

Eugenia F. Moglia and Paul Moglia

SEE ALSO: Codependency; Teens and Alcohol Abuse; Teens and Drug Abuse

Food addiction

Food addiction is characterized by the uncontrolled desire for and preoccupation with food. Food addicts are driven by obsessive-compulsive thoughts about food and eating despite knowing the negative effects of excess food intake, including obesity. Dependency on food, as with other dependent substances, occurs when destructive behavior persists despite the negative outcomes associated with repeated use.

CAUSES

Cited causes of food addiction include depression, loneliness, stress, hostility, boredom, childhood sexual or emotional trauma, and low self-esteem. Some scientists believe there is a biological explanation for food addiction that involves dopamine, a neurotransmitter in the brain.

Eating is typically a pleasurable experience, but food addiction is caused by a loss of control over the agent of abuse: food. Persons addicted to food may not recognize their addiction or may feel incapable of breaking the cycle of overeating. They have an undeniable preoccupation with food and are compelled to eat large amounts of food. For food addicts, this cycle eventually becomes the norm.

In an episode of binge eating it is not uncommon to consume in excess of 10,000 calories. These calories lead to obesity if not expended, yet it is not accurate to assume that all obese persons are food addicts. Food addicts continue to engage in compulsive overeating even when aware of its destructive effects. Those who eventually want to break the cycle often feel incapable of doing so, while others feel they can stop but continue to postpone doing so.

Eating habits are established during childhood. The development of poor eating habits, including binge eating, may result from ineffective coping mechanisms. Food serves as a barrier or substitute to dealing with emotionally difficult situations and relationships. Poor eating habits continue into adulthood and become ingrained in behavior.

RISK FACTORS

Binge eating disorder is the most common eating disorder in the United States. This and other forms of food addiction most commonly affect girls and women age fourteen to thirty-five years, perhaps because of society's emphasis on appearance and thinness. Both women and men can be food addicts, but women more often seek treatment. Food addiction affects persons of all body types and body weights.

Although food addiction most often results in obesity, not all obese persons are food addicts. Persons with a family history of overeating and persons who lack adequate coping mechanisms for stress, disappointment, and anger may be more at risk for the disorder. Persons with a genetic predisposition for binge eating are enabled by family members, who often allow the cycle to continue through their own actions and expectations.

SYMPTOMS

Binge eaters differ from bulimics in that they do not attempt to rid themselves of the consumed food after a binge. Binge eaters and food addicts spend overwhelming amounts of time planning and fulfilling food "frenzies," which occur publicly or privately. They may eat a reasonable portion in public yet overeat in private. They often eat when they are not hungry or when they are emotionally upset. Feelings of low self-worth and guilt often follow binges, yet these binges are followed by planning for the next episode of eating. Each encounter with food can perpetuate the cycle of destruction.

Though the majority of Americans eat more than what the US Department of Agriculture recommends, food addicts far exceed these same recommendations. Food addicts often feel full but may appear ravished, out of control, or on a high, or they may always claim to be hungry.

The insatiable appetite for food is a manifestation of other underlying problems. Food often becomes a substitute for other aspects of life that addicts do not perceive as fulfilled, including personal goals, finances, and personal and professional relationships. Food has filled these voids and temporarily provides the comfort, completeness, or pleasure that the addict so desperately seeks. Often, the addict makes food the object of obsession in attempts to delay or avoid dealing with uncomfortable situations or emotions.

Foods high in sugar and fat are thought to act as triggers for obsessive, compulsive eating. Therefore, withdrawal from these triggers is real and can cause cramps, tremors, and exaggerated feelings of depression and guilt.

SCREENING AND DIAGNOSIS
Screening tools in the form of questionnaires are available to determine if further evaluation may be necessary to aid in the diagnosis of a food addiction. However, these tools rely on self-reports. Food addicts are typically ashamed or in denial, or they feel they are too out of control to modify their behavior. These facts alter self-assessment tools.

Furthermore, food addiction is not a recognized diagnosis in the American Psychiatric Association's *Diagnostic and Statistical Manual of Mental Disorders*, although there is debate as to whether or not it should be included. Binge eating is a symptom of other well-known eating disorders, such as bulimia, yet the two have distinct differences.

Health care providers are in a unique position to help those who may suffer from food addiction. Obesity is often attributed to other medical problems, such as thyroid disorders. However, appropriate laboratory tests can determine if a causal relationship exists. Among other complications, binge eating may lead to depression, suicidal thoughts and tendencies, obesity, heart disease, hypertension, type 2 diabetes, hypercholesterolemia, and joint problems.

TREATMENT AND THERAPY
Other substances of abuse (such as cocaine and heroin) are harmful to the addict regardless of dose. Treatment and therapy for substance addicts involves the elimination of the abused substance, which not only is detrimental to the body but also is completely unnecessary to sustain life.

Treatment and therapy for food addiction is unique because eating is required for human survival. The abused substance cannot be entirely removed from the person's environment. Also noteworthy is that eating is a social behavior. Eating's social aspects make it more challenging to control, given that humans are immersed in activities involving food and eating. Whether compulsive or not, overeating is more acceptable when others are also engaging in this behavior.

To sever their dependency on food, addicts must first realize and accept that they have a problem and must willingly receive treatment and support from trained professionals, such as physicians, dieticians, and mental health specialists. Food addicts must reclaim power and learn to control food instead of allowing it to control them.

Obesity that often accompanies binge eating and food addiction should also be addressed. Weight loss and psychological counseling may occur separately or simultaneously, but both are required to optimize the addicts' future.

PREVENTION
Unhealthy foods tend to be more accessible and often are more affordable than sound, nutritious foods. Considering the predominance of hectic lifestyles in developed nations, this limited availability of healthy foods creates the perfect opportunity to make poor food choices. Obesity, the second leading cause of preventable death in the United States, can lead to premature death or disability. It is estimated that the United States spends more than $200 billion on obesity-related health care each year.

Behavioral changes are required to prevent and correct binge eating and obesity. Apart from eating healthy and exercising regularly, several other strategies are suggested. Education is necessary to increase awareness of the problem, and educational efforts should be provided worldwide. Ideally, healthier food choices will be made equally available and healthy eating habits will be taught and reinforced. Also, researchers will continue to explore the underlying reasons behind unnecessary eating or overeating.

FURTHER READING
Costin, Carolyn. *The Eating Disorder Sourcebook*. New York: McGraw-Hill, 2006. Provides information on recognizing eating disorders, on available treatments, and more.

Kessler, David A. *The End of Overeating: Taking Control of the Insatiable American Appetite*. New York: Rodale, 2009. Discusses how Americans have lost control over food and examines how they might regain that control.

Power, Michael L., and Jay Schulkin. *The Evolution of Obesity*. Baltimore: Johns Hopkins UP, 2009. Examines the "trend" of obesity, the reasons behind it, and why individualized methods are required to prevent and reverse it.

Wansink, Brian. *Mindless Eating: Why We Eat More Than We Think*. New York: Bantam, 2010. An exploration of "mindless" eating and how humans can be more cognizant of food intake.

WEBSITES OF INTEREST

HealthyPlace.com
http://www.healthyplace.com/eating disorders
Overeaters Anonymous
http://www.oa.org

Virginia C. Muckler

SEE ALSO: Compulsive Overeating; Overeaters Anonymous

Gambling

Gambling can be a recreational activity, a profession, or a psychopathology. Pathological gambling is an impulse-control disorder that often produces depression and anxiety as secondary conditions and also disrupts marital and family relationships. Psychopharmacological, behavioral, and twelve-step treatments are helpful.

INTRODUCTION

A gambler is a person who risks something of value based on an uncertain outcome for the possibility of reward: Typically, money is bet in the hope of making more money. Gamblers are classified as recreational, professional, or pathological. Recreational gambling is an enjoyable activity that has no evident adverse effects and may have possible mental-health benefits among certain groups, such as the elderly. A few individuals are professional gamblers, making their living by playing games of chance that involve some level of skill. Pathological gambling has a long history in the psychiatric literature, but it was not defined as a medical problem until 1980, when it was added to the diagnostic nomenclature. It is an impulse-control disorder and tends to lead to increasingly adverse consequences for individuals, their families, and others.

A diagnosis of pathological gambling requires the presence of five out of ten criteria:

1. becoming preoccupied with gambling,
2. exhibiting tolerance and withdrawal,
3. escaping from moods and life's problems,
4. chasing losses with more gambling,
5. lying about gambling,
6. losing control over the reduction of betting,
7. becoming irritable when trying to stop gambling,
8. committing illegal acts to obtain funds,
9. risking interpersonal relationships and vocation to gamble, and
10. seeking bailouts, such as turning to others for financial assistance. Mania must be ruled out when diagnosing pathological gambling.

PREVALENCE, RISK FACTORS, AND THEORIES

Most people who gamble in a given year are recreational gamblers. In the United States, only about 1 percent of adults (2.4 million people in 2012) become pathological gamblers—about the same percentage as are diagnosed with schizophrenia. Another 2 to 3 percent are considered problem gamblers, who experience detrimental consequences as a result of their betting but meet fewer than five of the diagnostic criteria. Slightly higher rates of pathological and problem gambling are found among adolescents.

Risk factors for developing pathological gambling include a parental history of gambling problems, alcohol and tobacco use, and membership in a minority. Males are more likely to be pathological gamblers than females. The most common comorbid conditions with pathological gambling are a personality disorder, which occurs in about half of those diagnosed (antisocial personality disorder is the most frequently found), and substance abuse, which is found in about one-third of pathological gamblers. Whether as a cause or a consequence, anxiety and depressive disorders are often diagnosed as well. When pathological gambling becomes chronic, a major depressive disorder may be present. Pathological gambling invariably affects the spouse and family of the gambler, making marital and family counseling necessary.

Theories explaining the development of pathological gambling are multivariate and address a range of factors, including biological, environmental, and parental. Studies during the first decade of the twenty-first century suggest a biological foundation for pathological gambling. The neurotransmitters serotonin and dopamine are implicated, as are endorphins. For example, some patients treated for Parkinson's disease with a dopamine agonist spontaneously developed urges to gamble and, in some instances, progressed to problem and pathological gambling. The urges remitted with cessation of medication.

Pathological gamblers show impulsivity, an inability to delay gratification, and higher levels of physiological arousal, such as increased heart rate, during gambling activity. There may be fundamental physiological differences in the neurological makeup of people who gamble to excess compared with those who can gamble in moderation.

Also associated with gambling are elaborate contingencies of reinforcement to create and sustain the behavior. The modern casino is a technological wonder designed to produce only one outcome: sustained gambling. In the 1970s, when the American gaming industry discovered that marketing to the middle class could significantly increase the pool of gamblers, industry members sought to increase the number of states in which gambling was legal. Eventually, gambling was legalized in some form in every state except Hawaii and Utah. The availability of gaming opportunities has led to an increase in pathological gamblers, which the industry has addressed with programs promoting responsible gambling. States that introduced lotteries have established programs to educate citizens about the dangers of gambling in excess.

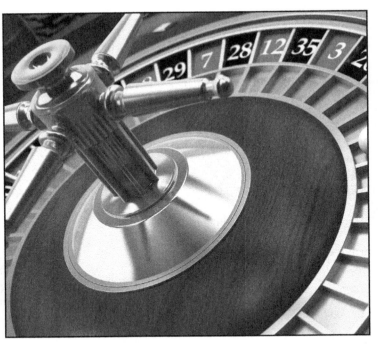

Photo: iStock

TREATMENT AND PREVENTION

A treatment program for pathological gambling begins with a comprehensive assessment that examines the individual's gambling frequency and duration, the extent of negative consequences, personality type, and psychological context. Common assessment tools include the South Oaks Gambling Screen (SOGS), a general psychiatric symptoms checklist, and careful questioning about substance abuse.

Treatment for pathological gambling can take a variety of forms. One effective method is cognitive behavior therapy, which focuses on changing patterns of thought and cognition related to gambling impulses. Another is Gamblers Anonymous, founded in 1957 and patterned after Alcoholics Anonymous, which provides a free twelve-step program with strong peer support. Daily meetings are held in many cities in the United States, and Gamblers Anonymous offers support and education for spouses, family, and friends of gamblers. Psychopharmacological treatments for gambling—including selective serotonin

reuptake inhibitors (SSRIs), opioid antagonists, and mood stabilizers—also have shown some promise.

Many states have websites that guide those who might have a problem with gambling to treatment locations. These sites also provide educational information and self-assessments. The National Council on Problem Gambling also provides educational information. Programs to prevent pathological gambling include state-mandated informational cards and plaques placed in casinos, state-supported television and billboard advertisements warning of the consequences of excessive gambling, and educational curricula designed to enlighten adolescents about the dangers of gambling.

FURTHER READING

Ariyabuddhiphongs, Vanchai. "Problem Gambling Prevention: Before, During, and After Measures." *International Journal of Mental Health and Addiction* 11.5 (2013): 568–82. Print.

Brewerton, Timothy D., and Amy Baker Dennis, eds. *Eating Disorders, Addictions and Substance Use Disorders.* Heidelberg: Springer, 2014. Print.

Castellani, Brian. *Pathological Gambling: The Making of a Medical Problem.* Albany: State U of New York P, 2000. Print.

Grant, Jon E., and Mark N. Potenza. *Pathological Gambling: A Clinical Guide to Treatment.* Arlington: Amer. Psychiatric, 2004. Print.

Knapp, Terry J., and Edward W. Crossman. "Pathways to Betting: Childhood, Adolescent, and Underage Gambling." *Gambling: Behavior Theory, Research, and Application.* Ed. Patrick M. Ghezzi et al. Reno: Context, 2006. 207–30. Print.

Koot, S., et al. "Compromised Decision-Making and Increased Gambling Proneness following Dietary Serotonin Depletion in Rats." *Neuropharmacology* 62.4 (2012): 1640–50. Print

Lesieur, Henry R., and Sheila B. Blume. "The South Oaks Gambling Screen (SOGS): A New Instrument for the Identification of Pathological Gamblers." *American Journal of Psychiatry* 144.9 (1987): 1184–89. Print.

Perkinson, Robert R., Arthur E. Jongsma Jr., and Timothy J. Bruce. *The Addiction Treatment Planner.* 5th ed. Hoboken: Wiley, 2014. Print.

Petry, Nancy M. *Pathological Gambling: Etiology, Comorbidity, and Treatment.* Washington: APA, 2004. Print.

Whelan, James P., Timothy A. Steenbergh, and Andrew W. Meyers. *Problem and Pathological Gambling.* Cambridge: Hogrefe, 2007. Print.

Terry J. Knapp

SEE ALSO: Addictive Personality and Behaviors

GHB (gamma-Hydroxybutyric acid)

GHB is a naturally occurring substance that resembles the neurotransmitter and energy metabolism regulator gamma-aminobutyric acid (GABA). GHB generally acts as an intoxicant and as a depressant of the central nervous system. Medically, GHB is used in general anesthesia and to treat narcolepsy, insomnia, clinical depression, and alcoholism. GHB is used illicitly as an intoxicant, euphoriant, "date rape" drug, and body-building supplement.

HISTORY OF USE

Russian chemist Alexander Mikhaylovich Zaytsev first reported the synthesis of GHB (gamma-hydroxybutyric acid) in 1874. French scientist Henri Laborit performed some of the first GHB research in the 1960s. In the late 1980s and 1990s, GHB was sold over-the-counter in the United States as a body-building supplement and sleep aid. Increased incidents of GHB intoxication moved the US Centers for Disease Control and Prevention and the US Food and Drug Administration (FDA) to issue warnings regarding its potential dangers.

In the late 1990s, GHB was used in several highly publicized drug-facilitated cases of sexual assault. Because of this, people labeled GHB a "date rape" drug. Because illicit formulations of GHB are commonly colorless, odorless liquids, surreptitious addition of GHB to drinks in bars and clubs is difficult to detect. Also, several GHB side effects (sedation, euphoria, decreased inhibitions, enhanced sex drive, and mild amnesia) enhance its effectiveness in drug-facilitated sexual assaults. In 2000, the FDA placed Xyrem on the list of schedule III controlled substances and listed nonmedical GHB as a schedule I controlled substance.

Also during the 1990s, GHB became widely used as a club drug. Club or party drugs are used by people who attend nightclubs, raves, and circuit parties. These drugs include methamphetamine, 3,4-methylenedioxymethamphetamine (MDMA, or ecstasy), lysergic acid diethylamide (LSD, or acid), and ketamine (special K). GHB, ecstasy, and ketamine are frequently used together, also in combination with alcohol, marijuana, and amphetamines.

The popularity of GHB as a club drug is largely due to the ease of its synthesis and its low cost. GHB is quite popular in dance clubs for persons younger than age twenty-one years, where alcohol is not sold; however, the youth in these clubs can drink water or other non-alcoholic beverages spiked with GHB. Club drugs related to GHB include gamma-butyrolactone (GBL) and 1,4-butanediol, both of which are liquids and found in paint strippers and varnish thinners. These chemicals are known as GHB "prodrugs" because they are converted to GHB by the body after ingestion.

EFFECTS AND POTENTIAL RISKS

In the brain, cells called neurons generate and propagate nerve impulses. GHB exerts its effects by binding to specific receptors on the surfaces of neurons. GHB binds to the GABAB and GHB receptors. When it binds the GABAB receptor, GHB causes sedation. Conversely, binding of the GHB receptor increases the release of the neurotransmitter glutamate, which is the principal excitatory neurotransmitter in the brain. Simultaneous activation of both the GHB and GABAB receptors at low GHB concentrations induces the release of the neurotransmitter dopaminedopamine in the ventral tegmental area (VTA). The VTA is one of the key reward regions of the brain, and dopamine release in the VTA produces a feeling of pleasure or satisfaction and is the reason for the addictive nature of GHB.

GHB induces sleep by binding GABAB receptors in the thalamo-cortical loop, which regulates sleep and arousal. Because GHB binds to the GHB receptor much more tightly than the GABAB receptor, decreases in the bodily concentration of GHB increase its stimulatory effects relative to its sedative effects. This causes people who have taken GHB to awaken abruptly after a particular time.

The effects of GHB are dose related. At 10 milligrams per kilogram body weight (mg/kg), GHB depresses the central nervous system and causes a general sense of calm and relaxation. GHB doses of 20 to 30 mg/kg induce sleep for two to three hours. A dose of 40 to 50 mg/kg induces even longer periods of sleep, but also causes amnesia, nausea and vomiting, dizziness, weakness, loss of peripheral vision, confusion, hallucinations, agitation, and low heart rate (bradycardia). Doses above 50 mg/kg cause seizures, unconsciousness, respiratory depression, and coma. GHB effects appear within fifteen minutes of oral ingestion, but the acute symptoms cease after seven hours.

Combining GHB with alcohol increases depression of breathing and can cause death. GHB is rather addictive, and long-term use can cause depression and suicidal tendencies. From 1995 to 2005 in the United Kingdom, the United States, and Canada, there were 226 GHB-related deaths.

FURTHER READING

Abadinsky, Howard. *Drug Use and Abuse: A Comprehensive Introduction.* 7th ed. Florence, KY: Wadsworth, 2010. A readable, but erudite, interdisciplinary introduction to drug abuse by a criminal justice academic who spent many years as a parole officer and inspector for the Cook County Sheriff's Office.

Gahlinger, Paul. *Illegal Drugs: A Complete Guide to Their History, Chemistry, Use, and Abuse.* New York: Plume, 2003. An informative compendium on the chemical, medical, and historical aspects of illegal drugs by a physician who is also a certified substance-abuse review officer.

Grim, Ryan. *This Is Your Country on Drugs: The Secret History of Getting High in America.* Hoboken, NJ: Wiley, 2010. A journalist examines illegal drugs, drug supply lines, the culture of drug abuse and drug abusers, the political and economic ramifications of drug abuse, and the problems facing drug enforcement in the United States.

Kuhn, Cynthia, Scott Swartzwelder, and Wilkie Wilson. *Buzzed: The Straight Facts about the Most Used and Abused Drugs from Alcohol to Ecstasy.* 3rd ed. New York: W. W. Norton, 2008. A popular and useful guide to illegal drugs by three professors from Duke University Medical Center.

WEBSITES OF INTEREST
National Institute on Drug Abuse
http://www.drugabuse.gov/infofacts/clubdrugs.html
Project GHB
http://www.projectghb.org
US Drug Enforcement Administration
http://www.justice.gov/dea/concern/ghb.html

Michael A. Buratovich

SEE ALSO: Date Rape Drugs; Depressants Abuse

Hallucinogens and their effects

Hallucinogens are substances that cause alterations of perception, including but not limited to changing what users see, hear, feel, taste, smell, and experience about themselves and their relationship to the world and others.

SIGNIFICANCE
Hallucinogenic drugs are widely used in the United States, despite the fact that such use can be dangerous and even life-threatening. Law-enforcement agencies expend significant resources in efforts to reduce the illegal manufacture, sale, and use of such drugs.

Hallucinogenic drugs, or hallucinogens, are capable of altering the perceptions of those who ingest them. Historically, some hallucinogens have been important parts of cultural rituals, particularly spiritual ceremonies and developmental rites of passage, and their use has been socially sanctioned because of these associations. Most hallucinogen use in the United States, however, is recreational in nature.

EFFECTS
As the name implies, hallucinations—internal perceptions that separate the individual from reality and that are not perceptible to others— are common effects of

hallucinogen usage. The hallucinatory experiences associated with these drugs may include increased awareness of surroundings and perceptual distortions, such as perceived heightened visual ability or changes in the way motion is perceived. Any and all of the senses may be affected simultaneously, creating often illogical and nonlinear observations. Some users of hallucinogens have reported experiencing synesthesia, a phenomenon in which one sense overlaps with another. For instance, the notes, melodies, and harmonies of music may be perceived both as sounds and as colors.

Users of hallucinogens may also experience a different sense of themselves as persons, with the drugs affecting their perceptions of consciousness and their bodies in relationship to others. Some experience greatly increased empathy and feelings of connection to others and the environment. In fact, in some users, the perceived dissolution of personal boundaries may proceed to such an extent that they cannot perceive any sense of self—in essence, they feel they become their surroundings.

The experience of taking a hallucinogen is often referred to as a trip. Some trips are brief; others are long. Experiences can vary substantially from one use session to the next in terms of length of time a person is affected, the quality of the experience (pleasurable or upsetting), the number of senses affected, and so on. Some of this variation may be accounted for by the specific drugs used, the dosages taken, the quality or purity of the drugs, and the physical and environmental circumstances or contexts under which the drugs are taken.

HOW HALLUCINOGENS WORK

In a 2001 research report, the National Institute on Drug Abuse describes the different ways in which hallucinogens and dissociative drugs work in the human body.

Hallucinogens cause their effects by disrupting the interaction of nerve cells and the neurotransmitter serotonin. Distributed throughout the brain and spinal cord, the serotonin system is involved in the control of behavioral, perceptual, and regulatory systems, including mood, hunger, body temperature, sexual behavior, muscle control, and sensory perception. . . . The dissociative drugs act by altering distribution of the neurotransmitter glutamate throughout the brain. Glutamate is involved in perception of pain, responses to the environment, and memory.

SUBSTANCES

Hallucinogens include human-made drugs, such as psychedelic "club drugs," as well as substances derived from certain plants and fungi. In the United States, these substances are classified as having no medical uses, although this is a matter of some debate. Some have argued that particular hallucinogens may be useful for treating trauma, psychopathology, and even conditions such as headaches.

Common hallucinogens include lysergic acid diethylamide (LSD), 2,5-dimethoxy-4-methylamphetamine (known as DOM or STP), and 3,4-methylenedioxymethamphetamine (also known as MDMA or ecstasy). Also popular are psilocybin, a hallucinogen derived from mushrooms (sometimes known as magic mushrooms), and peyote. Peyote, which is derived from the mescal cactus and contains mescaline, has a long history of being used in Native American spiritual ceremonies. Dimethyltryptamine (DMT), another substance found in plants and seeds but that also may be synthesized, is used for its hallucinogenic properties.

Users seeking hallucinogenic properties in their recreational drugs of choice also sometimes abuse substances that were originally seen as anesthetics, such as ketamine (known as special K) and phencyclidine (known as PCP or angel dust). These drugs' dissociative properties lead users to experience feelings of being detached from themselves or their experiences.

ASSOCIATED PROBLEMS

The experiences, or trips, that individuals have when they take hallucinogens can be pleasant or unpleasant. When pleasant, a trip can be a memorable experience, but when unpleasant, it can be like living trapped in a nightmare. Either circumstance can be dangerous, particularly if the individual under the influence is unsupervised. When experiencing pleasant hallucinations, users of hallucinogens may believe they can do things they cannot physically do (such as fly), and this may result in accidental injury or even death. Negative hallucinations may lead to aggression and paranoia that can spur attacks on others or objects, which may result in property damage, injuries, or—in extreme cases—deaths. In addition, users have reported the phenomenon of flashbacks—that is, the re-experiencing of trips well after the drugs' initial effects have passed. Such unexpected experiences may lead to confusion, aggression, and accidental injury.

STREET NAMES FOR HALLUCINOGENS AND DISSOCIATIVE DRUGS

LSD (lysergic acid diethylamide)
- acid
- blotter
- blotter acid
- boomers
- dots
- microdot
- pane
- paper acid
- sugar
- sugar cubes
- trip
- window glass
- windowpane
- yellow sunshine
- Zen

Ketamine
- bump
- cat Valium
- green
- honey oil
- jet
- K
- purple
- Special K
- special la coke
- super acid
- super C
- vitamin K

PCP
- angel
- angel dust
- boat
- dummy dust
- love boat
- peace
- superglass
- zombie

Hallucinogen use disorders follow the same pattern of problems as do use disorders associated with other substances of abuse. The use of hallucinogens may lead to daily functioning problems at work, home, or school, as trips and their associated recovery times may be lengthy. Hallucinogens can sometimes exacerbate preexisting psychological problems, and research indicates that they may even cause psychological problems, such as psychosis, in some users.

Like other substances of abuse, hallucinogens pose problems for law-enforcement agencies, which must expend significant resources to combat the illegal manufacture, sale, and use of these drugs as well as other crimes that stem from the actions of persons under the influence of hallucinogens. The production and distribution of hallucinogens and their components are particularly noteworthy growing problems, as manufacturers and drug traffickers increasingly conduct their business using the Internet.

FURTHER READING

Holland, Julie. Ecstasy: The Complete Guide— A Comprehensive Look at the Risks and Benefits of MDMA. Rochester, Vt.: Inner Traditions International, 2001. Presents data and arguments pertaining to the typical risks that may be expected from ecstasy and other club drugs. Includes discussion of research perspectives on the potential benefits of these drugs.

Jansen, Karl. Ketamine: Dreams and Realities. Ben Lomond, Calif.: Multidisciplinary Association for Psychedelic Studies, 2004. Provides a historical perspective on the uses of ketamine, a hallucinogenic substance, and addresses the risks and benefits related to the drug.

Julien, Robert M. A Primer of Drug Action: A Comprehensive Guide to the Actions, Uses, and Side Effects of Psychoactive Drugs. 10th ed. New York: Worth, 2005. Presents full coverage of the topic of hallucinogens, including information on these drugs' effects on mind and body and at the level of neurotransmitters.

Schultes, RichardEvans. Hallucinogenic Plants. New York: Golden Press, 1976. Illustrated field guide describes many different kinds of hallucinogenic plants and offers a historical perspective on their use.

Stafford, Peter. Psychedelics. Oakland, Calif.: Ronin, 2003. Provides broad descriptions of drugs that affect perception, focusing on what these substances may look like and how they may affect users. Also discusses the drugs' individual and societal impacts.

Weil, Andrew, and Winifred Rosen. From Chocolate to Morphine: Everything You Need to Know About Mind-Altering Drugs. Rev. ed. Boston: Houghton Mifflin, 2004. Presents a down-to-earth discussion of drugs that affect the mind. Easy to read.

Nancy A. Piotrowski

SEE ALSO: Designer Drugs; LSD; Mushrooms/Psilocybin; PCP

Heroin

Heroin is a highly addictive opioid drug derived from the poppy plant. As an opiate, it functions as a central nervous system depressant similar to morphine, opium, methadone, and hydromorphone (Dilaudid).

BUPRENORPHINE

Buprenorphine is an opioid analgesic approved for use in the treatment of moderate to severe pain and for treatment of opioid dependence. Buprenorphine has been investigated for treating symptoms associated with opioid and heroin withdrawal. It is available as a sublingual tablet for treating dependence, and it is classified as a schedule III controlled substance.

Buprenorphine therapy is divided into three phases: the induction phase, when treatment is initiated after a patient has abstained from opioid products for twelve to twenty-four hours; the stabilization phase, during which time a patient gradually reduces or discontinues the use of opioid products; and the maintenance phase, in which a patient continues a steady buprenorphine dose for an indefinite time to control cravings and withdrawal symptoms associated with opioid abstinence.

HISTORY OF USE

Diacetylmorphine, later named heroin, was originally synthesized in 1874 in London by the English chemist C. R. Alder Wright. However, it was not until 1898 that Bayer Pharmaceutical Company of Germany commercially introduced heroin as a new pain remedy and nonaddictive substitute for morphine. During the next several decades, heroin was sold legally worldwide and aggressively marketed as a cough medicine and as a safer, more potent form of morphine.

By the early twentieth century, heroin's intense euphoric effects were fully recognized, leading to widespread misuse. Numerous restrictions on the production, use, sale, and distribution of heroin were established to help prevent further abuse. These restrictions included the Harrison Narcotics Act of 1914, the Dangerous Drug Act of 1920, and the Heroin Act of 1924. As a result, heroin consumption briefly declined, but illicit production and trafficking grew. Heroin became one of the most sought after drugs in the world and, by 1970, the US Drug Enforcement Administration classified heroin as a schedule I controlled narcotic. Class I drugs are those with a high abuse potential and no legitimate medical use.

Various methods have been used to gain heroin highs over the years, depending on user preference and drug purity. The most common and economical method of heroin use is injection, or "shooting up." Popular forms of shooting up include "mainlining" (injecting directly into a vein) and "skin-popping" (injecting directly into a muscle or under the skin).

Snorting and smoking heroin became popular as a result of the availability of higher quality heroin, the fear of contracting blood-borne illnesses through needle sharing, and the erroneous belief that inhaling heroin would not lead to addiction. The best-known method of smoking heroin is "chasing the dragon." Originating in the 1950s in Hong Kong, this method involves heating and liquefying the drug on tin foil and inhaling the vapors.

Some users crave an even greater high and engage in "speedballing" or "crisscrossing," which involves simultaneously injecting or snorting alternate lines of heroin and cocaine, respectively. Heroin is considered one of the most dangerous and psychologically and physically addictive drugs available. It remains a serious health issue throughout the world.

EFFECTS AND POTENTIAL RISKS

Heroin is the fastest acting of the opiates; it is three times more potent than morphine. It acts by depressing the central nervous system through an endorphin-like mechanism. Heroin rapidly crosses the blood-brain barrier because of its high lipid solubility. It is quickly metabolized into morphine and binds to the opioid receptors responsible not only for suppressing pain sensation and relieving anxiety but also for critical life processes.

The short-term effects of heroin are attributed to its properties as an opiate. These effects have made heroin one of the most desirable drugs in the world. Heroin produces a warm surge of pleasure and euphoria referred to as a rush. This rush is followed by feelings of peacefulness, well-being, contentment, and physical relaxation. Users go "on the nod," alternating between wakeful and drowsy states while experiencing little sensitivity to pain.

Minor, negative, short-term effects of heroin use include nausea, vomiting, constipation, severe itching, dry mouth, difficulty urinating, heavy extremities, impaired mental functioning, and constricted pupils. Nonpleasurable sensations, such as irritability and depression, can occur as the high dissipates. However, the most serious side effect of heroin use is respiratory depression, which can be fatal.

The most immediate and intense heroin rush is achieved by intravenous injection. However, this transmission route is the most dangerous. The risk of contracting infectious diseases such as human immunodeficiency virus and hepatitis viruses is substantial. Furthermore, illegal street heroin can be contaminated with unknown additives and impurities such as sugar, starch, and poisons, which can cause blood vessel inflammation, blockage, and permanent damage.

Long-term heroin use can lead to adverse physical effects, including collapsed veins, heart and skin infections, liver and kidney disease, and pulmonary complications. Continuous heroin use may affect brain functioning as a result of repeated respiratory suppression and lack of oxygen. However, the most detrimental long-term effect of heroin use is physical and psychological dependence and addiction, which can occur quickly; users crave larger and larger doses of the drug to achieve the original high.

FURTHER READING

Brezina, Corona. *Heroin: The Deadly Addiction.* New York: Rosen, 2009. Discusses the health implications of abusing heroin.

Cobb, Allan B., and Ronald J. Brogan. *Heroin: Junior Drug Awareness.* New York: Chelsea House, 2009. Provides a basic overview of the history of heroin abuse and its addictive nature. Written for younger readers.

Elliot-Wright, Susan. *Heroin.* Chicago: Raintree, 2005. Examines the history, health effects, treatment, and prevention of heroin addiction and its dangerous effect on society.

Libby, Therissa A. *Heroin: The Basics.* Center City, MN: Hazelden, 2007. An introduction to the history, health effects, and addiction risks of heroin use.

Morales, Francis. *The Little Book of Heroin.* Berkeley, CA: Ronin, 2000. Discusses the history and chemistry of heroin and ways to avoid heroin addiction.

WEBSITES OF INTEREST

MedlinePlus: "Heroin"
http://www.nlm.nih.gov/medlineplus/heroin.html
National Institute on Drug Abuse
http://www.drugabuse.gov/infofacts/heroin.html
US Drug Enforcement Administration
http://www.justice.gov/dea/concern/heroin.html#1

Rose Cuilla-Bohling

SEE ALSO: Teens and Drug Abuse

Inhalants abuse

Inhalants abuse is the repeated inhalation of fumes, vapors, or gases from common household and commercial products despite evident negative effects.

GLUE

Like other abused inhalants, including cleaning compounds and petroleum products, many adhesives, including glue, contain a potent blend of chemicals, many of which can be intoxicating when inhaled in sufficient quantity. A common way of abusing adhesives is to squeeze an amount into a plastic bag, hold the bag against the nose and mouth, and then inhale the substance, which is made up of various chemicals; inhaling from a bag also limits oxygen intake and increases the effects of the inhalant.

Although their effects pass quickly, several of these chemicals, including toluene and hexane, affect gait and balance, movement, the brain's speech centers, and higher executive functions. In turn, these effects can lead to increased aggression or euphoria.

Many of these effects are augmented by low oxygen levels in the brain, leading to increased loss of balance and coordination and poor decision making. US government studies conducted in the early twenty-first century have shown an increase in inhalant abuse among older adolescents and young adults.

CAUSES

Inhalation of fumes, vapors, or gases leads to the rapid onset of a high that resembles alcohol intoxication. The chemicals in the inhalants are quickly absorbed from the lungs into the bloodstream and from there to the brain and other organs. The initial high lasts for only a few minutes, so most abusers inhale repeatedly over time to maintain a sustained high. Repeated use builds up tolerance, leading to the need for higher and more frequent dosing.

RISK FACTORS

Inhalant products, such as glues, nail polish removers, hairsprays, felt-tip markers, lighter fluids, and spray paints, are readily available in the home and the community. More than one thousand products containing inhalants can be obtained at a low cost and, for the most part, without legal restrictions on purchase or use. US state laws prohibiting the sale of products containing certain inhalants to minors are difficult to enforce. Legal consequences for abusing the few restricted inhalants are minimal.

Most first-time abusers are preteens or young adolescents who begin by experimenting with friends. Among the youngest users, girls are about as likely as boys to try inhalers. In contrast, among young adults, abuse is twice as common among men as among women. The National Institute on Drug Abuse estimates that about 15 percent of all eighth graders have had some experience with abusing inhalants and that 70 percent of abusers were younger than age eighteen years when their inhalants abuse began.

SYMPTOMS

The initial, brief high experienced with inhalants abuse is followed by drowsiness, lightheadedness, and agitation. Short-term adverse effects that can develop include headache, numbness and muscle weakness, nausea, and abdominal pain. Hearing loss and visual disturbances, even hallucinations, may occur.

Long-term use may result in weight loss, disorientation, incoordination, irritability, depression, and irreversible damage to the brain, heart, kidneys, liver, and other organs. Even a first-time user is at risk of death. The abuser can develop a rapid and erratic heartbeat, which can lead to cardiac arrest and death. Abuse also can reduce the body's oxygen level, leading to suffocation.

SCREENING AND DIAGNOSIS

Changes in an abuser's appearance and behavior are the primary indicators of abuse. An abuser may have red or runny eyes and nose, spots or sores around the mouth, paint or other products on the face, lips, nose, or fingers, or unusual breath odor or the odor of chemicals on clothing. The abuser may have slurred speech and appear to be dazed or drunk.

Behavioral changes include increased anxiety, excitability, and irritability. The abuser may become belligerent, even violent, with swings between extreme agitation and lethargy. Speech may be slurred. Disciplinary problems or truancy may develop. Extracurricular activities may be dropped in favor of socializing with friends or staying home. The abuser may develop a new set of friends or become a loner. Conflict with siblings and parents may increase.

No test, such as urinalysis, will detect inhalants abuse. The user has to be confronted and admit to the problem.

TREATMENT AND THERAPY

For most abusers, treatment is community-based and focuses on behavioral changes. One should listen to what an abuser has to say and remain calm and nonjudgmental. This may provide clues to underlying problems, such as peer pressure or problems at home, which can be resolved or redirected. One should focus on the serious health risks of inhalants abuse, not on such behavior being "bad," and should redirect an abuser to constructive, safe, and healthy activities.

A frequent or relapsing abuser will require professional help to identify and address underlying causes for the abuse and any concomitant physical or psychological problems. An initial step is a medical examination to determine if inhalants abuse has caused organ damage. Neurologic, psychological, and cognitive assessments should be part of the initial examination. Family stability, structure, and dynamics may contribute to the abuser's behavior. An effort should be made to obtain constructive participation in treatment by the abuser's family.

Few treatment centers address inhalants abuse. Detoxification may take up to thirty or forty days because inhaled chemicals stored in fatty tissue take a long time to break down and be flushed from the body.

During withdrawal, the abuser may experience headaches, nausea, excessive sweating and chills, tremors, muscle cramps, hallucinations, and even delirium. Relapse is common among heavy abusers, especially if underlying behavioral problems are not addressed.

PREVENTION

Children should be informed about the dangers of experimenting with inhalants, preferably before they try them. Inhalants abuse can be the gateway to further substance abuse. Parents, teachers, and other adults involved with children and young adolescents should know and be on guard for warning signs, including behavior changes, and should be prepared to discuss the dangers of inhalants abuse with the young person.

Parents should be aware of what inhalant products are in the home and how they can be used and stored so the risk of abuse is minimized. Similarly, school personnel should assess the use and storage of inhalant products in schools. Programs such as the Alliance for Consumer Education Inhalant Abuse Prevention Program can help parents, teachers, school administrators, and community leaders.

FURTHER READING

Abadinsky, Howard. *Drug Use and Abuse: A Comprehensive Introduction*. 7th ed. Belmont, CA: Wadsworth, 2011. Focuses on what drugs are abused, how they are abused, and how abuse is treated. Inhalants abuse is covered in chapter 6.

Julien, Robert M. *A Primer of Drug Actions*. 11th ed. New York: Worth, 2008. A concise, nontechnical guide to the mechanisms of action, side effects, uses, and abuses of psychoactive drugs. Chapter 4 is on inhalants.

Kuhn, Cynthia, Scott Swartwelder, and Wilkie Wilson. *Buzzed: The Straight Facts about the Most Used and Abused Drugs from Alcohol to Ecstasy*. 3rd ed. New York: W. W. Norton, 2008. Contains an informative, easy-to-read section on the risks involved in inhalants abuse.

Lowinson, Joyce W., et al., eds. *Substance Abuse: A Comprehensive Textbook*. 4th ed. Philadelphia: Lippincott, 2005. A comprehensive textbook on substance abuse. Chapter 20 covers inhalants abuse.

WEBSITES OF INTEREST

Alliance for Consumer Education, Inhalant Abuse Prevention Program
http://www.inhalant.org
National Inhalant Prevention Coalition
http://www.inhalants.com
National Institute on Drug Abuse
http://www.drugabuse.gov

Ernest Kohlmetz

SEE ALSO: Stimulants and Their Effects

Intervention

In the field of psychology, "intervention" is a term used to convey actions, therapeutic or experimental, to effect change. In many ways, the field of psychology is best known for its interventions in clinical treatment and research; therefore, this concept is a foundational one for the field.

INTRODUCTION

The word "intervention" is derived from the word "intervene," which means to come in between in a way that causes change. It is a term that is used in many profes-sions, including medicine, nursing, education, and law enforcement. The term is also used in the mental health field in several ways; one applies to clinicians and one applies to researchers. Across all professions, however, interventions are designed to be specific actions to deal with specific problems. In mental health, the typical target of intervention is psychopathology.

Among clinicians, the term "intervention" is generally used to refer to any application of a specific psychotherapy plan or technique. For instance, a clinician planning to work with a client who is depressed might describe the chosen intervention to combat the depression as a cognitive behavior therapy. Thus the therapy described was the way in which the therapist intended to make changes happen on the identified problem.

Researchers in mental health also use the term "intervention" but in a slightly different way. Those who do clinical research might also be looking to compare one treatment to another type of treatment or placebo (also known as an innocuous or inactive treatment). To discuss such research plans, professionals use special language that describes the mechanics of research methodology. Part of research methodology for any research project is the specific design chosen. In this case, where a researcher was comparing a treatment to a placebo condition, the methodology language would call this design a two-group comparison of intervention versus control, or, sometimes, treatment versus placebo. As such, among professionals working in mental health, the term "intervention" has at least two meanings. One is related to general clinical work. The second is related more to research. In some areas of mental health, the word also has specific implications. In the treatment for addictive behavior, for instance, intervention has a precise meaning.

USE IN ADDICTIONS AND SUBSTANCE USE TREATMENT

Beginning treatment for addiction generally requires that one either enter treatment voluntarily or otherwise be remanded to such care for legal reasons. Mental health professionals prefer that clients enter treatment voluntarily. Occasionally this does not happen because the person suffering fails to recognize the problem. With substance use and other problems related to addiction, this happens frequently because the range of problems demanding treatment can extend from mild to severe. With less-severe problems, social pressure to encourage a person to seek help might be scant. As problems become more severe and the presence of an addiction becomes more pronounced, however, social pressure to seek help does increase. Sometimes, family members and significant others may conclude that a loved one needs help before the loved one recognizes the problem. If the individual does not seek help, then others may seek out qualified professionals to help them perform an intervention.

Traditionally and predominantly used in the addictions field, the intervention approach expanded after the mid-1980s to address a wide range of self-destructive behaviors. In this technique, the attempt to effect change usually occurs in a circumscribed period of time and in a planned locale. These procedures should not be attempted without serious study and even consultation. In some cases, interventions can be simple, firm conversations that set boundaries with the intent of helping the person to change. In others, more sophisticated strategies may be needed, involving more people. In the latter case, the concerned party often enlists the help of professionals, usually called interventionists, to help them prepare for the event. Preparation typically involves identifying individuals whom the addicted person knows well and who have seen the effects of the addiction on that person's life. These individuals then convene for a structured confrontation that stresses concern for the welfare and safety of the confronted individual. The desired end result is usually for the person to decide to enter treatment.

FURTHER READING

Clough, Peter, and Cathy Nutbrown. *A Student's Guide to Methodology.* 3d ed. London: Sage, 2012. Print.

Corsini, Raymond J., and Danny Wedding. *Current Psychotherapies.* 10th ed. Belmont: Brooks-Cole, 2014. Print.

Health Library. "Intervention Trial." *Health Library.* EBSCO Information Services, 2014. Web. 27 May 2014.

Jay, Jeff, and Debra Jay. *Love First: A Family's Guide to Intervention.* 2d ed. Center City: Hazelden, 2008. Print.

Johnson, Vernon E. *Intervention: How to Help Someone Who Doesn't Want Help.* Center City: Hazelden, 2009. Digital file.

Mayo Clinic. "Intervention: Help a Loved One Overcome Addiction." *Mayo Clinic Diseases and Conditions: Mental Illness.* Mayo Foundation for Medical Education and Research, 23 Aug. 2011. Web. 27 May 2014.

Meier, Scott T. *Measuring Change in Counseling and Psychotherapy.* New York: Guilford, 2008. Print.

Nancy A. Piotrowski

SEE ALSO: Addictive Personality and Behaviors

Laxative abuse

Laxative abuse is the repeated and routine use of laxatives to lose weight, shed unwanted calories, feel thin, feel empty, manage bowel movements, or treat constipation. There are different types of laxatives, but stimulant and bulk agents are the most common. Stimulant laxatives and osmotic laxatives physically alter the bowel's ability to function, and with excessive use can cause permanent damage. Bulk agents do not have the same physical effects as stimulant laxatives if taken as directed, but the user may become psychologically dependent on these laxatives.

CAUSES

There are several causative factors associated with the abuse of laxatives. One is the mistaken belief that laxatives will prevent the absorption of calories and help with weight reduction. Another factor is the mistaken belief that daily bowel movements are a necessary part of good health and that laxative use is a harmless remedy to ensure this occurs. A third factor is the repeated use of laxatives to relieve constipation.

RISK FACTORS

There are four groups of people at risk for laxative abuse. The largest group to abuse laxatives includes persons who have an eating disordereating disordersand laxative abuse, such as anorexia or bulimia nervosa. Adolescents and young adults with low self-esteem and poor body image are particularly prone to disordered eating and laxative abuse. Anorexia nervosa is the severe restriction of food intake to bring about drastic weight loss, which in turn causes dehydration and subsequent constipation. Bulimia nervosa is characterized by a cycle of binge eating followed by behaviors such as vomiting or laxative abuse to compensate or reverse the effects of binge eating.

A second group to abuse laxatives includes athletes who need to stay within a specific weight range; these athletes include wrestlers, boxers, and jockeys. A third group is made up of middle-aged and older people with frequent bouts of constipation. In this group, excessive use often comes with the misperception that daily bowel movements are part of good health. The fourth group includes persons with a factitious disorder, wherein they abuse laxatives to intentionally cause diarrhea.

SYMPTOMS

Several physical warning signs and personality traits indicate laxative abuse. The physical signs include a history of alternating diarrhea and constipation or chronic diarrhea of an unknown origin; physical signs also include gastrointestinal complaints such as cramping or pain, dehydration, and retention of fluids that cause severe bloating and the feeling of being fat.

Certain personality traits are characteristic of those who abuse laxatives. These traits include an obsession with weight and body shape, low self-esteem, impulsiveness, and anxiousness. Exhibiting one of these traits does not mean a person is a laxative abuser, but having a combination of traits may increase the risk of laxative abuse. For example, if a person is obsessed with weight and has low self-esteem, they may binge eat. When this behavior does not make that person feel better, he or she may turn to laxatives to get rid of the calories just consumed.

SCREENING AND DIAGNOSIS

Screening and diagnosis of laxative abuse is tricky and oftentimes difficult because many abusers want to hide the behavior. The best screening tool is a clinician's suspicion. Once a clinician suspects laxative abuse, he or she can order blood tests to check for an electrolyte (potassium, magnesium, sodium, and chloride) imbalance, as chronic diarrhea will remove electrolytes through the stool and will prevent them from being absorbed into the body.

Persons with an eating disorder typically have low potassium levels in their blood (a condition called hypokalemia). Clinicians can check urine for the presence of a laxative. Another screening method is to perform a personality assessment by having the person complete surveys related to body dissatisfaction, low self-esteem, and level of drive to stay or be thin.

TREATMENT AND THERAPY

To overcome laxative abuse, users will need the medical expertise of a general physician, will need therapy with a psychologist or psychiatrist, and will need consultation with a registered dietician. The most immedi-

ate treatment is to stop taking laxatives and to seek a physician's care.

Many people will experience withdrawal symptoms that usually last from one to three weeks; in rare cases symptoms have lasted two days to two or three months. Side effects of withdrawal include constipation, fluid retention, feeling bloated, and temporary weight gain. To treat these side effects one should drink six to ten cups of water per day and decaffeinated beverages to hydrate one's body. (Caffeine is a diuretic and promotes fluid loss, and dehydration causes constipation.) One should eat regular meals and foods that promote normal bowel functioning, such as whole-grain or wheat bran foods with plenty of fluids, vegetables, and fruits.

Routine physical activity also helps regulate the bowel, but a physician should be consulted first because intense exercise can worsen constipation. Physicians may start their patients on fiber and osmotic supplements to help the bowel function properly and to establish normal bowel movements.

PREVENTION

No guaranteed mechanism prevents laxative abuse. However, education can be a powerful tool in helping people understand that laxatives will not prevent the body from absorbing food or losing weight. Moreover, routine laxative use will have a reverse effect on the body, causing dehydration and constipation. Also, social support from friends and family and being aware of the signs and symptoms of abuse are crucial; intervention could prevent long-term laxative abuse and irreversible physical and psychological consequences.

FURTHER READING

"How to Stop Abusing Laxatives." EatingDisordersReview. com. 1999. Web. 22 Feb. 2012. http://www.eatingdisordersreview.com/nl/nl_edr_10_5_14. Presents tips on how to stop abusing laxatives. Outlines common symptoms that will occur once laxatives are discontinued and discusses myths and medical complications about laxative use.

Le Grange, Daniel, and James Lock. *Eating Disorders in Children and Adolescents: A Clinical Handbook.* New York: Guilford, 2011. Chapters examine etiology and neurobiology, epidemiology, diagnosis and classification, medical issues and assessment, treatment, prevention, and parental roles.

Roerig, James L., et al. "Laxative Abuse: Epidemiology, Diagnosis, and Management." *Drugs* 70.12 (2010):

1487–503. Print. A comprehensive medical article about laxative abuse that describes persons at risk of this disorder, examines medical complications from laxative misuse, and discusses treatments for this disorder.

WEBSITES OF INTEREST
Bulimia.com
http://www.bulimia.com
National Eating Disorders Association
http://www.nationaleatingdisorders.org

Christine G. Holzmueller

SEE ALSO: Anorexia Nervosa and Bulimia Nervosa; Eating Disorders; Staying in a Healthy Weight Range

LSD

LSD, a synthetic amide of lysergic acid found in ergot, a fungus on grains, is a psychoactive intoxicant, similar to but stronger than psilocybin or mescaline. LSD has powerful mind-altering effects, usually called hallucinogenic or psychedelic.

HISTORY OF USE

LSD was synthesized in 1938 by Albert HoffmanAlbert Hoffman , of Sandoz Laboratories in Basel, Switzerland, as part of a research program seeking new medicines. LSD did not seem to offer such promise, but in 1943 Hoffman accidentally ingested a dose, experienced its psychoactive effects, and described these effects as being surprisingly transformational.

For the next twenty years, Sandoz Laboratories marketed LSD for research purposes. Among early research was that by the US Central Intelligence Agency, U.S.and LSD from the 1950s through the 1970s, in an attempt to discover whether LSD could be used for mind-control purposes. Mostly, however, psychiatry and psychology became involved, initially because LSD seemed to simulate a "model psychosis."

The perceptual distortions induced by LSD, however, are not experienced as hallucinations in the sense of something that is not there; rather, they transform what is given in the perceptual field. This distinction led Canadian psychiatrists Humphry Osmond, Abram Hoffer, and Duncan Blewett to use LSD as a treatment for psychosis. LSD was also studied as an adjunct in psychotherapy, especially by Stanislav Grof in Czechoslovakia. Before its criminalization, more than forty thousand patients were treated with LSD psychotherapy. Notable results occurred in alcoholics, felons, and the terminally ill, persons who normally are resistant to successful therapeutic outcomes.

In the United States, research was conducted at Harvard University by Timothy Leary, Ralph Metzner, and Richard Alpert (who later became Ram Dass). The trio's 1964 book *The Psychedelic Experience* popularized the view that LSD could be useful in enhancing human potential. Leary, in particular, became a public advocate for LSD with his slogan to "turn on, tune in, drop out."

Soon writers such as Aldous Huxley and Ken Kesey and musicians, most famously the Beatles, also reflected a view of LSD's possibilities. Cary Grant, a major film star, attributed a "new assessment of life" to his experience on LSD. By the 1960s, LSD had become a common drug for American youth, especially in California, where it spread among the burgeoning counterculture. Owsley Stanley, who made and distributed a large amount of LSD in San Francisco in the mid-1960s, is known for fueling the upsurge of interest there. Largely because of this sense that LSD contributed to a rejection of mainstream values, the drug became intensely controversial and the subject of much negative publicity. The manufacture and sale of LSD was made a crime in 1965 and possession was criminalized in 1966.

According to the US Substance Abuse and Mental Health Services Administration, LSD use peaked in the early 1970s, fell slowly to a low in 2003, and has been increasing since. The National Household Survey on Drug Abuse indicated that 20.2 million Americans age twelve years and older used LSD at least once in their lifetime. The most common age of first-time users is eighteen years.

EFFECTS AND POTENTIAL RISKS

The effects of LSD become noticeable within thirty to sixty minutes and last six to eight hours or more. The threshold dose is 25 micrograms (mcg), and 100 to 250 mcg is typical; beyond 400 mcg no further change seems to occur. A feature of LSD is how widely its effects vary. Researchers quickly realized the keys to this variability are the mental set (or state) of the user and the setting in which the drug is used.

The physiological effects of LSD include changes to the pulse rate, muscular tension, blood pressure, constriction of arteries in the periphery, and pupil dilation.

These effects tend to be mild and do not last beyond the psychoactive period. Longer term effects have been reported, most spectacularly chromosome breakage, but these claims have not survived rigorous research.

Negative experiential effects of LSD are cognitive and emotional. Judgment is impaired such that the user is not as concerned with safety. Emotionally, a user can become so disoriented as to feel anxiety or panic, a reaction augmented if the setting were conducive to disorientation. A rare longer-term negative effect is the unwelcome vivid memory of an emotionally charged moment from the LSD event, known as a flashback.

The experiential effects of LSD include positive aesthetic, psychological, and spiritual transformations. Aesthetically, the effects center on perceptual changes, especially to the visual field, which is intensely enhanced with greater mobility, colorfulness, transiency, luminosity, energy, swelling, vividness, and synesthesia. Psychologically, the effects of LSD include mood changes, particularly feelings of well-being and euphoria; a new and greater awareness of the world and of self; a deeper understanding of human relationships; a transcendence of time and space; and a sense of ineffability. Spiritually, the effects of LSD include a sense of rebirth; a sense of encounters with divinity; a sense of the world as sacred; and a sense of communion, unity, and nonduality.

These effects tend to be experienced as an inward journey; they are remembered and are felt by the user to be of lasting benefit. The effects are so unmistakable that blinded research studies are impossible. For this reason too, substances other than LSD are rarely sold as LSD.

LSD is not addictive. A tolerance is built up after a few days if used daily, but the tolerance is diminished quickly following cessation of use. Studies of lethal overdose levels in animals indicate it would require an extremely huge amount for humans, and no lethal overdoses have been shown in humans.

FURTHER READING

Dobkin de Rios, Marlene, and Oscar Janiger. *LSD, Spirituality, and the Creative Process.* Rochester, VT: Park Street, 2003. A research collection examining the impact of LSD on creativity before LSD was made illegal.

Grof, Stanislav. *LSD: Doorway to the Numinous.* Rochester, VT: Park Street, 2009. A good summary of the clinical research on LSD up to the point it was made illegal. Originally published in 1975.

Hoffman, Albert. *LSD: My Problem Child.* San Francisco: MAPS, 2005. The synthesizer of LSD reflects on its science and mysticism.

WEBSITES OF INTEREST

Multidisciplinary Association for Psychedelic Research
http://www.maps.org
National Institute on Drug Abuse
http://www.drugabuse.gov/infofacts/hallucinogens.html

Christopher M. Aanstoos

SEE ALSO: Hallucinogens and Their Effects; Mushrooms/ Psilocybin; PCP

Marijuana

A plant containing a psychoactive substance with the potential for both recreational abuse and medical use.

INTRODUCTION

The term "marijuana" refers to both the illegal drug and the plant itself. Marijuana is the most commonly used illicit drug (17.4 million past-month users) according to the 2010 National Survey on Drug Use and Health (NS-DUH). That year marijuana was used by 76.8 percent of current illicit drug users (defined as having used the drug at some time in the 30 days before the survey.

The hemp plant, Cannabis sativa, is a fast-growing (to fifteen feet) bushy annual with finely branched leaves further divided into lance-shaped, saw tooth-edged leaflets. The species was first classified in 1735 by the Swedish botanist Carolus Linnaeus. Both male and female plants produce tetrahydrocannabinol (THC), the psychoactive ingredient in the drug. THC collects in tiny droplets of sticky resin produced by glands located at the base of fine hairs covering most of the plant's surface, with the most highly concentrated THC found in the female flower heads. When pollinated, however, the female flower heads produce highly nutritious seeds containing no THC.

THE EFFECTS OF MARIJUANA

When marijuana is smoked, THC rapidly passes from the lungs to the bloodstream, which carries the chemical to organs throughout the body including the brain. The effects of smoked marijuana can last from 1 to 3 hours. If marijuana is consumed in foods or as beverage (e.g., tea)

the effect can appear between 30 to 60 minutes later. Interestingly, this effect can last up to one hour. Smoking by far delivers more THC to the bloodstream than eating or drinking. When it enters the brain, it binds to specific sites called cannabinoid receptors (CBRs) located on the surface of nerve cells, affecting the way those cells work. CBRs are abundant in parts of the brain that regulate movement, coordination, learning and memory, higher cognitive functions such as judgment and pleasure.

As THC enters the brain, it causes the user to feel euphoric or high by acting on the brain's reward system. This system controls the body's response to pleasurable things like sex and chocolate as well as to most drugs of abuse.

RECREATIONAL AND MEDICINAL USES
Responses vary according to dosage and experience using the drug, but most people experience a mild euphoria, or "high."

Mood, short-term memory, motor coordination, thought, sensation, and time sense can all be affected. Hunger, known as "the munchies," frequently occurs soon after exposure.

Marijuana can impede a person's ability to form new memories. In fact, people who have taken large doses of the drug may experience hallucinations, delusions, and loss of personal identity. All these symptoms encompass acute psychosis. The heart rate increases, the blood pressure increases while supine but drops when standing, and the eyes can become bloodshot. The most rapid onset with most temporary effect occurs with marijuana. Unlike alcohol or tobacco, no deaths have been directly attributed to marijuana use alone.

Marijuana has been cultivated and used as a medicine for thousands of years. The Food and Drug Administration (FDA) has approved a synthetic formulation of THC, Marinol (brand name of the generic drug dronabinol), that doctors can prescribe legally for the treatment of nausea and vomiting associated with cancer chemotherapy and the loss of appetite and weight loss characteristic of patients with acquired immunodeficiency syndrome (AIDS). In addition, both Marinol and marijuana are used to alleviate pain, muscle spasms, neurological disorders, and glaucoma. Many users of medicinal THC prefer to smoke marijuana despite its illegality rather than take the legal pill because orally delivered THC is not well absorbed by the body. Previously classified among drugs such as cocaine and morphine with a high potential for abuse, Marinol was moved to a less restricted category that includes anabolic steroids in July 1999.

Today, 25 years after Marinol was approved, the development of a THC-based mouth spray has been approved in the UK and Canada for relief of cancer associated pain and neuropathic pain in multiple sclerosis.

PERSPECTIVE AND PROSPECTS
Despite the FDA's tacit acknowledgment of the medicinal value of marijuana by the approval of Marinol, marijuana itself is classified as a substance with high potential for abuse and no accepted medical use under federal drug laws, stifling research into other potential medical benefits. Scientific evidence, including the 1990 report of the National Academy of Sciences Marijuana and Medicine: Assessing the Science Base, strongly supports further research.

FURTHER READING
Earleywine, Mitch. *Understanding Marijuana: A New Look at the Scientific Evidence.* New York: Oxford University Press, 2002.

ElSohly, Mahmoud A., ed. *Marijuana and the Cannabinoids.* Totowa, NJ: Humana Press, 2007.

Iversen, Leslie L. *The Science of Marijuana.* New York: Oxford University Press, 2000.

Mack, Alison, and Janet Joy. *Marijuana as Medicine? The Science Beyond the Controversy.* Washington, DC: National Academy Press, 2001.

National Institute on Drug Abuse. *NIH Research Report Series: Marijuana Abuse.* Rev. ed. Washington, DC: National Institutes of Health, 2012.

Onaivi, Emmanuel S., ed. *Marijuana and Cannabinoid Research: Methods and Protocols.* Totowa, NJ: Humana Press, 2006.

Shohov, Tatiana, ed. *Medical Use of Marijuana: Policy, Regulatory, and Legal Issues.* New York: Nova Science, 2003.

Sue Tarjan, updated by Stephen Henry

SEE ALSO: Teens and Drug Abuse

Marijuana legalization

Historically, Federal and most state law defined marijuana as a dangerous drug. Starting about 2000, state laws began to become liberalized. Today, there exists a crazy quilt of jurisdictional differences in which some states that shared borders had wildly different treatments of marijuana use.

INTRODUCTION

The liberalization of marijuana laws after 2000 sharply contrasts with popular attitudes earlier in the twentieth century. By 1900, regulations of medicines became more formalized at about the same time that cannabis itself was being outlawed. Cannabis sativa was regulated tightly in the United States beginning in 1906, and subject to prohibition during the 1920s. By the 1930s, it was regulated in all U.S. states; 35 states had adopted the U.S. Uniform State Narcotic Drug Act. During the late 1930s, Hearst newspapers and federal government agencies spurred a campaign to demonize cannabis as an incubator of violent crime.

By the 1970s, however, the legal pendulum had begun to swing toward liberalization. Awareness of marijuana's medical value spread in the 1990s, resulting in easing of laws in some jurisdictions. The federal Controlled Substances Act, however, still stated that cannabis has high potential for abuse, and no value as medicine. Resisting federal law, California voters chose to legalize medical marijuana by referendum in 1996. Hawaii approved medical marijuana, in 2000.

Two years after California voters supported medical marijuana, the Oakland Cannabis Buyers' Cooperative was sued by the U.S. government; May 14, 2001, the U.S. Supreme Court ruled that federal law did not allow an exception for medical cannabis because Congress had passed a law stating that it had no medical value. Many voters disagreed. Following Colorado's legalization of recreational cannabis use by popular vote in 2012, that state became, in 2013, the first fully regulated market in the world of this type.

HISTORY OF MARIJUANA USE, REGULATION, REPRESSION, AND LIBERALIZATION

In 1619, The Virginia Company, which regulated agriculture at Jamestown, enforced a decree by King James I that ordered every colonist to grow 100 marijuana plants for export as hemp. George Washington grew hemp as a cash crop at Mount Vernon. Hemp was widely used for fabric and rope in the United States until about 1900. Following the first use of cannabis in European medicine by William O'Shaughnnessy in 1839, it was introduced in pharmacies during the 1850s, often as a healing serum. Between 1850 and 1880 hashish "parlors" on

Oriental themes developed (as did opium dens) in many East Coast cities, including roughly 500 in New York City, some of which catered to an upper-class clientele.

Severe repression of marijuana use in the United States stems from the 1930s, when popular opinion was inflamed by such films as the federal government-sponsored *Reefer Madness*. By 1952, under the Boggs Act (as well as the Narcotics Act of 1956), first-time cannabis possession was subject to two to ten years in prison and a $20,000 fine (an amount of money worth several times today's value). The mandatory sentences were repealed in 1970.

In 1975, the Alaska Supreme Court decided in *Ravin v. State* that the state Constitution's right of privacy protected an adult's right to possess and use a small amount of marijuana at home for personal use. This was the first (and thus far, only) time that a state or federal court has upheld privacy as a defense from prosecution for cannabis use.

THE LEGAL SITUATION TODAY

By 2015, 23 states allowed use of marijuana for medicinal purposes. Colorado, Washington, Alaska, Oregon, and the District of Columbia allowed recreational use. Some states had decriminalized use, but not sale or possession. Minnesota, for example, has decriminalized recreational use, and medical use is legal. In New York State, use has been decriminalized in private, but remains illegal "in public view." By contrast, in Oklahoma, Wisconsin, and Texas, use, transport, or sale of any amount was illegal, as of May, 2015, for any reason.

Both Washington and Colorado have found that legal cannabis has reduced law-enforcement costs and increased tax revenue. The effects have been most notable in Washington, which has no state income tax. Tourism also has increased. Colorado has several bed and breakfasts that specialize in weed-related tourism. Some problems have arisen. For example, marijuana baked into food (cookies, lollipops, marshmallows, and the like) can deliver an especially potent, hallucination-laced high that lasts for several hours, especially with newly bred, very potent strains of cannabis. Also in Colorado, the percentage of fatal motor-vehicle accidents in which marijuana is a factor doubled within two years after it became legal for recreational purposes.

Treatment of marijuana use, possession, and sale differ widely in neighboring states. The border of Colorado and Nebraska has become a conflict zone as Nebraska's attorney general considered suing Colorado's state government because so much "weed" was flowing across the border, creating law enforcement problems. In Nebraska, use has been decriminalized for a first offense, but transport or sale of any amount remains illegal, a status not lost on State Patrol officers who have been busy intercepting large amounts of marijuana passing through the state on Interstate 90. At the same time, during 2015, the state's unicameral (single-chamber) legislature began hearings on tightly restricted use of medical marijuana with testimony from parents of children afflicted with uncontrolled epileptic seizures several times a day.

In Alabama, possession of marijuana was a felony in 2015 (except for a first offense). Across the border in Mississippi, the first offense (30 grams or less) has been decriminalized. Mississippi also has legalized non-psychoactive medical cannabis. In Florida, marijuana use is a misdemeanor (a felony if the user has more than 20 grams), and transportation and sale is a felony, but medical use is permitted in Georgia. In Idaho, possession of 85 grams (3 ounces) is a felony (as is transportation and sale of any amount), while across the border in Washington, medical and recreational use, possession, and sale are legal.

Portland and South Portland, Maine, had legalized use of cannabis for recreational and medical use by 2015 in a state where recreational use remained a civil infraction. Maine allows medical use. Washington, D.C. voters approved recreational and legal use, but recreational commercial activity was (as of 2015) forbidden by the U.S. Congress, which has extraordinary legal authority over governance of the Federal District. Some cities and Indian reservations also had passed their own legalization or decriminalization statutes or ordinances. However, the U.S. Justice Department has refrained in some cases from prosecuting offenders in jurisdictions where possession and use are now legal.

Within the context of wildly varying state laws, possession and sale remains illegal under U.S. federal law. Cannabis in 2015 remained a Schedule I controlled substance, the most serious classification. Meanwhile, in Seattle, a legal marijuana culture evolved. A full color, glossy magazine titled *Dope* was being published that described boutique cannabis cultivation (some "buds" had been bred that were as potent as 40 per cent THC, the active ingredient that makes people high). Competitions were being held in a "Cannabis Cup," and tasters examined new strains as if they were fine wine. Bums in Seattle's Pike Street Market asked passersby for a toke.

In many Midwestern and Southern states, meanwhile, people were still going to prison for doing things that were legal in some other states.

Sometimes, laws passed to penalize drug trafficking in more repressive times come into conflict with businesses that are now legal. Jack Healy described such an instance in the *New York Times*:

"Money was pouring into Bruce Nassau's five Colorado marijuana shops when his accountant called with the bad news: The 2014 tax season was approaching, and Mr. Nassau could not rely on the galaxy of deductions that other businesses use to reduce their tax bills. He was going to owe the Internal Revenue Service a small fortune. "I had to write a check for $275,000," Mr. Nassau said. 'Unbelievable.'"

The law under which he was being assessed was passed to prevent drug dealers from claiming their business expenses when marijuana was illegal everywhere. The law was passed by Congress in 1982, and signed by President Ronald Reagan, after a methamphetamine and cocaine dealer in Minneapolis went to tax court seeking to write off all of his expenses as a business. In 2015, with marijuana at least partially legal in many states, the IRS was banning all tax credits and deductions from "the illegal trafficking in drugs." Under U.S. tax law, marijuana business transactions are still illegal in any form.

FURTHER READING

Deitch, R. (2003). *Hemp - American History Revisited*. New York: Algora Publishing. This is a detailed history of hemp's history, use, and legal status through American history.

Healy, J. (2015, May 10). "Legal marijuana faces another federal hurdle: taxes." *New York Times*. http://www. nytimes.com/2015/05/10/us/politics/legal-marijuana-faces-another-federal-hurdle-taxes.html Laws passed during more repressive times have been crippling marijuana businesses in states where it is now legal.

Jones, N. (2004). *Spliffs: A Celebration of Cannabis Culture*. New York: Black Dock Publishing. This book describes and endorses cannabis use.

Musto, D. F. (1999). *The American Disease: Origins of Narcotic Control* (3rd ed.). New York: Oxford University Press. This book provides a history and a critique of marijuana regulation through history in the United States.

Sides, H. (2015, June). "Weed: The Science of Marijuana". *National Geographic*, 30-57. This article is one of few comprehensive descriptions of marijuana's medical effects.

Bruce E. Johansen

SEE ALSO: Marijuana; Media and Substance Abuse

Media and smoking

The depiction of smoking in film, television, and news programs powerfully shapes attitudes and beliefs about smoking. This depiction significantly affects individual decisions about whether or not to smoke.

TELEVISION AND YOUTH SMOKING

Because of the prevalence of smoking depicted on television, researchers conducted a study to determine if youths with greater exposure to television viewing were more apt to start smoking. These results were published in the journal *Pediatrics*.

Researchers from the Center for Child Health Outcomes at Children's Hospital and Health Center in San Diego, California, studied data on 592 youths (age ten to fifteen years) from the National Longitudinal Survey of Youth, Child Cohort. Specifically, researchers examined the association between television viewing in 1990 and smoking initiation from 1990 to 1992.

After controlling for baseline factors, researchers found an increasing association between the duration of TV viewing and the likelihood of starting smoking. Compared with children who watched less than two hours of TV per day, children who watched more than two to three hours of TV per day were 2 times more likely to begin smoking. Those who watched three to four hours of TV per day were 3.2 times more likely to begin smoking, those who watched four to five hours of TV per day were 5.2 times more likely to begin smoking, and those who watched five hours of TV per day were 6 times more likely to begin smoking.

The results of the study suggest that the more television that youths watch, the more likely they are to begin smoking. However, the study had major limitations because it did not consider the type of television programs the youths had been watching.

SMOKING IN FILM

In 2009, a furor of public disapproval followed actor Sigourney Weaver's smoking scenes in the PG-13 rated blockbuster film *Avatar*. The smoking scenes involving the character Dr. Augustine were lambasted not only as illogical for portraying a smoking doctor but also as gratuitous, inasmuch as the scenes contributed nothing to the storyline. Director James Cameron responded to the criticism by saying that portraying Weaver as a smoking scientist revealed her as a conflicted and flawed character.

The American public takes for granted that smoking is likely in R-rated films, but it becomes increasingly difficult for directors to justify smoking scenes in films rated G, PG, or PG-13, given that minors make up the most likely audience for these films. In 2007, after decades of prompting by antismoking activists, the Motion Picture Association of America (MPAA) acquiesced and said that it would take into account during the ratings process all superfluous smoking scenes, those scenes deemed unnecessary in creating historical authenticity or in the telling of the film's narrative. Regardless, the MPAA is still criticized by parents and antismoking activists for not taking smoking in films and its negative influence on young people more seriously.

Although smoking had always been portrayed on screen to some degree, it was in the early 1940s, during World War II, that smoking in film experienced an explosion in popularity, which accelerated throughout the 1950s. With smoking's health risks still largely unknown by the public at the time, and with free cigarettes being distributed to US troops by the military, smoking came to be regarded more and more as an affordable luxury, hedonistic and provocative and sensually gratifying.

Women, newly representative of the American workforce, were depicted onscreen as seductive, liberated, sexual, and erotic smokers. Hollywood studios received compensation from tobacco companies for on-screen endorsements. Female stars such as Bette Davis, Joan Crawford, and Betty Grable exuded glamour and sex appeal while smoking on screen. Leading men such as Clark Gable, Humphrey Bogart, and Spencer Tracy personified masculinity as they smoked their way through scene after scene.

By the 1990s, however, some Hollywood stars, recognizing their responsibility as role models for young people, began to resist. Pierce Brosnan, for instance, who had smoked repeatedly as the character James Bond in previous films, vowed that he would never again smoke on screen playing that role; producers conceded, and Brosnan continued to play the role of James Bond, but newly smoke-free. This is significant because researchers have found a direct correlation between seeing tobacco use depicted in films and trying cigarettes among adolescents. Higher levels of exposure to smoking in films are associated with an increased likelihood of trying cigarettes, even when researchers controlled for age, school performance, gender, and the smoking habits of family members or friends.

SMOKING ON TELEVISION

Before the passage by the US Congress of the Public Health Cigarette Smoking Act in 1970, which banned all television and radio advertising of cigarettes, cigarette advertisements were a pervasive feature of American television programming. Winston, Camel, Marlboro, and Tareyton were just a few of the ubiquitous tobacco sponsors of television shows throughout the 1950s and 1960s.

For many years, the longest running Western on television, *Gunsmoke*, which was sponsored by Winston cigarettes, was introduced with the slogan "Winston tastes good, like a cigarette should." The Marlboro Man television advertising campaign, in particular, is often cited as the single most successful advertising campaign in history. At a time when Westerns like *Gunsmoke*, *Bonanza*, *Wagon Train*, and *The Rifleman* dominated television ratings, the image of the Marlboro Man, a cowboy figure from the Old West, resonated with the American public in a profound sense like no other image. Consequently, Marlboro cigarettes became the best-selling brand, not only in the United States but also in countries with consumers who connected with the cowboy archetype.

The two actors who portrayed the Marlboro Man, Wayne McLaren and David McLean, both developed cancer and died as a result of smoking. After being diagnosed with cancer, both men launched antismoking public-service campaigns, informing the public that their illness was directly attributable to smoking. After his death from lung cancer in 1995, McLean's family filed a wrongful death lawsuit against Philip Morris, the manufacturer and distributor of Marlboro cigarettes.

Commercials were the primary advertisers of cigarettes and smoking, but television shows did their part too. Ashtrays and cigarettes were omnipresent props on set, including those of talk shows and game shows. This type of advertising is now called product placement.

In the early 1960s, members of the most popular entertainment group, dubbed The Rat Pack, held a lit cigarette in one hand and a glass of alcohol in the other, while they sang, danced, joked, and acted their way to stardom. Frank Sinatra, Dean Martin, Sammy Davis Jr., Peter Lawford, and Joey Bishop were emblematic of their time. Almost ten years later, attitudes had changed little, as evidenced by the television show Rowan and Martin's Laugh-In. The show's hosts and characters each week held lit cigarettes and alcoholic beverages throughout the show.

With the advent of the cigarette brand Virginia Slims in 1968, whose slogan announced to women, "You've come a long way, baby," more and more women similarly were depicted on television as smokers. Smoking became a sign of female equality, liberation, and independence. After January 2, 1971, when cigarette advertising was banned on television and radio, Virginia Slims, Marlboro, and other brands were relegated primarily to print media and billboards.

Television, especially in later decades, began to provide a venue for public service and antismoking campaigns. Television and film stars, such as Yul Brynner and many others in the mid-1980s, made powerful and moving antismoking commercials for the American Cancer Society. Brynner, throughout his career, was seen on television either smoking or holding a cigarette. Shortly after his death from lung cancer, a commercial revealing a frail and ravaged Brynner urged American audiences to avoid smoking, attributing his premature death from lung cancer to cigarettes.

SMOKING AND THE NEWS MEDIA

The news media reports on issues of smoking and tobacco. Sometimes, the news media itself is the source of that news.

In 1995 the CBS news magazine show 60 Minutes became a source of controversy after learning from Jeffrey Wigand, the vice president of research and development at Brown and Williamson tobacco company, that Brown and Williamson had consistently lied about the dangerous threats posed to health by tobacco and had deliberately deceived the public for decades. In April 2005, ABC World News Tonight anchor Peter Jennings announced on the air that he had been diagnosed with lung cancer. Viewers reacted with shock and disbelief. Jennings, who had smoked for years and then quit, confessed to his viewers that after the enormous stress of the terrorist attacks of September 11, 2001, he had been "weak" and had resumed smoking. Less than four months after making this revelation on air, Jennings died of lung cancer.

Jennings's story marked one of the latest in a long line of television journalists to succumb to the effects of smoking. For decades, news anchors read the news with cigarette in hand, as an ashtray rested conveniently near the microphone. Legendary journalist Edward R. Murrow, who was rarely seen without a cigarette, died in 1965 of lung cancer. NBC national news anchor Chet Huntley, also seen nightly smoking a cigarette while delivering the news, died of lung cancer in 1974. More recently, in 2007, television news anchor Tom Snyder, who also had appeared on television holding a cigarette, died of leukemia.

FURTHER READING

Egendorf, Laura. *Issues That Concern You: Smoking.* Farmington Hills, MI: Greenhaven, 2008. Examines the specific ways that Hollywood and the film industry inspire young people to smoke.

Hyde, Margaret, and John Setaro. *Smoking 101: An Overview for Teens.* Minneapolis, MN: Twenty-First Century, 2006. Discusses the commonplace policy of tobacco companies providing free cigarettes to Hollywood stars, and the lucrative endorsement contracts to stars who filmed tobacco commercials to be aired in foreign countries.

Lehu, Jean-Marc. *Branded Entertainment: Product Placement and Brand Strategy in the Entertainment Business.* London: Kogan, 2007. Analyzes the historical practice of product placement of branded tobacco products on television and in film, often as a way to fund production.

O'Reilly, Terry, and Mike Tennant. *The Age of Persuasion: How Marketing Ate Our Culture.* Berkeley, CA: Counterpoint, 2009. Discusses the Marlboro Man and Virginia Slims advertising campaigns as the most successful targeted advertising strategies in marketing history.

Rabinoff, Michael. *Ending the Tobacco Holocaust.* Santa Rosa, CA: Elite, 2007. Argues that the number-one determining influence on fourteen-year-old peer groups regarding smoking is the Hollywood film industry and actors who smoke on screen.

WEBSITES OF INTEREST

Action on Smoking and Health
http://www.ash.org
Americans for Nonsmokers' Rights
http://no-smoke.org
Campaign for Tobacco-Free Kids
http://www.tobaccofreekids.org
Smoke Free Movies
http://smokefreemovies.ucsf.edu

Mary E. Markland

SEE ALSO: Smoking and Its Effects

Media and substance abuse

Mass media has been used as a tool to inform the public of the dangers of substance abuse since the early twentieth century. Conversely, mass media has been studied since the 1970s as a potential influence of the cultural proliferation of substance abuse.

HISTORY OF MEDIA AND SUBSTANCE ABUSE

While much is known about the influences of genetics, psychosocial development, peer interactions, and communal surroundings in a person's decision to begin drug and alcohol abuse, little is known about the ability of media to contribute to or detract from these factors. Similarly, while media campaigns in both print and television have been utilized by local, state, and federal governments to highlight the dangers of drug and alcohol abuse, their effectiveness is difficult to define.

The 1936 film *Tell Your Children* is largely recognized as the first antidrug film in American cinema. Originally created as a propaganda-style production by a church group, the film depicted the dangers of marijuana use in overtly dramatic and exaggerated fashion to spread fear of the drug. The film did not gain a large viewership until its rerelease in 1971 as *Reefer Madness* (1971), where the film's outrageous claims that marijuana induced insanity and homicidal tendencies were perceived as comical by modern audiences, transforming the film into a pro-marijuana piece by the National Organization for the Reform of Marijuana Laws (now called NORML).

The alteration of *Reefer Madness* from cautionary tale to hyperbolized farce in thirty-five years is representative of a long-standing trend in the relationship between substance abuse and media. Namely, that media in most forms is rarely capable of being produced with the speed at which the cultural perceptions and attitudes of drugs and alcohol fluctuate. The use of media as a tool against the abuse of drugs and alcohol always has been hampered by another historical disadvantage: Nearly all forms of major mass media, from music to film, television, and art, all originally portrayed substance abuse in a casual manner devoid of association with its potential danger.

As alluded to in an October 2010 study by the American Academy of Pediatrics, drug and alcohol abuse have been portrayed as normative behaviors in American culture in nearly all facets of media since the early twentieth century, depictions that may be the result of lax attitudes toward such portrayals. This tradition has made the challenge of creating effective antidrug media campaigns that much more difficult.

MEDIA AS A CAUSE OF SUBSTANCE ABUSE

The notion of media as an influential factor in the prevalence of substance abuse has been examined by sociologists since the 1970s. Media studies began to identify the frequency with which alcohol was depicted in television programming. This research found that alcohol use was predominantly portrayed as socially acceptable across the entertainment-television landscape, and that depictions of use were rarely portrayed negatively.

Hard drugs such as heroin and cocaine have rarely been portrayed glamorously in American media, and studies dating to 1974 began to decry the depiction of marijuana on television as a humorous, harmless escape or even a rite of passage. This notion of harmlessness has remained through contemporary American television series such as *That 70's Show*, a Fox situation comedy that aired from 1998 to 2006 and that regularly depicted scenes alluding to marijuana use by its main characters, all of whom are high school students.

A landmark 2012 study by Dartmouth College examined the influence of film on the predictors of adolescent alcohol consumption. A two-year survey sample revealed that 80 percent of the films watched by American teenagers depicted alcohol consumption, while 65 percent contained product placements for alcoholic beverages for advertising purposes. The study concluded that widespread exposure to cinematic depictions of substance abuse does act as a predictor for adolescent binge drinking and cigarette smoking.

Activist groups and civic organizations of all kinds have condemned a perception of pervasive themes like sexual promiscuity, rebellion, and violence since the beginnings of popular music. The prevalence of substance abuse in popular music also has been widely criticized. A 1999 report by the US Department of Health and Human Services indicated that of the one thousand most popular songs between the years 1996 and 1997

that were surveyed, more than one-quarter of those songs made reference to either alcohol or illicit drug use.

Perhaps no form of media is more responsible for persuasive messages aimed at promoting substance abuse as advertising. According to the US Department of Justice, the alcohol industry spends close to $2 billion annually on television, radio, print, and outdoor advertisements, while figures for advertising expenditures for the tobacco industry are often three times that amount. These vast expenditures are likely reasons for the increase in youth exposure to alcohol advertising; ads increased by as much as 71 percent between 2001 and 2009, according to figures from the Johns Hopkins School of Public Health. While limited evidence has resulted in legislation and in voluntary advertising codes to restrict the advertisement of alcohol near such places as schools, it has remained difficult to extract the precise effect an increasing prevalence of alcohol advertising exposure has on society.

Contradictory research contends that no large-scale scientific evidence exists that concretely attributes the proliferation of alcohol- and substance abuse-related portrayals in advertising and mass media as a pathway to abuse. These findings marginalize the effect of such media, stating that they act merely as any other commercialized persuasive device, such as those for food, soft drinks, and cosmetics, aimed at the market of a particular group of consumers.

USE OF MEDIA TO PREVENT SUBSTANCE ABUSE

New rounds of criticism aimed at the film and music industries decrying their legacy of positively portraying drug, alcohol, and tobacco use have corresponded with a new immersion by anti-substance-abuse advocacy groups into contemporary forms of media such as social networking. Programs initiated by groups such as the National Youth Anti-Drug Media Campaign have created youth-centric websites like AbovetheInfluence.com and theAntiDrug.com to warn young people about the dangers of substance abuse. Other groups have produced public service announcements for television.

Similar sites such as the American Legacy Foundation's TheTruth.com attempt to tackle issues such as tobacco smoking with a rebellious flair, voicing not only the health dangers of tobacco use but also rage at the perceived duplicity of the tobacco industry. The site even sells clothing with antitobacco messages. Academic journals such as *Prevention Science* and the *American Journal of Public Health* have explicated the success of the National Youth Anti-Drug Media Campaign among young people.

The newly pervasive nature of custom-tailored media and social networking will solidify its already established arena in which both the ills and successes of society are portrayed. The prevailing belief among sociologists contends that until the values and goals of society place the education of the dangers of substance abuse at higher regard, their presence in media will not be abolished. Only through dismantling the misconceptions surrounding drinking, smoking, and drug use built by previous generations can substance abuse be regarded as negative and dangerous behaviors by popular culture as a whole.

FURTHER READING

Ericson, Nels. "Substance Abuse: The Nation's Number One Health Problem." *OJJDP Fact Sheet* 17 (2001). Web. 27 Apr. 2012. https://www.ncjrs.gov/pdffiles1/ojjdp/fs200117.pdf.

Flay, Brian R., and Judith L. Sobel. "The Role of Mass Media in Preventing Adolescent Substance Abuse." *NIDA Research Monograph* 47 (1983): 5–35. Print.

Newman, Lori M., ed. *Does Advertising Promote Substance Abuse?* Detroit: Greenhaven, 2005.

Office of National Drug Control Policy. "Substance Use in Popular Music Videos." Jun. 2002. Web. 27 Apr. 2012. http://www.scenesmoking.org/research/SubstanceUseIinMusic.pdf.

Stoolmiller, Mike, et al. "Comparing Media and Family Predictors of Alcohol Use: A Cohort Study of US Adolescents." *BMJ Open* 2.1 (2012). Web. 27 Apr. 2012. http://bmjopen.bmj.com/content/2/1/e000543.full.

Strasburger, Victor C. "Children, Adolescents, Substance Abuse, and the Media." *Pediatrics* 126.4 (2010). Web. 27 Apr. 2012. http://pediatrics.aappublications.org/content/126/4/791.full.

WEBSITES OF INTEREST

Above the Influence
http://www.abovetheinfluence.com
Center on Alcohol Marketing and Youth
http://www.camy.org
Parents: The Anti-Drug
http://www.antidrug.com
TheTruth.com
http://www.thetruth.com

John Pritchard

SEE ALSO: Families and Substance Abuse; Media and Smoking

Mescaline

Mescaline is a naturally occurring psychedelic with mind-altering properties. It is structurally related to amphetamine but has mental effects similar to lysergic acid diethylamide (LSD).

HISTORY OF USE

Mescaline, named after the Mescalero Apaches, is a classic psychedelic drug with a long history of use worldwide. It was first isolated from the peyote cactus by a German chemist named Arthur Heffter in 1897.

Mescaline-containing cacti were traditionally used by Native American tribes in religious ceremoniesceremonial drug usemescaline to treat physical and spiritual ailments, to alter states of consciousness, to generate mystical visions, and to induce spiritual cleansing through nausea and vomiting. In the early twentieth century the establishment of the Native American ChurchNative American Church and mescaline (NAC) legitimized the use of psychoactive cacti in ritual ceremonies.

In 1919, mescaline became one of the first natural hallucinogens to be produced synthetically. During the hippie movement in the 1960s and 1970s, the use of mescaline as a recreational drug became extensive because of its mind-expanding properties. Mescaline use has been illegal in the United States since the early 1970s, with the exception of use in NAC ritual ceremonies. Mescaline is a schedule I hallucinogen because of its high abuse potential and its lack of legitimate medical use.

EFFECTS AND POTENTIAL RISKS

Mescaline is most commonly known for its powerful psychotropic effects. Although its chemical structure does not resemble that of LSD, it acts similarly. Its hallucinogenic effects are caused by its binding to serotonin receptors in the brain and inducing numerous behavioral and perceptual changes.

Mescaline's short-term psychological effects are related to increased serotonin levels. Mescaline alters sensory, time, and space perceptions and thought processes and mood. It induces intense visual hallucinations of enhanced color and detail followed by euphoric dreamlike states, giving the illusion of having an out-of-body experience. Negative short-term physical effects include nausea, vomiting, sweating, dizziness, headache, anxiety, and tachycardia (rapid heartbeat).

Mescaline's hallucinogenic effects are known as trips. Users experience good trips resulting from pleasurable images or bad trips resulting from disturbing images. Some users experience a blending of the senses called synesthesia. Long-term use can potentially lead to mental health problems, including drug-induced psychosis and hallucinogen-persisting perception disorder known as flashbacks.

FURTHER READING

Brands, Bruna, Beth Sproule, and Joan Marshman. *Drugs and Drug Abuse*. Toronto: Addiction Research, 1998.

Cunningham, Nicola. "Hallucinogenic Plants of Abuse." *Emergency Medicine Australasia* 20.2 (2008): 167–74. Print.

Fantegrossi, William E., Kevin S. Murnane, and Chad J. Reissig. "The Behavioral Pharmacology of Hallucinogens." *Biochemical Pharmacology* 75.1 (2008): 17–33. Print.

WEBSITES OF INTEREST

National Institute on Drug Abuse
http://www.drugabuse.gov/Infofacts/hallucinogens.html
Native American Church
http://www.nativeamericanchurches.org

Rose Ciulla-Bohling

SEE ALSO: Amphetamine Abuse; Hallucinogens and Their Effects; LSD

Methamphetamine

Methamphetamine is a psychostimulant in the phenoethylamine and amphetamine class of drugs. It is a white, odorless, bitter-tasting crystalline powder that is highly addictive. It is used medically to treat attention deficit hyperactivity disorder, exogenous obesity, and narcolepsy.

METH MOUTH

Meth mouth is a popular term for the extensive tooth decay and oral hygiene issues associated with heavy use of methamphetamine, a potent central nervous system stimulant. The acidic nature of methamphetamine may contribute to meth mouth, but the condition largely re-sults from drug-induced changes that profoundly affect oral health.

These changes include decreased production of saliva, which fosters bacterial growth and tooth decay; repetitive jaw clenching and tooth grinding, which damages enamel and causes teeth to fracture; and frequent cravings for sugary, carbonated beverages, with extended periods of poor oral hygiene.

A common sign of meth mouth is extreme tooth decay, with stained, blackened, or rotting teeth that often cannot be salvaged. Often, the only remedy is tooth extraction, with full-mouth reconstruction or a dental prosthesis as treatment. The effects on the oral cavity include dry mouth, cracked teeth, and sore and bleeding gums.

HISTORY OF USE

A Japanese scientist first synthesized methamphetamine in 1919. Along with amphetamines, methamphetamine was given to both Axis and Allied soldiers during World War II as performance aids and to counteract sleep deprivation. Illegal use of methamphetamine rose in the United States in the 1960s, originating in the Southwest. Methamphetamine was supplied by labs in Mexico and smuggled into the United States through US border states. By the 1980s, methamphetamine had become increasingly popular in the Midwest and in the southern states, partially because of the availability of fertilizer that could be used as an ingredient in methamphetamine production.

Although the National Institute on Drug Abuse reports that methamphetamine use among teenagers is in decline, studies show that there are between 15 and 16 million methamphetamine abusers worldwide, a number some experts say is second only to marijuana use. Admission rates to rehabilitation centers for methamphetamine addiction are higher in some states than for cocaine or even alcohol abuse.

One of the methods of coping with the rising methamphetamine problem has been a slow but progressive change in treating addicts. Prison officials, psychologists, and legislators have made changes in the prison system so that prisoners addicted to methamphetamine can safely go through detoxification and receive further treatment.

Treatment for methamphetamine addiction has become specialized. The matrix model includes cognitive-behavioral therapy, family education, positive reinforcement for behavior change and treatment compliance, and a twelve-step program. No ideal medication has been found for treatment, although some studies have examined the use of the tricyclic antidepressant imiprazine (Tofranil).

EFFECTS AND POTENTIAL RISKS

The physical effects of a methamphetamine high resemble those of the body in a fight-or-flight, hyperarousal response. Heart rate and blood pressure increases, and awareness is heightened with increased self-confidence.

Chronic methamphetamine use and methamphetamine overdose lead to extremely dangerous physical conditions, including myocardial infarction, cardiopulmonary arrest, seizures, hypoxic brain damage, hyperthermia, and intracranial bleeds. Psychiatric symptoms are extremely common and include insomnia, mood disorders, violent behavior, paranoia, and hallucinations.

Methamphetamine increases the release of and blocks the body's reuptake of dopaminedopamine, which increases the levels of dopamine in the brain. The inability of the brain to release the excess dopamine creates the user's rush or high. Chronic methamphetamine use leads to a change in the activity of the dopamine system, specifically a decrease in motor skills and impaired verbal learning skills. Chronic use also affects emotions, memory, and general cognitive abilities. Because methamphetamine is highly lipophilic, it enables a rapid and extensive transport across the blood-brain barrier. It is highly neurotoxic and can stay in the body's system for eight to thirteen hours.

Even after a methamphetamine user stops using the drug, the damage to his or her brain continues. There is evidence of impairment of the anterior cingulated cortex, the area of the brain that influences cognitive functions and emotions and regulates behavior. The drug disables the ability to choose between healthy and unhealthy behaviors. Enhanced cortical gray matter volume also declines with age, leading to an accelerated rate of mental functioning, primarily because of a reduction in the number of neurons rather than shrinkage of gray matter. Methamphetamine users are at a greater risk for degenerative or cognitive diseases, and persons who are comorbid with depression are at a higher risk for dementia.

Methamphetamine use also increases the risk of transmission of the human immunodeficiency virus (HIV) and the hepatitis virus. Shared-needle use and higher risk sexual behavior increase the chances that a user will be infected with a sexually transmitted disease. Methamphetamine users who are HIV positive tend to suffer more neuronal injury and cognitive impairment.

A common physical trait of a chronic methamphetamine user is poor oral hygiene, or meth mouth. Methamphetamine use can cause a decrease in saliva output, leading to chronic dry mouth. Users will often drink large amounts of sugary carbonated soft drinks, which leads to severe dental decay. Many methamphetamine users also may grind or clench their teeth, causing tooth fractures.

FURTHER READING

Nakama, Helena, et al. "Methamphetamine Users Show Greater Than Normal Age-Related Cortical Gray Matter Loss." *Addiction* 106.8 (2011): 1474–83. Print. A cross-sectional study that suggests that methamphetamine users suffer a decline in cognitive health at earlier ages than those who do not use methamphetamine.

Padilla, Ricardo, and Andre V. Ritter. "Meth Mouth: Methamphetamine and Oral Health." *Journal of Esthetic and Restorative Dentistry* 20.2 (2008): 148–49. Print. Examines the occurrence of meth mouth.

Schep, Leo, Robin J. Slaughter, and D. Michael G. Beasley. "The Clinical Toxicology of Methamfetamine." *Clinical Toxicology* 48 (2010): 675–84. Print. An overview of the biochemical mechanisms of methamphetamine on the brain and an extensive list of toxicokinetics and clinical features of methamphetamine abuse.

WEBSITES OF INTEREST

Drug Information Portal. National Library of Medicine
http://druginfo.nlm.nih.gov/drugportal
National Institute on Drug Abuse
http://www.drugabuse.gov/drugs-abuse/methamphetamine

S. M. Willis

SEE ALSO: Amphetamine Abuse

Mushrooms/psilocybin

The drug substances in "magic" mushrooms, psilocybin (4-phosphoryloxy-N,N-dimethyltryptamine) and psilocin (4-hydroxy-N,N-dimethyltryptamine), are hallucinogenic. They have properties similar to LSD, or acid, and produce alterations of digestive and cardiac function, motor reflexes, behavior, and perception.

HISTORY OF USE

Hallucinogenic mushrooms containing psilocybin are thought to have existed as long or longer than the human race. Historically, artwork such as pictures, statues, and carvings depicting the mushrooms have been seen near tribal settlements. In Central and South America, psilocybin-containing mushrooms were commonly used in religious ceremonies until Spanish settlers spread Catholicism and banned their use. Mushrooms are sacred to indigenous peoples and are considered entheogens, psychoactive substances that guide their religious path through the spirit world.

In the early twentieth century ethnobotanists Richard Evans Schultes and Blas Pablo Reko traveled to Mexico and sought out these mushrooms. Schultes published a report of his findings in 1939. After hearing of this work, ethnomycologists Roger Heim and R. Gordon Wasson and pediatrician Valentina Wasson traveled to Central America to investigate the use and effects of the mushrooms. In 1957 the Wassons published the article "Seeking the Magic Mushroom" in *Life* magazine.

Mushrooms symbolized hippie counterculture in the 1960s and 1970s and were commonly used in the United States and Great Britain. The mushrooms led to the discovery of LSD, a synthetic hallucinogen.

It is difficult to determine the level of use of psilocybin-containing mushrooms because most studies of drug use neglect to include this drug. The *Monitoring the Future* survey published in 2008 reported that 7.8 percent of high school seniors had used hallucinogens other than LSD. This group of drugs includes peyote and psilocybin. Use in the previous year by participants was reported as 5 percent.

EFFECTS AND POTENTIAL RISKS

Psilocybin and its active form, psilocin, are not inactivated by heating or freezing. To mask its bitter flavor, the mushroom is brewed into tea or cooked with other foods. Digestion and absorption of the psilocybin take about twenty minutes, and the effects last from four to six hours.

Psilocybin can produce relaxation or weakness of the muscles, lack of coordination, excessive pupil dilation, nausea, vomiting, and drowsiness. Mushroom abusers are at risk of poisoning if poisonous mushrooms are accidentally ingested with psilocybin mushrooms.

The psychological effects of psilocybin use include hallucinations, an altered perception of the passage of time, and confusion between fantasy and reality. Panic and psychosis also may occur, especially with high doses. Persistent use comes with flashbacks, risk of psychiatric disease, memory impairment, and tolerance.

FURTHER READING

Laing, Richard R., ed. *Hallucinogens: A Forensic Drug Handbook.* San Francisco: Elsevier, 2003.

National Institute on Drug Abuse. "Hallucinogens: LSD, Peyote, Psilocybin, and PCP." 2009. Web. 10 Mar. 2012. http://www.nida.nih.gov/infofacts/hallucinogens.html.

"Psilocybin Mushrooms." Web. 26 Mar. 2012. http://www.erowid.org/plants/mushrooms/mushrooms.shtml.

WEBSITES OF INTEREST

AbovetheInfluence.com
http://www.abovetheinfluence.com/facts/drugshallucinogens
National Drug Intelligence Center
http://www.justice.gov/ndic/pubs6/6038
National Institute on Drug Abuse
http://www.drugabuse.gov

Kimberly A. Napoli

SEE ALSO: Hallucinogens and Their Effects; LSD

Overeaters Anonymous

Overeaters Anonymous (OA) is a twelve-step recovery program based on the methods and philosophy of Alcoholics Anonymous. OA members profess that they are "powerless over food" and that their "lives have become unmanageable." The purpose of the group is not to promote weight loss and dieting but to support inner changes and daily actions that remove the feeling that one must consume excess and addictive foods.

BACKGROUND

Overeaters Anonymous (OA) was founded by Rozanne S., Jo S., and Bernice S. in 1960 after Rozanne had attended a Gamblers Anonymous (GA) meeting to support a friend. Rozanne discovered that the members' stories of compulsive gambling mirrored her own story of compulsive overeating. She recognized that the twelve steps and twelve traditions of recovery that were the foundation of Alcoholics Anonymous (AA) and adopted by GA could be applied to recovery from compulsive overeating.

The OA program is based on twelve steps, twelve traditions, and eight tools of recovery. The twelve steps are almost identical to those of AA. In AA literature, the word alcohol can be replaced with trigger food and the word drinking can be replaced with compulsive overeating to make the principles applicable to OA members. However, an important distinction between the two groups is that although AA members can abstain from all alcohol, OA members cannot abstain from all food.

Persons who wish to disengage from compulsive overeating must identify and refrain from ingesting specific food ingredients that trigger the compulsion. The most common trigger foods are wheat and sugar. In addition, compulsive overeating may be triggered by compulsive food behaviors, such as the need to empty a package of food or the need to finish food on a plate rather than leaving a portion or discarding food. In 2009, OA defined abstinence as "the action of refraining from compulsive eating and compulsive food behaviors."

The twelve traditions, nearly identical to those of AA, are guidelines for conducting meetings and sustaining the principles of the organization. Each of the twelve traditions has a related spiritual principle: unity, trust, identity, autonomy, purpose, solidarity, responsibility, fellowship, structure, neutrality, anonymity, and spirituality.

By using the eight tools of recovery, members are better able to achieve and maintain abstinence from compulsive overeating. The first tool is a plan of eating. (OA does not promote a specific dietary plan but encourages members to develop a personal eating plan after consulting a physician or dietitian and identifying trigger foods to avoid.) The second tool is sponsorship. A sponsor is an experienced OA member who helps a new member understand and work the twelve steps. The third tool is the OA meeting, which provides regular support from other OA members and helps members to overcome the isolation and shame that impede recovery.

The fourth tool of recovery is the telephone. Members are encouraged to ask for help from one another, especially when emotions are overwhelming. The fifth tool is writing as a way of examining one's reactions to difficult situations and discovering alternative coping mechanisms. The sixth tool is literature, particularly the publications of OA and the *Big Book* of AA. Such reading material provides insight into the nature and consequences of compulsive overeating and provides hope for recovery.

The seventh tool is anonymity, which protects members from gossip as they express their pain and struggles and also asserts equality among members. The eighth tool is service. Members are asked to sustain the organization with acts such as welcoming new members, setting up and cleaning up meeting rooms, and sharing news of upcoming OA events.

OA is a nonprofit organization. All funding comes from the sale of OA literature and voluntary contributions collected at meetings. The program has not changed over time. The demographics of its members have changed only as a reflection of trends in the general population. More participants today have college degrees, more work full-time, and more are divorced.

MISSION AND GOALS

The official literature of OA states that "Our primary purpose is to abstain from compulsive overeating and to carry this message of recovery to those who still suffer." OA has an estimated fifty-four thousand members in more than seventy-five countries, with sixty-five hundred groups meeting each week. Most members are white females who have been in the program an average of 5.7 years. They began the program with moderate obesity.

Although OA does not focus on diet and calorie counting, members of OA experience an average weight loss of 21.8 pounds as a result of working the program. Like other twelve-step programs, OA seeks to improve the physical, mental, and spiritual facets of the lives of its members. A 2002 survey found that 90 percent of OA members reported improvements in these areas.

Specific OA practices have a demonstrated significant relationship with the maintenance of abstinence from foods that trigger compulsive overeating: weighing and measuring foods on a deliberate food plan; regular communication with other OA members, specifically a sponsor; spending time in introspection; writing as a form of personal expression and investigation; attending OA meetings regularly; reading OA literature for inspiration; and working the steps, particularly the fourth and ninth steps. Abstinence and spirituality were strongly correlated with self-reported success.

FURTHER READING

Alcoholics Anonymous. *Alcoholics Anonymous Big Book*. 4th ed. New York: Author, 2007. The bible of twelve-step recovery programs, including Overeaters Anonymous.

Costin, Carolyn. *The Eating Disorder Sourcebook*. New York: McGraw-Hill, 2006.

Overeaters Anonymous. *For Today*. Torrance, CA: Author, 1982. Daily affirmations and readings to inspire compulsive overeaters and food addicts in recovery.

---. *Overeaters Anonymous*. 2nd ed. Torrance, CA: Author, 2001. A collection of short personal accounts of persons who have successfully worked the OA program.

WEBSITES OF INTEREST

HealthyPlace.com
http://www.healthyplace.com/eating-disorders
Overeaters Anonymous
http://www.oa.org

Bethany Thivierge

SEE ALSO: Eating Disorders; Obesity; Support Groups

Over-the-counter (OTC) drugs

Pills, capsules, tablets, or syrups that can be purchased without prescription for the self-treatment of common illnesses, such as colds, fever, and headache.

INDICATIONS AND PROCEDURES

Drugs or medications that can be purchased directly, without a prescription, are called over-the-counter (OTC) medications or drugs. These medications may be suggested by physicians or simply purchased for consumption as a result of self-diagnosis and self-prescription. Most of the common OTC medications are used to treat common ailments such as cold and fever symptoms, headache, coughs, and similar complaints. Such self-treatment may be initiated at will and discontinued at any time.

Dozens of pharmaceutical companies produce and market hundreds of drugs for sale as over-the-counter medications, but they fall into only a few categories. The basic types of OTC medications, along with some brand examples, include analgesics (Advil, Tylenol), antacids (Milk of Magnesia), antidiarrheal medications (Imodium), antifungal agents (Tinactin), antihistamines (Benadryl), antiacne treatments (Clearasil), anti-inflammatory drugs (Motrin), decongestants (Sudafed), motion sickness (Meclizine), laxatives (Metamucil, Dulcolax), dandruff treatments (Selsun Blue), expectorants (Robitussin), hair growth formulas (Rogaine), and sleep aids (L-Tryptophan).

The most frequently used category of OTC medications is analgesics, which are more popularly known as painkillers. Analgesics include a diverse group of drugs that are used to relieve soreness, general body pain, and headaches. Probably the most common analgesic is aspirin, which is part of a group of medications termed nonsteroidal anti-inflammatory drugs (NSAIDs) that chemically affect the central and possibly the peripheral nervous system by leading to a decrease in prostaglandin production. Many analgesics are used in combination with other drugs such as vasoconstriction drugs that contain pseudoephedrine, which is especially important for the relief of sinus congestion, and in combination with antihistamine drugs, which relieve the worst symptoms of allergy.

Decongestants must certainly rank as the second most common category of OTC medications. Generally, decongestants are taken to relieve nasal congestion and allied symptoms of colds and flu by acting to reduce swelling of the mucous membranes of the nasal passageways. A recurring problem with most nasal decongestants is that they increase hypertension, but this effect is lessened by including one or more antihistamines in the preparation. The brand name drug Dimetapp, for example, is both an antihistamine and a decongestant, while various Tylenol products may contain drugs that collectively work to soothe sore throat, relieve nasal congestion, or suppress coughing.

Despite the fact that over-the-counter drugs are available to everyone, their marketing and use is restricted by the Food and Drug Administration (FDA) in the United States and similar agencies with regulatory powers in many other countries. The FDA mandates ingredients and labeling of OTC drugs and specifies rigid testing and safety standards that must be met prior to marketing. Pharmaceutical companies must apply to the New Drug Agency (NDA) for the approval of drugs. The NDA specifies testing requirements prior to issuing a license for the sales and marketing of the proposed new drug. Following approval, the FDA regularly reviews and maintains the right to remove or restrict marketing and sales of OTC drugs that create adverse side affects or are potentially addictive.

Following discovery, testing, and FDA approval of a new drug, it is given a unique trade name or brand name. The pharmaceutical company is awarded an exclusive patent to manufacture and market the drug for a specified period of time, usually seventeen years in the United States but of variable length in other countries. At the end of this time, the company no longer has proprietary rights to the drug, which may then be manufactured and marketed by other pharmaceutical companies. These drug companies may choose to market the drug under a new brand name of their choosing but not under the original label, which may still be manufactured by the original pharmaceutical company that designed and patented the drug. Spin-off products of these companies must still pass rigid FDA quality control standards which demonstrate that their product contains sufficient amounts of the active ingredients to promote bioequivalency before it can be marketed as an OTC medication—that is, the new drug has to be the therapeutic equal of the original drug.

Drugs manufactured by other pharmaceutical companies following patent expiration are typically called generic drugs and are strictly regulated by the U.S. Drug Price Competition and Patent Term Restoration Act (also known as the Hatch-Waxman Act), which was enacted in 1984. Tylenol, for example, is the exclusive brand name of an analgesic over-thecounter medication that contains the active chemical ingredient acetaminophen. Following the release of its patent, many other pharmaceutical companies started marketing pain relief drugs containing products for pain relief under the their own trade name or brand name. These copies are considered generic drugs and provide the consumer with a wide choice of the most popular drugs, usually at greatly reduced cost.

Manufacture and marketing of a generic drug by new companies usually means that their product costs considerably less, partly because of competition but mostly because the new drug companies did not bear the initial costs of development, marketing, and promotion that were part of the original financial investment of the parent company. Furthermore, manufacturers of generic drugs enjoy all the benefits of prior marketing, public acceptance, and possibly dependence on the most popular OTC medications. Generally, however, the parent company enjoys a certain competitive advantage of brand name recognition that promotes continued use of their marketed product, thereby reducing the impact of cheaper competition.

Over-the-counter medications may take the form of packets, tablets, capsules, pills, drops or droplets, ointments, inhalants, lotions, creams, suppositories, or syrups. Except for creams and topical ointments, OTC medications are administered orally, in contrast to drugs that are taken by injection. This mode of delivery places natural limits on their therapeutic effectiveness in several ways.

After being swallowed, OTC medications pass down the esophagus, through the stomach, and into the small intestine, bwhere they are digested and absorbed. This mode of delivery requires a certain time interval between oral intake of the drug and its arrival in the bloodstream that transports it to target cells, tissues, and organs, thus delaying the effects of the drug. Tablets or capsules sometimes get stuck in the back of the mouth or on the lining of the esophagus, where they start to dissolve. When this happens, the ingredients may cause irritation, nausea, and sometimes vomiting, and the therapeutic value is lost. Furthermore, a certain amount of each key ingredient will be destroyed by the digestive enzymes of the gastrointestinal system, may be metabolized by cells of the intestinal epithelia, or may simply pass through the gut without being absorbed. Even following absorption into the blood, a certain amount of the drug may be lost because liver and other body cells set about removing foreign substances in the blood almost as soon as they are detected, generally by metabolizing the ingredient into a harmless chemical that will be excreted into the bile or be removed by the kidneys. This process explains why all drugs, including OTC medications, must be taken in repeated doses at regularly prescribed intervals in order to obtain maximum therapeutic value.

A final factor complicating delivery efficiency and thus the therapeutic value of OTC medications involves their packaging. Capsules, tablets, and pills in particular all contain substances in addition to the chemical ingredient, such as coatings, fillers, stabilizers, and often color additives. These substances, called excipients, do not contribute to the actual working of the drug itself, but they often modify both the rate and the extent of dissolution of the drug as it travels the gastrointestinal tract. While most excipients ultimately reduce the overall degree of delivery, some have important functions of permitting them to transit through the stomach, which has limited absorption ability, and into the small intestine, where chemical dissolution and absorption occurs at an optimum rate. For some drugs, the natural limits placed on delivery efficiency by gastrointestinal processes and excipient components can be sharply reduced by placing the capsule or tablet directly under the tongue, thus entirely bypassing the alimentary tract.

USES AND COMPLICATIONS

Primarily because of liability issues, all OTC medications include labels that are sometimes extensive. Label components typically consist of a list of one or more symptoms addressed by the medication, active ingredients contained in the drug, warnings, directions for use, and the date after which the medication should be discarded. For example, the label on a common OTC medication used to treat severe colds notes that it is to be used to relieve symptoms of nasal congestion, cough, sore throat, runny nose, headache and body ache, and fever. Directions for use are specific as to number of times a day, hours between use, and factors involving taking the medication, such as with or without glasses of water prior to or following administration and limits regarding food intake.

Most labels also carry prominent warnings regarding use with respect to age, alcohol consumption, sedatives or tranquilizers, and combinations of medications. Most over-thecounter medications also state that use should be continued only for a specified time and that, if symptoms persist, the user should stop taking the medication and consult a physician. Finally, the user is usually cautioned to stop taking the OTC medication immediately if headache, rash, nausea, or similar symptoms appear. Despite these warnings, even commonly used OTC medications pose certain health hazards, and the user is advised to take these medications with full recognition of potential problems.

In the United States, while the FDA periodically issues warnings regarding OTC medications, their actual use by consumers normally is not regulated, documented, or monitored. This has led to a number of concerns regarding real and potential overuse of OTC drugs, particularly for reasons unrelated to their medicinal intent. It has also led directly to the modification of certain OTC medications to engineer drugs that are highly addictive.

Because their use is unregulated—or, more correctly, cannot be regulated—over-the-counter medications can be deliberately abused. Overdosing with certain types of painkillers, for example, has become a frequent method of suicide attempt. The use of Tylenol in suicide attempts is increasing. Tylenol overdosing causes the destruction of liver cells that synthesize blood coagulants. Loss of these blood coagulants results in uncontrolled bleeding, most evidently through the eyes, nose, and mouth but also internally. Internal bleeding continues until death occurs, usually within a few days following onset.

Perhaps the most egregious misuse of OTC medications is to induce or achieve temporary "highs" that parallel those obtained by use of street or hard drugs. Cough suppressants that contain the drug dextromethorphan, for example, affect the central nervous system and can be used as mood-altering drugs that cause brain damage and even death at high doses. An even more serious abuse is the cooking of common drugs to obtain the highly addictive drug methamphetamine, popularly called meth. Also known as ice or speed, meth is a highly addictive drug that is often devastating and sometimes deadly. In some regions of the United States, it ranks with heroin and cocaine as the popular drug of choice. Record growth in use and the ability to cook meth from readily obtained OTC drugs has led to the creation of National Methamphetamine Awareness Day to draw attention at all levels to this problem.

This cooking process involves the conversion of certain OTC medications into meth. Some other sources for cooking meth include diet aids, tincture of iodine or other iodine solutions, and household cleaning solutions. In response to the widespread home manufacture of meth, a national federal law was enacted to require pharmacies to check photo identification and keep records of over-the-counter sales of cold medications that contain pseudoephedrine and ephedrine, which are the two popular ingredients in many cold medications. By-products of in-home meth cooking labs are garbage cans filled with Sudafed packages and a distinct odor of cat urine. The cooking process itself releases potentially harmful toxic chemicals that can pose serious health hazards to lungs and the respiratory system and also poses the risk of fire.

PERSPECTIVE AND PROSPECTS

Originally, OTC medications were available for purchase only at pharmacies, along with physician-prescribed drugs. Today, a varied selection of OTC medications is available at many retail outlets, including supermarkets, food stores, and even convenience stores, although pharmacies still continue to offer the greatest selection. This can lead to a confusion of terms, as such medications or drugs are often no longer sold "over the counter" but instead can be found on shelves alongside other items for sale.

To complicate matters, certain drugs are offered as OTC medications at low dosages but must be obtained by prescription at higher dosages. For example, the popular analgesic ibuprofen (Advil, Motrin) can be purchased as an OTC medication at dosages of less than

200 milligrams, but higher dosages can be obtained only via prescription. Similarly, the antidiarrheal medication Imodium, an opiate, is available as an OTC medication in liquid form, while tablets of Imodium are available only by prescription.

The status of over-the-counter medications may change over time, depending on effectiveness and safety issues. While some OTC drugs are removed from the general market following various concerns regarding safety, other drugs are transferred from prescription drugs to OTC medications. Examples include the antihistamine drug Benadryl, which is used to relieve symptoms of allergy and guard against allergic reactions, and the painkiller ibuprofen, both of which were, until recently, sold as prescription drugs only but are nnow available as OTC medications.

While the distribution and sale of over-the-counter medications is strictly regulated by state and federal laws in the United States, certain drugs that are deemed harmless may be offered for sale as medical cures for many ailments and thereby compete with OTC medications. These so-called miracle drugs have become increasingly popular because of the Web, which opens the door to purchases without prescription. Media promotions also sometimes offer these medications, complete with testimonials that dramatically describe their success as a cure-all for ailments. These types of medications are often labeled "quack" drugs. They pose a threat to users of prescription and OTC medications in several ways. First, they are generally useless, offering a nonexistent cure for health problems. Second, they are manufactured without regard to quality control measures that legitimate drug manufacturers must follow. Third, time may be lost in using the quack drug, especially if the condition is chronic and the symptoms need to be treated immediately. Finally, while some may be harmless, other quack drugs contain chemical ingredients that are potentially dangerous when used in combination with genuine over-the-counter medications.

FURTHER READING

"Careful: Acetaminophen in pain relief medicines can cause liver damage." *fda.gov*, January 13, 2011.

Griffith, H. Winter, and Stephen Moore. *Complete Guide to Prescription and Non-Prescription Drugs*. Rev. ed. New York: Penguin Group, 2010.

Litin, Scott C., ed. *Mayo Clinic Family Health Book*. 4th ed. New York: HarperResource, 2009.

"Over-the-Counter Medicines." *MedlinePlus*, June 24, 2013.

Prescription and Over-the-Counter Drugs. Rev. ed. Pleasant View, N.Y.: *Reader's Digest*, 2001.

Sanberg, Paul, and Richard M. T. Krema. *Over-the-Counter Drugs: Harmless or Hazardous?* New York: Chelsea House, 1986.

"Use Caution with Over-the-Counter Creams, Ointments." *fda.gov*, April 1, 2008.

Dwight G. Smith

SEE ALSO: Cough and Cold Medication; Painkiller Abuse

Painkiller abuse

A painkiller is an opioid medication used to reduce or alleviate pain. Painkiller abuse is the excessive use of painkilling drugs or use for nonmedical purposes. Painkiller addiction is the condition of physical or psychological dependence on a painkiller. The drugs are obtained legally through prescription, purchased as an over-the-counter medication, or bought illegally.

CAUSES

Opioids come in two forms: natural and synthetic. Natural opioids are derived from the opium plant; synthetic (artificial) and partially synthetic opioids are structurally similar to natural opioids. Morphinemorphine and codeinecodeine are purified from the crude opium latex. Partially synthetic drugs derived from morphine include heroin, oxycodoneoxycodone (OxyContin), hydromorphone (Dilaudid), and oxymorphone (Numorphan). Synthetic compounds that resemble morphine in their chemical structure include fentanyl (Duragesic), levorphanol (Levo-Dromoran), meperidine (Demerol), methadonemethadone, and dextropropoxyphene (Darvon).

All opioids exert their effect by modifying the transmission of the nerve impulse between neurons (nerve cells). Neurons are separated from each other through short spaces called synapses. When the nerve impulse reaches the terminal end of one neuron, neurotransmitters are released into the synapse. The neurotransmitter travels across the synapse and binds to receptors on the terminal of the next neuron to allow continuation of the nerve impulse. In the case of opioids, this neurotransmitter is dopaminedopamine.

Opioids act to increase and maintain the concentration of dopamine in the synapse by two methods. Some drugs prevent the reuptake of dopamine from the synapse by binding to proteins that normally transport dopamine. Other drugs act to increase the release of more dopamine from the presynaptic neuron terminal. The result is the maintenance and enhancement of the pleasurable effect promoted by dopamine.

Opium and its synthetic counterparts have structural similarities to natural pain relievers in the body called endorphinsendorphins. Endorphins are secreted by the pituitary gland in response to pain stimuli, resulting in the relief of pain by binding to pain receptors and preventing transmission of the pain impulse. Endorphins are also secreted in response to pleasurable activities, such as eating and sex, resulting in a high that is similar to that caused by morphine. Endorphins are more potent than morphine, but they do not lead to addiction because they are broken down by enzymes and do not accumulate.

Nonsteroidal anti-inflammatory drugs (NSAIDs) are painkillers that act in the body by a different mechanism. The most common NSAIDs are acetaminophen, acetylsalicylic acid (aspirin), and ibuprofen and are readily available over the counter. NSAIDs act by inhibiting the cyclooxygenase enzymes 1 and 2 that are involved in the synthesis of prostaglandins. Prostaglandins are involved in a variety of body processes, including sensitization of nerve endings.

NSAIDs are most commonly used for headache relief; however, they are often used to treat symptoms for which they are not recommended, such as anxiety, sleep problems, and stress. Authorities generally agree that the use of NSAIDs rarely leads to physical dependence.

OxyContin and heroin have similar chemical structures and bind to the same receptors in the brain.

RISK FACTORS

Painkiller abuse may include self-medication, or the use of the drugs without a prescription to relieve pain or other symptoms. Chronic pain is a common cause of painkiller abuse. A person with chronic pain may begin to take painkiller medication beyond the physician's prescription in larger doses or more frequently. People also use drugs for recreational purposes to produce euphoria, an emotional state of intensely pleasurable feelings.

More painkillers are available than ever before because of an increasing awareness and desire of physicians to reduce severe pain in their patients. In many cases, only opioid drugs can reduce severe pain. Physicians need to balance the need for relieving a patient's pain versus the chance that the patient's opiate use may lead to addiction. The ready availability of painkiller drugs can lead the patient to ignore alternative means of pain control. Additionally, many new pain medications first became available in the 1990s.

Social factors can be important in painkiller abuse. Exposing drugs to adolescents and young adults is a critical factor, as it can lead to a lifetime of drug abuse. A family structure lacking stability or that is disruptive and violent can result in a lack of good role models and a poor sense of direction for children. Pain medications may be readily available at home, leading teens to take them to relieve pain or stress without a doctor's prescription.

Peer pressure, the influence of friends and acquaintances in school and on the street, can be an important driving force, too. Adolescents often seek acceptance within particular groups, and adolescents may be prone to drug experimentation within these groups. Some persons of any age are more likely to become drug dependent, especially those who lack confidence or self-esteem, who may look to drugs to fill a void or to overcome loneliness or depression.

Genetic susceptibility can be a factor in painkiller abuse, although it is difficult to separate genetic from environmental influences. An estimated 40 to 60 percent of the variability of addiction is caused by genetic factors or by combined genetic and environmental interactions.

SYMPTOMS

Signs of painkiller abuse can be psychological or physical. Psychologically, the person abusing drugs is focused on obtaining more drugs. He or she may increase the dose over time and often continues to use drugs after his or her medical condition has improved. Physical appearance often declines, and the person may show shifts in energy, mood, and concentration. He or she may withdraw from family and friends and might neglect household and work responsibilities.

Typical symptoms of painkiller addiction are feelings of euphoria, lethargy, mental confusion, nausea, and poor judgment. Less specific symptoms include slurred speech, shallow breathing, bloodshot eyes, constipation, and unusual drowsiness. The addict eventually develops a tolerance for the drug, requiring higher doses to obtain the same effect. Withdrawal symptoms often occur if the addict abruptly stops using the drug. Withdrawal symptoms may include agitation, muscle aches, insomnia, anxiety, cramps, and nausea and vomiting.

SCREENING AND DIAGNOSIS

A physician will take a complete history of the patient, perform a physical examination, and send blood or urine samples to a laboratory to test for the presence of suspected drugs. Although blood tests are more likely than urine tests to detect drugs, urine tests are more common. Opiates are usually found in the urine within twelve to thirty-six hours of last use. A particular drug abuse screening test was developed in 1982, and it consists of questions to be answered by persons concerned about their involvement with drugs.

TREATMENT AND THERAPY

Treatment of painkiller addiction requires the person to stop using the drug. Abrupt discontinuation of drugs by long-term users, that is, going "cold turkey," results in severe withdrawal symptoms. A more practical treatment involves slowly decreasing the use of the drug (through a process known as detoxification); complete abstinence follows.

Newer drugs, such as buprenorphine and nal-trex-onenalrexone, block the effect of opiates on the body, thereby reducing withdrawal symptoms and the length of withdrawal. Patients taking buprenorphine also can become mildly addicted to that drug. A newer version of the drug has been introduced; it is combined with another drug, naloxonenaloxone. When this drug combination is injected, the person goes into withdrawal, thus preventing abuse in use.

Psychological addiction may continue long after physical withdrawal from the drug. The recovering addict can experience difficulties in coping with daily activities, and there is a great danger the user will return to drug use. Each patient needs to be treated on an individualized basis. The detrimental mental and emotional states that led to drug use need to be identified and addressed, and the patient needs to be taught how to avoid drugs and drug culture. These changes may include new activities and new social and relational contacts.

PREVENTION

Prevention is based on removing the risk factors. Education of children by family and teachers about the dangers of painkiller abuse is paramount. Parents need to keep prescription pain medications away from children, and sharing information about drug use can become part of a school's science curriculum. Additionally, for persons taking prescription painkillers to manage chronic pain, it is important to use the medication only at the prescribed dosages to avoid developing a dependency.

FURTHER READING

Abbott, Francis, and Mary Fraser. "Use and Abuse of Over-the-Counter Analgesic Drugs." *Journal of Psychiatry and Neuroscience* 23.1 (1998): 13–34. Print. Examines the widespread use and abuse of over-the-counter painkillers from the perspective of psychiatry.

Byrne, Marilyn, Laura Lander, and Martha Ferris. "The Changing Face of Opioid Addiction: Prescription Pain Pill Dependence and Treatment." *Health Social Work* 34.1 (2009): 53–56. Print. A clinical-health perspective on changes in social work to address the abuse of painkillers and other opioids.

Twombly, Eric, and Kristen Holtz. "Teens and the Misuse of Prescription Drugs: Evidence-Based Recommendations to Curb a Growing Societal Problem." *Journal of Primary Prevention* 29.6 (2008): 503–16. Print. Discusses the abuse of prescription drugs, including painkillers, among youth.

WEBSITES OF INTEREST

Drug Dependence. PubMed Health
http://www.ncbi.nlm.nih.gov/pubmedhealth/PMH0002490
National Institute on Drug Abuse
http://www.drugabuse.gov

David A. Olle

SEE ALSO: Over-The-Counter (OTC) Drugs; Teens and Drug Abuse

PCP

PCP is a recreational drug with hallucinogenic and dissociative properties. It was first produced as a potential agent for anesthesia but was later recognized as a dangerous substance of abuse that can significantly alter mental status.

HISTORY OF USE

Phencyclidine (PCP) was originally synthesized in 1926 as 1-(1-phenylcyclohexyl)piperidine. It was intended for use as an intravenous surgical anesthetic during World War II because it caused decreased sensitivity to pain (analgesia) without decreasing heart and lung function or muscle tone. Its use was discontinued for this purpose after patients had adverse psychological side effects that included increased agitation and psychosis.

PCP was patented 1963 as the anesthetic Sernyl by Parke-Davis Pharmaceutical but was taken off the market two years later because of the drug's negative psychological effects and long half-life. PCP reappeared for veterinary use in 1967 as an animal tranquilizer.

PCP gained popularity as a recreational substance in the late 1960s because of the psychological effects. In 1969, however, PCP was made an illegal substance to possess, sell, or manufacture. In the early 1970s, the drug was categorized as a schedule III controlled substance. It was moved from schedule III to schedule II in 1978.

Since the 1970s, PCP's popularity has substantially decreased, but the drug remains readily available. Initial data from the peak of PCP use in 1979 revealed that 7 percent of high school students had used the drug. Data in 2009 from the National Survey on Drug Use and Health showed that only 122,000 Americans had used PCP within the previous calendar year; 1 percent of these persons were high school students.

Many persons are exposed to PCP without their knowledge. One study found that almost 25 percent of marijuana also contained trace levels of PCP. Additionally, PCP and other recreational drugs are gaining popularity as alternative drugs for treating chronic pain.

EFFECTS AND POTENTIAL RISKS

PCP acts as an N-methyl d-aspartate (NMDA) receptor antagonist by blocking NMDA receptor activity. It also inhibits the nicotinic acetylcholine receptor channels. By both of these mechanisms, PCP interferes with the brain's natural neurotransmitter responses. The actions of PCP on the brain are complex, causing both stimulation and depression of the central nervous system. This explains why some users may have a calming response to PCP exposure, while others may have an agitated or aggressive reaction.

The timing of drug effects depends on the mode of administration. Inhalation of PCP is the most common route because the drug works quite rapidly if inhaled; symptoms can be observed within about five minutes. With oral ingestion, symptoms can take up to one hour to be realized. The first effects of PCP last for approximately four to seven hours, but the long-lasting consequences continue for several days or even one week.

Initial effects of low doses (3 to 5 milligrams [mg]) resemble those of alcohol intoxication, including slurred speech and an unsteady gait (ataxia), and a numbing of the arms and legs. There is a significant increase in blood pressure (hypertension), pulse rate (tachycardia), and analgesia.

At increased doses (of more than 5 mg) PCP causes a decrease in respiratory rate, an irregular heart beat (arrhythmia), increased muscle tone (hypertonia), and seizures. In addition to the physiological effects, PCP also produces significant alterations in mental status at high doses. The psychological effects include hallucinations, delusions, an "out-of body" experience, amnesia, paranoia, a catatonic state, and disorganized thinking. Depression and psychosis may persist for an extended time after withdrawal.

The risk of permanent schizophrenic-like symptoms exists with PCP abuse rather than with occasional recreational use. PCP is unpredictable in how mood and mental status will be changed, and some users have negative experiences that lead to an increased tendency for suicidal thoughts or committing violent acts. Hospitalization may be required to closely monitor symptoms while recovering.

Coma and deaths have been reported from cardiac arrest, strokes from hypertension, increased body temperature (hyperthermia), breakdown of muscle (rhabdomyolysis), and increased potassium levels (hyperkalemia). Suicides and accidents secondary to violent behavior also are commonly reported. Deaths also occur because of the consumption of an unknown dosage, the presence of contaminated materials in substances that have been illegally manufactured and distributed, underlying medical issues, and the use of other drugs simultaneously.

FURTHER READING

Bey, Tareg, and Anar Patel. "Phencyclidine Intoxication and Adverse Effects: A Clinical and Pharmacological Review of an Illicit Drug." *California Journal of Emergency Medicine* 8.1 (2007): 9–14. Print. Comprehensive review of the biochemistry, physiological and psychological effects, and medical management of PCP.

Deroux, Stephen, Anthony Sgarlato, and Elizabeth Marker. "Phencyclidine: A 5-Year Retrospective Review from the New York City Medical Examiner's Office." *Journal of Forensic Sciences* 56.3 (2011): 656–59. Print. Results of a study that found that lower doses of PCP can be fatal if a user has additional medical concerns.

Liu, F., et al. "Changes in Gene Expression after Phencyclidine Administration in Developing Rats: A Potential Animal Model for Schizophrenia." *International Journal of Developmental Neuroscience* 29.3 (2011): 351–58. Print. Results of a study of rats that found PCP alters gene expression and thus increases neuronal cell death, with discussion of the implications for potential treatment of schizophrenia symptoms in humans.

WEBSITES OF INTEREST
National Institute on Drug Abuse
http://www.drugabuse.gov/infofacts/hallucinogens.html
The Partnership at DrugFree.org
http://www.drugfree.org/drug-guide/pcp

Janet Ober Berman

SEE ALSO: Hallucinogens and Their Effects

Pornography addiction

As pornography becomes more readily available, it is important to establish whether or not it is truly addictive. Researchers in both the psychological and medical communities have not come to a consensus about whether or not pornography is addictive, but research has found that pornography does play a role in relationships. Clinically, it is important to pay attention to how pornography affects the relationship and the self-esteem of each partner.

INTRODUCTION
With the rise in the availability of technology, pornography is easier to access than ever before. Consumers no longer have to go to specialty stores to buy magazines or videos. Pornography is accessible at the click of a button through the Internet and television. With the availability of pornography, researchers and lay people have begun to question whether there is a limit or threshold for when recreational use becomes an addiction. Some say that pornography addiction is similar to drug addiction. Others argue that pornography is not addictive, but compulsive. Research has yet to provide a definitive answer to the question of whether or not pornography is truly addictive. However, research has found significant results in regards to how pornography affects relationships.

WHAT IS PORNOGRAPHY ADDICTION?
Oftentimes sexual addiction and pornography addiction are defined similarly and the definitions are interwoven. The American Psychological Association (APA) asserts that sexual behavior becomes an illness "if you spend so much time pursuing intercourse or masturbation so as to interfere with your job or other important activities." They extend a similar definition to pornography addiction. APA also states that "repetitively engaging in sexual behaviors when you are anxious, depressed, or stressed," including pornography consumption, qualifies as maladaptive.

The American Psychological Association uses the Diagnostic Statistical Manual (DSM) to assess mental health and to classify behavioral disorders within the population. In the creation of the DSM 5, experts considered adding sexual addiction to the list of behavioral disorders. While it was under consideration, APA labeled sexual addiction as "hypersexual disorder" with a pornography subtype. APA stated that a male with hypersexual disorder would have seven or more orgasms per week for at least six months after age 15. However, APA did not have enough data on women's sexual behaviors. Ultimately, when the DSM 5 was printed in 2013, hypersexual disorder was not included. Hypersexual disorder is controversial, and professionals in the fields of psychology and medicine have not come to a consensus about the existence of pornography addiction.

PORNOGRAPHY AS AN ADDICTION
Dr. Valerie Voon conducted a study looking at the brain scans of people who identified as sexual addicts. Dr. Voon scanned individuals' brains as they watched pornography and found that they had the same brain scans as people who abuse alcohol when they view advertisements for alcoholic beverages. Some use Voon's research to equate pornography addiction with drug and alcohol abuse. However, Dr. Voon says it is too soon to say if pornography addiction is the same as addiction to drugs or alcohol.

Another study conducted at Binghamton University with 181 young adults found that there were differences in DNA that explained differences in sexual behavior. Researchers found that the DRD4 gene was activated in individuals with hypersexual behaviors. The DRD4 gene controls the amount of dopamine that is released. Researchers believe that the DRD4 affects dopamine in the same ways that drugs affect dopamine. The DRD4 study has not yet been replicated. No study has shown a connection between sex and opiate receptors, which are involved in drug and alcohol addictions.

Researchers at the University of California, Los Angeles looked at the brain's electrical activity with people who had trouble controlling porn use. Their brain scans were no different for images of porn than for neutral images, such as people skiing. The study found that their brain activity was not similar to that of addicts. Researchers have not come to a conclusion about whether or not pornography is addictive.

COMPULSION OR ADDICTION?

In 2013, a study was conducted with 226 men that identified a high use of porn. The men had a high correlation between pornography use and certain personality traits. The personality traits that correlated with pornography use were considered compulsive personality traits, such as obsessive checking. The researchers posited that perhaps using pornography is compulsive rather than addictive. Therefore, users of pornography felt compelled to use pornography but not addicted to pornography. The research study was correlational, not causal, and further research is needed.

EFFECTS OF PORNOGRAPHY ON RELATIONSHIPS

The research is inconclusive about whether or not pornography or sex addictions are legitimate diagnoses. However, research has been conducted that speaks to the effects of porn use on relationships and intimacy. Pornography can play a role in relationships.

Researchers Bridges and Morokoff found that when men used pornography, intimacy levels in relationships were lowered. However, when women used pornography, intimacy levels increased. The researchers hypothesized the difference between men and women are due to how men and women consume pornography. Men typically watch pornography alone while women typically watch it with their partner. It is included in the "lovemaking ritual" with women and not as a solitary activity. Researchers at Brigham Young University and the University of Missouri found similar results. Men's use of pornography lowered sexual quality however women's use of pornography increased sexual quality.

Perception of pornography use can also affect relationship quality. Researchers Stewart and Szymanski found that girlfriends who perceived their boyfriend's use of pornography as problematic had lower self-esteem, poorer relationship quality, and lower sexual satisfaction. Researchers also found that if the non-using partner found out about pornography use and thought it was harmful to the relationship, then sexual frequency was reduced and intimacy was reduced. The same was not true of partners who did not think pornography was harmful.

CLINICAL IMPLICATIONS

It is not clear yet in the research whether pornography addiction is a true diagnosis or if it is merely a compulsive behavior. Future research may better be able to speak to the similarities and differences between pornography addiction and addiction to drugs and alcohol. What is clear in the research is that pornography affects relationships. For some couples, it does not affect intimacy or sexual frequency. For others, it can lower sexual frequency and intimacy.

Oftentimes it is believed that individuals seek out pornography due to a lack of sex in the relationship. Researchers found that couples engaged in sex as often as the average for all couples in the United States. Pornography users did not seek out pornography due to a lack of sexual activity in the relationship. Communication about pornography use may help couples avoid the possible negative effects of pornography on relationships.

FUTURE DIRECTIONS

Further research is needed in the area of pornography addiction. The medical and psychological communities have not come to a conclusion about whether or not pornography use can become addictive. Research in these areas will help inform treatment for individuals who identify as sex or pornography addicts. Research currently addresses heterosexual relationships but research is needed about same-sex relationships and the effects of pornography use.

FURTHER READING:

Cloud, J. (2011). "Sex Addiction: A Disease Or A Convenient Excuse?" *Time*. Retrieved from: http://content.time.com/time/magazine/article/0,9171,2050027-1,00.html. This article provides an overview of research on pornography addiction. It also includes a firsthand account from a self-identified sex addict.

Downs, M. (n.d.). "Is Pornography Addictive?" *WebMD*. Retrieved from http://www.webmd.com/men/features/is-pornography-addictive. This article presents opinions from members of the medical community. It also addresses the debate between pornography addiction and pornography compulsion.

Skinner, K. B. (2014). "Is Pornography (Sexual) Addiction Real? *Psychology Today*. Retrieved from https://www.psychologytoday.com/blog/inside-porn-addiction/201411/is-pornography-sexual-addiction-real. This article presents the perspective of a marriage and family therapist and author on the topic of pornography addiction. Skinner believes that it is truly an addiction.

Skinner, K.B. (2012). "Pornography's Influence On Sexual Intimacy". *Psychology Today*. Retrieved from https://www.psychologytoday.com/blog/inside-porn-addiction/201201/pornographys-influence-sexual-intimacy. This article includes studies on how pornography affects intimacy, sexual frequency, and sexual satisfaction. It encourages individuals to take pornography addiction seriously because people are suffering from its consequences.

Weir, K. (2014). "Is Pornography Addictive?" *Monitor on Psychology*, 45. Retrieved from http://www.apa.org/monitor/2014/04/pornography.aspx. This article includes a summary of psychological research on whether or not pornography is addictive. It also addresses how pornography affects relationships and the characteristics of pornography users.

Amanda Backer Lappin

SEE ALSO: Masturbation; Sex Addiction

Pregnancy and alcohol

Alcohol use during pregnancy has been associated with fetal alcohol syndrome, fetal death, spontaneous abortion, and stillbirth. In 2008 and 2009, 10 percent of pregnant women age fifteen to forty-four years reported alcohol use, including binge drinkers and heavy drinkers. Although no limit on alcohol consumption has been established for pregnant women, major negative effects on the fetus have been observed with chronic alcohol use (six drinks per day), with binge drinking (five or more drinks in succession), or with drinking a total of forty-five alcoholic beverages per month.

FETAL ALCOHOL SYNDROME

Fetal alcohol syndrome (FAS) in children is the most widely recognized consequence of alcohol use during pregnancy. The syndrome was first recognized in the late 1960s as a pattern of physical abnormalities and mental impairment in children of alcoholic women.

Since the 1960s, other terms have been developed to encompass the broad spectrum of milder disorders associated with the effects of alcohol use on the fetus during pregnancy. These terms include fetal alcohol effects (FAE), fetal alcohol spectrum disorders (FASD), and alcohol-related neurological disorders.

FAS affects approximately 4 to 6 percent of infants of mothers who drink heavily while pregnant. The estimates of children with neurological impairment from prenatal alcohol exposure (not classified as FAS) are much higher. The statistics on the numbers of children with FAS may be underestimates, because the diagnosis of FASD is largely dependent on disclosure from the mother of her own alcohol abuse. Thus, the diagnosis of FAS is difficult to make and is determined primarily through reports of the mother's alcohol use during pregnancy in conjunction with a group of identifiable abnormalities in the child. The condition is characterized in a child by abnormal prenatal and postnatal growth, dysmorphic facial features, and central nervous system damage.

Alcohol use by pregnant women has been associated with growth deficiencies in both the fetus and the child after birth. Newborns have lower birth weights, and children with FAS demonstrate growth retardation even with sufficient nutrition. Weight and height remains in the lower one-tenth percentile for the child's age group. Additionally, the child may have a low weight-to-height ratio and a short stature.

There are characteristic abnormal facial features in children with FAS, most noticeably small head size. Also present is maxillary hypoplasia, the underdevelopment of the jawbones that, when combined with an underdeveloped midface, gives the illusion of a protruding lower jaw. This may also be accompanied by a small separation between the upper and lower eyelids (palpebral fissures); a small, flat, upturned nose; thin upper lip; and characteristically folded "railroad track" ears. These facial features may become less obvious as the child matures.

Neurological deficiencies are the most severe consequence of FAS. Fetuses of women who drink heavily have been found to have a lower prenatal cranial-to-body growth ratio, with brain abnormalities continuing throughout early childhood. It is believed that every episode of consumption of two or more alcoholic drinks by the pregnant woman leads to the death of a quantity of fetal brain cells. Children with FAS generally have IQs about ten points lower than average; those with the most extreme FAS symptomology can have IQs of 60 to 70. Delayed speech and speech and language difficulties may be present throughout childhood.

Maternal alcohol use during pregnancy has been associated with attention deficit hyperactivity disorder (ADHD) in children, with the degree of severity of the ADHD directly related to the amount of alcohol consumed by the mother while pregnant. Impaired or delayed development of fine motor skills has also been observed in toddlers with FAS. Psychiatric disorders such as substance abuse, paranoia, personality disorder, aggressiveness, and behavioral dysfunction occur at increased rates in children with FAS. Unlike the abnormal facial features that improve as the child matures, neurological deficiencies persist into adulthood and throughout life.

Less apparent effects of maternal alcohol abuse on the child after birth include abnormalities of the hand. The pinky finger is bent inward toward the other fingers, and the upper crease of the palm is prominent, ending between the index and ring fingers. Other possible symptoms of FAS are cardiac defects and excessive hair growth. Various types of hearing loss have also been attributed to FAS and may contribute to the developmental and social delays that children with FAS often experience.

The manifestations of FAS symptoms are highly variable among children and dependent upon the amount of alcohol consumed by the mother while pregnant. Relationships have been observed between the amount and frequency of alcohol consumed and the gestational age of the fetus. The first six weeks are critical to embryonic development, as are the last few months of pregnancy, when the fetus undergoes a period of extensive growth. Therefore, alcohol consumption during these periods of pregnancy poses a higher risk to the fetus.

Binge drinking appears to be particularly deleterious to the fetus, as it is exposed to a high level of alcohol. During binge drinking, the pregnant woman's liver takes longer to metabolize the large amount of alcohol, thereby also exposing the fetus to alcohol for an extended time.

Other factors may influence the severity of FAS symptoms exhibited by a child. It is theorized that the unique sensitivity of the pregnant woman to alcohol may moderate the effects of alcohol on the developing fetus. Variations in genes have been identified that influence the inclination to abuse alcohol, the rate of alcohol metabolism, and the tendency to develop FAS. Other factors present during pregnancy, such as maternal age, use of other drugs, nutrition, and even birth order, may influence the severity of FAS symptoms.

PREVENTION

Because no level of alcohol consumption by pregnant women has been determined to be safe for the developing fetus, the US surgeon general has recommended that women who are pregnant or intend to become pregnant in the near future, and those who are not using birth control, abstain from drinking alcohol entirely. This guidance is based on statistics showing that many pregnancies are unintentional, and women may drink alcohol before they realize they are pregnant.

The early weeks of pregnancy, including the time from conception to recognition of the first missed menstrual period, are critical to neurological development. Although alcohol use has been shown to decline after a woman realizes she is pregnant, the use of any alcohol during this time may be especially harmful to the embryo.

FAS is caused only by alcohol consumption by pregnant women and is a completely preventable cause of birth defects. Although FAS is not hereditary, the tendency to abuse alcohol may be. Health care providers can perform alcohol screening as part of routine prenatal care and can provide alcohol abuse information for their patients.

Alcohol use in the three months prior to pregnancy is also a good predictor of the pattern of alcohol use during the first three months of pregnancy. This information can be used to provide pregnant women with information on early intervention and abstinence programs. Women at high risk for alcohol abuse during pregnancy, however, frequently do not receive adequate prenatal care.

FURTHER READING

Centers for Disease Control and Prevention. "A 2005 Message to Women from the US Surgeon General: Advisory on Alcohol Use in Pregnancy." 2005. Web. 22 Mar. 2012. http://www.cdc.gov/ncbddd/fasd/documents/SurgeonGenbookmark.pdf. Guidelines on the use of alcohol during pregnancy.

Ethen, Mary K., et al. "Alcohol Consumption by Women Before and During Pregnancy." *Maternal and Child Health Journal* 13 (2009): 274–85. Print. A study of the prevalence, patterns, and predictors of alcohol use before and during pregnancy in the United States.

Gray, Ron, Raja A. S. Mukjerjee, and Michaek Rutter. "Alcohol Consumption During Pregnancy and Its Known Effects on Neurodevelopment: What Is Known and What Remains Uncertain." *Addiction* 104 (2009): 1270–73. Print. A brief, high-level summary of potential risks to the fetus when exposed to alcohol in utero.

O'Leary, Colleen M. "Fetal Alcohol Syndrome: Diagnosis, Epidemiology, and Developmental Outcomes." *Journal of Paediatric and Child Health* 40 (2004): 2–7. Print. A review of the literature on FAS to increase awareness of the diagnostic features and epidemiology of FAS and the developmental deficiencies associated with this syndrome.

Ornoy, Asher, and Zivanit Ergaz. "Alcohol Abuse in Pregnant Women: Effects on the Fetus and Newborn, Mode of Action and Maternal Treatment." *International Journal of Environmental Research and Public Health* 7 (2010): 364–79. Print. Results of investigations of the effects of alcohol use on the developing embryo and fetus in both animal models and humans.

Wattendorf, Daniel J., and Maximillian Muenke. "Fetal Alcohol Spectrum Disorders." American Family Physician 72 (2005): 279–82. Print. A review of the epidemiology, clinical presentation, diagnosis, and management of fetal alcohol spectrum disorders.

WEBSITES OF INTEREST

Fetal Alcohol Spectrum Disorders, Center for Excellence
http://fascenter.samhsa.gov
National Organization on Fetal Alcohol Syndrome
http://www.nofas.org

Debra A. Appello

SEE ALSO: Fetal Alcohol Syndrome; Teen Pregnancy

Pregnancy and drug use

Drug abuse during pregnancy frequently leads to spontaneous abortion, premature birth, stillbirth, low birthweight infants, and an increased risk of sudden infant death syndrome. Birth defects caused by drug abuse during pregnancy are rare, however. Drugs considered to have abuse potential during pregnancy include marijuana, cocaine, heroin, hallucinogens, and prescription pain medications.

DRUG USE DURING PREGNANCY

For the years 2008 and 2009, 4.5 percent of pregnant girls and women age fifteen to forty-four years, including 7.1 percent of women age eighteen to twenty-five years, admitted to some kind of illicit drug use in the past month. Drug use was highest during the first trimester of pregnancy and decreased in the second and third trimesters. The most commonly reported illicit drugs used were heroin, cocaine, and benzodiazepines.

Certain factors in the life of a drug-abusing woman contribute to her reluctance to seek help, obtain prenatal care, or to stop using drugs during pregnancy. Many women who exhibit a pattern of drug use have mental, social, and financial problems. These situations contribute to an overall unhealthy routine that may include smoking, poor diet, stress, violence, and unpredictable living conditions, resulting in adverse pregnancy outcomes.

Drug-addicted women frequently are much more likely to smoke cigarettes and to use intravenous drugs during pregnancy, potentially exposing themselves to blood-borne infections. The high rates of mental illness in women who abuse drugs and illnesses that include anxiety, depression, and personality disorders contribute to a high rate of relapse among women who attempt to discontinue drug use while pregnant.

Women who abuse drugs may fail to obtain prenatal care for several reasons. For example, amenorrhea is a common side effect of drug abuse, so a woman may not realize she is pregnant. Drug use can be particularly risky to the fetus during the first eight weeks of pregnancy, a critical period of fetal development. Drug addiction also may lead to forgotten or missed appointments or to a lack of concern regarding the health of the fetus. Women who abuse drugs also endanger their own health through unhealthy lifestyles and relationships that may involve physical abuse, which also risks harm to the fetus.

COCAINE

The 1980s witnessed a significant increase in the use of cocainecocaineand pregnancy and crack cocaine in the United States. Cocaine remains a serious public health issue in the United States, with the majority of cocaine-using women in their childbearing years.

It has been determined that when a pregnant woman uses cocaine, the drug crosses the blood-brain barrier and the placenta, becoming readily available to the developing fetus. Animal models have shown that cocaine interferes with fetal brain development because it interacts with neurotransmitters and affects gene expression, but the mechanisms for this are unknown. Children exposed to cocaine prenatally have demonstrated deficits in attention span and impulse control, which may be attributed to the effects of cocaine on areas of the brain regulating these functions.

Cocaine is known to be a vasoconstrictor and may contribute to spontaneous abortion and low birth weight from a lack of blood flow to the fetus. Cocaine use during pregnancy, especially crack cocaine, has been linked to deformed arms, legs, and internal organs because of this vasoconstriction effect during fetal development. Lack of blood flow across the placenta also prevents the transport of oxygen and nutrients to the fetus. Infants born to cocaine-addicted women also are more likely to be hospitalized in a neonatal intensive care unit.

Infants are also affected indirectly by their mother's cocaine use through the effects that use has on the area of the brain that controls maternal behavior. Cocaine disrupts the pathways in the brain that control maternal-infant bonding behavior and disrupts the production of oxytocin, a hormone that is key to triggering response behaviors in mothers.

OTHER SUBSTANCES

In addition to cocaine, other frequently misused substances, such as methamphetamine, marijuana, hallucinogens, and opiates, have demonstrated increased risk of premature labor and low birth-weight infants. Methamphetaminemethamphetamineand pregnancy use has grown substantially in the United States, particularly in the western half of the country. Thus far, however, there have been few studies of the effect of methamphetamine use on the developing fetus.

It is known that methamphetamine interacts with biochemical transporters in the brain and is transported directly into cells. Once inside nerve cells, methamphetamine disrupts the release and metabolism of neurotransmitter molecules in the brain, impairing the development of the neurotransmitter system. Methamphetamine is a vasoconstrictor, similar to cocaine, and can have the same effect on the fetus through lack of blood flow.

Magnetic resonance imaging studies of children exposed to methamphetamine in utero have revealed abnormal brain structure in association with neurological developmental deficiencies. Newborn babies prenatally

exposed to methamphetamine are usually underweight and have shown similar neurological effects as those exposed to cocaine. Animal models have demonstrated learning deficiencies, behavioral problems, and hyperactivity.

Heroin is a short-acting opiate that, with repeated use and withdrawal, can cause muscle contractions, leading to premature labor. However, no studies have shown that heroin use during pregnancy causes central nervous system damage in the developing fetus. Opiates cross the placenta, so opiate abusers may give birth to addicted newborns who must subsequently undergo withdrawal. These newborns experience irritability, central nervous system difficulties, gastrointestinal disorders, and respiratory symptoms for up to eight days after birth. As in the case of cocaine, it is difficult to determine if these symptoms are caused by the mother's heroin use or are consequences of other factors associated with the mother's lifestyle.

REMEDIAL ACTIONS

It is difficult to attribute specific fetal deficiencies to illicit drug use because of the many other confounding factors in the drug-addicted woman's life. These factors include smoking and poor nutrition, both of which may adversely affect the pregnancy too.

Residential treatment during pregnancy has demonstrated positive outcomes, but it is unclear if this outcome is from stabilization of the drug use or from an overall healthier lifestyle. Studies have shown that drug-addicted women who receive early intervention and extensive prenatal care and supervision can have pregnancy outcomes equivalent to women who do not use drugs. Comprehensive prenatal care can substantially reduce the risk of premature labor and low birth-weight infants among drug abusers.

It is recommended that pregnant women stop using cocaine during pregnancy, but the cocaine must be reduced in a measured fashion to avoid side effects, such as maternal seizures. Methadone treatment has been found to stabilize opiate abusers during pregnancy by allowing the women to gradually diminish opiate abuse through the pregnancy without the repeated use and withdrawal of heroin. The effect of drug abuse on infant mortality remains to be studied and delineated.

FURTHER READING

Burgdorf, Kenneth, et al. "Birth Outcomes for Pregnant Women in Residential Substance Abuse Treatment." *Evaluation and Program Planning* 27 (2004): 199–204. Print. An exploratory study investigating the effect of residential substance abuse treatment on pregnancy outcomes.

Hepburn, Mary. "Substance Abuse in Pregnancy." *Current Obstetrics and Gynaecology* 14 (2004): 419–25. Print. An overview of the management of high-risk pregnancies caused by drug or alcohol abuse.

Pinto, Shanthi M., et al. "Substance Abuse During Pregnancy: Effect on Pregnancy Outcomes." *European Journal of Obstetrics and Gynecology and Reproductive Biology* 150 (2010): 137–41. Print. A retrospective study of drug-abusing women in the United Kingdom in a four-year period to determine the effect of drug use on maternal and perinatal complications.

Prentice, Sheena. "Substance Misuse in Pregnancy." *Obstetrics, Gynaecology, and Reproductive Medicine* 20 (2010): 278–83. Print. A study of substance misuse during pregnancy and the role of the specialist midwife.

Roussotte, Florence, Lindsay Soderberg, and Elizabeth Sowell. "Structural, Metabolic, and Functional Brain Abnormalities as a Result of Prenatal Exposure to Drugs of Abuse: Evidence from Neuroimaging." *Neuropsychology Review* 20 (2010): 376–97. Print. A study of the effects on the fetal brains of humans and animals, using MRIs, of mothers who abused alcohol, cocaine, or methamphetamine during pregnancy.

Salisbury, Amy L., et al. "Fetal Effects of Psychoactive Drugs." *Clinical Perinatology* 36 (2009): 595–619. Print. A study of the effects of cocaine, methamphetamine, and selective serotonin reuptake inhibitors on the developing brain and central nervous system of the fetus.

Strathearn, Lane, and Linda C. Mayes. "Cocaine Addiction in Mothers: Potential Effects on Maternal Care and Infant Development." *Annals of the New York Academy of Science* 1187 (2010): 172–83. Print. A study of how cocaine use affects maternal care and infant development in both humans and animal models.

WEBSITES OF INTEREST

Fetal Alcohol Spectrum Disorders, Center for Excellence
http://fascenter.samhsa.gov

National Institute on Drug Abuse
http://www.drugabuse.gov

Debra A. Appello

SEE ALSO: Cocaine and Its Effects; Teen Pregnancy

Prescription drug abuse

Prescription drug abuse is the use of prescribed medications for reasons other than intended by a medical professional. Prescription drugs are taken in excess quantity, more frequently, or for a longer time than prescribed in order to produce changes in mental or physical status. The abuse of prescription drugs is now considered an epidemic in both the United States and in Canada.

DATA COLLECTION

The collection of accurate data on prescription drug abuse is of paramount importance, as prescription drugs constitute the second most abused class of substances behind marijuana. The National Survey on Drug Use and Health (1992) reported that 4 million people in the United States abused or misused prescription pain relievers; this figure rose to 5 million in 1998, 6.5 million in 1999, and 8.4 million in 2001. Furthermore, there was an overall increase in the prevalence of prescription drug abuse (0.17 percent in 1991–1992 to 0.28 percent in 2001–2002).

The abuse of prescription drugs causes a great burden on individuals and on the health care system. The Drug Abuse Warning Network found a significant increase of 98.4 percent in emergency room visits related to prescription medication abuse from 2004 to 2009, from approximately 627,000 cases in 2004 to more than 1.2 million. A rise in deaths secondary to this abuse, specifically with opioids, also was observed. The amount of opioid-related deaths increased by 68 percent from 1999 to 2004. The economic impact is significant, with 2001 estimates for abuse of opioid medications revealing a $2.6 billion cost to the health care system for treatment, $1.4 billion cost to the criminal justice system, and $4.6 billion cost in the workplace of affected persons. Therefore, the collection of statistics on other prescription drugs of abuse and research on prevention and treatment are becoming public health priorities.

Statistics reveal that the majority of persons who abuse prescription drugs still do not receive proper medical or mental health treatment for the problem. While one study in the United States found that treatment admissions rose by one-third from 2001 to 2003, another study found that fewer persons enrolled in treatment in 2001–2002 than in 1991–1992 (by 36.4 percent); this translates into 86 percent of prescription drug abusers not receiving proper care in 2001–2002.

In Canada, the Centre for Addiction and Mental Health similarly found that only 11 percent of admissions to treatment programs for substance abuse were for prescription drug abuse. When persons sought treatment, they most commonly attended twelve-step programs such as Narcotics Anonymous. Some also attended drug rehabilitation programs or were aided by a psychologist, physician, or social worker. The under-utilization of treatment demonstrates how greater effort is needed to understand why this population does not receive the same detoxification and psychological treatment as illicit substance and alcohol abusers.

DATA COLLECTION CHALLENGES

Until recently, there has been a paucity of reliable and valid medical literature on prescription drug abuse because the problem went either unrecognized or under-recognized by physicians and researchers. Health care providers and researchers often inquire only about illicit substances and neglect to ask patients about abusing prescription medications. Several national and international agencies and networks have since been established to obtain statistics and track trends of prescription drug abuse.

Additionally, there is no agreed-upon, standardized definition of what constitutes prescription drug abuse, and the medical literature does not agree on whether to classify the problem as abuse or misuse. This poses a challenge when attempting to collect and analyze data. It remains difficult to determine from an examination of medical records if a person took medication secondary to self-treating an actual medical diagnosis, such as chronic pain, anxiety, or sleep disorders, or if that person abused the drug to get high.

RISK FACTORS FOR PRESCRIPTION DRUG ABUSE

Teenagers and young adults age eighteen to twenty-five are typically considered the highest risk population for prescription drug abuse for two reasons: the ease of access to medications from family or friends and the general social acceptability of using prescription medications, instead of illicit drugs, to get high. One study of college

students estimated that 20 percent of this population had misused prescription drugs; this figure has risen since about 1995. While men, overall, are more likely than women to abuse prescription drugs, women often misuse prescriptions to self-medicate rather than to get high.

Prescription drug abuse is more common among non-Hispanic Caucasians than among persons of other ethnic backgrounds. Data from 1999 hospital records revealed that 87 percent of persons admitted for prescription drug abuse were of Caucasian ancestry; later studies have confirmed this population as the greatest risk.

Furthermore, persons who abuse prescription drugs are more likely to consume alcohol and be diagnosed with other illicit substance disorders. The data have not found a change in this statistic over time, with most persons in this population being young and unmarried men. However, the population characteristics have been further elucidated. Persons of African American ancestry and those age forty-five years and older showed a significant increase in being diagnosed with both a prescription drug abuse and substance abuse or alcohol disorder. The reasons for the rise of concurrent disorders in other demographics need to be determined through further study.

TRENDS AND STATISTICS BY DRUG CATEGORY

Prescription drugs are divided into four categories for purposes of studying their abuse patterns: opioids; sedatives, hypnotics, and tranquilizers; stimulants; and anesthetics. However, the categories are not always mutually exclusive, as many persons abuse medications in multiple classes. One study found that 19.3 percent of persons abused medications from two classes, 11.1 percent from three classes, and 5 percent from all four classes.

Opioids. Opioids, such as oxycodone, methadone, hydrocodone, and codeine, constitute the most commonly abused class of prescription drugs and are intended to act as pain relievers. Data between 1991–1992 and 2001–2002 shows that the prevalence of opioid abuse increased significantly. This rise is attributable, in part, to opioids being the most frequently prescribed class of medications. Physicians prescribed hydrocodone-acetaminophen for pain management more than any other pain medication in 2008, a 6.9 percent increase from 2006. The use of fentanyl, which is an opioid patch, showed a similar increase in prescriptions and accounted for approximately six thousand more emergency room visits secondary to abuse in 2008 when compared with 2006.

Sedatives, hypnotics, and tranquilizers. Another popular class of prescription drugs includes sedatives, hypnotics, and tranquilizers. Commonly abused medications in this category include phenobarbital, methaqualone, clonazepam, and alprazolam. Physicians are more frequently prescribing these medications to reduce symptoms of insomnia, anxiety, and panic disorders. Women are more likely to be admitted for treatment with this category. Data from a ten-year span (1991–1992 to 2001–2002) shows an increase in the prevalence of sedative abuse. While tranquilizer abuse accounted for more emergency room visits in 2006 than in 2004 (36 percent), another large study did not find any significant increases in the prevalence of tranquilizer abuse in that same ten-year period.

Stimulants. Common stimulants include amphetamine, dextroamphetamine, and methamphetamine. The abuse of stimulants is on the rise because of the increasing amount of prescriptions written to treat attention deficit hyperactivity disorder (ADHD). The US Drug Enforcement Administration found a 600 percent increase in ADHD prescriptions between 1990 and 1995, many of which were then sold to others for nonmedical purposes. Not all studies, however, have found an increase in stimulant abuse. Because more prescriptions are given to younger school-age persons to treat ADHD, the age of hospital admission for this category is younger than for other classes of prescription drug abuse.

Anesthetics. The least commonly abused class of prescription drugs is anesthetics, as most of these require administration by a physician and are not generally prescribed. However, health care professionals who have access to these medications, especially anesthesiologists, are at risk.

FURTHER READING

Birnbaum, Howard, et al. "Estimated Costs of Prescription Opioid Analgesic Abuse in the United States in 2001." *Clinical Journal of Pain* 22.8 (2006): 667–76. Print. Study provides figures on the increasing costs of prescription drug abuse to both the medical and criminal justice fields.

Hernandez, S., and L. Nelson. "Prescription Drug Abuse: Insight into the Epidemic." *Clinical Pharmacology and Therapeutics* 88.3 (2010): 307–17. Print. Article lists a summary of current networks and studies that collect data on prescription drug abuse as well as some of the commonly misused substances.

McCabe, Sean, Carol Boyd, and Christian Teter. "Subtypes of Nonmedical Prescription Drug Misuse." *Drug and Alcohol Dependence* 102 (2009): 63–70. Print. Research data on prevalence of prescription drug abuse by type of drug and race and gender demographics.

McCabe, Sean, James Cranford, and Brady West. "Trends in Prescription Drug Abuse and Dependence, Co-Occurrence with Other Substance Use Disorders, and Treatment Utilization: Results from Two National Surveys." *Addictive Behaviors* 33 (2008): 1297–1305. Print. Study reports trends in prescription drug abuse and treatment from 1991–1992 and 2001–2002.

WEBSITES OF INTEREST

Canadian Centre on Substance Abuse
http://ccsa.ca
Center for Behavioral Health Statistics and Quality
http://www.samhsa.gov/about/cbhsq.aspx
National Institute on Drug Abuse
http://drugabuse.gov

Janet Ober Berman

SEE ALSO: Painkiller Abuse; Stimulants and Their Effects

Recognizing the symptoms

Substance abuse is characterized by the overuse of alcohol or drugs that leads to compulsive urges to consume the substance of choice. Substance abuse affects the user's quality of life and the ability to make good decisions. In addition to negative behavioral symptoms, substance abuse generates harmful physical symptoms—unseen physiological damage to internal organs and visible deterioration in the user's appearance.

RISK FACTORS

Experimentation with alcohol and drugs is the most prominent risk to becoming a substance abuser. Whether the reward of the high is physical pleasure, the temporary removal of a traumatic memory from the mind, or simply acceptance by a peer group, experimenting with substances is always risky. Symptoms of the substance use and its effects begin to appear immediately.

Many neuroscientists and mental health professionals assert that some persons are more susceptible than others to becoming addicted to alcohol or drugs because of genetic, biological, or environmental tendencies or exposure. Risk factors include a family history of substance abuse, mental disorders, childhood trauma, and early experimentation with substances. For persons with or without these risk factors, experimentation with certain substances could lead to addiction.

The earlier a substance abuser recognizes the symptoms of substance abuse and acknowledges the dangers of continued use, the earlier he or she can advance toward treatment and recovery. At any point between a substance abuser's experimentation and addiction, signs of dependency increasingly become apparent. Friends and family members may recognize the symptoms and then intervene to break a substance abuser's destructive patterns. By not confronting a person suspected of substance abuse, the problem will likely worsen.

Though a substance abuser is likely to admit to using a substance, he or she is less likely to admit to abusing that substance, which makes the process of intervention difficult. Still, the more proficient a loved one or friend is in recognizing the symptoms of substance abuse, the more confident he or she can be in intervening.

PHYSICAL SYMPTOMS

The most profound physiological symptoms of substance abuse stem from how substances radically alter the biochemical processes of the brain. Alcohol and drugs affect how the brain's nerve receptors receive, process, and send information by overtaking the brain's neurotransmitters and by overstimulating the brain's pleasure center.

This effect on the brain is manifested in a substance abuser's mood. He or she will seem cheerful or "normal" when feeling the initial effects, or the high, of the substance. Once the high wears off, he or she will be noticeably agitated or depressed. A substance abuser also requires increasingly higher and more frequent dosing of the substance of choice to achieve the same effects after physical dependence develops.

Without increasing dosage and frequency, the abuser will experience disruptive withdrawal symptoms. Other common physical warning signs of substance abuse include bloodshot and glassy eyes, sudden weight loss or weight gain, change in appetite, deteriorating personal appearance and hygiene, odor of alcohol or smoke emanating from the person's breath or clothing, tremors, lack of coordination, and changes in speech patterns like slurring.

Though all substances can generate short-term or long-term effects on the body, different substances affect the body differently and manifest different symptoms. Alcohol, for example, increases dopamine in the brain, and when abused it impedes the natural production and transmission of dopamine. As the brain's organic ability to generate pleasure chemicals is impeded by chronic alcohol consumption, the alcoholic develops a tolerance for alcohol and has difficulty functioning in daily life without it. Physical signs of alcoholism are the odor of alcohol on the breath and skin, bloodshot eyes, redness in the face, a bloated stomach, slurred speech, and a lack of coordination and focus.

Marijuana's main active chemical, delta-9-tetrahydrocannabinol (THC), impacts sites in the brain known as cannabinoid receptors. A marijuana user will have bloodshot and glassy eyes, impaired coordination, difficulty with thinking, and memory loss. Because THC weakens the immune system, a chronic marijuana smoker frequently contracts respiratory infections.

Cocaine stimulates the nervous system by increasing the level of dopamine in the brain, and it adversely affects the ability of the brain to transmit dopamine organically. A cocaine user is hyperactive and talkative when high and appears fatigued and melancholy later, when the high has worn off. Chronic cocaine snorting causes a chronic cough, frequent nose bleeds, and even permanent damage to the nasal cavity, including a loss of the sense of smell and loss of appetite. Those who smoke crack cocaine or methamphetamine (meth) experience blemishes on the skin, weight loss from decreased appetite, and rotting teeth. Stimulants, such as cocaine, crack cocaine, and meth, also will manifest physical signs of dilated pupils, dry mouth, unusual sleeping and eating patterns, and increased heart rate and blood pressure.

Nonstimulant drugs generate different symptoms. Abusers of heroin, for example, exhibit weight loss; tremors and twitching; track marks on the arms, legs, or feet; paleness; sweating; and reduced heart rate and respiration. Abusers of narcotic depressants, including prescription painkillers, appear drunk and exhibit poor judgment, clumsiness, sleepiness, and an inability to concentrate.

BEHAVIORAL SYMPTOMS

Substance abuse inflicts long-term changes to the brain; the neuroadaptations the brain produces to control the release of dopaminedopamine and regulate emotions remain with the addict even after treatment and abstinence. Substance addiction also alters the prefrontal cortex of the user, causing the reduction in neuron activity in this part of the brain.

These changes to the brain also lead to the release of the neurotransmitter glutamate, which impairs the addict's decision-making ability. Glutamate facilitates impulsiveness and intense focus on achieving the immediate reward of pleasure. Consequently, addicts often engage in reckless behavior, and rehabilitated addicts are prone to relapse when faced with substance-related stimuli. In the amygdala, the part of the brain involved in memory formation, emotional memories associated with being high are enhanced, thereby making it difficult for the addict to resist stimuli that trigger these memories.

Because substance abuse radically affects the physiology of the brain, abuse also profoundly affects behavior. The need to consume the substance of choice increasingly dominates a substance abuser's sense of judgment and daily actions.

Substance abuse may be attributed to several disruptive and harmful behavioral patterns, such as family disintegration, loss of employment, domestic violence, and child abuse. Common behavioral symptoms include the inability to refrain from consuming the substance, an obsession with achieving the next high, an abandonment of important responsibilities and interpersonal relationships, and a disregard for the obvious harm the substance is causing to the body.

Consistent with the effect that substance abuse has on the brain, a substance abuser is more likely to drop out of school or quit a job, may change peer groups often, may experience conflicts with the law, and may experience mood swings, recklessness, laziness, and paranoia.

The classic behavioral symptom of persons with a substance abuse problem is that they sever important relationships by betraying those closest to them. Because the quest for the next high is so prominent in their mind, substance abusers will lie, cheat, and steal from strangers and loved ones alike to get the next fix.

FURTHER READING

Fisher, Gary, and Nancy Roget. *Encyclopedia of Substance Abuse Prevention, Treatment, and Recovery*. Thousand Oaks, CA: Sage, 2009. An encyclopedia of key concepts and approaches used in the field of substance abuse.

Hoffman, John, and Susan Froemke, eds. *Addiction: Why Can't They Just Stop?* New York: HBO, 2007. The companion book to the HBO documentary of the same name, presenting information and testimonies about addiction in the United States.

Lawford, Christopher Kennedy. *Moments of Clarity*. New York: Morrow, 2009. First-person accounts of addiction and recovery.

"The Science of Drug Abuse and Addiction." Dec. 2011. Web. 9 Apr. 2012. http://www.drugabuse.gov/publications/media-guide/science-drug-abuse-addiction. An easy-to-read overview of substance abuse, including its symptoms.

WEBSITES

American Council for Drug Education
http://www.acde.org
American Society of Addiction Medicine
http://www.asam.org
National Institute on Drug Abuse
http://drugabuse.gov

Melissa Walsh

SEE ALSO: Addictive Personality and Behaviors; Intervention

Recovery

Recovery is a process of breaking one's addiction to an abusive substance, behavior, or other compulsion. Recovery involves maintaining abstinence from that addiction through behavior change and active effort. Recovery is not a single event but is a process of change and a new, sober way of living. Recovery takes practice, effort, and focus on daily living with support from health professionals, counselors, community members, and peer groups.

METHODS AND GOALS

The goal of sober living is not out of reach for any addict who can admit that his or her addiction has become a chronic illness. Recovery is intended to treat the illness of addiction and to break the habitual behaviors and viewpoints that fostered chronic abuse. Recovery is not a straightforward process for anyone; treatment plans differ for each addict, and the steps involved vary for each person.

Recovery typically involves long-term health care planning. Treatment might encompass substance detoxification and medication to reduce symptoms of drug withdrawal, integrated treatment of mental health issues by psychologists or addiction counselors, and development of a self-care routine with general practitioners to bolster physical health. New behavior skills and extended support systems that act as positive influences for a sober life also are frequently set in place during this treatment and recovery process.

Recovery often can involve a drastic change of life skills and beliefs from those expressed during addiction. For example, friendships, work settings, and homes that do not foster positive support of sobriety are not helpful and should be avoided during recovery. These components of the old lifestyle are best replaced with stable, sober living settings.

Recovery groups, such as twelve-step programstwelve-step programs, help recovering addicts to identify a new set of colleagues and peers. Twelve-step and other recovery programs teach supportive behavior therapy, introduce new traditions for living, encourage reevaluation of ethics and fault, and identify risk behaviors or situations to avoid, all with a supportive sponsor and a community of peers with shared experiences.

Participation in social programs within the community boosts independence and expands sober relationships. Common populations that support societal involvement during recovery include neighborhood associations, lay counselors, clergy at religious institutions, physicians, and recovered peers within twelve-step programs or transitional living environments. Sober family members also provide crucial encouragement of sober living and recovery.

Temptations for substance use exist in society. Recovery depends upon minimizing and countering inevitable stressors, such as social events that involve alcohol or cigarettes. Balancing the temptation for substance abuse and triggers of cravings with sober alternatives, such as gum chewing, is a constant goal of recovery.

Psychological counseling can strengthen an addict's resolve to maintain abstinence during recovery, especially in early recovery periods in which withdrawal and cravings remain especially strong. Trust in the relationships and social system built during recovery care, rather than in those from addiction living, is essential to maintaining abstinence and fully experiencing sober society.

Developing new interests and hobbies not only expands recovery options by introducing new people into a support network; it also provides skills and commitments that can distract from inevitable temptations. For example, enrollment in a team sport or community center class provides a recovered addict a safe setting to

mentally redirect anxiety, focus on positive skills, and interact with peers. Recovery is possible only with a commitment to some or all of these behavior-change and counseling methods.

By integrating positive habits and involvement with work, family, and neighborhood groups, a recovering addict develops coping skills and a solid network to minimize the inevitable stresses that increase the likelihood of relapse. The varied treatment and support programs offer different benefits to different people, but all options include goals of renewed commitment to physical and psychological health and to social and community participation. Long-term follow-through and continued development of reinforcements of sober living are crucial, ongoing goals of maintained recovery.

RECOVERY AS A PROCESS

A person begins to use a particular substance voluntarily, but the physical and psychological changes that result from substances of abuse formulate an addiction (which is nonvoluntary) that becomes a chronic disease. Like numerous other chronic diseases, addiction may never be fully cured. Instead, recovery is a prolonged arc that involves daily choices, decisions, and actions to minimize compulsions.

Successes alternate with challenges in an evolving process of growth. Multiple transitions are necessary to achieve sobriety. First, recovering addicts need to admit their problem and evaluate the choices that led to addiction; then, they need to address the problem with active medical treatment; finally, they need to learn to live without the substance or compulsive behavior to reenter society.

Recovered addicts must become focused and functional because they are constantly managing high levels of temptations, stress, and cravings. Repeated care during recovery is often required to prevent relapse and to sustain abstinence. Relapserelapse is the recurrence of addiction symptoms (for example, drug use and compulsive behaviors) after recovery has been established—the slip in the climb toward unbroken periods of abstinence.

Typically, a recovered addict will experience multiple phases of relapse when his or her coping skills or other psychosocial supports falter. Thus, recovery is not a singular, one-time goal but instead comprises progressive struggles and achievements. By acknowledging recovery attempts and learning from past relapse experiences, future recovery goals are more likely to be achieved. Relapse is not failure or a sign of weakness.

It is a common occurrence for many recovering addicts, and it frequently becomes a learning experience and an educational tool.

ADVOCACY AND SUPPORT

Because recovery is a way of life, not a static goal, and because recovered addicts are fully immersed in conventional society, support for sustained recovery is beneficial to public health and the wider community. Stigmas associated with substance abuse and addiction treatments can impede full involvement in work and community settings. Addiction and treatments are financial burdens to the recovered addict also.

Advocacy and support from government and private organizations improve public awareness of addiction as a disease and encourage public support for successful recovery and sobriety. The Substance Abuse and Mental Health Services Administration's Recovery Support Strategic Initiative, for example, educates recovered addicts and the public about four major dimensions of life in recovery: health, home, purpose, and community.

Recovered addicts not only overcome a disease; they also focus on living in a physically and emotionally healthy way. Their sobriety is best supported by a stable, safe living environment and by purposeful daily activities, such as work, school, family, and volunteer endeavors. Finally, through building new social networks and relationships in a positive community, a recovered addict experiences hope and support that foster daily recovery.

FURTHER READING

Coombs, Robert H., ed. *Addiction Recovery Tools: A Practical Handbook.* Thousand Oaks, CA: Sage, 2001. A text for addiction counselors and others who provide services for substance abuse recovery. Includes directions for multiple treatment methods and guidance principles that vary from traditional medical care to holistic support.

Kelly, John F., and William L. White, eds. *Addiction Recovery Management: Theory, Research, and Practice.* New York: Humana, 2011. Describes a health professional's direct approach to recovery, including evidence-based guidance about successful methods to support recovery at multiple stages of the process.

National Institute on Drug Abuse. Drugs, Brains, and Behavior: *The Science of Addiction.* Bethesda, MD: NIDA, 2010. A clinical review of how addictions develop and how to use that knowledge to break

addictive behaviors, in part by combining medical treatment with behavior change and support systems for recovery.

WEBSITES OF INTEREST

HelpGuide.org
http://www.helpguide.org/mental/drug_abuse_addiction_rehab_treatment.htm
National Institute on Drug Abuse
http://www.drugabuse.gov/publications/infofacts/treatment-approaches-drug-addiction
Substance Abuse and Mental Health Services Administration
http://www.samhsa.gov/recovery

Nicole M. Van Hoey

SEE ALSO: Addictive Personality and Behaviors; Intervention; Support Groups

Ritalin

Ritalin is a central nervous system stimulant that shares many characteristics with amphetamines. It is a controlled substance that is most often prescribed for attention-deficit hyperactivity disorder.

HISTORY OF USE

Although originally synthesized in 1944, Ritalin was not studied for its therapeutic effects in humans until the mid-1950s. Early on, Ritalin was used to treat narcolepsy (a sleep disorder), depression, and chronic fatigue. By the 1960s it was discovered to produce a calming effect in children who had been diagnosed with symptoms of attention-deficit hyperactivity disorder (ADHD).

When Ritalin is administered orally, its effects are slowed by the gastrointestinal tract, which effectively prevents the user from experiencing a euphoric high. However, when the drug is crushed and snorted or used intravenously, it can lead to intense feelings of pleasure that some have equated with cocaine usage.

Ritalin abuse has been on the rise. This increase has been driven by two primary factors. First, there has been an increase in the number of people diagnosed with ADHD. Second, persons without ADHD have learned that Ritalin can be used as a cognitive enhancer for improving academic performance on tasks that require sustained, focused attention.

Estimates indicate that between 3 and 10 percent of school-aged children in the United States meet the diagnostic criteria for ADHD. This trend has increased the overall availability of the drug. Adolescents and young adults more often abuse Ritalin by snorting it or by ingesting larger quantities to experience exhilaration. In 2010, researcher Eric Racine and his colleague and co-author Cynthia Forlini looked into rates of lifetime non-medical stimulant use and found that the prevalence for using stimulants, including Ritalin, to augment cognition ranged from 3 to 11 percent of college students.

EFFECTS AND POTENTIAL RISKS

Ritalin increases the presence of the neurotransmitter dopamine in the brain by blocking its reuptake by the cells that release it. Short-term adverse effects include headache, nausea, irregular heartbeat, wakefulness, agitation, anxiety, increased blood pressure, and, in rare instances, seizures. Long-term adverse effects include anxiety and sleeplessness. Initial reports of suppression of growth have been placed in doubt by later studies. Physical and psychological dependence can occur with chronic abuse.

FURTHER READING

Iversen, Leslie. *Speed, Ecstasy, Ritalin: The Science of Amphetamines.* New York: Oxford UP, 2008. Provides information on the medical and nonmedical history of amphetamine use, including Ritalin.

Levinthall, Charles F. *Drugs, Behavior, and Modern Society.* 7th ed. Boston: Pearson, 2012. An informative text describing the effects and history of a wide range of substances of abuse.

Racine, Eric, and C. Forlini. "Cognitive Enhancement, Lifestyle Choice, or Misuse of Prescription Drugs?" *Neuroethics* 3 (2010): 1–4. Discusses the medical and nonmedical use of stimulant drugs and explores ethical issues involving the use and prescription of cognition-enhancing products.

WEBSITES OF INTEREST

Center for Substance Abuse Research
http://www.cesar.umd.edu/cesar/drugs/ritalin.asp
National Center for Biotechnology Information
http://www.ncbi.nlm.nih.gov/pubmedhealth/PMH0000606

Bryan C. Auday

SEE ALSO: Stimulants and Their Effects

Secondhand smoke

Secondhand smoke is a combination of two types of exposure to tobacco smoke in the environment: mainstream and sidestream. Mainstream smoke involves exposure to smoke that has been exhaled by a smoker. Sidestream smoke is that smoke emitted from a lit tobacco product, such as a cigarette, cigar, or pipe. Sidestream smoke is the more dangerous of the two because it contains a much larger concentration of cancer-causing (carcinogenic) and toxic agents, which are small enough to easily enter the body and damage a variety of cells.

SECONDHAND SMOKE

Even for persons who do not smoke, exposure to tobacco smoke is dangerous. Consider the following:

- Secondhand smoke causes disease and premature death in children and adults who do not smoke.
- Children exposed to secondhand smoke are at risk for sudden infant death syndrome, lung infections, ear problems, and severe asthma.
- Being exposed to secondhand smoke while pregnant can increase the risk of stillbirth and birth disorders and defects.
- Parents who smoke can cause breathing problems and slow lung-growth in their children.
- Secondhand smoke affects the heart and causes coronary heart disease and lung cancer in adults.

HEALTH EFFECTS

The effects of secondhand smoke on persons who share an environment with smokers are similar to the effects on smokers themselves. In 2006, US Surgeon General Richard Carmona issued a statement on secondhand smoke that concluded that both children and adults who have never smoked can get sick and die as a result of exposure to secondhand smoke.

Secondhand smoke is categorized as a type A carcinogen, meaning there is strong evidence of its cancer-causing effects in human beings. Cancer is only one of the effects that secondhand smoke can have on the body. Secondhand smoke also has been found to increase the incidence of heart disease, respiratory infections (such as bronchitis, pneumonitis, and pneumonia), asthma, middle ear infections, and sudden infant death syndrome, among other disorders. Even brief exposure to secondhand smoke can damage the lining of blood vessels and cause clumping of platelets, both of which can result in heart disease.

TOXINS

Smoke (whether primary or secondhand) consists of several thousand different chemicals, hundreds of which are toxic and more than fifty of which are known to be carcinogenic. Toxins that are found in secondhand smoke include formaldehyde, benzene, vinyl chloride, carbon monoxide, hydrogen cyanide, butane, ammonia, arsenic, and lead. These toxins can directly and indirectly affect almost any organ in the body. According to most research, any exposure to secondhand smoke can be harmful, even minimum exposure.

Studies indicate that the greatest amount of secondhand smoke exposure takes place in enclosed spaces, such as in the home or in vehicles. The US Environmental Protection Agency has urged people who smoke to refrain from doing so in their homes or automobiles.

FURTHER READING

Barnoya, Joaquin, and Stanton A. Glantz. "Cardiovascular Effects of Secondhand Smoke: Nearly as Large as Smoking." *Circulation* 111 (2005): 2684–98. Print. Describes the dangers of secondhand smoke exposure to cardiovascular health.

Glantz, Stanton A., and William W. Parmley. "Even a Little Secondhand Smoke Is Dangerous." *Journal of the American Medical Association* 286 (2001): 462–63. Print. Provides information regarding the damage to the body caused by secondhand smoke.

Parker, Philip M., and James N. Parker, eds. *Second-Hand Smoke: A Medical Dictionary, Bibliography, and Annotated Research Guide to Internet References*. San Diego, CA: Icon Health, 2004. An informative medical dictionary providing detailed information on the properties and effects of secondhand smoke.

WEBSITES OF INTEREST

Mayo Clinic
http://www.mayoclinic.com/health/secondhand-smoke/CC00023
Medline Plus: Secondhand Smoke
http://www.nlm.nih.gov/medlineplus/secondhandsmoke.html

National Cancer Institute
http://www.cancer.gov/cancertopics/factsheet/Tobacco/ETS
US Environmental Protection Agency
http://www.epa.gov/smokefree/healtheffects.html

Robin Kamienny Montvilo

SEE ALSO: Smoking and Its Effects

Sexual assault and alcohol use

Sexual assault is physical attack by means of forced, or nonconsensual, sex. Alcohol consumption does not cause sexual assault, but they are highly correlated. Alcohol-induced cognitive impairment disinhibits inappropriate behavior by making it more difficult to process inhibitory cues.

PREVALENCE

The prevalence of sexual assault, involving or not involving alcohol intoxication, cannot be accurately determined because it is often unreported. Estimates are based on reports from law enforcement and on random samples of crime victims, interviews with incarcerated rapists and others imprisoned for assault, interviews with victims who seek hospital treatment, general population surveys of women, and surveys of male and female college students.

This research suggests that approximately one-half of all sexual assaults involve alcohol consumption by the perpetrator, the victim, or both; 34 to 74 percent occur when the perpetrator is under the influence of alcohol; and 30 to 79 percent are associated with the victim's alcohol consumption.

Findings suggest two distinct subtypes of sexual assault involving substance abuse: those involving mutual substance use and those in which only the perpetrator abused a substance. Assaults involving mutual substance abuse tend to occur between acquaintances rather than intimates, to originate outside the home, and to result in rape or attempted rape rather than sexual coercion. Women who were assaulted by a substance-using perpetrator but who did not use a substance themselves reported lower income, lower rates of employment, and the highest rates of partner physical aggression and injury. When assault occurs in close relationships, women whose partners abuse alcohol are 3.6 times more likely than other women to be assaulted by their partners.

Sexual assaults involving alcohol are more likely than other sexual assaults to occur between men and women who know each other but not well (for example, dates, acquaintances, and friends). These assaults also tend to occur at parties or in bars. The typical scenario involves a woman who is assaulted by a single man who uses verbal and physical pressure, which the woman attempts to resist.

PSYCHOLOGICAL CORRELATIONS

Men who report that they drink heavily are more likely than other men to report having committed sexual assault. A man's behavior can be influenced by certain situations, such as when consensual sex is a possible outcome. Research demonstrates that when people have an expectation about a situation, they tend to more heavily observe cues that fit that expectation. Studies confirm that a man's misperception of a woman's degree of sexual interest is a significant predictor of sexual assault.

Many men expect to feel more powerful, disinhibited, and aggressive after drinking alcohol. Men with these expectations may feel more comfortable forcing sex when they are drinking because they can later justify that the alcohol made them act accordingly. Heavy drinkers may routinely use intoxication as an excuse for engaging in socially unacceptable behavior, including sexual assault. Alcohol also is used by a perpetrator to incapacitate the person assaulted. Furthermore, certain personality characteristics (such as impulsivity and antisocial behavior) may increase a man's propensity both to drink heavily and to commit sexual assault.

Women who drink alcohol are often perceived as being more sexually available and promiscuous, compared with women who do not drink, which may put them at an increased risk for being targeted for assault. Although a woman's alcohol consumption may increase her risk of sexual assault, she is in no way responsible for the assault.

PHARMACOLOGIC CORRELATIONS

Laboratory studies that examine alcohol's effects on responses to sexual and aggressive stimuli have shown that alcohol consumption disrupts higher-order cognitive processes, including abstraction, conceptualization, planning, and problem-solving. As a result, alcohol consumption may lessen a perpetrator's ability to generate nonaggressive solutions to sexual satisfaction.

Intoxication narrows the perceptual field of drinkers so that they focus on what is most important to them in a given situation. Hence, a perpetrator will focus only on social cues that indicate interest in sexual activity. Cognitive deficits lead to a focus on gratification, sense of entitlement, and anger, rather than on empathy and consequences. Once aggression is begun, it is difficult to stop. Alcohol's effects on motor skills may limit the victim's ability to resist effectively, thus heightening the likelihood of a completed assault.

MITIGATION

Sexual assault and heavy drinking are separate issues. A perpetrator must recognize that sexual contact without consent is sexual violence, whether alcohol is involved or not. However, it is useful to focus on the use of alcohol in dating and sexual situations in models of alcohol's role in sexual assault, rather than on general drinking patterns, because the level of alcohol consumption does not differ between perpetrators and nonperpetrators.

Effective sex offender programs teach four principles of sexual consent: privilege, permission, justification/intent, and responsibility.

1. Privilege: Sex is never a right; it is always a privilege.
2. Permission: A person needs to be sober enough to know whether or not they have been given permission; and the other person must be capable, at the time, of giving permission. If someone is passed out, unconscious, or asleep, they are legally incapable of giving consent.
3. Justification/Intent: No minimization of the use of aggression as a result of alcohol or drug use, stress, deviant arousal patterns, loss of control or misunderstandings.
4. Responsibility: The only person who ever is responsible for a sexual assault is the perpetrator.

FURTHER READING

Abbey, Antonia, et al. "Alcohol and Sexual Assault." *Alcohol Health and Research World* 25.1 (2001). Web. 28Mar. 2012. https://www1.columbia.edu/sec/cu/health/pdfs/alcohol_sexual_assault.pdf. An overview of the evidence correlating alcohol consumption and sexual assault.

Dawgert, Sarah. *Substance Use and Sexual Violence: Building Prevention and Intervention Responses, A Guide for Counselors and Advocates.* Enola: Pennsylvania Coalition Against Rape, 2009. Examines drug and alcohol use, abuse, and addiction as it relates to sexual violence.

LeBeau, Marc A., and Ashraf Mozayani, eds. *Drug-Facilitated Sexual Assault: A Forensic Handbook*. San Diego, CA: Academic, 2001. A handbook for investigators of sexual crimes that covers how drugs are used to facilitate sexual assaults.

WEBSITES OF INTEREST

Centers for Disease Control and Prevention
http://www.cdc.gov/ViolencePrevention/sexualviolence
Men Can Stop Rape
http://www.mencanstoprape.org
Sexual Assault Awareness Month
http://www.nsvrc.org/saam

Stephanie Eckenrode

SEE ALSO: Rape and Sexual Assault; Teen s and Alcohol Abuse

Sexual assault and drug use

Sexual assault is any form of sexual activity, including rape and sexual harassment, where consent is not freely given. Drug use is defined as the use or misuse of any legal or illicit psychoactive, mood-altering chemical, including alcohol, marijuana, stimulants, hallucinogens, benzodiazepines, sedatives, and opiates.

DRUG-FACILITATED SEXUAL ASSAULT

According to the US Department of Health and Human Services, sexual assault includes the nonconsensual acts of inappropriate touching; vaginal, anal, or oral penetration (rape); attempted rape; and child molestation. Sexual assault can be verbal, visual, or involve coercive physical attempts to engage another person in unwanted sexual contact or attention.

Sexual assault often involves the use of psychoactive mood-altering drugs and alcohol. According to the US Department of Justice, close to 40 percent of all rapes and other forms of sexual assault in a given year in the United States involve alcohol use by the offender. Drug use in addition to the alcohol use accounted for 18 percent of sexual assaults.

Drug-facilitated sexual assault involves the administration of drugs that usually induce amnesia in the victim. This type of assault often occurs in bars or nightclubs.

The drug is usually slipped into an alcoholic beverage without the victim's knowledge. These drugs are often referred to as date rape drugs, the most common of which are sedative hypnotics such as gamma hydroxybutyrate, Rohypnol, ketamine, and Soma.

Date rape is common during college years. Drugs and alcohol play significant roles in date rape, with as much as 75 percent of men and 50 percent of women in college involved in a sexual assault reporting having been under the influence at the time of the assault. In eighty percent of sexual assaults the victim and perpetrator are known to each other, and more than 50 percent of sexual assaults occur close to the victim's home. The most common profile of the sex offender is white, male, and age thirty-one years.

Neither drugs nor alcohol excuses a perpetrator seeking sexual relations without consent. Programs to rehabilitate sex offenders attempt to help the offenders make the distinction that drugs and alcohol do not give license for sexual abuse. Drug and alcohol problems are considered separate from deviant sexual behavior.

VICTIMS OF SEXUAL ASSAULT

The profile of an assault victimvictimization and drug use is generally female, age twelve to thirty-four years. Girls and women age sixteen to nineteen are at highest risk. Boys also can be victims of sexual assault. By the age of eight years, one in four girls and one in six boys has been sexually assaulted.

Crime rates are often misleading when it comes to the statistical reportage of sexual assault and drug use. These crimes are vastly underreported because of a deep sense of shame, embarrassment, and guilt induced in the victim. Another factor leading to underreporting of sexual assault occurs because of the effect of drugs or alcohol on memory. Often the drugs interfere with the recall of the assault, leaving victims unable to remember if they consented to engage in sex.

POST-TRAUMATIC STRESS AND SELF-MEDICATION

Sexual assault, including rape, is a leading cause of post-traumatic stress disorderpost-traumatic stress disorder-sexual assault and (PTSD). In general, women are two to three times more likely than men to develop PTSD. One of the leading risk factors of PTSD is sexual assault that causes the victim to feel powerless.

Studies consistently demonstrate high rates of co-morbidity between PTSD and substance abuse disorder.

Specifically, there exists a strong relationship between drug use and victimization through sexual assault. Often, the victim of a sexual assault will use drugs and alcohol to self-medicate the symptoms of the trauma. Rates of substance abuse disorder are as high as 30 to 50 percent of the population of women diagnosed with PTSD, according to the National Comorbidity Study. An Office of Justice Programs report on substance abuse and victimization notes that victims of sexual assault are 5.3 percent more likely than nonvictims to use prescription drugs, 3.4 times more likely to use marijuana, and 10 times more likely to use hard drugs to cope with their assault.

However, there is a tendency to blame the victim because drugs are often involved at the time of sexual assault for both the perpetrator and the victim. This also is true when victimization leads to substance abuse, and the victim is further stigmatized. Research shows that being sexually assaulted puts one at higher risk for a repeated assault. For these reasons, research points to the need for gender-sensitive treatment to address sexual assault, PTSD, victimization, and empowerment.

FURTHER READING

Breslau, N., et al. "Vulnerability to Assaultive Violence: Further Specification for the Sex Difference in Post-Traumatic Stress Disorder." *Psychological Medicine* 29 (1999): 813–21.

Jackson-Cherry, Lisa R., and Bradley T. Erford. *Crisis Intervention and Prevention.* Upper Saddle River, NJ: Pearson, 2010.

Koss, M. P. "Hidden Rape: Incident, Prevalence, and Descriptive Characteristics of Sexual Aggression and Victimization in a National Sample of College Students." *Rape and Sexual Assault II.* Ed. Ann W. Burgess. New York: Garland, 1988.

"Sexual Assault and Substance Abuse." *Research and Advocacy Digest* 8.1 (2005): 1–15. Web. 6 Apr. 2012. http://www.mecasa.org/joomla/images/pdfs/substance_use/sexual_assault_and_sub_abuse.pdf.

US Bureau of Justice Statistics. Sexual Assault of Young Children as Reported to Law Enforcement. Washington, DC: DOJ, 2000.

WEBSITES OF INTEREST

National Center for PTSD
http://www.ptsd.va.gov
National Violence Against Women Prevention Research Center

http://www.musc.edu/vawprevention
Rape, Abuse, and Incest National Network
http://www.rainn.org

Amanda Lefkowitz

SEE ALSO: Rape and Sexual Assault; Teens and Drug Abuse

Smoking and its effects

The inhalation of tobacco in the form of cigarettes or cigars, which poses important health risks; those risks can be significantly decreased by smoking cessation, even in older age.

CAUSES AND EFFECTS

Cigarette smoking has long been known to have adverse effects. Smokers get more wrinkles than nonsmokers and brown/black discoloration of teeth so they tend to look older than their chronological age. They also are more likely to develop worsening of age-related problems such as gum disease, loss of teeth, and alteration in sense of smell and taste. Loss of teeth leads to difficulty chewing, which in turn leads to difficulties with digestion. Most people who lose teeth eventually develop loss of the bone that should support their teeth, making it increasingly difficult to fit dentures.

Smokers are ten times more likely to get lung cancer than nonsmokers. Lung cancer is now the number one cause of cancer death in women, as well as in men. In addition to lung cancer, smokers have a higher incidence of cancers of the head and neck, esophagus, colon, rectum, kidney, bladder, and cervix. Smokers are three to six times more likely to have a heart attack than are nonsmokers. In older people, the major risk factor for disease of the coronary arteries is hypertension, but smoking is still significant, especially when combined with other risk factors for heart disease, such as diabetes or high cholesterol. Smoking and diabetes are also the two most important risk factors for diseases of the veins and arteries of the lower leg. Those who continue to smoke once these diseases develop are much more likely to require limb amputation than those who quit. Smokers may develop chronic obstructive pulmonary disease (COPD), which includes emphysema and chronic bronchitis, and are eighteen times more likely than nonsmokers to die of diseases of the lungs other than cancer. Older smokers also show a decrease in muscle strength, agility, coordination, gait, and balance. The changes in these areas make them seem older than their actual age.

Smoking has long been thought to be associated with peptic ulcer disease. In addition, smoking makes the symptoms of many diseases worsen or increases the risk of complications in patients with allergies, diabetes, hypertension, and vascular disease. Male smokers are at greater risk of experiencing sexual impotence. Female smokers tend to experience an earlier menopause, bone loss called osteoporosis and are therefore at increased risk for hip fracture than nonsmokers. Smokers are more likely to develop glaucoma than nonsmokers. (Studies completed in 1996 indicated an increased risk with smoking for macular degeneration, the leading cause of blindness in older adults. The evidence is mixed on smoking and Alzheimer's disease, but a 1998 study contradicted earlier work and found that the risk is greater in smokers than in nonsmokers.) Finally, smokers are at greater risk of death or injury caused by cigarette-related fires.

Cigarette smoking tends to speed up the processes in the liver for breaking down, using, and eliminating medications, both nonprescription and prescription. This means that medications may not perform as expected in the body. Smokers may need to take medications more frequently or in greater doses than nonsmokers, so it is important for health care providers to know that a person smokes. The drugs known to be affected by smoking include sedatives, narcotic and synthetic narcotic painkillers, certain antidepressants, anticoagulant medications, asthma medications, and certain blood pressure medications. These changes are of particular concern in the older population for a number of reasons. First, older people (whether smokers or nonsmokers) tend to need more medications than younger people.With each additional drug, the risk of serious drug interaction and other adverse effects increases. Second, changes in body composition and function that alter the metabolism of drugs come with age, making medication use somewhat riskier in older persons, in terms of adverse effects and complications. The additional changes associated with smoking increase these risks significantly.

The dangers of passive smoking are well documented. More than fifty compounds in secondhand smoke are identified as carcinogens in humans. The effects seem to be more harmful in children than in adults, but adults who are affected are at increased risk for cancer, heart disease, noncancerous lung diseases, and allergies.

TREATMENT AND THERAPY

Numerous studies have shown that smoking cessation has health benefits in as little as one year, such as reducing the risk of heart attack and coronary artery disease. Within two years of smoking cessation, the risks of stroke and diseases of the blood vessels in the lower leg are reduced as well. Even though chronic lung disease is not reversible, those who quit smoking slow the decline in lung function considerably. Risks for cancers also decrease significantly with smoking cessation and are similar to the cancer risk for nonsmokers in ten to thirteen years. These findings indicate that it is worthwhile even for older people to give up smoking. An average forty-year-old gains approximately nine additional years of life by quitting smoking, and a sixty-year-old gains approximately three additional years.

Because smoking is an addiction, it may be difficult to quit, particularly after years of cigarette use. Most smokers have to stop several times before quitting permanently. Setting a quit date, attending support group meetings, taking it one day at a time, undergoing hypnosis,making a contract with a friend or a health care provider, substituting carrot sticks for cigarettes, increasing exercise (particularly swimming), and breathing deeply all seem to be helpful techniques. Nicotine replacement systems are available in the United States on a nonprescription basis, but it is important for older people, particularly those with health problems or who are taking multiple medications, to consult a health care professional prior to using them. It is also important that anyone using these aids stop smoking completely. Continuing to smoke while using nicotine replacement could potentially cause toxicity, and it decreases the success of cessation attempts, since the behavior of smoking is still present. Two non-nicotine-containing medications are available by prescription for smoking cessation: bupropion SR (Wellbutrin, Zyban) and varenicline (Chantix). Both medications significantly increase the success rates at the end of treatment and one year later. Themechanism of action is by stimulating chemical messengers in the brain that are affected by nicotine.

Electronic cigarettes are used as a tool for smoking cessation. It is a battery-powered device that can deliver nicotine without the combustion or smoke. Use and awareness of ecigarettes has dramatically increased over the past few years. Studies have suggested that physical and behavioral stimuli, such as holding a cigarette, can reduce the craving to smoke. Recent findings suggest that individuals who used e-cigarettes reduced the number of tobacco cigarettes they smoked. These findings suggest that the e-cigarettes may be an important tool for reducing the harm that tobacco cigarettes can cause. Unfortunately, the benefits and risks of electronic cigarette as of 2013 are still uncertain. More studies are needed for further investigation of their safety and efficacy.

PERSPECTIVE AND PROSPECTS

Smoking is the main avoidable cause of death in the United States and many other developed nations. More than 10 percent of North Americans over the age of sixty-five smoke cigarettes This put them, and those with whom they live, at risk for significant health problems. These risks appear to increase both with age and with the number of years of smoking.

After World War II, more women began smoking. Because the diseases related to smoking usually take years to develop, it was only in the last part of the twentieth century that rates of smoking-related disease among women began to approach those of men. Research indicates that smoking cessation appears to be beneficial, even in a person who has smoked for many years.

FURTHER READING

Britton, John. *ABC of Smoking Cessation*. Malden, MA: Blackwell, 2004. This guide provides practical information for smoking cessation and discusses the public health and individual health problems associated with smoking.

Hales, Dianne. *An Invitation to Health Brief*. Updated ed. Belmont, CA: Wadsworth/Cengage Learning, 2010. This updated, helpful resource covers many aspects of health, including mental health, physical fitness, stress management, and preventive medicine.

Jorenby, Douglas E., et al. "Efficacy of Varenicline, an α2β4 Nicotinic Acetylcholine Receptor Partial Agonist, versus Placebo or Sustained-Release Bupropion for Smoking Cessation." *Journal of the American Medical Association* 296, no. 1 (July 5, 2006): 56-63. This article compares two non-nicotine smoking-cessation products to a placebo in a smoking-cessation study with evaluation at the end of treatment and at fifty-two weeks. Varenicline was found to be significantly more effective than bupropion. Both agents were more effective than a placebo.

Marcus, Bess H., Jeffrey S. Hampl, and Edwin B. Fisher. *How to Quit Smoking without Gaining Weight*. New York: Simon & Schuster, 2004. This paperback book from the American Lung Association provides expert advice on quitting smoking without gaining substantial weight. It provides motivation and discusses physical activity and many strategies to help with cravings. Includes recipes and meal plans.

Parles, Karen, and J. H. Schiller. *One Hundred Questions and Answers about Lung Cancer*. 2nd ed. Sudbury, MA: Jones and Bartlett, 2010. A patient-oriented guide that covers a range of topics related to lung cancer, including risk factors and causes; methods of prevention, screening, and diagnosis; available treatments and how to choose among them; and ways of coping with common emotional and physical difficulties associated with the diagnosis and treatment.

Pirozynski, Michael. "One Hundred Years of Lung Cancer." *Respiratory Medicine* 100, no. 12 (December, 2006): 2073-2084. Lung cancer is the most commoncause of cancer death in the world, and cigarette smoking remains the major risk factor. Discusses treatment and prognosis.

Sloan, Frank A., et al. *The Price of Smoking*. Cambridge, MA: MIT Press, 2006. This book contains a thorough analysis of the costs of smoking, which have often been ignored. These costs are carefully and comprehensively discussed by a group of economists

Rebecca Lovell Scott, updated by Bianca Garcia, and Luzanna Plancarte

SEE ALSO: Secondhand Smoke

Steroids: HGH and PEDS

Performance-enhancing drugs (PEDs) are substances taken to improve strength, speed, endurance, or mental focus. Many PEDs have legitimate medical uses, but when taken by individuals to improve performance rather than to treat a medical condition, these drugs can have serious side effects such as decreasing fertility and an increasing the risk of heart damage. Anti-doping agencies that regulate sports organizations routinely test for banned PEDs. There is also a thriving industry in "designer" PEDs that claim to be undetectable by standard drug tests, and are used to increase mental sharpness instead of physical prowess. This essay deals only with common drugs of abuse used to enhance athletic performance.

INTRODUCTION

Trying to gain an edge in athletic competitions is nothing new. The first recorded use of a PED in the Olympic Games occurred in 1904 when a marathon runner injected himself with strychnine, a poison that acts as a muscle stimulant. Before 1935, almost all PEDs were stimulants similar to amphetamines and cocaine. That changed in the 1940s after a chemist learned how to make the male hormone testosterone in the laboratory.

Testosterone is a type of anabolic-androgenic steroid (AAS). Steroids are a class of compounds that include both male and female sex hormones. Anabolic refers to the muscle-building properties of the hormone. Androgenic indicates that the hormone increases male sexual characteristics. There are other types of steroid hormones such estrogen, progesterone, and cortisol, but only AASs increase muscle mass. In athletic circles, AAS drugs are commonly just called steroids or 'roids.

By 1960, chemists had figured out how to synthesize a number of synthetic AASs not normally produced by the body but that had an effect similar to testosterone. These drugs were embraced by competitive athletes and body builders. AASs were banned by the International Olympic Committee in 1975, and, as drug-testing technology improved, many competitors were stripped of their medals for abusing these drugs. The United States added AASs to the list of controlled substances in 1990. This made providing steroids for non-medical uses a felony, but athletes, even down to the high school level, continued to use them. Today illicit laboratories and unethical physicians work to provide a constantly changing stream of synthetic AASs that either mimic the actions of testosterone or stimulate the body to produce excess amounts of the hormone. Makers of these drugs are always looking for ways to stay one step ahead of drug testing agencies such as the World Anti-Doping Agency (WADA).

The use of human growth hormone (HGH) has a much shorter history. In the body, it is made by the pituitary gland. Chemists were able to synthesize HGH in the laboratory in the 1980s and used it to treat children with genetic defects who failed to produce enough of the hormone naturally. Later HGH was embraced by healthy adult athletes in the belief that it would increase strength and slow aging. HGH is especially attractive to illegal users because it cannot be detected in urine tests; a blood test is required to document its presence. As of 2015, there is little evidence that HGH has any effect in adults.

HOW ANABOLIC-ANDROGENIC STEROIDS WORK

Testosterone is in the class of hormones called androgens that includes a number of related compounds sold with names such as Androstenedione, Oxandrin, Dianabol, Winstrol, Deca-durabolin, and Equipoise. Street names include gym candy, pumpers, halo, stackers, var, drol, the clear, and primo. Testosterone is naturally produced by the testes in men. It stimulates increased protein production. Levels of the hormone normally increase at puberty leading to the development of male sexual characteristics such as growth in muscle mass, development of denser bones, body hair, thickening of the vocal cords leading to a lower-pitched voice, the distinctive male profile of broad shoulders and a narrow waist, and an increased sex drive.

Testosterone production peaks in the early twenties and decreases with age. However, despite advertisements to the contrary, low testosterone, or low T, is not a common disorder among healthy men. Legitimate medical uses of the hormone include treatment for delayed puberty and muscle wasting in diseases such as cancer and AIDS. Bodybuilders and athletes abuse testosterone and related AASs in an effort to become larger, stronger, and have better-defined muscles.

EFFECTS OF ANABOLIC-ANDROGENIC STEROIDS

AASs do increase muscle mass and bone density, but to achieve this, individuals must take levels of the drug ten to one hundred times greater than the therapeutic dose. Testosterone and its relatives can be taken as an injection, a pill, or as a gel applied to the skin. HGH is given as an injection.

Using AASs in excess and over time can cause serious negative health side effects. Men who use AASs can become sterile. This occurs because the testes stop producing testosterone when high levels of artificial testosterone are circulating in the body. The testes atrophy (shrivel), and sperm fail to mature. In addition, excess testosterone in men may be converted into estrogen, a female sex hormone. This causes men to develop breasts, a condition called gynecomastia. Other side effects of AAS abuse include acne and baldness.

Because the heart is a muscle, it increases in size when stimulated by AASs. As the heart enlarges, its pumping capacity decreases, and heart rhythm irregularities can develop leading to a heart attack, even in young people. Other side effects include an increased risk of liver damage or liver cancer, kidney failure, high blood pressure, and high cholesterol levels. HGH abusers can develop abnormal hearts and thin, weak bones (osteoporosis). Women who abuse AASs often develop male characteristics such as a deepened voice, broad shoulders, facial hair, a disrupted menstrual cycle, and the internal effects on the heart, liver, and kidney seen in men.

AASs also affect mood and behavior. Continued use can lead to aggression and explosions of temper and violence often called "roid rage." Extended use can also cause paranoia, irritability, and impaired judgment. These behavioral changes tend to interfere with normal social relationships.

In order to minimize side effects, many athletes practice cycling, or taking AASs for a set period and then quitting for a period. Stopping often leads to depression, mood swings, restlessness, insomnia, loss of appetite, decreased sex drive, and cravings for the drugs.

Along with AAS drugs, abusers often take excessive quantities of dietary supplements. This practice is called stacking. Dietary supplements are products such as vitamins, minerals, herbs, amino acids, and enzymes. Supplements are not regulated with the same rigor and do not require testing as pharmaceutical drugs. Multiple studies have found that many dietary supplements, especially those sold over the Internet, do not conform to their labeling. Either they fail to contain the advertised ingredient in the amount specified or they contain unlisted ingredients. Some of these supplements contain banned substances while others can enhance the side effects of AASs.

In recent years, testing for PEDs has increased and improved. Many professional athletes such as Barry Bonds, Mark McGwire, Bill Romanowski and Lyle Alzado have been involved in steroid-use scandals. Cyclist Lance Armstrong was stripped of his seven Tour-de-France titles and banned for life from professional cycling after his PED use was revealed.

FURTHER READING

Kille, L. W. (2013, May 9). "Performance-enhancing Drugs In Athletics: Research Roundup". Retrieved from: http://journalistsresource.org/studies/society/culture/athletic-academic-performance-enhancing-drugs-research-roundup. This site has reprinted summaries of research on various PEDs. It also contains links to stories about PED use in the military, among fire fighters and police officers, in professional and amateur sports.

United States Anti-Doping Agency (USADA). (2015, May 13). "Effects of PEDs". Retrieved from: http://www.usada.org/substances/effects-of-performance-enhancing-drugs. This is a government-sponsored website that describes and has videos of physical and psychological effects of various PEDs by gender. The site also has links to lists of banned drugs and supplements.

United States National Library of Medicine. (2014, September 18). Anabolic steroids. Retrieved from: http://www.nlm.nih.gov/medlineplus/anabolic-steroids.html. This gateway website that provides links to all aspects of anabolic steroid use including current research. One set of links connects to information specifically for teens.

Wedro, B. (2014, July 29). Steroids. Retrieved from: http://www.emedicinehealth.com/steroids/article_em.htm. This comprehensive article by a physician outlines various types of steroids and their legitimate and illicit uses. A slide show depicting some of the side effects of abuse accompanies the article.

Woolston, C. (2015, March 11). *Human Growth Hormone*. Retrieved from: http://consumer.healthday.com/encyclopedia/substance-abuse-38/illicit-drugs-news-217/human-growth-hormone-647257.html. This article discusses the legal status of HGH, the drug's side effects, and problems with getting impure or non-existent HGH on the black market.

Tish Davidson

SEE ALSO: Acne; Stimulants and their Effects

Stimulants and their effects

Stimulants are drugs such as caffeine, cocaine, and amphetamine that alter physiological responses by increasing blood pressure, heart rate, and motor activity. Changes in psychological states include euphoria, increased focus, alertness, and energy. Using higher quantities for a long time can lead to both physical and psychological dependence.

CAUSES

The most frequently ingested stimulant is caffeine, which is used by 80 percent of the adult population of the United States. Caffeine, a member of a class of chemicals known as xanthines, is found not only in coffee, tea, and soda beverages but also in a number of foods. Caffeine affects the nervous system by inhibiting the neurotransmitter substance adenosine.

Adenosine is an inhibitory brain chemical that brings on sleepiness, slows the heart rate, and lowers blood pressure and body temperature. Because caffeine interferes with the inhibitory action of adenosine, the resulting effect is an increase in brain activity, which leads to heightened alertness and a lack of fatigue. Consuming too much caffeine can lead to caffeinismcaffeinism, which is a temporary condition characterized by insomnia, restlessness, nervousness, and anxiety.

Two other stimulants, cocaine and amphetamine, exert their effects by increasing the availability of three primary neurotransmitter substances: dopamine, norepinephrine, and serotonin. Although the mechanisms through which each drug alters the presence of these brain chemicals differ, the end product—having an abundance of a particular neurotransmitter in the synapse—is responsible for the behavioral and physiological changes that occur. Although the connection between cocaine and excessive amounts of dopamine is believed to be responsible for the rapid and strong dependency that can form, the latest research reveals a more complex picture that implicates interactions among several additional neurotransmitters.

RISK FACTORS

Stimulant overuse and abuse is more likely to occur in adults younger than age forty years, with the majority being males. Most persons who experiment with cocaine do so to experience a euphoric high; however, competitive athletes and college students are more likely to use stimulants to enhance physical or cognitive performance. Of all the stimulants, cocaine and methamphetamine pose the greatest risk of dependency.

SYMPTOMS

Physiological and psychological symptoms associated with the ingestion of stimulants are determined by several factors. These factors include the method of drug delivery (snorting, taking a pill), the specific dosage, and the length of time that the drug has been used.

Low-dosage, short-term side effects associated with stimulant usage include such changes as appetite suppression; increased alertness, particularly for persons diagnosed with attention deficit disorder; euphoria; an increased confidence in task performance; hypertension; pupil dilation; and delayed onset of sleep. With acute use of cocaine and methamphetamine, even at low dosages,

initial feelings of euphoria and elation will dissipate and frequently result in depression, anxiety, and a desire or craving to ingest more of the drug.

Higher dosages of stimulants used for a long time can lead to drug tolerance. Essentially, increased amounts of the drug are needed to produce the same psychoactive effects. This condition sets the stage for chronic abuse. Long-term effects of stimulants can result in anxiety, depression, paranoia, seizure, pulmonary edema, stroke, gastrointestinal complications, and sudden death from cardiac complications.

Cocaine and methamphetamine abuse can lead to a drug-induced psychosis, which is characterized by visual and auditory hallucinations, incoherent speech, paranoia, and abnormal sleeping patterns. In addition, chronic usage of stimulants can lead to dependence, which results in drug craving. This intense craving can lead to behavioral changes, in which a drug user may forego social, family, and work responsibilities to acquire the drug.

SCREENING AND DIAGNOSIS

A licensed clinical psychologist or medical doctor will ask a battery of questions that assess previous drug history, family history, and the degree to which current use of stimulants is affecting the person's physical, social, and psychological health.

TREATMENT AND THERAPY

For stimulants that produce dependency, no pharmacological treatment exists that directly targets the mechanisms that brought on the addiction. Antidepressant drugs are used in persons who experience depression during detoxification. Cognitive-behavioral therapies are used to help persons acquire new coping strategies to refrain from going back to using a stimulant.

PREVENTION

In terms of caffeinism, adverse symptoms can be resolved by simply reducing the amount of caffeine one normally consumes. For prescribed medications such as amphetamines, it is important to monitor any potential adverse side effects. If these emerge, one should contact the medical doctor who authorized the prescription. Cocaine use should be avoided because of its potential for harmful side effects.

FURTHER READING

Iversen, Leslie. *Speed, Ecstasy, Ritalin: The Science of Amphetamines.* New York: Oxford UP, 2008. This book is devoted to discussing what is understood about amphetamines and nonamphetamine drugs, such as Ritalin.

Levinthall, Charles F. *Drugs, Behavior, and Modern Society.* 7th ed. Boston: Pearson, 2012. A highly readable account of the major categories of psychoactive drugs, such as the stimulants, to better understand how these substances travel within the body, affect the central nervous system, and exert their behavioral effects.

Maisto, Stephen A., Mark Galizio, and Gerard J. Connors. *Drug Use and Abuse.* 6th ed. Florence, KY: Cengage, 2010. Introduces the reader to the central substance abuse and treatment issues. Includes good information on cognitive and behavioral treatment approaches that are used to treat drug abuse.

Meyer, Jerrold S., and Linda F. Quenzer. *Psychopharmacology: Drugs, the Brain, and Behavior.* Sunderland, MA: Sinauer, 2005. The chapters on stimulants are well documented with examples from research that address results from brain imaging studies and clinical trials for therapeutic applications.

Rasmussen, Nicolas. *On Speed: The Many Lives of Amphetamine.* New York: New York UP, 2008. Features one of the best historical introductions to the use of amphetamines as a behavioral and cognitive enhancer primarily by military personnel in the United States and Great Britain.

WEBSITES OF INTEREST

Behavioral Biology Research Center, Johns Hopkins University
http://www.caffeinedependence.org/caffeine_dependence.html
Center for Substance Abuse Research
http://www.cesar.umd.edu/cesar/drugs/ritalin.asp
Cocaine Anonymous
http://www.ca.org
NIDA for Teens: Stimulants
http://www.teens.drugabuse.gov/facts/facts_stim1.php

Bryan C. Auday

SEE ALSO: Amphetamine Abuse; Caffeine and Mental Health; Cocaine and Its Effects

Students Against Destructive Decisions (SADD)

Students Against Destructive Decisions is a peer-to-peer education and prevention organization that provides children and young adults with resources and activities that encourage them to reject illegal substances, including alcohol and drugs, and detrimental behaviors, such as drunk driving, binge drinking, bullying, and violence.

BACKGROUND

Robert Anastas, a health educator and counselor at Wayland High School in Massachusetts, had the idea to create an organization called Students Against Driving Drunk (SADD) in 1981 after the deaths of two athletes he had coached. Both boys had been inebriated when they were in separate fatal automobile accidents. Anastas soon developed and taught a class focusing on the ramifications of driving drunk.

Anastas and fifteen of his students then established SADD. The students served as peer leaders and role models who created and presented projects that focused on changing teenagers' attitudes about driving and intoxication. The peer leaders stressed that drinking is not essential for students to attain popularity and acceptance by classmates. In 1997, as the organization's goals and missions expanded beyond a sole focus on drunk-driving prevention, the group changed its name to Students Against Destructive Decisions, reflecting its commitment to reducing other dangerous behaviors, including binge drinking, drug use, and violence.

SADD, now based in Marlborough, Massachusetts, expanded nationally, as students formed chapters throughout the United States. Soon after the organization's creation, SADD leaders introduced the Contract for Life, which involves both youths and their parents. Advice columnists Dear Abby and Ann Landers republished SADD's Contract for Life in their columns. CBS television followed by broadcasting the film Contract for Life: The SADD Story (1983). By this time SADD chapters also were being established internationally, and the organization extended its membership to include college and middle school students and youth at summer camps, churches, and community clubs.

Since 1991, SADD has designated a student of the year. Many members attend SADD's annual national conference. Government, business, and nonprofit organizations help to fund SADD programs. SADD provides helpful information on its website and on social networks such as Facebook and Twitter and it publishes the electronic newsletter SADDvocate. SADD's public service messages are televised nationally.

The US Department of Health and Human Services (HHS) presented Anastas with an appreciation award for his service to SADD and selected Carl Olsen, who was the first SADD president while at Wayland High School, to serve on a government panel studying alcoholism. SADD members have represented the organization at international meetings focused on driving safety, hosted by the World Health Organization and the United Nations.

MISSION AND GOALS

SADD's mission is exemplified by its Contract for Life. Signers of the contract state they are aware of risks associated with driving drunk and agree not to drink, use drugs, drive impaired, or ride in vehicles operated by substance-impaired drivers. They promise to wear seatbelts and contact parents when exposed to alcohol or drug hazards.

Illegal alcohol consumption is consistently the greatest problem affecting adolescents, so the organization's primary goal has been to prevent fatalities associated with drunk drivers. SADD chapters present programs covering accident simulations that show emergency responders removing bodies from vehicles and law enforcement personnel arresting inebriated drivers.

SADD supplements its general programs with discussion of the dangers of cell-phone use while driving. The organization also supports mental health programs for students in kindergarten through high school that focus on preventing stress, depression, and suicide. SADD programs also address obesity, eating disorders, bullying, hazing, and youth violence.

Youth are discouraged from using tobacco products, steroids, and prescription drugs not prescribed to them. Organization materials address teenage sexuality, pregnancy, and sexually transmitted infections. Leaders urge students to remain in school and graduate.

Partnering with other organizations, including the National Highway Traffic Safety Administration, SADD assists in devising programs to address issues of drinking and substance use at graduations and proms. Liberty Mutual Insurance helps SADD by acquiring information from teenagers about their experiences with illegal substances and their attitudes toward risky behaviors.

SADD supports legislation that enforces and maintains the nationwide drinking age of twenty-one years.

The organization also endorses legislation requiring seatbelt use and the implementation of graduated driver's licenses, which are obtained by youth who undergo several stages with varying restrictions as they gain driving experience and awareness of driving-associated responsibilities. SADD also promotes the proposed Students Taking Action for Road Safety Act.

By the early twenty-first century, SADD has guided approximately seven million youth. Researchers estimate that SADD has helped to reduce teenage drunk-driving fatalities as much as 60 percent since the organization's founding in 1981.

FURTHER READING

Anastas, Robert, and Kalia Lulow. *The Contract for Life*. New York: Pocket, 1986. SADD's founder discusses why he created the organization and looks at its accomplishments in the group's first five years.

"Prom, Graduation Season, and the SADD Pledge." *Alcoholism and Drug Abuse Weekly* 18.16 (2006): 5. Print. Present methods that SADD chapters can implement to present information to students and seek assistance from adults, including teachers, to combat drunk driving, especially in relation to traditional student celebrations.

Rosenberg, Merri. "Kids as Messengers on Teenage Drinking." *New York Times*, 20 Apr. 2003, p. 2. Discusses SADD activities at several high schools and includes quotations from students and school counselors concerning their experiences. Explains how SADD differs from other antidrinking strategies.

Wallace, Stephen. *Reality Gap: Alcohol, Drugs, and Sex—What Parents Don't Know and Teens Aren't Telling*. New York: Union Square, 2008. A SADD official and counselor analyzes youths' and adults' attitudes, behaviors, and misperceptions about alcohol, drugs, and other social issues.

WEBSITES OF INTEREST

National Organizations for Youth Safety
http://www.noys.org
National Student Safety Program
http://www.adtsea.org/nssp
Students Against Destructive Decisions
http://www.sadd.org

Elizabeth D. Schafer

SEE ALSO: Support Groups; Teens and Alcohol Abuse; Teens and Drug Abuse

Sugar addiction

Sugar addiction is the compulsive physiological need for sugar. This compulsive need constitutes a behavioral addiction, an interpretation that is reinforced when sugar addicts, long habituated to large amounts of sugar, experience classic withdrawal symptoms when their sugar intake is reduced.

CAUSES

Just as the search for explanations of addiction to alcohol and other drugs has been complicated by the nature-nurture debate, so too have been the controversies over sugar addiction. Some medical researchers and physicians believe that sugar addiction might be genetic, that is, that the biological nature of certain humans or, more specifically, the information programmed into their deoxyribonucleic acid (DNA), can explain why some people become addicted to sugar (in a way similar to how others become addicted to, for example, alcohol, nicotine, or heroin).

Other researchers have traced the pleasurable physiological state (popularly known as a sugar high) induced by an intake of sugar to the activation of certain receptors in the brain. Sugar is said to affect the same neurotransmitters in the brain associated with the pleasure produced by such substances as nicotine in cigarette smoke.

Those who emphasize the cultural rather than the genetic causes of physiological addiction to sugar point out that refined sugar (or sucrose, largely derived from sugar cane and sugar beets) has been a relatively recent addition to the human diet. Throughout most of the evolution of Homo sapiens and the early history of civilized humans, the dietary need for glucose was satisfied by the ingestion of fruits, vegetables, and fats, which could, as needed, be metabolized into glucose.

Even after techniques were discovered allowing sugar to be extracted from plants, most humans were unable to use this sugar because of its expense. Sugar did not become an inexpensive commodity until the eighteenth century, when doctors began to discover some of its negative effects on the human body. For some historians, the origin of sugar addiction can be traced to this period, when laborers could be inexpensively fed with sweetened foods and drinks rather than with costly meats, fruits, and vegetables.

Contemporary analysts now believe that sugar addiction has both genetic and cultural causes. However, because of the uniqueness of every person's biochemistry, it is difficult if not impossible to precisely divide causality for this relatively recent medical phenomenon into its biological and environmental sources.

RISK FACTORS

Scientists have discovered a number of medical conditions that predispose a person to sugar addiction. For example, a weak adrenal gland results in an insufficient quantity of glucocorticoid hormones to properly regulate glucose levels in the blood, leading to an intense craving for sugar. Furthermore, persons with a penchant for overeating are often susceptible to sugar addiction.

Cultural factors also can pose risks. For instance, in many advanced societies the processed food industries add massive amounts of refined sugar to numerous products, thus allowing for large numbers of suitably predisposed persons to become sugar addicts.

SYMPTOMS

A common symptom of sugar addiction is the overpowering urge, several times a day, to consume something sweet. If afflicted persons are unable to satisfy these urges, they often feel weak, apathetic, and dizzy. These symptoms may be relieved by the ingestion of sugar-containing foods and sweetened beverages, but continued dependence on sugar results in tolerance with increased consumption needed to relieve symptoms and re-experience the pleasurable feelings that sugar consumption initially created.

With the removal of sugar from the addict's diet, withdrawal symptoms often occur, such as tremors of the extremities, painful headaches, and digestive difficulties, including nausea. Psychological symptoms include irritability, depression, and drastic mood changes.

Researchers have noted numerous long-term health problems associated with sugar addiction, including such well-known consequences as obesity and dental decay. The American Diabetes Association regards the overconsumption of sugar as a major cause of degenerative diseases in the United States, including diabetes, heart disease, and cancer. Sugar also has a negative effect on the body's immune system by depleting white blood cells, thus reducing this system's ability to fight infectious agents.

SCREENING AND DIAGNOSIS

Screening for sugar addiction has not been a part of most routine physical examinations, with the exception of physical exams of the obese and of persons showing clear symptoms. For those who believe that sugar addiction is endemic to Western society, this neglect to screen for the addiction imperils the health of many people.

This lack of monitoring for sugar addiction has led to numerous books on this disorder, many of which contain guidelines for self-diagnosis. However, self-diagnoses can be inaccurate, even dangerous. Blood tests exist to monitor symptoms before and after the ingestion of sugar, and these tests can provide reliable evidence leading to a diagnosis of sugar addiction.

TREATMENT AND THERAPY
According to some advocates, the world is facing a crisis centered on the treatment of sugar addiction that faces several cultural barriers. Sugar has become "a legalized recreational drug" that is "socially acceptable to consume." Sugar addiction is considered an acceptable addiction, one wholly separate from other addictions; this is an alarming perspective to those calling for prevention and treatment of sugar addiction.

The treatment of sugar addicts is also hindered by the denial of their dependence in a manner reminiscent of classic drug addicts. Also, similar to another addictive product—tobacco—countries frequently subsidize sugar production because of its importance to their economies. Furthermore, it is common for sugar and its presence in numerous foods and drinks to receive much more legal immunity than tobacco.

Therapy for sugar addiction can be a long and difficult process. Sugar addicts should not expect their sugar cravings to vanish in a few weeks or months. Most physicians and nutritionists begin treatment with diet modification. After tests, doctors generally attempt to stabilize blood sugar levels by getting their sugar-addicted patients to eat modest meals rich in protein. A nutritious breakfast is especially important, as is the elimination of sugar and artificial sweeteners from all meals and snacks.

Some doctors insist on treating sugar addiction the way they treat alcohol and other drug addictions, that is, by insisting their patients avoid all refined sugars and sugar-containing foods and drinks from their diet. This can be daunting because so many processed foods contain fructose, dextrose, maltose, and other sugary additives such as corn syrup. Some nutritionists even suggest a drastic reduction in the consumption of fresh fruits and fruit juices, which contain sugar. Others, though, allow some fruit in the diet during the transition to a totally sugar-free diet.

Doctors also can prescribe medicines that may help reduce the craving for sugar, and nutritionists may advise recovering sugar addicts to take amino acids, such as glutamine and tyrosine, to help reduce cravings. Others have found that chromium supplements help to balance blood sugar.

Orthomolecular physicians believe that good health can be achieved by balancing substances normally present in the body or by adding essential vitamins and minerals to the diet. These practitioners tend to agree with believers in sugar addiction that this sweet substance is alien to the body and poses a danger to health. For orthomolecular physicians, megavitamin therapy, along with the elimination of sugars and other processed foods that are incompatible with the body's normal and natural array of molecules, is optimum for health.

Other therapies add behavioral modifications for the treatment of sugar addiction. These therapies include exercise, especially relaxed walking, and eight hours of sleep every night. For serious cases, some professionals recommend psychotherapy, because certain patients become addicted to sugar to assuage feelings of loneliness or self-hatred. Therapists often try to discover why patients crave sugar; oftentimes, this craving is caused by past trauma.

With increasing awareness of sugar addiction, many treatment options have become available. Professionals now promote their services in treating this disorder. Treatment centers that include group therapy for sugar addiction also are available.

PREVENTION
Curbing sugar addiction involves both the individual and society. Even those skeptical of this addiction agree that most persons consume far too much sugar and that this overconsumption contributes to many health problems. Evolution has not prepared the human body to handle an average intake of 150 to 300 pounds of sugar each year. Several states in the United States have failed in their attempts to put a tax on sugary soft drinks. In concept, the prevention of sugar addiction is simple: Drastically reduce sugar consumption. In reality, though, individuals and societies rarely are willing to accomplish this.

FURTHER READING
Appleton, Nancy, and G. N. Jacobs. *Suicide by Sugar: A Startling Look at Our #1 National Addiction.* Garden City, NY: Square One, 2009. Written by a long-time believer in the dangerous reality of sugar addiction,

Appleton and her coauthor have collected data linking sugar consumption to a range of disorders, from dementia to cancer.

Avena, Nicole M., Pedro Rada, and Bartley G. Hoebel. "Evidence for Sugar Addiction: Behavioral and Neurochemical Effects of Intermittent, Excessive Sugar Intake." *Neuroscience and Biobehavioral Reviews* 32.1 (2008): 20–39. Print. Results of a study using rats to determine whether or not sugar can be a substance of abuse and lead to a natural form of addiction. Concludes that the evidence supports the hypothesis that under certain circumstances rats can become sugar dependent.

Bennett, Connie, and Stephen T. Sinatra. *Sugar Shock! How Sweets and Simple Carbs Can Derail Your Life—and How You Can Get Back on Track.* New York: Berkley, 2006. This popular paperback, intended for a wide readership, marshals much evidence for how eating massive amounts of sugar has harmed the health of millions of people. Offers advice on ending one's sugar habit. Index.

Macinnis, Peter. *Bittersweet: The Story of Sugar.* Boston: Allyn & Bacon, 2002. This narrative of how sugar processing became big business contains "very few heroes and many villains." Some who made sugar hoped to save lives, others to make money, but they all ended up harming the common good, the health of sugar consumers. Glossary, references, and index.

Minitz, Sidney W. *Sweetness and Power: The Place of Sugar in Modern History.* New York: Viking, 1985. An anthropologist explains how politics and slavery transformed sugar from "a rare foreign luxury" to a necessary commodity in industrialized societies. Bibliography, notes, and index.

Yudkin, John. *Sweet and Dangerous.* New York: Bantam, 1974. A pioneer in analyzing the connections between sugar and many health problems summarizes research on sugar. An account that many have found "prophetic" and as relevant today as it was when first published. Yudkin's research had a strong influence on Linus Pauling and the other founders of orthomolecular medicine.

WEBSITES OF INTEREST

Academy of Nutrition and Dietetics
http://www.eatright.org

American Diabetes Association
http://www.diabetes.org

Food Addicts Anonymous
http://www.foodaddictsanonymous.org

Robert J. Paradowski

SEE ALSO: Food Addiction; Sugar Substitutes

Support groups

The history of support groups in modern times begins with the formation of the Oxford Group in 1908 and the subsequent development of Alcoholics Anonymous. For the participants, support groups reduce feelings of isolation, offer information, instill hope, provide feedback and social support, and teach new social skills. In the early twenty-first century, support groups exist for persons suffering from all kinds of medical and psychological conditions and for victims of violent crime.

INTRODUCTION

Humans are social animals in that they live in groups. These networks among people are powerful in shaping behavior, feelings, and judgments. Groups can lead to destructive behavior, such as mob violence and aggression, but they can also encourage loyalty, nurturing of others, and achievement, as found in cancer-support groups. Scientific investigation of how groups affect human behavior began as early as 1898, but the main body of research on group functioning began only in the 1940s and 1950s. The study of groups is still a major topic of scientific enquiry.

D. R. Forsyth defined a group as "two or more individuals who influence each other through social interaction." A group may be permanent or temporary, formal or informal, structured or unstructured. Those groups known as support groups may share any of these characteristics.

Why do human beings seek out groups? Social learning theorists believe that humans learn to depend on other people because most are raised within families, where they learn to look to other people for support, validation, amusement, and advice. Exchange theorists, on the other hand, reason that groups provide both rewards (such as love and approval) and costs (such as time and effort). Membership in a group will "profit" the individual if the rewards are greater than the costs. Yet another set of theorists, the sociobiologists, argue that humans form groups because this has a survival benefit for the species.

They hypothesize a genetic predisposition toward affiliation with others. It is within groups that the fittest have the greatest chance of survival.

Whatever the reason for forming groups, all groups have important characteristics that must be addressed in seeking to understand why support groups work. First of all, group size is important. Larger groups allow more anonymity, while smaller groups facilitate communication, for example. Group structure includes such elements as status differences, norms of conduct, leaders and followers, and subgroups. Individuals in groups develop social roles—those expected behaviors associated with the individual's position within the group. Roles are powerful in influencing behavior and can even cause individuals to act contrary to their private feelings or their own interests. These roles carry varying degrees of status within the group—who is influential and respected and who is less so. Groups may have subgroups, based on age, residence, roles, interests, or other factors. These subgroups may contribute to the success of the whole or may become cliquish and undermine the main group's effectiveness.

Groups also have varying degrees of cohesion. Cohesion reflects the strength of attachments within the group. Sometimes cohesion is a factor of how well group members like one another, sometimes a factor of the need to achieve an important goal, and sometimes a factor of the rewards that group membership confers. All groups have communication networks, or patterns of openness and restrictions on communication among members.

Group norms are those attitudes and behaviors that are expected of members. These norms are needed for the group's success because they make life more predictable and efficient for the members. Leadership may be formal or informal, may be task oriented or people oriented, and may change over time. Finally, all groups go through fairly predictable stages as they form, do their work, and conclude. The comprehensive term for the way a group functions is group dynamics.

HOW GROUPS INFLUENCE INDIVIDUALS

Researchers have found that for all animals, including human beings, the mere presence of other members of the same species may enhance performance on individual tasks. This phenomenon is known as social facilitation. However, with more complex tasks the presence of others may decrease performance. This is known as social inhibition or impairment. It is not clear whether

this occurs because the presence of others arouses the individual, leads individuals to expect rewards or punishments based on past experience, makes people self-conscious, creates challenges to self-image, or affects the individual's ability to process information. Most theorists agree that the nature of the task is important in the success of a group. For example, the group is more likely to succeed if the individual members' welfare is closely tied to the task of the group.

Groups provide modeling of behavior deemed appropriate in a given situation. The more similar the individuals doing the modeling are to the individual who wants to learn a behavior, the more powerful the models are. Groups reward members for behavior that conforms to group norms or standards and punish behaviors that do not conform. Groups provide a means of social comparison—how one's own behavior compares to others' in a similar situation. Groups are valuable sources of support during times of stress. Some specific factors that enhance the ability of groups to help individuals reduce stress are attachment, guidance, tangible assistance, and embeddedness. Attachment has to do with caring and attention among group members. Guidance may be provision of information or it may be advice and feedback provided by the group to its members. Tangible assistance may take the form of money or of other kinds of service. Embeddedness refers to the sense the individual has of belonging to the group. Some researchers have shown that a strong support system actually increases the body's immune functioning.

ALCOHOLICS ANONYMOUS

The most well-known support group is Alcoholics Anonymous (AA), formed in Akron, Ohio, in the late 1930s. AA groups now number in the tens of thousands and are found across the globe. What is less well known is that AA is an outgrowth of the Oxford Group, an evangelical Christian student and athlete group formed at Oxford University in England in 1908. The Oxford Group's ideals of self-examination, acknowledgment of character defects, restitution for harm done, and working with others directly influenced the steps to recovery practiced by members of AA and other so-called twelve-step groups, including Al-Anon, Narcotics Anonymous, and Smokers Anonymous.

For addicts, support groups are important for a number of reasons. They provide peer support for the effort to become "clean and sober." They provide peer pressure against relapsing into substance use. They assure addicts that they are not alone—that others have suffered the destruction brought about by drinking or drug use. Addicts in twelve-step groups learn to interact with others on an emotional level. Importantly, members of AA and other support groups for addicts are able to confront the individual's maladaptive behaviors and provide models for more functional behavior. The norm for AA is sobriety, and sobriety is reinforced by clear directions on how to live as a sober person. Another important aspect of AA is the hope that it is able to inspire in persons who, while using, saw no hope for the future. This hope comes not only from seeing individuals who have successfully learned to live as sober persons but also from the group's emphasis on dependence on a higher power and the importance of a spiritual life.

OTHER SUPPORT GROUPS

Not all support groups are for addicts. Support groups exist for family and friends of addicts as well as for adoptive parents, children who have been adopted, persons with acquired immunodeficiency syndrome (AIDS), caregivers for patients with Alzheimer's disease, amputees—and that is just the beginning. Why are these groups so popular? Some writers believe that Americans have turned away from the "rugged individualism" that has characterized the national psyche in the past and are searching for meaning in groups to replace the extended families found in other societies. However, this does not explain why support groups are also popular in other parts of the world. The answer probably lies in the characteristics of groups.

Support groups are generally composed of small numbers of people who are facing similar challenges in their lives. They meet, with or without a trained facilitator, to explore their reactions, problems, solutions, feelings, frustrations, successes, and needs in relation to those challenges. They build bonds of trust. Members show compassion for one another. Groups may provide material support or simply assure the individual member he or she is not alone. They help minimize stress and maximize coping. They model strategies for dealing with the given challenge. They provide information. They nurture their members. They encourage application of new learning. Through this sharing, each member grows, and through individual growth, the group matures.

Support groups have traditionally met in person, but the Internet has altered this expectation. Many support groups now meet online. These may take the form of synchronous or asynchronous chat groups, bulletin boards, Web sites with multiple links to information sources, referrals, and collaboration with professionals. These groups, while not well studied, seem to serve the same purposes as in-person groups. In addition, they provide a possible advantage: The anonymity of the Web makes it possible to observe and to learn from observing without actually participating until one is comfortable doing so.

Support groups may not be sufficient in and of themselves to solve individual problems. They are probably most effective as a part of an integrated plan for addressing the challenge in the individual's life that involves other resources as appropriate. For example, the caregiver of a person with Alzheimer's disease may also need social services support, adult daycare or respite care facilities, medical assistance for control of problem behaviors, and home health services to deal successfully with the day-to-day challenges of caring for the patient. The support group can facilitate access to these other resources in addition to serving as an important stress reducer and support system for the caregiver.

FURTHER READING

Carlson, Hannah. *The Courage to Lead: Start Your Own Mutual Help Support Group—Mental Illnesses and Addictions*. Madison: Bick, 2001. Print.

Galinsky, Maeda J., and Janice H. Schopler, eds. *Support Groups: Current Perspectives on Theory and Practice*. New York: Routledge, 2013. Print.

Klein, Linda L. *The Support Group Sourcebook: What They Are, How You Can Find One, and How They Can Help You*. New York: Wiley, 2000. Print.

Kleinberg, Jeffrey L., ed. *The Wiley-Blackwell Handbook of Group Psychotherapy*. Malden: Wiley, 2012. Print.

Mowat, Joan. *Using Support Groups to Improve Behaviour*. Thousand Oaks: PCP/Sage, 2007. Print.

Nichols, Keith, and John Jenkinson. *Leading a Support Group: A Practical Guide*. New York: Open UP, 2006. Print.

O'Halloran, Sean. *Talking Oneself Sober: The Discourse of Alcoholics Anonymous*. Amherst: Cambria, 2008. Print.

"Support Groups: Make Connections, Get Help." *Mayo Clinic*. Mayo Foundation for Medical Education and Research, 1 Aug. 2012. Web. 15 July 2014.

Rebecca Lovell Scott

SEE ALSO: Intervention; Overeaters Anonymous; Recovery

Tanorexia

Can the search for a perfect, enduring tan become a deadly addiction, or just a cultural compulsion? Most people like a tan, but some become addicted to the point where they use artificial tanning beds in all seasons, and risk skin cancer. Some doctors have given such an unhealthy drive to tan a name—Tanorexia—and have begun to study it as a medical malady and a mental illness. "Like anything else, an unhealthy preoccupation with tanning takes a recreational pastime to an obsession. It has yet to be scientifically determined if there is a physical or psychological drive behind this addiction, but with tanning salons so readily available, tanorexia should not be ignored," wrote Susan Evans, a physician, for a website sponsored by the popular Dr. Oz television show.

INTRODUCTION

The term "Tanorexic" originated with humor writer David Sedaris, who used it to describe his well-tanned sister in his memoir, *Me Talk Pretty One Day*, (2000). The experts have not yet agreed on exactly how much exposure to the sun (or artificial tanning) is really unhealthy, but most dermatologists have agreed that tanning to excess produces skin damage. At the same time, a deep tan is popularly believed to be an indicator of health and beauty, at least among people of plain complexion in European-descended cultures. Those who tan to excess may think it makes them look young, but in the long run tanning ages skin, causing perceived beauty to decline, "eventually lead[ing] to premature wrinkles, blotchy patches, dry skin, and melanoma (skin cancer)" (Evans, 2010).

TANNING AS ADDICTIVE BEHAVIOR

Fifteen to 20 minutes of direct exposure to sunlight meets the body's needs for vitamin D. Excessive tanning has nothing to do with nutrition, however. "Addicts live in constant fear of fading," said Amy Wechsler, a dermatologist and psychiatrist in New York City. "Suddenly they feel fatter, older, even sicker. It explains the extremes they go to keep it up" (Flahive, n.d.). According to Susan Evans and Dr. Oz, "Studies indicate that people who suffer from tanorexia display the same addictive behavior as smokers or people with other addictive habits. Just as in an addiction to plastic surgery, there is no point where the person reaches a goal. It's an elusive point they strive for, with no end in sight" (Evans, 2010).

In 2005, a team of dermatologists published a study indicating that frequent users of tanning beds experience a pattern of addiction similar to that of smokers and alcoholics (Warthan, et al., 2005). Another study (Kaur, et al., 2006) found that "Biochemical evidence indicates that tanning addicts are addicted to an opioid release experienced during tanning. When frequent tanners took an endorphin blocker in a 2006 study, they experienced severe withdrawal symptoms, while infrequent tanners experienced no withdrawal symptoms under the same conditions" (Kaur, et al., 2006). Even with such studies, Tanning addiction or tanorexia are not yet mentioned in the *Diagnostic and Statistical Manual of Mental Disorders*.

"Their minds distort the truth," said Glenn Kolansky, a New Jersey dermatologist. "Anorexia is a serious eating disorder. Anorexia is a refusal to maintain a normal body weight, and intense fear of gaining weight as well as a distorted body image. No matter how skinny you become, it is never enough. They are both distorted body image disorders but one is the misconception of one's thinness, and the other is misconception of the color or tan look of the skin" (Walters, 2012).

People who become addicted to tanning may continue to expose themselves no matter how dark they become, according to Evans, as they endure exposure to ultraviolet rays beyond safe limits. The behavior becomes obsessive-compulsive. Just as anorexics lose a sense of proportion about his or her body mass, an obsessive tanorexic loses a sense of how much he or she already has tanned. Addicted to tanning they will continue the behavior no matter how dark they already are, increasing their risk of cancer due to the prolonged exposure to the UV rays. Tanning addicts who use only spray tans are not at a physical risk but they are still dealing with an obsessive-compulsive disorder. "Increasingly," wrote Madeline Hunt in UCLA Her Campus (2012), "Women in their 20s are being diagnosed with melanoma and other types of skin cancer.... Ever since the leathered face of New Jersey mother, Patricia Krentcil, shocked audiences on the news this spring, the question has been thrown out there: Are we tan obsessed?"

Flahive wrote that "Even addicts can occasionally be scared straight. Michael Kors, whose bronzed skin is synonymous with his upscale brand, recently declared that he's switching to self-tanners after discovering a basal-cell carcinoma on his face. " Damage caused by the UV radiation exposure cannot be reversed.

FURTHER READING

Evans, S. (2010, July 26). "Tanorexia: are you obsessed with your tan?" The Dr. Oz Show. http://www.doctoroz.com/blog/susan-evans-md/tanorexia-are-you-obsessed-your-tan. Is tanning to excess a compulsion that can kill you? Dr. Oz entertains the question.

Flahive, E. (n.d.) Are you tanorexic? Web MD. Accessed June 9, 2015. http://www.webmd.com/beauty/sun/you-tanorexic. This article from *Marie Claire* magazine discusses how to determine dangers of excessive tanning.

Hunt, M. (2012, May 22). Tanorexia—has tanning gone too far? 5 facts all tanoholics (and everyone else!) should know about the sun.

UCLA Her Campus. http://www.hercampus.com/school/ucla/tanorexia-has-tanning-gone-too-far-5-facts-all-tanoholics-and-everyone-else-should-know. This blog contains practical advice about keeping tanning from becoming an addiction.

Kaur, M., A. Liguori, W. Lang, Rapp, S., Fleischer, A., Jr., Feldman, S. (2006). Induction of withdrawal-like symptoms in a small randomized, controlled trial of opioid blockade in frequent tanners. *Journal of the American Academy of Dermatology,* 54(4):709-711. This study found that found biochemical evidence that tanning addicts are addicted to an opioid release.

Walters, J. (2012, May 15). What you need to know about tanorexia. *Shape Magazine.* http://www.shape.com/blogs/shape-your-life/what-you-need-know-about-tanorexia. This brief article outlines the addictive nature of excessive tanning.

Warthan, M., T. Uchida, Wagner,R., Jr. (2005, August). UV light tanning as a type of substance-related disorder. *Archives of Dermatology,* 141:963-966. A team of dermatologists published a study indicating that frequent users of tanning beds experience a pattern of addiction similar to smokers and alcoholics.

Bruce E. Johansen

SEE ALSO: Obsessive-Compulsive Disorder

Teens and alcohol abuse

Alcohol abuse is a pattern of heavy drinking that significantly compromises a person's physical health and social functioning. In the United States, six percent of fourteen-year-old children, about one-third of eighteen year olds, and one-half of college students age eighteen to twenty-four years are binge or heavy drinkers. Despite intensive government efforts to curb the problem, the prevalence of underage alcohol abuse has remained constant since about 1990.

BEER: A HISTORY OF ITS CONSUMPTION AND EFFECTS

Beer is one of the world's oldest beverages, dating to 3500 bce or earlier for common usage. It is produced in varying levels of alcohol concentration during the fermentation process.

Today, beer as a product and its advertising are highly visible to persons of all ages. Being readily available and inexpensive, beer is a frequent beverage in initial alcohol consumption. Its abuse derives from overconsumption or a habitual pattern of use. Some studies have found that as many as one-half of thirteen-year-olds in the United States have consumed alcohol. Early consumption increases risk of alcohol dependence in adulthood. Adolescent risks include damage to the developing brain, physical or sexual assault, and reduced academic performance.

The alcohol in beer is rapidly absorbed into the bloodstream; short-term effects are proportional to consumption. Beer is a central nervous system depressant, and every organ is affected; reaction time, judgment, speech, and movement abilities may be compromised, contributing to the frequency of motor vehicle accidents.

Gender, age, weight, food consumption, and tolerance levels affect blood alcohol content (BAC), generally the best measure of short-term use and effects. Though initial feelings of euphoria, decreased inhibition, and extroversion may be present in moderate use, significant impairment, coma, or death may result when the BAC exceeds .30. No safe level of consumption has been established for girls and women who are pregnant or nursing.

Alcohol-related disorders may result from long-term use of beer, as with other alcoholic beverages. Chronic usage can damage the liver, heart, gastrointestinal tract, nervous system, bone marrow, and endocrine system, and it is associated with an increased cancer risk. In addition, vitamin deficiencies, alterations in blood sugar and fat levels, hepatitis, fatty liver, cirrhosis, esophagitis, gastritis, and dementia may develop. The physical and emotional effects of addiction can result in behavioral disorders, including violence and mood and anxiety disorders.

SCOPE OF THE PROBLEM

Alcohol use and abuse among young people in the United States is pervasive and destructive. Despite minimum legal drinking ages of between eighteen and twenty-one years since World War II, and despite a nationwide minimum legal age of twenty-one years since about 2000, 80 percent of Americans began drinking alcohol by age eighteen years; the peak age for binge drinking is eighteen to twenty-one years. A 2008 National Institutes of Health survey estimated that 1.4 million youth age twelve to seventeen years experienced alcohol abuse or dependence in the past year and that 2.3 million twelve to twenty year olds drank five or more drinks on an occasion, five or more times per month.

At age twelve, 11 percent of boys and 9 percent of girls have commenced drinking, and 1 percent of them are classified as binge and heavy users. By age fourteen years, the numbers are 31 and 33 percent for use, respectively, and 6 percent of them are binge or heavy users. At age eighteen years, 73 percent have commenced drinking, 42 percent have used alcohol in the past month, and 39 percent are heavy users. Girls age fourteen to eighteen years are somewhat more likely than boys to use alcohol regularly, probably because they are more mature physically and because they often associate with older boys. After age eighteen years, levels of problem drinking are higher among young men, although the gender differential has been steadily narrowing since the 1970s.

Alcohol dependence, characterized by maintenance drinking and an inability to regulate intake, affects 2 percent of twelve to seventeen year olds who drink, 12.2 percent of eighteen to twenty year olds, and 11 percent of young adults age twenty-one to twenty-four years. In contrast, only 3.8 percent of forty to forty-four year olds and less than 2 percent of persons older than age fifty years are dependent on alcohol.

People who commence heavy or episodic binge drinking before age sixteen years are more than twice as likely as people who start drinking after age eighteen years to develop alcohol dependence. This statistic is often cited as justification for higher drinking ages and for more diligent enforcement of laws against underage drinking. There is some controversy whether this is a matter of cause and effect. Early heavy drinkers usually have alcoholic parents or siblings and are probably genetically susceptible to alcoholism; as well, they probably are subject to environmental influences favoring alcohol abuse.

Rates of both alcohol abuse and alcohol dependence decline steadily after age twenty-five years, a pattern that has been consistent for many decades despite changing social attitudes. Among drinkers with a normal trajectory, work and family responsibilities reduce the opportunities for, and acceptability of, frequent intoxication. For those who develop alcohol dependence, a point is eventually reached in which the person either receives treatment and abstains, or dies of the disease.

Rates of teen and young-adult alcohol abuse in northern Europe are similar to those in the United States, except that the average age of onset of heavy drinking is lower; this is in part due to lower minimum legal drinking ages. A survey of fifteen to sixteen year olds in thirty-four European countries in 2007 showed more than 80 percent had drunk alcohol in the past year and 43 percent had been intoxicated or consumed more than five drinks on one occasion in the past thirty days. There is considerable variation from country to country, with abuse being less frequent in southern Europe.

In Great Britain, drinking among schoolchildren is a serious national problem of recent origin. Up until 1960, persons age sixteen to twenty-four years had the lowest per capita alcohol consumption of any adult group; since 1990, the situation has reversed. Some of this pattern (which is seen to a lesser extent in the United States) may be attributed to the rising age of workforce participation. Few sixteen to eighteen year olds are employed full time, and an increasing proportion of eighteen to twenty-four year olds are students with more leisure time and fewer responsibilities than working counterparts. In general, high rates of unemployment that are not accompanied by extreme economic privation produce high levels of alcohol abuse.

EFFECTS OF EARLY ALCOHOL USE AND ABUSE

Alcohol abuse exacts a heavy toll among young people. In 2007, 1,825 college students in the United States died in alcohol-related accidents, 599,000 were injured, 696,000 were involved in nonsexual assaults, 97,000 were sexually assaulted, 400,000 had unsafe sex while intoxicated, 3,360,000 reported driving drunk, about 5 percent were arrested for alcohol-related offenses, and 25 percent reported adverse academic consequences because of drinking. Twenty-five percent of "low-alcohol use" campuses and 50 percent of "high use" campuses reported property damage.

The negative effects on a person's life range from short-lived and inconsequential to profound. Drinking leads to a massive loss of productivity, both in poor academic performance and in the resources that college administrators divert from academics toward combating alcohol problems on campuses.

Statistics on alcohol use for persons eighteen to twenty-five years of age who are not enrolled in a college or university are not as comprehensive; in general, rates of binge drinking are lower but still significant. For both college and university students and people in the workforce, an early and persistent pattern of alcohol abuse tends to translate into poorer career prospects and family instability, even if the drinker never becomes alcohol dependent or if the drinker later successfully enters a recovery program.

Alcohol can serve as a gateway drug. A high proportion of younger heavy drinkers also use marijuana, and the culture surrounding binge drinking among young people for whom it is illegal provides opportunities for experimenting with more dangerous street drugs. Many methamphetamine addicts report that they began using the drug to counteract the effects of alcohol on the job.

REDUCING UNDERAGE DRINKING

Federal, state, and local governments devote a great deal of energy to combat underage drinking through education and increased enforcement. Federal law in the United States now mandates a minimum state drinking age of twenty-one years as a condition of receiving federal highway funds. This law has reduced the availability of alcohol to middle and high school students but has had little effect on levels of consumption among eighteen to twenty-one year olds.

A comparison of the United States with European countries, where a drinking age of sixteen or eighteen years is typical, calls into question whether the approach in the United States is effective. In no European country is the level of problem drinking among eighteen to twenty-one year olds higher than in the United States. It can be argued that turning any alcohol consumption into a criminal activity increases the chances of excessive use and alcohol-associated risky behaviors, such as unsafe sex, without reducing the proportion of young adults whose use adversely affects their lives and the lives of those around them.

Revenue considerations often complicate efforts to curtail alcohol abuse among young people. Underage drinkers comprise a major market sector. Advertising campaigns continue to target this demographic despite government regulation. Flavored alcoholic beverages are

of particular concern to regulators and to opponents of alcohol use among youth. Also, in college and university towns, the revenue stream generated by sporadic enforcement of liquor laws tends to undermine efforts at truly effective enforcement.

If statistics on traffic accidents are any indication, efforts made toward curbing underage drinking and reducing alcohol abuse among high school and college students do seem to have had a significant effect on driving behavior, but not on consumption. Effects of heightened education and enforcement on the population as a whole and on older age groups are not dramatic and can be partially explained by other factors, including an aging population and a persistent recession that tends to depress luxury consumption among people who are not alcohol dependent. Also unknown, but probably significant, is the degree to which marginalized youth, who a generation ago would have abused alcohol, are turning to street drugs instead.

FURTHER READING

Bellenir, Karen, and Amy Sutton. *Alcoholism Sourcebook.* Detroit: Omnigraphics, 2007. Consumer information about alcohol use, abuse, and dependence. Includes statistics on physical and social pathology.

A Developmental Perspective on Underage Alcohol Use. Spec. issue of *Alcohol Research and Health* 33.1 (2009): 1–76. Print. Seven research papers focusing on alcohol use in physical and social contexts.

Grant, Bridget, et al. "The 12-Month Prevalence and Trends in DSM-IV Alcohol Abuse and Dependence, United States, 1991–1992 and 2001–2002." *Drug and Alcohol Dependence* 74.3 (2004): 223–34. Print. A detailed statistical report and analysis.

Hingson, Ralph W., Wenxing Zha, and Elissa R. Weitzman. "Magnitude and Trends in Alcohol-Related Mortality and Morbidity among U.S. College Students Ages 18–24, 1998–2005." *Journal of Studies on Alcohol and Drugs* 16 (2009): 12–20. Print. A statistical paper, underscoring the need for intervention and counseling.

Monti, Peter M., Suzanne M. Colby, and Tracy O'Leary, eds. *Adolescents, Alcohol, and Substance Abuse: Reaching Teens through Brief Interventions.* New York: Guilford, 2001. A multiauthored volume with emphasis on clinical practice.

WEBSITES OF INTEREST

College Drinking: Changing the Culture
http://www.collegedrinkingprevention.gov
Institute of Alcohol Studies
http://www.ias.org.uk/resources/factsheets/adolescents.pdf
Mothers Against Drunk Driving
http://www.madd.org/underage-drinking
National Institute on Alcohol Abuse and Alcoholism
http://www.niaaa.nih.gov
National Institutes of Health Fact Sheets
http://report.nih.gov/NIHfactsheets

Martha A. Sherwood

SEE ALSO: Alcohol and Its Effects; Alcohol Poisoning; Binge Drinking; Drunk Driving

Teens and drug abuse

Drug abuse is a complex disease that leads to changes in the structure and function of the brain in teenagers and young adults.

TOUGH LOVE

Organizations that prescribe a tough-love perspective hold teenagers responsible for their behavior by helping them become aware of the consequences of their actions. Strategies often focus on confrontation and ultimatums and are considered a last response to behaviors that are self-destructive or dangerous to others.

In the 1960s, the tough-love approach was prescribed to parents who felt powerless because of their unruly, out-of-control children, many of whom were using drugs. Some persons credit David and Phyllis York as popularizers of this parenting approach in the 1980s. Many residential rehabilitation programs that provide addiction treatment represent this approach, some in the form of behavior modification centers or wilderness programs. The assumption is that certain rules and strategies will produce well-behaved, well-ordered teens.

The tough-love perspective has its critics, however. Opponents believe that parents can prevent children from "bottoming out" through a relationship that communicates understanding and support, rather than confrontation and ultimatums.

DRUG ABUSE

Teenagers and young adults who abuse drugs often display problem behaviors such as poor academic performance and dropping out of school. They also are at an increased risk of unplanned pregnancies, violence, and infectious diseases.

For most young people, the initial decision to take drugs is voluntary. However, the repeated use of substances such as drugs, alcohol, and tobacco causes changes in the brain that affect one's self-control and ability to make sound decisions. Drugs also cause the brain to send intense impulses that compel the user to take more drugs. Because of this, drug abuse can result in addiction.

The teen brain is still developing, making the effects of drug abuse even more complex for this population. One area of the brain still maturing during adolescence is the prefrontal cortex, which enables a person to consider situations fully, make solid decisions, and keep emotions and desires under control. Because this critical part of an adolescent's brain is still a work in progress, adolescents are at greater risk for poor decision-making (such as trying drugs or continued use). Also, using drugs while the brain is still developing may lead to profound and long-lasting consequences.

No single factor determines whether a person will become addicted to drugs. The overall risk for addiction is affected by the person's biological makeup and his or her environment. It can even be influenced by gender or ethnicity, a person's developmental stage, and the surrounding social environment (such as conditions at home, at school, and in the neighborhood). Scientists estimate that genetic factors account for 40 to 60 percent of a person's vulnerability to addiction, including the effects of environment on gene expression and function.

Adolescents and persons with mental disorders are at greater risk of drug abuse and addiction than the general population, making drug abuse prevention programs for teens critically important. Alcohol, tobacco, and illicit drug abuse are reduced when science-validated drug-abuse prevention programs are properly implemented by schools and communities. Such programs help teachers, parents, and health care professionals shape teens' perceptions about the dangers of drug abuse. While many events and cultural factors affect drug abuse trends, levels of abuse are reduced when teens and young adults learn that such abuse is harmful.

COMMONLY ABUSED DRUGS

Drug use in teenagers and young adults varies between ages thirteen and nineteen years. Younger teens are less likely to use most drugs than older teens. An exception is the use of inhalants, which is seen more in younger teens and less in older ones, in part because inhalants are readily accessible to teens. An average home has between thirty and fifty products with abuse potential. Also, inhalants are inexpensive and are legal to buy and possess. Additionally, the perceived risk of use is low.

More and more teens are abusing prescription drugs. Use of marijuana has remained stable but is more common. About 15 percent of high school seniors report having abused prescription drugs and about 32 percent report having used marijuana in the last year. According to the 2010 Monitoring the Future survey, prescription and over-the-counter drugs are among the most commonly abused drugs by twelfth graders; only alcohol, marijuana, and tobacco are used more often. Youth who abuse prescription medications also are more likely to report using other drugs.

Other drugs that are abused by teens and young adults include opioids (heroin, opium), stimulants (cocaine, amphetamine, methamphetamine), club drugs (methylenedioxy-methamphetamine, flunitrazepam, gamma-hydroxybutyrate), dissociative drugs (ketamine, PCP and analogs, Salvia divinorum, dextromethorphan), hallucinogens (lysergic acid diethylamide, mescaline, psilocybin), and anabolic steroids.

DRUG ABUSE AND ITS EFFECTS ON THE BRAIN

Drugs contain chemicals that interfere with the brain's communication system and change the way nerve cells normally send, receive, and process information. Drugs cause this interruption by imitating the brain's natural chemical messengers and by overstimulating the reward circuit of the brain.

Some drugs (such as marijuana and heroin) have a structure that is similar to chemical messengers called neurotransmitters, which are naturally produced by the brain. This similarity allows the drugs to fool the brain's receptors and activate nerve cells to send abnormal messages.

Other drugs, such as cocaine or methamphetamine, can cause the nerve cells to release large amounts of natural neurotransmitters (mainly dopamine) or to prevent the normal recycling of these brain chemicals, which is needed to shut off the signaling between neurons. The result is a brain full of dopamine, a neurotransmitter present in brain regions that controls movement, emotion, motivation, and feelings of pleasure. The overstimulation of this reward system, which normally responds to natural behaviors linked to survival (for example, eating and spending time with loved ones), produces euphoric effects in response to psychoactive drugs. This reaction sets in motion a reinforcing pattern that "teaches" a person to repeat the rewarding behavior of abusing drugs.

As a person continues to abuse drugs, the brain adapts to the overwhelming surges in dopamine by producing less dopamine or by reducing the number of dopamine receptors in the reward circuit. The result is a lessening of dopamine's effect on the rew Primary Secondary card circuit, which reduces the abuser's ability to enjoy the drugs, as well as the events in life that previously brought pleasure. This decrease compels the addict to keep abusing drugs to bring the dopamine function back to normal; however, larger amounts of the drug will be required to achieve the same dopamine high—an effect known as tolerance.

Long-term abuse also causes changes in other brain-chemical systems and circuits. Glutamate is a neurotransmitter that influences the reward circuit and the ability to learn. When the optimal concentration of glutamate is altered by drug abuse, the brain attempts to compensate, which can impair cognitive function.

Brain imaging studies of drug addicts show changes in areas of the brain that are critical to judgment, decision making, learning and memory, and behavior control. Together, these changes can drive an abuser to seek and take drugs compulsively despite adverse, even devastating consequences; this is the nature of addiction.

TREATMENT

Drug abuse is a treatable disease with many effective treatments available. Some important points about drug abuse treatment include the following: Medical and behavioral therapy, alone or together, are used to treat drug abuse. Treatment can sometimes be done on an outpatient basis, but severe drug abuse usually requires residential treatment, in which the patient sleeps at the treatment center.

Treatment can take place within the criminal justice system, which can help to prevent a convicted person from returning to criminal behavior. Furthermore, studies show that treatment does not need to be voluntary to work.

Addiction is a difficult disorder to treat, especially if diagnosed late into the condition, although remissions can be achieved in up to 60 percent of patients. Whether or not treatment works depends on the patient's level of functioning at entry into treatment, premorbid functioning, comorbid conditions, and the support systems and resources available to the patient. Treating a substance abuser is not a hopeless process, but it can be a long and difficult one, similar to the treatment of any chronic disorder.

FURTHER READING

Gogtay, N., et al. "Dynamic Mapping of Human Cortical Development during Childhood through Early Adulthood." *Proceedings of the National Academy of Sciences* 101 (2004): 8174–79. Print.

Graham, A. W., and T. K. Shultz, eds. *Principles of Addiction Medicine*. 3rd ed. Chevy Chase, MD: American Society of Addiction Medicine, 2003.

National Institute on Drug Abuse. *Drugs, Brains, and Behavior: The Science of Addiction.* Bethesda, MD: NIDA, 2010.

---. *Preventing Drug Use among Children and Adolescents: A Research-Based Guide for Parents, Educators, and Community Leaders.* Bethesda, MD: NIDA, 2003.

Rehm, J., et al. "Global Burden of Disease and Injury and Economic Cost Attributable to Alcohol Use and Alcohol-Use Disorders." *Lancet* 373 (2009): 2223–33. Print.

WEBSITES OF INTEREST

GirlsHealth.gov
http://www.girlshealth.gov/substance
National Institute on Drug Abuse
http://www.drugabuse.gov
National Institute on Drug Abuse for Teens
http://teens.drugabuse.gov

Claudia Daileader Ruland

SEE ALSO: Amphetamine Abuse; Antidepressants; Barbituates; Cough and Cold Medications; Cocaine and Its Effects; Date Rape Drugs; Depressants Abuse; Designer Drugs; Hallucinogens and Their Effects; Heroin; LSD; Marijuana; Methamphetamine; Mushrooms/Psilocybin; Over-The-Counter (OTC) Drugs; PCP; Pregnancy and Drug Use; Ritalin; Steroids: HGH and PEDS; Stimulants and Their Effects

Going Green

Alternative fuels (wind, solar, ethanol)

In 2013, for the first time, electric utilities world-wide installed more new capacity from renewable sources (143 gigawatts, GW) than fossil fuels (141 GW), according to an analysis presented April 14, 2014 at the Bloomberg New Energy Finance annual summit in New York City. BNEF analysts expect that "The shift will continue to accelerate, and by 2030 more than four times as much renewable capacity will be added" (Randall, 2014).

INTRODUCTION

The costs of solar and wind power have been declining rapidly, to the point where wind competes favorably under some conditions with fossil fuels. This is an important reason why wind has suddenly become very popular as a source of electrical generation in many of the United States, especially in the Midwest. The Omaha Public Power District, for example, heretofore wholly coal and nuclear generated, by 2016 will be about one-third wind. By that time, one-half of Iowa's electricity will be generated by wind power. The cost of wind power is now being quoted as low as 1 to 2 cents per kilowatt hour, often lower than coal, oil, or natural gas. In 2014, California's government had a target of 33 percent renewable power by 2020.

Solar technology is undergoing a revolution that may eventually allow power to be acquired from nearly any surface on which the sun shines. One such technology is the "artificial leaf." At Caltech's Jorgensen Laboratory, a team of more than 190 people have been using silicon, nickel, iron, and other materials in the Joint Center for Artificial Photosynthesis (JCAP), a $16-million, five-year program funded by the U.S. Department of Energy that is attempting to replicate photosynthesis as an energy source. At the same time, the "green" credentials of biofuel (ethanol) are being questioned, for reasons described below.

WIND POWER'S SPREADING WEB

Wind-power advocates now watch the share of electricity generated by turbines rise day by day. "A glorious wind blows on the prairie," remarked one such observer in Omaha in mid-April, 2015, as the share of wind power in the Southwest Power Pool (the Regional Transmission Organization that balances demand and supply) passed 25 per cent on April 11 at 1:10 p.m. Central Daylight Time, during a warm, breezy afternoon in a region from North Dakota southward through northern Texas. Wind has been gaining power share so quickly that we can watch it happen. It passed 28 per cent later the same day.

Advances in wind-turbine technology adapted from the aerospace industry have reduced the cost of wind power from 38 cents per kilowatt-hour (during the early 1980s) to 3 cents or less under some conditions. This rate is competitive with costs of power generation from fossil fuels, but costs vary according to site. Major corporations, including Shell International and British Petroleum, have been moving into wind power.

Global installations of wind power increased by 35,467 and 51,447 megawatts in 2013 and 2014, respectively, according to the Global Wind Energy Council. As of the end of 2014, worldwide, total cumulative installed capacity from wind power totaled 369,553 MW, an increase of 16 per cent in one year. In 2014, China was adding half of the world's new capacity and, at 114,763 MW, was the world's leader, with 31.7 per cent of the world total. The United States was second at 65,879 (17.8 per cent), followed by Germany (39,165 MW, 10.6%); Spain: 22,987 MW (6.2 per cent); India: 22,465 MW (6.1 per cent) ; United Kingdom: 12,440 MW (3.4 per cent), and Canada: 9,694 MW, 2.6 per cent). (Global Wind, 2015).

The Netherlands in 2015 was building a large array of wind turbines 50 miles offshore in the North Sea at a cost of $3 billion that will provide power for 1.5 million homes beginning in 2017. Wind power from sea-based platforms costs as much as three times that of land-based wind farms because of relatively high constriction, maintenance, and transmission costs, but government subsidies have been used to support the Dutch program.

Spain's tiny industrial state of Navarre, which generated no wind power in 1996, by 2002 generated 25 per cent of its electricity that way. By 2007, 60 per cent of its electricity was from renewable sources (mainly wind, with some solar), and plans are in place to raise that proportion to 75 per cent by 2010.

THE COMING REVOLUTION IN SOLAR POWER

A breakthrough in solar power has been sought since the days of Thomas Edison. In a conversation with Henry Ford and the tire tycoon Harvey Firestone in 1931, shortly before Edison died, he said: "I'd put my money on the sun and solar energy. What a source of power! I hope we don't have to wait until oil and coal run out before we tackle that" (Revkin, October 30, 2006).

Solar power has advanced significantly since the days of inefficient photovoltaics. In California, solar power is being built into roof tiles, and talk is that nanotechnology will eventually make any surface the sun hits a source of power—windows, for example. Experiments have been undertaken with a new form of solar energy —*Concentrating Solar Power (CSP)*, "a mirror in the shape of a parabola to focus light onto a black pipe with a heat-transfer fluid inside. The fluid is used to boil water into steam, which turns a generator that can produce 64 megawatts. The newest solar-thermal technology involves building a 'power tower,' a tall structure flanked by thousands of mirrors, each of which pivots to focus light on the tower, heating fluid. That design can work even in places with weaker sunlight than a desert" (Wald, 2008). Private homes using alternative energy sources now feed power into the electrical grid, as meters run backward, paying householders for contributed power.

With residential solar power capacity growing at more than 30 per cent a year in some places (including Hawaii, California, Arizona, and Japan) by 2015, so much power is being feed back into the grid that it is wreaking havoc with the budgets of some utility companies, as it cuts into their revenues. In Hawaii, for example, about 12 per cent of private homes by 2015 were producing enough solar power to feed some back into the grid and receive payment for it. " "Hawaii is a postcard from the future," said Adam Browning, executive director of Vote Solar, a California-based advocacy organization. Some utilities have been adding fees for use of solar on their grids. "Hawaii's case is not isolated," said Massoud Amin, University of Minnesota electrical and computer engineering professor. "When we push year-on-year 30 to 40 percent growth in this market, with the number of installations doubling, quickly — every two years or so — there's going to be problems" (Cardwell, 2015).

"Solar power has captured the public imagination," wrote Andrew C. Revkin and Matthew L. Wald in the *New York Times*, "Panels that convert sunlight to electricity are winning supporters around the world — from Europe, where gleaming arrays cloak skyscrapers and farmers' fields, to Wall Street, where stock offerings for panel makers have had a great ride, to California, where Gov. Arnold Schwarzenegger's Million Solar Roofs initiative is promoted as building a homegrown industry and fighting global warming" (Revkin and Wald, 2007). For all the excitement, however, solar power in 2006

contributed only 0.01 per cent of the United States' electricity supply. "Most of the environmental stuff out there now is toys compared to the scale we need to really solve the planet's problems," said Vinod Khosla, a prominent Silicon Valley entrepreneur who focuses on energy (Revkin and Wald, 2007).

By 2011, major builders were beginning to sell midrange tract houses with installed solar power and utility bills close to zero. In some sunny areas, including Tucson, Arizona and Las Vegas, Nevada, houses were being sold by Arizona-based Meritage Homes, the ninth-largest residential construction company in the United States, for $140,000 to $170,000, which produce as much energy as they consume. The homes come with a nine-panel solar array that reduces electric bills by about one-third. For $10,000 more, 24 more panels reduce power bills to zero, more or less, depending on consumption.

With solar power still usually more expensive than coal per kilowatt hour inventors are working on new technologies to reduce that gap. As a measure of the interest in solar in California, the U.S. Bureau of Land Management received applications for projects that could cover 78,490 acres adjacent to the Joshua Tree National Park—125 projects that, if they are built, could replace 70 industrial-sized coal-fired power plants.

The silicon solar panels that dominate the industry today may be replaced by new technologies that combine several light-absorbing materials that capture different portions of the solar spectrum, or solar cells manufactured in rolls of thin copper-indium film gallium selenide atop a metal foil. Nanotechnology plays a role in some designs for future solar generating technology that is been theorized, but not yet commercialized. While today's silicon cells convert about 15 to 20 per cent of sunlight to electricity in the field (up to 24 per cent under perfect laboratory conditions), new technologies that have broached the realm of theory (and some in design, but not commercialization) raise that figure to 40, 60, even 80 per cent. Photovoltaics made of plastic may dramatically reduce manufacturing costs.

CORN ETHANOL: HOW "GREEN" IS IT?

Corn ethanol is a carbon-based fossil fuel when it is burned to propel cars and trucks. Depending on its source (and whose statistics are considered), ethanol emits only 10 to 34 per cent less greenhouse gases than gasoline. Even that savings isn't what it seems. Corn must be grown on factory farms, a very energy-intensive business. Under some circumstances (if a biomass field replaced a forest, for example) this type of fuel might actually produce a net increase in emissions of greenhouse gases, considering the entire production process. Thus, corn ethanol and other forms of "biofuel" are not very "green." Corn just does not contain enough energy to make it efficient. Ethanol from sugar cane (widely used in Brazil) contains eight to ten times as much energy per unit of mass as corn, and may be a better bet as an environmentally conscious fuel.

FURTHER READING

Cardwell, Diane. (2015, April18) "Solar Power Battle Puts Hawaii at Forefront of Worldwide Changes." *New York Times* http://www.nytimes.com/2015/04/19/business/energy-environment/solar-power-battle-puts-hawaii-at-forefront-of-worldwide-changes.html This report examines the problems that established power sources have encountered as a rapid rise in solar power cuts into their budgets.

Flannery, Tim. (2005) *The weather makers: how man is changing the climate and what it means for life on Earth*. New York: Atlantic Monthly Press. Describes how human beings have been changing climate since the days when the main fuel was firewood.

Randall, Tom. (2015, April 14). Fossil fuels just lost the race against renewables:

This is the beginning of the end. *Bloomberg Business*. http://www.bloomberg.com/news/articles/2015-04-14/fossil-fuels-just-lost-the-race-against-renewables Installed new capacity for electricity generation with solar and wind passed that of fossil fuels in 2013, according to this report.

Revkin, Andrew C. (2006, October 30). "Budgets falling in race to fight global warming. *New York Times*. http://www.nytimes.com/2006/10/30/business/worldbusiness/30energy.html Thomas Edison and Henry Ford favored solar power. The world is now catching up with them.

Revkin, Andrew C. and Matthew L. Wald. (2007, July 16). Solar power captures imagination, not money. *New York Times*. http://www.nytimes.com/2007/07/16/business/16solar.html Solar power had reached the planning stage in 2007, but funding for technological innovation was lagging.

Wald, Matthew. (2008, March 6). "Turning glare Into watts." *New York Times*. http://www.nytimes.com/2008/03/06/business/06solar.html Wald reports

on ways in which solar power is being widely adapted around the United States.

Bruce E Johansen

SEE ALSO: Becoming a Green Consumer; Conservation; Nonrenewable Energy Resources; Renewable Energy Resources.

Battery recycling

Battery recycling is increasing in the US; the Rechargeable Battery Recycling Corporation (RBRC) saw a 10% growth in its rechargeable battery collections in 2008 (6.9 million pounds) over 2007. A new, $100 million Johnson Controls, Inc battery recycling plant in Florence County, South Carolina will create an estimated 250 new jobs by 2010. The Detroit 3 automakers contracted with OnTo Technology LLC of Bend, Oregon to develop more efficient processes for recycling lithium-ion (li-ion) and nickel-metal hydride (NiMH) batteries, to power current and upcoming hybrid vehicles. In 2007, over 13,000 tons of cobalt was sold globally for manufacturing li-ion batteries. This figure will likely rise since li-ion batteries are expected to gain in use over the next decade.

ECONOMIC & ENVIRONMENTAL BENEFITS OF BATTERY RECYCLING CHANGE INDUSTRY: WATCH LIST

- The federal Mercury-Containing Rechargeable Battery Management Act (Battery Act) calls for state regulatory agencies and the Environmental Protection Agency (EPA) to facilitate battery recycling and to reduce the quantity of toxins in the environment from discarded batteries.
- The EPA's Universal Waste Rule created a new "universal waste" category that includes batteries. The Rule makes it easier for businesses and private citizens to recycle spent batteries.
- Battery recycling nonprofits and for-profits thrive in the US today; serving every economic sector and recycling all battery types.
- The Rechargeable Battery Association (PRBA) has played an active role in creating the national regulations for collecting and recycling rechargeable batteries.
- RBRC has recycled approximately 50 million pounds of rechargeable batteries since its inception in 1996.

- More lead-acid batteries are recycled each year in the US than any other type of battery.

- Worldwide, a large untapped market exists for recycling spent batteries, as indicated by figures such as those from the UK where less than 2% of disposable consumer batteries and only 5% of rechargeable batteries are currently recycled.

- Corporations across the nation demonstrate an awareness of the economic, environmental, and public relations benefits of recycling batteries.

Businesses, consumers, and governments increasingly recognize the environmental and economic benefits that can be derived by recycling batteries. This is due in part to the growing awareness that batteries play a significant role in powering the use of everyday products. Indeed, billions of batteries help to power economies across the world by making it possible to use vast numbers of portable electronics from cell phones to pacemakers, laptops to backup generators.

The chemicals that comprise battery electrodes are usually toxic, as well as non-renewable and often difficult to mine. Therefore, their recovery through recycling brings cost-containment and environmental benefits: Reducing the amount and therefore the expense of mining to acquire raw materials, and protecting public health by keeping toxic metals out of the land and water. Other battery components, such as polypropylene, can also be repackaged and sold for a variety of manufacturing uses.

Since 1995, federal and state regulations have emerged to encourage proper disposal and recycling of batteries. These regulations can create new business opportunities. Anaheim-based TOXCO responded to a 2004 California law by targeting its recycling efforts to capture the individual market, where prior to this it had focused mainly on large industrial clients. Nonprofit and for-profit organizations have sprung up to provide battery recycling services. These groups and companies point out in their marketing collateral that they help corporations meet regulatory requirements related to properly recycling spent batteries and meeting landfill rules.

Technologies to recycle batteries continue to develop, and the resulting products are resold to battery manufacturers and other industries. Corporations across several retail sectors, including the hospitality and electronics retail industries, have expanded their battery recycling programs in recent years. The three major US automakers recently contracted with OnTo Technology LLC to conduct research and development for recycling li-ion and NiMH batteries.

BUSINESS OPTIONS & BEST PRACTICES: BATTERY RECYCLING BENEFITS

Batteries power portable products worldwide, from cell phones and laptops to backup generators. The chemicals that make up battery electrodes can be rare and difficult to mine, so there is a growing awareness that recycling batteries and reusing their components makes sense economically. The benefits gained by recycling batteries include reducing the amount of mining required to obtain raw materials and preventing toxic metals from leaching into water supplies and the earth. Environmental protections are mandated by federal and state laws, and the public has grown more aware that tossing batteries in the trash harms the environment.

Businesses show increasing interest in reaping the economic and public relations benefits of running sustainable operations. Further, recycling rechargeable batteries has been touted as an easy and relatively low-cost method for improving facilities' green bottom line. Reasonable battery recycling expenses are fostered by such organizations as the nonprofit RBRC (please see the Battery recycling organizations section). RBRC's Call2Recycle program offers all economic sectors no-cost rechargeable battery recycling. Other organizations provide battery recycling services as well, and market themselves as helping corporations to meet regulatory requirements related to properly recycling spent batteries.

BATTERY RECYCLING ORGANIZATIONS & CORPORATIONS

Nonprofit and for-profit battery recycling organizations in the United States serve all economic sectors, from individual consumers to large industries, and recycle every type of battery in use today. In the nonprofit realm, PRBA—The Rechargeable Battery Association (formerly called the Portable Rechargeable Battery Association)—was started in 1991 by five rechargeable battery manufacturers: Energizer, Panasonic Battery Corporation, SAFT America, SANYO Energy Corporation, and Varta Batteries. This Washington, DC-based trade association, which works on issues affecting manufacturers and consumers of li-ion and NiMH batteries, helped to create a regulatory environment that is more amenable to collecting and recycling rechargeable batteries by participating in the creation of the Universal Waste Rule, and by supporting the Battery Act (please see the Regulations section). The PRBA also represents the Rechargeable Power Industry at all governing levels—state, federal, and international—regarding legislative, regulatory and standards issues. In 2004, the group received official observer status by the United Nations Committee of Experts on the Transport of Dangerous Goods and on the Globally Harmonised System of Chemical Classification and Labeling.

PRBA sought to make battery collection and recycling more practical and widespread by testing pilot projects in several states, and then developed the nationwide nonprofit RBRC in 1994. Based in Atlanta, RBRC provides public education as well as no-fee recycling programs for retailers. RBRC began recycling operations in 1996 and since that time has recycled nearly 50 million pounds of rechargeable batteries in the US and Canada. Healthy increases have been seen from year to year. For example, there was a 7.7% increase from 2003 to 2004, a nearly 10% increase from 2004 to '05, and 9.6% growth between 2007 and 2008.

The for-profit battery recycling industry is also quite active. The Ellwood City, Pennsylvania-based International Metals Reclamation Company (INMETCO) is the recycling resource for RBRC. INMETCO opened its facility in December, 1995 to recycle nickel-cadmium (NiCd) and other battery types. In addition to small rechargeable batteries from the consumer market, INMETCO recycles large NiCd batteries used in military, railroad, and telecommunications industries for back-up power. The company also recycles NiCd batteries used in such products as portable power tools and medical equipment. The 99.5% pure cadmium that results from INMETCO's processing is resold for use in new NiCd batteries. Recovered nickel and iron are melted into an alloy that is used in manufacturing stainless steel. The batteries' electrolyte is used as a chemical reactant in INMETCO's wastewater treatment plant. No materials are landfilled, which benefits the company's industrial customers by eliminating their landfill-related liabilities.

The Howell, Missouri-based Battery Solutions recycles all battery types for any US location. The company provides a full array of battery recycling services and relieves clients of compliance burdens by keeping track of and adhering to regulatory requirements, and maintaining state and federal certifications. In addition, the company issues the Certificate of Reclamation so that clients can document their adherence to battery recycling standards.

Anaheim, California-based TOXCO, which opened its doors in 1984, has developed a patented lithium recycling process that gives it a competitive advantage. The company claims to be the only operation in the world capable of recycling any kind of lithium battery regardless of size. Its operations have expanded to handle most battery chemistries. TOXCO also runs The Big Green Box, a global, low-cost program that helps cities, towns, individuals, and corporations to recycle batteries and other electronics. A one-time fee covers all costs associated with the recycling process, including a transportation container, shipping to TOXCO's recycling site, and recycling fees. TOXCO is allied with two other Anaheim, California-based corporations, SA Recycling and Kinsbursky Brothers Inc. Both companies are international metals recyclers. Kinsbursky Brothers Inc. is also a dominant but non-lithium battery recycler on the west coast.

SIZE OF THE BATTERY RECYCLING MARKET

The EPA estimates the annual sale of rechargeable batteries in the US is more than 350 million units, and that volume is expected to rise as portable electronics continue to grow in popularity for business and personal uses. Even greater numbers of non-rechargeable batteries are sold each year. For instance, in 2003, more than 3 billion alkaline batteries were sold in the US (most alkaline batteries are not rechargeable). The RBRC collected and recycled 6.9 million pounds of rechargeable batteries in 2008.

More lead-acid batteries are recycled each year in the US than any other type of battery. Recent industry figures estimate that 2.52 million tons of the batteries' lead was recycled, representing 99% of the mineral in spent batteries. The batteries' casings and acid are also recycled.

Belgium-based battery recycling corporation Umicore, which predicts that li-ion batteries will dominate portable energy sources for the coming decade, sees business opportunities in adopting cutting-edge recycling technology for these batteries. Umicore noted that in 2007, over 13,000 tons of cobalt were sold globally for manufacturing li-ion batteries. The healthy growth of battery recycling operations in the US has been cited in news reports. For example, RBRC reported that it enjoyed a 10% growth in its rechargeable battery collections in 2008. But it is generally recognized that only a small percentage of all batteries manufactured each year are currently recycled. For example, in the UK, less than 2% of consumers' disposable batteries and just 5% of rechargeable batteries are recycled. These figures indicate that, worldwide, a large untapped market exists.

BEST PRACTICES

The automotive industry's closed-loop recycling process for lead-acid batteries- inspired primarily by regulatory mandates   has resulted in considerable spent-battery reuse. Advancing recycling technology continues to improve yields for those batteries that are recycled. Lead, for example, is recaptured at rates of up to 99%. As costs escalate for raw materials such as sulfuric acid, economic benefits feed back into automakers' operations. US know-how in closed-loop lead-acid battery recycling is recognized as cutting-edge, and is being exported to China by US company Johnson Controls. Also in the auto industry, the Detroit 3 in 2007 contracted with Bend, Oregon-based OnTo Technology LLC to develop processes for recycling li-ion and NiMH batteries. The automakers are interested in recovering costly raw materials such as cobalt and lithium, especially as the use of hybrid and other fuel-efficient vehicles rises. NiMH batteries are currently used in hybrid vehicles, and li-ion batteries are likely to power vehicles of the future. Johnson Controls Inc broke ground on a new $100 million automobile battery recycling plant in Florence County, South Carolina in 2009, which is expected to create 250 new jobs by 2010.

Corporations across several retail sectors have expanded their battery recycling programs in recent years. In 2007, Circuit City upped its involvement in RBRC's Call2Recycle program by distributing battery recycling bags to its customers. The company, which began working with RBRC in 2006 by placing Call2Recycle boxes in its stores, said the new initiative made it the nation's first retailer to increase its collaboration with RBRC. Also in 2007, Motel 6 became the first operation in the hospitality industry to recycle batteries and install efficient fluorescent light bulbs without a federal mandate to do so. In 2008, DeWalt unveiled a National Battery Recycling Month for October, inviting individuals to bring their spent power tool batteries into their stores for recycling, and in return receive a $10 battery discount.

BATTERY RECYCLING TECHNOLOGY

A variety of technologies are employed to recycle batteries, and the resulting products feed new battery manufacture and other industries. TOXCO's 70,000-plus square foot physical plant in British Columbia recycles li-ion batteries. The company uses a patented cryogenic process to render the lithium inert, as it can be explosive at room temperatures. The lithium batteries are first stored beneath the earth in concrete bunkers. Any lingering electrical energy is drained from large batteries. The cryogenic process lowers the lithium temperature to -325°F. At that point the batteries can be shredded. Lithium is converted to the resalable state of lithium carbonate, which is a fine powder. Cobalt is retrieved for resale as well. Battery Solutions shreds or hammers the lithium batteries and submerges the pieces in a caustic water solution, which neutralizes the lithium. Products sold by this facility include clean scrap metal (which goes to metal recyclers) and lithium carbonate (for new batteries and battery parts).

Howell, Missouri-based Battery Solutions recycles batteries of a variety of chemistries. For instance, it sends lead acid batteries to a hammer mill where they are broken apart. The pieces are fed to a vat, in which the plastics float while the lead and other heavier components sink. A scooper removes the polypropylene, which is then washed, dried, melted down, and fed through an extruder that creates plastic pellets suitable for re-manufacture. The lead is cleaned, melted, and poured into ingot molds. As impurities naturally float to the surface while the lead is still molten, they are scraped off. Once cooled, the lead ingots are sold to battery manufacturers. Battery acid is neutralized with a baking soda-like compound, and this process transforms the acid to water. Once treated, this water meets regulatory standards for purity. The acid can also be converted to sodium sulfate, which is used in glass, laundry detergents, and for making textiles.

Alkaline batteries can be shredded, and their chemicals of zinc and manganese are sold once they are recovered and separated from one another in the recycling process. Batteries that use non-reactive materials such as cadmium, lead, nickel, and silver can also be shredded, and the minerals can be sold.

A Belgium company, Umicore, recycles rechargeable li-ion and NiMH batteries in a process involving a furnace and plasma technology to prevent the formation of toxins such as dioxin. The result is a clean slag from which various materials can be separated for reuse or to help heat the furnace. For example, the melted aluminum is sold for use as aggregate in concrete or other construction materials. Most of the cobalt in the li-ion batteries is converted back to lithium cobalt dioxide (LiCoO2), which can then be used to manufacture new li-ion batteries. The nickel is also recovered separately for reuse in new rechargeable NiMH batteries.

In China, a bioleaching technique has been used successfully to recycle NiCd batteries. In this process, sulfuric acid is produced in bioreactors with a combination of sewage sludge bacteria and sulfur. A settling tank receives the overflow from the bioreactor. The nickel and cadmium rises to the top of the settling tank and is sent to a leaching reactor for reuse in new NiCd batteries. The sludge from the settling reactor is clean enough for agricultural use.

REGULATIONS

The EPA's Universal Waste Rule (40 C.F.R. Part 273), which was finalized in April of 1995, simplified the management standards for federally-defined "hazardous wastes." Wastes are considered "universal" if they are hazardous but present less risk to humans and the overall environment than other hazardous wastes. This category includes batteries as well as mercury-containing items (such as thermostats), lamps, and pesticides. The rules are intended to make it easier for businesses and private citizens to recycle spent batteries and other products. States are allowed to change the Universal Waste Rules and add new wastes to the list. In addition, the EPA offers assistance in implementing the rules.

Each state can adapt the Universal Waste Rule to most effectively comply with the federal standards. A resource for checking on individual states can be found at http://www.epa.gov/osw/wyl/stateprograms.htm. California, for example, passed the Rechargeable Battery Act of 2006. This law mandates the free collection of rechargeable batteries by retailers that sell them, except for those operations with gross yearly sales of under $1 million, and stores that sell mainly food. Most states have regulations requiring retailers to accept spent lead-acid batteries from consumers.

In May 1996, the federal government passed the Battery Act, which calls for state regulatory agencies and the EPA to reduce the quantity of toxins in the environment from discarded batteries. The Battery Act focuses particularly on stopping the use of mercury in battery manufacture, and facilitating battery recycling. As mentioned in the Battery recycling organizations & corporations section, the Battery Act was shepherded by the recycling battery industry's PBRA. Through its participation in creating the Battery Act, PBRA helped make it possible for RBRC to collect and recycle nickel-cadmium (Ni-Cd) rechargeable batteries nationwide.

Corporations sometimes find that state regulations can open doors to business opportunities. For instance, TOXCO responded to a California law passed in 2004 and expanded in 2006 by targeting its recycling efforts to capture the individual market, where prior to this it had focused mainly on large industrial clients. The California law requires all residents and businesses to recycle alkaline batteries. It was this law that inspired TOXCO to launch its Big Green Box program as mentioned in the Battery recycling organizations & corporations section.

RELATED ENTITIES

EPA, universal wastes information: http://www.epa.gov/osw/hazard/wastetypes/universal/batteries.htm

EPA, online tool for researching individual states' adaptations of the Universal Waste Rule: http://www.epa.gov/osw/wyl/stateprograms.htm.

Rechargeable Battery Recycling Corporation: http://www.rbrc.org/start.php

Portable Rechargeable Battery Association: http://www.prba.org/

European Portable Battery Association http://www.epbaeurope.net/

ACRONYMS

EPA - Environmental Protection Agency

RBRC - Rechargeable Battery Recycling Corporation

Li-ion - Lithium-ion batteries

Ni-cd - Nickel-cadmium batteries

NiMH - Nickel-metal hydride

INMETCO - International Metals Reclamation Company

BIB-References

FURTHER READING

"Approximately 90% of our lithium recycling process is remote controlled - keeping personnel at safe distances". (2003). *Toxco*. Retrieved July 15, 2009, from http://www.toxco.com/processes.html

"Battery recycling and disposal guide for households". (2009). *Environment, Health & Safety Online*. Retrieved June 30, 2009, from http://www.ehso.com/ehshome/batteries.php

"Battery recycling at Inmetco". (n.d.). *INMETCO Services: Battery Recycling*. Retrieved July 16, 2009, from http://www.inmetco.com/services_battery.htm

"Battery recycling information sheet". (2005). *Waste Online*. Retrieved on July 17, 2009, from http://www.

wasteonline.org.uk/resources/InformationSheets/Batteries.htm

Bertuol, D., Bernardes, A., & Tenório, J. (2006). "Spent NiMH batteries: Characterization and metal recovery through mechanical processing". *Journal of Power Sources,* 160(2), 1465-1470. Retrieved July 3, 2009, from EBSCO Online

Database Academic Search Complete. http://search.ebscohost.com/login.aspx?direct=true&db=a9h&AN=22582753&site =ehost-live

Bridges, T. (2009, June 2). "$100 million facility to bring 250 jobs to Florence County". *Florence Morning News* (SC). Retrieved July 16, 2009, from EBSCO Online Database Newspaper Source Plus. http://search.ebscohost.com/login.aspx?direct=true&db=n5h&AN=2W61838241049&site=ehost-live

Carlson, C. (2009). "Bucking trends". *Waste Age,* 40(3), 10-10. Retrieved July 16, 2009, from EBSCO Online Database Business Source Complete. http://search.ebscohost.com/login.aspx?direct=true&db=bth&AN=37170905&site=ehost-live

"Circuit City expands battery recycling commitment". (2007). *TWICE: This Week in Consumer Electronics,* 22(21), 60. Retrieved July 16, 2009, from EBSCO Online Database Academic Search Complete. http://search.ebscohost.com/login.aspx?direct=true&db=a9h&AN=27133493&site=ehost-live

"Company introduces battery recycling month". (2008). *Surface Fabrication,* 14(10), 9. Retrieved July 16, 2009, from EBSCO Online Database Business Source Complete. http://search.ebscohost.com/login.aspx?direct=true&db=bth&AN=34586543&site=ehost-live

"Easy battery recycling with the big green box". (2009). *The Big Green Box.* Retrieved July 3, 2009, from http://www.biggreenbox.com/index.php

"End sites recycling process". (2009). *Battery Solutions: Smart Recycling Made Easy.* Retrieved July 3, 2009, from http://www.batteryrecycling.com/Battery+Recycling+Process

Rechargeable Battery Recycling Corporation. (2009). Frequently asked questions. Retrieved on July 1, 2009, from http://www.rbrc.org/consumer/howitallworks_faq.shtml

Helping protect the environment since 1971. (2009). *Battery Solutions: Smart recycling made easy.* Retrieved on July 3, 2009 from http://www.batteryrecycling.com/contact+us

Jusko, J. (2008). "Putting waste to work". *Industry Week/IW,* 257(10), 41-44. Retrieved July 16, 2009,

from EBSCO Online Database Academic Search Complete. http://search.ebscohost.com/login.aspx?direct=true&db=a9h&AN=34697071&site =ehost-live

Miller, C. (2009). "Lead-acid batteries". *Waste Age,* 40(4), 42-42. Retrieved July 16, 2009, from EBSCO Online Database Business Source Complete. http://search.ebscohost.com/login.aspx?direct=true&db=bth&AN=38012625&site= ehost-live

Motel 6 develops national recycling program. (2007). *Buildings,* 101(8), 12. Retrieved July 16, 2009, from EBSCO Online Database Business Source Complete. http://search.ebscohost.com/login.aspx?direct=true&db=bth&AN=26324804&site=ehost-live

NiCAD battery recycler opens for business. (1996). *BioCycle,* 37(7), 26. Retrieved July 3, 2009, from *EBSCO Online Database Academic* Search Complete. http://search.ebscohost.com/login.aspx?direct=true&db=a9h&AN=9608060309&site=ehost-live

Portable Rechargeable Battery Association. (n.d.) About PRBA. Retrieved July 1, 2009, from http://www.prba.org/About_PRBA/Default.ashx

Regulations. (2009). *Battery Solutions: Smart recycling made easy.* Retrieved July 3, 2009, from http://www.batteryrecycling.com/regulations

Smith, C. (2008). Recycling rechargeable batteries. *Sustainable Facility,* 33(6), 36-36. Retrieved July 16, 2009, from EBSCO Online Database Business Source Complete. http://search.ebscohost.com/login.aspx?direct=true&db=bth&AN=35372982&site=ehost-live

Stoffer, H. (2007). Detroit 3 research advanced battery recycling. *Automotive News,* 81(6259), 28J-28J. Retrieved July 16, 2009, from EBSCO Online Database Business Source Complete. http://search.ebscohost.com/login.aspx?direct=true&db=bth&AN=25463985&site= ehost-live

Streamlined rule for `universal' waste. (1995). *BioCycle,* 36(7), 10. Retrieved June 30, 2009, from EBSCO Online Database Academic Search Complete. http://search.ebscohost.com/login.aspx?direct=true&db=a9h&AN=9508091548&site =ehost-live

Toxco Inc. Retrieved July 15, 2009, from Toxco website. http://www.toxco.com

Truini, J. (2005). Calif. requires retailers to take back batteries. *Waste News,* 11(13), 18-18. Retrieved July 15, 2009, from EBSCO Online Database Business Source Complete. http://search.ebscohost.com/login.aspx?direct=true&db=bth&AN=18745744&site=ehost-live

Truini, J. (2005). Retailers must accept batteries. *Waste News*, 11(17), 3-3. Retrieved July 15, 2009, from EBSCO Online Database Business Source Complete. http://search.ebscohost.com/login.aspx?direct=true&db=bth&AN=19319762&site= ehost-live

Umicore buying German catalyst recycler as Europe growth eyed. (2003). *American Metal Market*, 111(48), 15. Retrieved July 15, 2009, from EBSCO Online Database   Business Source Complete. http://search.ebscohost.com/login.aspx?direct=true&db=bth&AN=11581951&site= ehost-live

Umicore battery recycling. (2005). *Umicore*. Retrieved July 16, 2009, from http://www.batteryrecycling.umicore.com/batteryRecycling/

United States Environmental Protection Agency. (2008). Wastes - hazardous waste- universal waste. Retrieved July 1, 2009, from http://www.epa.gov/osw/hazard/wastetypes/universal/

Universal wastes. (2005). *ECAR*. Retrieved July 14, 2009, from http://www.ecarcenter.org/EPAUWNewRule.html

Zhu, N., Zhang, L., Li, C., & Cai, C. (2003). Recycling of spent nickel-cadmium batteries based on bio-leaching process. *Waste Management*, 23(8), 703. Retrieved July 3, 2009, from EBSCO Online Database Academic Search Complete. http://search.ebscohost.com/login.aspx?direct=true&db=a9h&AN=11255601&site =ehost-live..BIX-

The Editors

SEE ALSO: Recycling Technology

Becoming a green consumer

Food production in the United States today requires six calories of energy to produce one calorie of food. Much of this is expended in transport, but also in energy-intensive cultivation of factory farms, as well as through many people's preference for energy intensive food, such as meats, most notably beef (Hillman and Fawcett, 2007).

INTRODUCTION

The United Nations Food and Agriculture Organization has stated that the livestock business generates more greenhouse-gas emissions than all forms of transportation combined. "Environmentalists are still pointing their fingers at Hummers and S.U.V.'s when they should be pointing at the dinner plate," said Matt A. Prescott, manager of vegan campaigns for People for the Ethical Treatment of Animals (Deutsch, 2007). To make the point, PETA acquired a Hummer, installed a driver in a chicken suit, and draped over it a vinyl banner naming meat as the top cause of global warming. The Hummer is now a mobile billboard for the carbon footprint of animal protein. "You just cannot be a meat-eating environmentalist," said Prescott (Deutsch, 2007).

The Humane Society of the United States ran advertising in environmental magazines on the same theme. The ads depict a car key and a fork. "Which one of these contributes more to global warming?" the ads ask. They answer the question with "It's not the one that starts a car," (Deutsch, 2007). Judging by statistics, the folks at PETA have some work to do. The average United States citizen today eats more than 200 pounds of red meat, poultry, and fish per year, an increase of 23 pounds compared to 1970.

THE CARBON FOOTPRINT OF MEAT

Many people are now going vegetarian as part of a personal climate-change strategy. Billions of chickens, cattle, turkeys, pigs, and cows being raised in factory farms produce methane from digestion and feces. The raising of animals for human consumption is the single largest source of methane emissions in the United States, and a methane molecule is 23 times as effective at retaining heat as one of carbon dioxide.

Animal agriculture is also a major source of carbon dioxide. Production of animal protein requires about ten times the fossil-fuel input (producing ten times the carbon-dioxide) compared to edible plants. The feeding, killing, and processing of meat is enormously energy-intensive. Taking such things into account, a study by University of Chicago professors Gidon Eshel and Pamela Martin argues that a completely vegetarian diet (avoiding eggs and dairy products as well as meat, fish, and fowl) can remove as much carbon dioxide and methane from the air (or, in some cases, more) than driving a hybrid car (compared to one with an internal-combustion engine). They calculated that the difference between a meat-centered diet and vegetarianism had the same effect on greenhouse gas production as switching from an SUV to a standard sedan. Nitrous oxide in manure (warming effect: 296 times greater per molecule than that of carbon dioxide) and methane from animal flatulence (23 times greater) mean that "a 16-oz. T-bone is comparable to a Hummer on a plate" (Will, 2007).

FAR-FETCHED FOOD

A walk through an average United States supermarket is a tour of the world, a cornucopia of food choices. The carbon-conscious sometimes take pride in eating low on the food chain, substituting vegetables and fruits for meat. What, however, if our fruits and vegetables come from Chile, Nicaragua, and New Zealand out of season? In that case, most of their carbon calories come in the form of transportation, most of it powered by oil. Food sold in U.S. grocery stores travels an average of 1,500 miles to reach consumers, according to David Pimentel, professor of ecology and agricultural science at Cornell University. The food industry burns almost one-fifth of all the petroleum consumed in the United States, about as much as automobiles, according to Michael Pollan's Omnivore's Dilemma (Knoblauch, 2007).

A tour of a typical U.S. supermarket also reveals that modern transport and various free-trade agreements [the North American Free Trade Agreement (NAFTA) and others] have rendered distance nearly irrelevant to our food supply. The idea of "seasonal" produce has nearly lost its meaning. During winter, in the United States, many fruits and vegetables are now routinely imported from the Southern Hemisphere. Geography (and energy expenditure) has become so irrelevant in today's American grocery stores that some salmon are raised in the Pacific Northwest, shipped to China to be cut (where labor is cheap), and shipped back to North America to be sold.

Cruising the aisles of an Omaha Hy-Vee (a regional grocery chain), within an hour provided a long list of long-distance imports. The first figure below is miles; the second is kilometers. Distances are in air miles from New York City. For surface miles via ocean transport add 10 per cent. Some of these goods probably have been air-shipped, but most have reached Hy-Vee via surface, ships, trucks, and trains, which involve longer distances but is much more energy-efficient. These are only a few examples of what is available.

Alaska: salmon (Anchorage: 3,371/5,425)

Australia: winter nectarines (Sydney: 9,935/15,989)

Chile: grapes and other winter fruits (Santiago: 5,107/8,219)

China: beer (Beijing: 6,843/11,012)

Costa Rica: pineapples and bananas (San Jose: 2,509/4,039)

Ecuador: cut flowers; tilapia (Quito: 2,834/4,560)

Germany: beer (Frankfurt: 3,858/6,208)

Honduras: shrimp (Tegucigalpa 2,004/3,225)

Hong Kong: Jasmine rice (8,059/12,968)

Italy : premium pasta (Rome: 4,283/6,891)

Kenya: tilapia (fish), shrimp (Nairobi: 7,358/11,842)

Mexico: mangoes and papayas, watermelon (all seasons), cantaloupe, winter strawberries (Mexico City: 2,090/3,363)

Nicaragua: winter watermelon, shrimp (Managua: 2,310 miles/3, 719 kilometers)

Peru: winter asparagus (Lima: 3,640/5,857)

Philippines: mangoes (Manila 8,509/13,693)

Russia: caviar (Moscow: 4,668/7,511)

Spain: Olives; Artichoke Hearts (Madrid: 3,591/5,779)

United Kingdom: Coleman's mustard (London: 3,463/5,772)

Within the United States, many fruits and vegetables are shipped nationwide from California (Los Angeles: 2,451/3,944), at what would be international distances in many other countries. In summer, however, produce is more localized. The area around Omaha produces some of the best watermelon on Earth, but for only two to three months (August – October).

The fish counter of one Omaha supermarket alone could serve as a virtual United Nations of seafood. A neighborhood Hy-Vee in Omaha sells fish and shellfish of about 80 varieties (alphabetically, from Arctic Char to Whitefish) from 35 countries: the United States, Canada, Mexico, Costa Rica, Chile, Ecuador, Colombia, U.S. Virgin Islands, China, Honduras, Panama, Bahamas, Suriname, Belize, Guatemala, Venezuela, Nicaragua, Brazil, the Philippines, Namibia, Indonesia, Australia, New Zealand, India, Thailand, the United Kingdom, France, Peru, India, Vietnam, Bangladesh, Malaysia, Pakistan. Sri Lanka, and Brazil. The only types of fish obtained solely from the United States (usually many hundreds of miles from land-locked Omaha) are Carp, Alaskan Cod, Oysters, White Wild Shrimp (the chain sells 17 varieties of shrimp), Catfish, and Idaho Rainbow Trout (Hy-Vee Seafood, 2007).

LOCALIZING THE FOOD CHAIN

Concern about global warming has helped to spur a movement toward locally grown food. Even as the supply lines of many grocery chains lengthen, more urban residents are raising food on vacant lots. By 2014, 3,000 community gardens were operating in United States urban areas. In 2007 novelist Barbara Kingsolver landed a title (*Animal, Vegetable, Miracle*, HarperCollins) describing how her family spent a year eating local ore home-grown food on the New York Times hardcover best-seller list (at number 9, August 12). The web site Sustainable Table (www.sustainabletable.org), which addresses food and energy issues, tracks such things.

The shortest distance of all, of course, is from one's backyard (or rooftop) to the kitchen. Some New York City residents, who have access to rooftops, have been making a purposeful effort to localize their eating habits by raising all manner of vegetables, and even honey (with attendant bees), and the occasional chicken, for laying and eating.

More city dwellers are raising their own chickens. Urban chickens have become the rationale for cottage industries. Internet pages have proliferated (see: thecitychicken.com or backyardchickens.com). In Los Angeles, Phoenix and Austin, Tex., residents have organized chicken-centric social events, and, according to one report, "dozens of books — a whole new form of chick lit — on raising chickens, including Barbara Kilarski's *Keep Chickens! Tending Small Flocks in Cities, Suburbs and Other Small Spaces,* and related titles like *Anyone Can Build a Tub-Style Mechanical Chicken Plucker,* by Herrick Kimball" (Price, 2007). The movement even has its own magazine, *Backyard Poultry,* founded in 2006. Some cities ban in-city chickens, especially crowing roosters, but New York City, Oakland, San Francisco, Houston, Chicago, Seattle, and Portland, Ore., among others, have laws permitting them.

Some United States food chains that specialize in organic foods, such as Whole Foods Market, among others, make an effort to purchase locally grown fruits and vegetables. Local grocery chains also purchase locally in season, some of the time in areas with extensive agricultural bases (corn in Nebraska and Iowa, for example). Even Wal-mart, as part of its never-ending search of ways to save money, recently has been finding ways to localize its supply chain.

FURTHER READING

Deutsch, C.H. (2007, August 29). Trying to connect the dinner plate to climate change." *New York Times.* This article describes how food choices affect global warming. http://www.nytimes.com/2007/08/29/business/media/29adco.html

Hillman, M. and Fawcett, T. (2007). *The suicidal planet: How to prevent global climate catastrophe.* New York:

St. Martin's Press/Thomas Dunne Books. This global survey of global-warming solutions includes many related to food and other consumer choices.

"Hy-Vee seafood: Country of origin." (2007). Peony Park Hi-Vee, Omaha, NE. September 27, 2007. Photocopy. This supermarket list provides an eye-opening list of seafood sources.

Knoblauch, J. A. (2007, Spring) Have it your (the sustainable) way. *EJ* (*Environmental Journalism*), 28-30, 46. This primer for journalists focuses on environmental aspects of food consumption.

Price, C. (2007, September 19). A chicken on every plot, a coop in every backyard." *New York Times.* http://www.nytimes.com/2007/09/19/dining/19yard.html. Save the planet one urban chicken coup at a time.

Will, G.F. (2007, April 12). Fuzzy climate math. Washington Post. A conservative columnist takes aim at green food choices. http://www.washingtonpost.com/wp-dyn/content/article/2007/04/11/AR2007041102109_pf.html

Bruce E. Johansen

SEE ALSO: Buying Local; Genetically Modified Foods; Vegetarian Diet

Biofuels

Biofuels such as ethanol and biodiesel are excellent transportation fuels that are used as substitutes or supplements for gasoline and diesel fuels. Biofuels can also be burned in electrical generators to produce electricity. Two biofuels are used in vehicles: ethanol and biodiesel. Biogas and methane are used mainly to generate electricity. Biomass was used traditionally to heat houses.

INTRODUCTION

Biofuels are made mainly from plant material such as corn, sugarcane, or rapeseed. Theoretically, biofuels can be generated anywhere on Earth where living organisms can grow.

PRIMARY USES

Biofuels such as ethanol and biodiesel are excellent transportation fuels that are used as substitutes or supplements for gasoline and diesel fuels. Biofuels can also be burned in electrical generators to produce electricity. Two biofuels are used in vehicles: ethanol and biodiesel.

Biogas and methane are used mainly to generate electricity. Biomass was used traditionally to heat houses.

TECHNICAL DEFINITION

Biofuels are renewable fuels generated from or by organisms. They can be manufactured from this organic matter and, unlike fossil fuels, do not require millennia to be produced. Since they are renewable, biofuels are considered by many as potential future substitutes for fossil fuels, which are nonrenewable and dwindling. Moreover, pollution from Fossil fuelsunsustainabilityfossil fuels affects public health and has been associated with global climate change, because burning them in engines releases Carbon dioxidecarbon dioxide (CO_2) into the atmosphere. Using biofuels as an energy source generates fewer pollutants and little or no carbon dioxide. In addition, the utilization of biofuels reduces U.S. dependence on foreign oil.

DESCRIPTION, DISTRIBUTION, AND FORMS

Over millions of years, dead organic matter—both plant and animal organisms—played a crucial role in the formation of fossil fuels such as oil, natural gas, and coal. Since the nineteenth century, humans have increasingly depended on fossil fuels to meet energy needs. As the supply of fossil fuels has diminished, humankind has begun looking for alternative energy sources. Thus, the use of biofuels—including ethanol, biodiesel, methane, biogas, biomass, biohydrogen, and butanol—is increasing.

Ethanol is a colorless liquid with the chemical formula C_2H_5OH. Another name for ethanol is ethyl alcohol, grain alcohol, or simply alcohol.

Biodiesel is a diesel substitute obtained mainly from vegetable oils, such as soybean oil or restaurant greases. It is produced by the transesterification of oils, a simple chemical reaction with alcohol (ethanol or methanol), catalyzed by acids or bases (such as sodium hydroxide). Transesterification produces alkyl esters of fatty acids that are biodiesel and glycerol (also known as glycerin).

Methane is a colorless, odorless, nontoxic gas with the molecular formula CH_4. It is the main chemical component (70 to 90 percent) of natural gas, which accounts for about 20 percent of the U.S. energy supply. Methane was discovered by the Italian scientist, Alessandro Alessandro Volta, who collected it from marsh sediments and showed that it was flammable. He called it "combustible air."

Biogas is a gas produced by the metabolism of microorganisms. There are different types of biogas. One type contains a mixture of methane (50 to 75 percent) and carbon dioxide. Another type comprises primarily nitrogen, hydrogen, and carbon monoxide (CO) with trace amounts of methane.

Biomass is a mass of organisms, mainly plants, that can be used as an energy source. Plants and algae convert the energy of the Sun and carbon dioxide into energy that is stored in their biomass. Biomass, burning in the form of wood, is the oldest form of energy used by humans. Using biomass as a fuel source does not result in net CO_2 emissions, because biomass burning will release only the amount of CO_2 it has absorbed during plant growth (provided its production and harvesting are sustainable).

Molecular fuel from hydrogen (H_2) is a colorless, odorless, and tasteless gas. It is an ideal alternative fuel to be used for transportation because the energy content of hydrogen is three times greater than in gasoline. Also, it is virtually nonpolluting and a renewable fuel. Using H_2 as an energy source produces only water; H_2 can be made from water again. A great number of microorganisms produce H_2 from inorganic materials, such as water, or from organic materials, such as sugar, in reactions catalyzed by enzymes. Hydrogen produced by microorganisms is called biohydrogen.

Butanol (butyl alcohol) is a four-carbon alcohol with the molecular formula C_4H_9OH. Among other types of biofuels, butanol has been the most promising in terms of commercialization. It is another alcohol fuel but has higher energy content than ethanol. It does not pick up water as ethanol does and is not as corrosive as ethanol but is more suitable for distribution through existing pipelines for gasoline. However, compared to ethanol, butanol is considered toxic. It can cause severe eye and skin irritation and suppression of the nervous system.

HISTORY

The concept of biofuels is not new. People have been using biomass such as plant material to heat their houses for thousands of years. The idea of using hydrogen as fuel was expressed by Jules Verne in his novel *L'Île mystérieuse* (1874-1875; *The Mysterious Island*, 1875). In 1900, Rudolf Rudolf Diesel, the inventor of the diesel engine, used peanut oil for his engine during the World Exhibition in Paris, France. Henry Ford's first (1908) car, the Model T, was made to run on pure ethanol. Later, the popularity of biofuels as a fuel source followed the "oil trouble times." For example, biofuels were considered during the 1970's oil embargo. Early in the twenty-first century, concerns about global warming and oil-price increases reignited interest in biofuels. In 2005, the U.S. Congress passed the Energy Policy Act, which included several sections related to biofuels. In particular, this energy bill required more research on biofuels, mixing ethanol with gasoline, and an increase in the production of cellulosic biofuels.

OBTAINING BIOFUELS

Ethanol is produced mainly by the microbial fermentation of starch crops (such as corn, wheat, and barley) or sugarcane. In the United States, most of the ethanol is produced by the yeast (fungal) fermentation of sugar from cornstarch. Ethanol can be produced from cellulose, the most plentiful biological material on Earth; however, current methods of converting cellulosic material into ethanol are inefficient and require intensive research and development efforts. Ethanol can also be produced by chemical means from petroleum. Therefore, ethanol that is produced by microbial fermentation is commonly referred to as "bioethanol."

In the United States, biodiesel comes mainly from soybean plants; in Europe, the world's top producer of biodiesel, it comes from canola oil. Other vegetative oils that have been used in biodiesel production are corn, sunflower, cottonseed, jatropha, palm oil, and rapeseed. Another possible source for biodiesel production is microscopic algae (microalgae), the microorganisms similar to plants.

Methane is produced by microorganisms and is an integral part of their metabolism. BiogasBiogas is produced during the anaerobic fermentation of organic matter by a community of microorganisms (bacteria and archaea). For practical use, methane and biogas are generated from wastewater, animal waste, and "gas wells" in landfills. Biomass is produced naturally, in the forest, and agriculturally, from agricultural residues and dung.

No fuel from commercial biohydrogen production process exists. The most attractive for industrial applications is H2 production by photosynthetic microbes. These microorganisms, such as microscopic algae, cyanobacteria, and photosynthetic bacteria, use sunlight as an energy source and water to generate hydrogen.

Butanol can be produced by the fermentation of sugars similar to the ethanol production. The most well-known pathway of butanol generation is fermentation by bacterium Clostridium acetobutylicum. Substrates utilized for butanol production—starch, molasses, cheese whey, and lignocellulosic materials—are exactly the same as for ethanol fermentation. The biological production by fermentation is not economically attractive because of low levels of product concentrations and high cost of product recovery compared to the chemical process.

USES OF BIOFUELS

With increasing energy demands and oil prices, ethanol has become a valuable option as an alternative transportation fuel. The Energy Policy Act of 2005 included a requirement to increase the production of ethanol from 15 to 28 billion liters by 2012. Beginning in 2008, a majority of fuel stations in the United States were selling gasoline with 10 percent ethanol in it. Nearly all cars can use E10, fuel that is 10 percent ethanol. Blending ethanol with gasoline oxygenates the fuel mixture, which burns more completely and produces fewer harmful CO emissions. Another environmental benefit of ethanol is that it degrades in the soil, whereas petroleum-based fuels are more resistant to degradation and have many damaging effects when accidentally discharged into the environment. However, a liter of ethanol has significantly less energy content than a liter of gasoline, so vehicles must be refueled more often. Ethanol is also more expensive than gasoline, although rising prices of gasoline could cancel that disadvantage. In addition, carcinogenic aldehydes, such as formaldehyde, are produced when ethanol is burned in internal combustion engines. Carbon dioxide, a major greenhouse gas, forms as well. Moreover, the widely used fuel mix that is 85 percent ethanol and 15 percent gasoline (the E85 blend) requires specially equipped "flexible fuel" engines. In the United States, only a fraction of all cars are considered "flex fuel" vehicles. By comparison, however, most cars in Brazil have flex engines. Beginning in 1977, the Brazilian government made using ethanol as a fuel for cars mandatory. Brazil has the largest and most successful "ethanol for fuel" program in the world. As a result of this successful program, the country reached complete self-sufficiency in energy supply in 2006.

Biodiesel performs similarly to diesel and can be used in unmodified diesel engines of trucks, tractors, and other vehicles, and it is better for the environment. Burning biodiesel produces fewer emissions than petroleum-based diesel; it is essentially free of sulfur and aromatics and emits less CO. Additionally, biodiesel is less toxic to the soil. Biodiesel is often blended with petroleum diesel in different ratios of 2, 5, or 20 percent. The most common blend is B20, or 20 percent biodiesel to 80 percent diesel fuel. Biodiesel can be used as a pure fuel (100 percent or B100), but pure fuel is not suitable for winter because it thickens in cold temperatures. In addition, B100 is a solvent that degrades engines' rubber hoses and gaskets. Moreover, biodiesel energy content is less than in diesel. In general, biodiesel is not used as widely as ethanol. However, biodiesel users include the United States Postal Service; the U.S. Departments of Defense, Energy, and Agriculture; national parks; school districts; transit authorities; and public-utilities, waste-management, and recycling companies across the United States. In January, 2009, Continental Airlines successfully demonstrated the use of a biodiesel mixture from plants and algae (50 percent to 50 percent) to fly its Boeing 737-800.

In the 1985 Mel Gibson movie *Mad Max Beyond Thunderdome*, a futuristic city was run on methane that was generated by pig manure. In reality, methane can be a very good alternative fuel. It has a number of advantages over other fuels produced by microorganisms. First, it is easy to make and can be generated locally, which does not require distribution. Extensive natural gas infrastructure is already in place to be utilized. Second, the utilization of methane as a fuel is an attractive way to reduce wastes such as manure, wastewater, or municipal and industrial wastes. In local farms, manure is fed into digesters (bioreactors) where microorganisms metabolize it into methane. Methane can be used to fuel electrical generators to produce electricity. In China, millions of small farms have simple small underground digesters near the farm houses. There are several landfill gas facilities in the United States that generate electricity using methane. San Francisco has extended its recycling program to include conversion of dog waste into methane to produce electricity and to heat homes. With a dog population of 120,000 this initiative promises to generate a significant amount of fuel with a huge reduction of waste at the same time. Methane was used as a fuel for vehicles for a number of years. Several Volvo car models with bi-fuel engines were made to run on compressed methane with gasoline as a backup. Biogas can also be compressed, like methane, and used to power motor vehicles.

In many countries, millions of small farms maintain a simple digester for biogas production to generate energy. Currently, there are more than five million household digesters in China, used by people mainly for cooking and lighting, and there are more than one million biogas plants of various capacities in India.

Utilization of methane and biogas as an energy source in place of fossil fuels is providing significant environmental and economic benefits. Biofuels are essentially nonpolluting, although their utilization results in production of CO_2 and contributes to global warming, though with less impact on Earth's climate than methane itself as a greenhouse gas. Even though the use of methane and biogas as energy sources releases CO_2, the process as a whole can be considered "CO_2 neutral" in that the released CO_2 can be assimilated by their producers, archaea and bacteria.

Some examples of biomass use as an alternative energy source include burning wood or agricultural residue to heat homes. This is an inefficient use of energy—typically only 5-15 percent of the biomass energy is actually utilized. Using biomass that way produces harmful indoor air pollutants such as carbon monoxide. Yet biomass is an almost "free" resource costing only labor to collect. Biomass supplies more than 15 percent of the world's energy consumption. Biomass is the top source of energy in developing countries; in some countries it provides more than 90 percent of the energy used.

Hydrogen powered U.S. rockets for many years. Today, a growing number of automobile manufacturers around the world are making prototype hydrogen-powered vehicles. Only water is emitted from the tailpipe—no greenhouse gases. The car is moved by a motor that runs on electricity generated in the fuel cell via a chemical reaction between H_2 and O_2. Hydrogen vehicles offer quiet operation, rapid acceleration, and low maintenance costs. During peak time, when electricity is expensive, fuel-cell hydrogen cars could provide power for homes and offices. Hydrogen for these applications is obtained mainly from natural gas (methane and propane) via steam reforming. Biohydrogen is used in experimental applications only. Many problems need to be overcome before biohydrogen can be easily available. One of the reasons for the delayed acceptance of biohydrogen is the difficulty of its production on a cost-effective basis. For biohydrogen power to become a reality, tremendous research and investment efforts are necessary.

Butanol can be used as transportation fuel. It contains almost as much energy as gasoline and more energy than ethanol for a particular volume. Unlike 85 percent ethanol, a butanol/gasoline mix (E85 blend) can be used in cars designed for gasoline without making any changes to the engine.

FURTHER READING

Chisti, Yusuf. "Biodiesel from Microalgae." *Biotechnology Advances* 25, no. 3 (2007): 294-306.

Glazer, Alexander N., and Hiroshi Nikaido. *Microbial Biotechnology: Fundamentals of Applied Microbiology.* New York: W. H. Freeman, 2007.

Service, Robert F. "The Hydrogen Backlash." *Science* 305, no. 5686 (August 13, 2004): 958-961.

Wald, Matthew L. "Is Ethanol for the Long Haul?" *Scientific American* 296, no. 1 (January, 2007): 42-49.

Wright, Richard T. *Environmental Science: Towards a Sustainable Future.* 9th ed. Englewood Cliffs, N.J.: Prentice Hall, 2004.

AE Biofuels. http://www.alternative-energy-news.info/technology/biofuels/

Sergei A. Markov

SEE ALSO: Alternative Fuels (Wind, Solar, Ethanol); Hybrid Vehicles; Renewable Energy Sources

Buying local

There are many different reasons why buying local is important. The first reason centers on economics. Money spent in your community buying local products and food stays in your community, creating employment opportunities and a thriving local economy. The second reason centers on health and wellness. Products, especially food and farm products purchased locally tend to be better for you. Freshly picked fruits and vegetables are high in nutrients and taste significantly better than produce that has been shipped to a grocery store from a distance. Finally, buying local creates a sense of community engagement. Relationships with local shopkeepers and farmers benefit both you and the business being supported.

INTRODUCTION

Buying local is so important for your community, the environment, and your health. When you buy products or food from local merchants or local farms, the money you spend stays in your community. Some of that money goes toward paying local workers, and keeping those in your community (or maybe even yourself) employed. A percentage of that money also goes toward purchasing more local goods for consumers to enjoy. These local goods are better for the environment, as buying local means that goods are imported from an area close by, or even from your own neighborhood. Because these goods are purchased or made a short distance away, less gas or fuel is used to transport the goods, lowering transport emission rates and protecting the environment.

Buying locally also allows for increased personal relationships with those in the community. When you buy locally, you get to know the shopkeeper, artisan, or farmer whom you are purchasing from. Many times, the greater the personal relationship, the more the shopkeeper, artisan, or farmer will keep you abreast of information, deals, or discounts related to their product. This relationship can also lead to employment or business opportunities for you. Many teens and young adults have received jobs from local shopkeepers or famers with whom they are familiar with, and purchase from.

There are three main ways an individual can buy locally: buying from local/neighborhood businesses (as opposed to big box stores or online retailers), shopping at one's local farmer's market, or purchasing a share from a community supported agriculture (CSA) program.

As stated previously, buying from an independent, local business strengthens the economic base of the community. It also allows you to directly get to know the business owners within your community. Purchasing items through local businesses also keeps your community a unique and fun place to be. Many local items are also of higher quality than national chain items. Think of your favorite pizza shop, for example. Is your favorite pizza shop part of a national chain, or is it a local shop? Does the owner of your local pizza shop know you by name? Can you see or taste the difference in the quality of ingredients? Local pizza tends to be tastier (and better for you) than pizza from a national chain. That is because the ingredients used in pizza from a national chain tend to be shipped from further away. Because these ingredients are transported, many times preservatives need to be added to the dough, cheese, and sauce to keep them from spoiling.

Shopping at a farmers market is another way to support local merchants. Farmers markets are a once a week gathering of farmers, small businesses, and local food purveyors, usually centrally located in a town square, town park, or local parking lot. Some markets only exist during the growing season (for example, April to November in the Northeast region of the United States), or they can be open all year long. Many farmers markets contain local information booths, and even have live entertainment by local musicians. Attending a farmers market is an easy and enjoyable way to buy local.

Many farmers markets have a bring-your-own-bag policy, so make sure to bring a reusable bag and/or cooler to the market you plan to attend. The bring-your-own-bag policy eliminates overhead for the farmer, but more importantly helps the environment, as plastic bags are not biodegradable, and may take hundreds of years to break down in landfills. At the farmer's market, make sure to talk to the farmers and merchants. They love telling you how they grew their food or created their product. They also will tell you how to best use their product, and share recipes and ideas. If you are buying in quantity, farmers and merchants will usually give you a discount or free items at the market. Also, note that towards the end of the farmers market, when there is less variety to choose from, prices tend to be reduced. Therefore, if you are on a budget, the last hour of the farmer's market may be the best hour to arrive. Being a "regular" at the farmer's market has many perks. When you are a regular, the market becomes your community center, where you can socialize and eat delicious, local food. Being a regular at the farmers market can also be your ticket to your next summer job, as many farmers/merchants hire their regulars as farm hands or market help.

Community supported agriculture programs (or CSAs) are another way to buy locally. CSAs allow you to buy local, seasonal food directly from a farmer. CSAs work like this: At the beginning of the growing season, a farmer or farm offers a certain number of "shares" to the public. These shares are like memberships/subscriptions to the farm, and allow the farmer to market his/her farm early in the year (before the long days on the field begin). As the purchaser, you buy a share at the beginning of the growing season, and in return, you receive a box of seasonal produce each week throughout the farming season (approximately six months of the year). Some farms even offer "working shares", where you work on the farm for a specific number of hours in exchange for a discount on your share price. The produce received typically includes many different types of vegetables and fruits, but some CSAs also offer local honey, eggs, dairy products, and meat.

Shares can cost between 300 – 700 US dollars depending on the farm and region, and the types of products offered. Usually, when you join a CSA, you end up getting more product for money you have invested than you would from purchasing your fruits and vegetables from a local grocery store. Plus, the vegetables and fruits in your weekly share were usually picked that morning. Fresh picked vegetables and fruits have amazing flavor,

high vitamin and mineral content, and a longer shelf life than produce from a grocery store. Because you receive so many different types of produce in your box, a membership to a CSA allows you to become exposed to new fruits and vegetables, and new ways of cooking/preparing those fruits and vegetables. You also get to visit the farm on a weekly basis when you pick up your share, and get to establish a relationship with the people who grow and care for your food.

In this age of online purchasing, sprawling commercial malls, and big box stores, it becomes more and more important to support your local community by making sure your money goes to local products and merchants. Buying local not only supports individuals in your community, but also helps you feel more a part of your community, and allows you to live a healthier and more environmentally connected life. The relationships you create with local merchants and farmers can also assist you in finding employment that can help you make money throughout your years in high school and college. Buying local not only benefits local merchants and the overall environment, but it also benefits you!

FURTHER READING

Local Harvest. (2015). Retrieved from http://www.local-harvest.org/. A helpful website with a database listing of over 4000 farms in the United States. Typing your city, state, and zip code onto the database will provide the user with a listing of farms, farmer's markets, CSA's, produce stands, and restaurants specializing in local foods.

Sustainable Connections. (2014). Retrieved from https://sustainableconnections.org/about/vision. Sustainable Connections is a non-profit organization whose mission is to support and encourage local business development, green building, farms, and energy efficient building projects. It is a think tank and resource center for those who support local businesses and sustainable agriculture.

U.S.D.A Farmers Market Directory. (2015). Retrieved from http://search.ams.usda.gov/farmersmarkets/. This is a website sponsored by the United States Department of Agriculture. It is updated monthly. This website provides a listing of farmer's markets by zip code and geographical region. It also provides information regarding vendor payment options, products available, and whether there is a winter market available in your town or city.

Gina Riley,

SEE ALSO: Becoming a Green Consumer; Genetically Modified Foods; Nutrition; Organic Food Industry

Carbon footprint

Measuring one's carbon footprint is a useful tool for evaluating the effect upon the climate of one's GHG emissions and for ascertaining the results of specific changes in laws, regulations, or behavior.

BACKGROUND

The carbon footprint of an entity or an activity is its total annual contribution to the greenhouse effect. It is measured in units of mass of carbon dioxide (CO_2) per year, but it includes the entity's output of all greenhouse gases (GHGs) into the atmosphere. The effects of other GHGs are measured in terms of the equivalent amount of CO_2 necessary to produce the same effect, the gases' carbon dioxide equivalent (CO_2e).Carbon footprint-Carbon dioxidefootprintGreenhouse gas emissionscarbon footprintCarbon footprintCarbon dioxidefootprint-Greenhouse gas emissionscarbon footprint[c]Pollution and waste;Carbon footprint

The United States emission of CO_2 into the atmosphere increased at an average rate of 1.1 percent per year during the 1990's, but at an average of 3.1 percent per year in the early twenty-first century. This rate of increase is attributable to a higher intensity of energy use per unit of domestic product. The carbon footprint of a person is expressed as the CO_2e, in kilograms, of GHG emissions caused by that individual's lifestyle.

One portion of a person's carbon footprint is constituted directly by the CO_2 emitted by such activities as home heating, cooking, and driving an automobile. Other portions are less direct, as they comprise the CO_2 emissions of manufacturers whose products the person purchases or benefits from, vehicles used to ship those products, power plants whose electricity the person uses, and so forth. Carbon footprint measurements are being developed to educate individuals, organizations, and nations as to how to reduce the global warming effect of their activities. A given carbon footprint is a subset of the overall ecological footprint of the totality of human activities.

CARBON FOOTPRINT BY INDIVIDUAL ACTIVITY

When measuring the carbon footprint of an individual, one generally excludes breathing and other bodily functions and focuses on a person's discretionary lifestyle, although people will disagree as to what is and is not discretionary. The primary factors that contribute to an individual's carbon footprint are the amount of travel performed, the energy consumed in heating and cooling homes, and the amount of trash generated. Several "calculators" have been developed that take into account various factors.

As an example, 1 liter of gasoline contains 637 grams of carbon. Burning that gasoline in air generates 2,334 grams of CO_2. Thus, a car running 19,200 kilometers per year at an average of 10.5 kilometers per liter of gasoline emits about 4.26 metric tons of CO_2 per year. The carbon footprint of an average American family of four might include the emission of 12.7 metric tons of CO_2 from home energy use, 11.6 metric tons from driving two cars, 10.7 metric tons from food (including its growth or husbandry, processing, packaging, transportation, and preparation), and 3.2 metric tons from air travel, for a total of 38.2 metric tons of CO_2 emissions per year.

The carbon footprint of food is a complex and controversial issue. It depends strongly on where one lives (because of the cost and energy used by transportation and storage) and the type of food product. Some food products go through numerous processing steps that consume large amounts of energy. On average, one unit of energy gained from food consumed in the United States requires as many as seven to ten units of energy to produce. Some of this inefficiency is due to the macroeconomics of agriculture in a nation like the United States. For example, it was estimated in the late 1990's that over 90 percent of all fresh vegetables consumed in the United States came from the San Joaquin Valley of California, implying large transportation costs. Breakfast cereal requires thirty-two times as much energy to produce as does an equivalent amount of blended flour.

The energy cost of packaging food is also very large. The aluminum container of a prepackaged frozen dinner, which has no nutritive value, requires 3 times as much energy to produce as does 1 kilogram of blended flour. Producing a 36-centiliter aluminum soda can requires 3.4 times as much energy. All of this energy comes with attendant costs in CO_2 emissions. Thus, several lifestyle choices made for convenience lead to the creation of much larger carbon footprints than are necessary.

People who live in some metropolitan areas may appear to have smaller carbon footprints if they use public transportation or enjoy shorter commutes rather than driving themselves long distances to work. The per capita carbon footprints of residents of many U.S. cities can be compared to one another, taking into account only the contributions from transportation and residential energy use. Among the cities with the smallest footprints is Honolulu, Hawaii, at 1.356 metric tons per year. Los Angeles; New York; Portland, Oregon; Seattle, and San Francisco all have per capita carbon footprints between 1.4 and 1.6 metric tons. At the other extreme, smaller but spread-out, semirural towns in the Snow Belt have footprints of around 3.4 metric tons.

The average per capita carbon footprint for the one hundred largest U.S. metropolitan areas is 2.235 metric tons. However, this calculation is based primarily on personal transportation and heating costs. It does not include the significant costs of transporting food and other supplies to these cities. For some people, a large carbon footprint is calculated simply because they have to take long airplane trips occasionally. Although the fuel mileage of modern airliners per person is considerably better than that of most cars, airline travel can easily exceed twice the automobile miles driven per year, and emissions of airplanes are more damaging than are those of automobiles, because they are released so much higher up in the atmosphere.

Food, air transportation, and the energy involved in making personal technology products contribute vastly to individuals' carbon footprints. When these are included, the average per capita footprint of a U.S. resident is 20 metric tons, compared to a worldwide average of 4.4 metric tons. Much of the difference lies in the energy intensity of the products that are used in developed nations, as is demonstrated by the previous discussion of food. Industrialized nations have built very efficient systems for minimizing the monetary cost of consumer goods, but these systems operate at a high cost in energy use. They are able to obtain and employ energy at low prices through efficient power plants and transmission grids. However, the cost in CO_2 emissions of this heavy energy use shows up as a large national carbon footprint. Because of these features of the U.S. economy, even the least privileged and the most conservation-minded Americans appear to have carbon footprints that are double that global average. Thus, measures to reduce U.S. carbon footprints must be accompanied by national policy decisions and major systemic changes in order to be successful.

CARBON FOOTPRINTS OF BUSINESSES AND ORGANIZATIONS

Businesses and organizations have large carbon footprints, because they use fleets of vehicles and large buildings that have to be lit and climate-controlled every day. The emissions due to transportation and incidental energy use accrue in addition to direct emissions from manufacturing. On the other hand, larger organizations can implement dramatic reductions in their carbon footprints through means that are not yet available to individual homes. Examples include the installation of large areas of rooftop photovoltaic panels by companies such as Google and WalMart.

Facilities located in areas with predictable weather, such as California, are able to produce much of the electricity they require with solar technology that does not generate emissions. Producing the solar panels themselves requires a significant amount of energy and emissions, but once installed they operate with zero emissions for a long time. Likewise, many large organizations have switched to vehicles that are operated on natural gas (mostly methane) instead of gasoline or diesel fuel. Since methane released into the atmosphere has a global warming potential more than twenty times that of CO_2, burning methane achieves a net reduction in equivalent CO_2 emission. Large buildings are also able to use combined solar heating, power generation, and even air conditioning using appropriate building surface systems.

Many organizations are working to become carbon neutral. Such entities buy offsetting credits from low-emission projects such as wind farms and apply the credits toward their own emissions. It is often impossible to reduce actual emissions to zero, or in some cases at all. For example, air travel cannot be avoided completely. In such cases, trading emission credits to achieve carbon neutrality is a viable solution, as it supports the development of green technologies in the future.

MEASURES TO REDUCE CARBON FOOTPRINTS

Individuals' carbon footprints may be reduced by recycling plastics, glass, paper, and magazines; using more fuel efficient cars; reducing the number of miles driven per year per person by either car pooling, using public transportation, or simply reducing travel; changing to fluorescent lightbulbs; and turning thermostats up during summer and down during winter. National carbon footprints can be reduced through appropriate policies. The signatories to the Kyoto Protocol have adopted a complex system of certified emissions reduction credits (or carbon credits) that can be traded on the open market, allowing a large marketplace to develop for emission reduction schemes. In the United States, federal tax credits have offset the higher initial costs of installing modern, low-emission water heaters, home heaters, air conditioners, and energy-saving windows in homes, as well as the costs of hybrid and fuel-cell automobiles. Some nations are phasing out the use of incandescent lightbulbs, forcing their replacement with more efficient, longer-lasting compact fluorescent bulbs. Policies that encourage telecommuting at work also contribute strongly to emission reductions.

Rapid increases in the cost of fossil fuels have induced dramatic changes in the economics of energy use. For instance, as mass-produced food prices increase, locally grown food from smaller farms becomes competitive. When consumers purchase more local foods, the emissions from food shipments decrease.

Policies that improve transportation options for people and help them live closer to population centers have been shown to reduce carbon footprints. In the United States, individuals are moving farther away from cities in order to enjoy better living environments, and when jobs change, people may choose to remain in the same homes rather than move closer to their new workplace. This results in long-distance commuting. Moreover, more houses are built to meet the increasing demand for rural accommodation, and these houses require heating using mainly natural gas. Thus, the individual's desire for better living can have a negative effect on the environment with increased emission of CO_2. Other activities, such as the frivolous use of fire extinguishers, can have huge carbon footprints, because fire suppressants such as halon 1310 can have CO2e's thousands of times greater than that of CO_2.

CONTEXT

The carbon footprint has become an increasingly important concept as decisions at the personal, community, industry, state, and national levels are guided by the need to reduce GHG emissions. Changes in energy policy that reward utilities for the efficiency of their overall operation, rather than just for delivering ever-larger amounts of power, can greatly help reduce carbon footprints. Finally, shifting to increased use of "clean coal" power plant technology and to nuclear power can substantially reduce carbon footprints by rendering the power generation underlying much industrial human activity carbon neutral.

FURTHER READING

Brown, M. A., F. Southworth, and A. Sarzynski. *Emission Facts: Average Carbon Dioxide Emissions Resulting from Gasoline and Diesel Fuel*. Washington, D.C.: Author, 2005. Short note showing examples of how to calculate the CO2 emissions from motor fuels.

_____. *Shrinking the Carbon Footprint of Metropolitan America*. Washington, D.C.: Brookings Institution, 2008. This report gives data on the carbon footprints in U.S. metropolitan areas, with breakdowns by type of activity. It discusses policy issues in reducing carbon footprints and argues for improved coordination between different federal agencies.

Environmental Protection Agency. U.S. Office of Transportation and Air Quality. Greenhouse Gas Emissions from the U.S. Transportation Sector, 1990-2003. Washington, D.C.: Author, 2006. This sixty-eight-page report documents the emissions from different modes of transportation, including road, air, rail, and water travel. Appendix B gives data on different components of transportation.

Padma Komerath

SEE ALSO: Conservation

Composting

Composting facilities can be prone to a number of problems, most notably odor control. However, research continues to develop new and better ways to control odor and produce compost in an efficient manner.

COST REDUCTIONS & EFFICIENCY ARE THE NAME OF THE GAME: WATCH LIST

Composting on a commercial or institutional scale, while beneficial for both an organization and its members, typically requires applications and permits.

An increasing number of local authorities are requiring the separation of yard and garden waste from other waste. Trash and recycling companies that do not comply with local laws may be subject to fines.

KEY TAKEAWAYS

Composting organic waste is an environmentally-sound strategy that keeps organic material out of the landfill and recovers it for other uses.

On-site composting is typically less expensive than paying for a waste collection company to haul the organic waste to a landfill.

The more tons of organic waste that are composted by an organization, the less expensive it is to operate the facility per ton of waste.

The demand for compost in such industries as agriculture, silviculture, residential retail, nursery sod production, and landscaping is typically greater than the supply of available compost.

Not all approaches to composting are equally suitable to all commercial and institutional applications. Before instituting a composting strategy or investing in composting technology, a business or institution should first determine what its needs are and what strategy will most cost-effectively help it meet these needs.

According to the United States Environmental Protection Agency, two-thirds of the municipal solid waste discarded into the waste stream in the United States comprises organic materials (EPA, 1999). Some of these materials (e.g., newspaper, office paper, corrugated cardboard), have a high recovery rate. Other types of organic material, however, do not (e.g., yard trimmings, food scraps, certain grades of paper), and tend to be disposed of in landfills rather than recycled despite the fact that they, too, can be recycled and recovered. In 1999, the EPA estimated that between $9 and $37 per ton could be saved by recycling organic material. At that time, there was an estimated 62 million tons comprising the municipal solid waste stream. The EPA estimates that approximately 36 percent of this solid waste could be composted using existing strategies and technologies.

There are a number of strategies used in the United States for composting organic material. These include familial residential strategies (e.g., grasscycling, backyard composting, residential source-separated composting) as well as industrial strategies.

The most popular industrial strategies for composting include: Yard trimmings composting, in which leaves, grass, brush and other organic yard and gardening debris are collected and composted at central facilities

On-site institutional composting, in which large institutions (e.g., universities, schools, hospitals) process food scraps, paper, and yard trimmings on-site at their own facilities

Commercial composting, in which organic waste at large commercial or institutional facilities (e.g.,

supermarkets, restaurants, schools) is collected and separated for collection and composting.

Mixed waste composting, in which municipal solid waste is separated into component streams for composting, recycling, or refuse disposal.

Of the industrial strategies for organic waste composting, on-site institutional composting is the most cost-effective when compared to other industrial composting options due to its low program costs, which are typically more than offset by the concomitant savings in disposal costs. In addition, large organizations and institutions that compost can realize other financial benefits as well. The EPA estimates that the demand for compost is much greater than the supply of available compost. There is a ready market for compost in the agriculture, silviculture, residential retail, nursery sod production, and landscaping industries. In addition, the more tons of organic material that are composted, the lower the cost to operate the technology or strategy necessary to process them. However, not every composting strategy works for every commercial or institutional organization. A composting strategy should be chosen based on the needs of the organization.

BUSINESS OPTIONS & BEST PRACTICES

According to the United States Environmental Protection Agency (1999), there are four commonly used strategies for commercial and institutional composting: Yard trimmings composting, on-site institutional composting, commercial composting, and mixed waste composting.

Yard Trimmings Composting. In this approach to composting, leaves, grass, brush and other organic yard and gardening debris are collected and composted at central facilities. Typically, organic yard and garden waste are collected curbside either through bag collection (in which homeowners or other recyclers place bagged yard and garden waste at the curb for pickup by the recycling company) or through bulk collection (in which vacuum machines, front-and loaders, mobile chippers, or similar equipment is used to collect loose yard waste that has been raked to the curb or into the street. Bulk collection of this type typically requires three to five workers per vehicle, while bag collection typically relies on existing packer fleets and crews of two to three workers.

Composting facilities for the processing of collected yard trimmings can range from low-technology strategies in which large piles of leaves or yard trimmings are periodically turned with front-end loaders, to high-technology operations in which more sophisticated equipment such as size reduction equipment, dedicated windrow turners, or screening equipment is used. For some composting operations, low-technology approaches are sufficient. Such approaches can be viable options particularly if sufficient land is available for long-term composting of organic material.

However, high-technology processing methods produce higher-quality compost that can be used for other purposes sooner than low-technology approaches, thereby making room for more organic material the following year and yielding more financial benefits to the organization. Other considerations to be taken into account when considering whether to use a high-technology or low-technology approach to composting include the cost of equipment. For example, many public works departments already use front-end loaders for a variety of purposes, and require no additional capital investment for equipment in order to operate a low-technology composting facility. On the other hand, the cost of the windrow turner increases with its capacity, and the cost of operating a composting facility increases with the complexity of the strategy being used. The range of equipment needed for yard trimmings composting is also dependent on the specific composting model being used.

For example, if brush is accepted at the composting site, it must first be run through a chipper to reduce its size. However, expensive equipment (e.g., tub grinders, compost screens) can sometimes be jointly purchased and shared among communities.

Centralized composting facilities can emit odors that make it an undesirable neighbor. Odor at composting facilities can be generated due to the types of materials collected, management issues, siting, and climactic conditions. For example, because of their high moisture and nitrogen contents, grass clippings can quickly become anaerobic and emit offensive odors. Therefore, it is important for a composting facility to process grass clippings expediently to avoid both odor problems and groundwater contamination. Storm water management, litter control, siting, and permitting issues may also be of concern when setting up and running a centralized composting facility.

In addition, organic material that is swept to the curb or into the street for bulk collection systems can become contaminated by street trash or oil, or blow into the streets and, therefore, is uncollectible until it is put back at the curb, or can cause leaf fires in hot catalytic converters. Logistically, bulk collection can also be cumbersome, requiring scheduled pickups and residents to park elsewhere on collection days.

On-site Institutional Composting. Many large institutions (e.g., universities, schools, hospitals, correctional facilities, military installations) process food scraps, paper, and yard trimmings on-site at their own facilities rather than at a central facility. Such organizations are typically well-suited for implementing their own on-site composting program because of the availability of land to do so. By composting on-site, large institutions can reduce the costs of trash disposal or provide a working lab for research in composting techniques and technology (e.g., for universities). Ohio University, for example, has instituted an on-site composting program (Ohio University, 2009). The system has a total capacity of 28 tons of organic material, which can be composted in 14 days without odor and with minimal human input. Between the introduction of the system in late January and the end of May 2009, the system has composed 34.5 tons of food waste and biodegradable serviceware and 19 tons of yard waste. Organic material to be composted is collected in 64 gallon bins at the central foodservice facility, although the university hopes to expand its collection of organic waste to all campus eateries in the near future. In order to help train both the patrons and food service employees on how to separate organic from inorganic material (e.g., chip bags, catsup packages), the university has posted several different posters in the kitchens and near where the patrons sort their waste. The university plans on using the resulting compost to amend the soil in the landscaping beds around campus, thereby not only saving money on trash collection and hauling costs, but on landscaping costs as well.

Commercial Composting. In commercial composting programs, organizations that generate large amounts of commercial organic materials (e.g., supermarkets, restaurants, schools) use commercial services to collect and separate their waster for composting. Such organizations can generate a large amount of organic waste on a continuing basis, including not only food scraps, but other organic waste such as soiled and waxed cardboard and paper. For example, it has been found that between 75 and 90 percent of the waste stream in such organizations can be organic. If a great deal of organic waste is generated, it is typically placed in roll-off compactors that are filled on site and then hauled to a composting facility. Some institutions that generate smaller amounts of organic waste may collect their material in outside containers (e.g., toters, dumpsters) that are collected at frequent intervals by packer trucks or by a collection service that swaps empty containers for full ones.

Commercial composting strategies are not without their technical difficulties. Equipment can leak and create odors and messy conditions, although this is typically correctable by replacing the watertight gaskets on compactors and packer trucks. In addition, to reduce odor, toters and dumpsters need to be rinsed out and cleaned regularly. The resultant waste water needs to be properly handled so that it does not contaminate the site. This can be done, for example, through the capture of the waste water in a separate collection vehicle container which then dumps the water into the sewage system (which typically requires a permit). Or, waste water can be stored with the organics, although this practice may increase collection costs. New technologies (e.g., degradable liners for the containers) are being researched.

Mixed Waste Composting. In this approach to the composting of organic materials, municipal solid waste is separated at composting facilities into separate streams for composting, recycling, or refuse disposal. Most mixed waste composting facilities are equipped with preprocessing equipment such as trammels or shear shredders, and composting technology used in mixed waste facilities can range from simple windrows to expensive digester drums. This range of options allows mixed waste composting facilities to better control odor and the quality of the finished compost in addition to effectively maximizing the composting speed in order to facilitate the processing of more throughput for the facility.

Although early mixed waste composting facilities often had no provisions for odor control, this is no longer true. Odors from mixed waste composting facilities can be controlled in a number of ways including facility enclosure, material handling procedures, processing technologies, process control, and end-of-pipe odor control technologies (usually biofilters). Most mixed waste composting facilities use a combination of these approaches.

Another frequent concern with mixed waste composting facilities is the quality of the finished compost. Organic materials separated from the waste stream may be contaminated with such things as heavy metals and organic chemicals from batteries, electronics, or hazardous household waste. Waste material such as glass or plastic fragments destined for other waste streams in the facility can get into the organic material stream, making the resulting compost less marketable. However, the composting industry is currently working on better ways to control these potential problems.

Composting is not limited to industrial and institutional settings, however. Agricultural facilities produce another kind of organic waste: Manure. This is not a minor matter. One dairy cow generates approximately 120 pounds of manure per day. California produces an estimated 70 billion pounds of manure per year from its dairy farms. This is the equivalent of the waste of a city of 22 million people (EPA, 2009). However, properly composted, manure can be a valuable commodity for farmers, landscapers, and gardeners.

The EPA recently funded a pilot project to investigate the benefits of combining dairy manure with urban green waste (e.g., yard and garden debris). The co-composted mixture was found to be a good soil amendment for farming and gardening and helped regenerate poor soils and reduced or eliminated the need for chemical fertilizers. This composted mixture is much better for the environment and human health than raw manure, which contains high levels of nutrients and pathogens. Co-composted manure has been found to be safer for crops, cheaper than commercial fertilizers, and better for plants.

REGULATORY ENVIRONMENT
The management of organic material, including facility siting and permits, is regulated at the state rather than the local level, with the exception of biosolids and animal manures. Although the requirements for obtaining a composting facility permit vary from state to state, they frequently involve the submission of a detailed facility design, operating plans, description of incoming materials, the amount and types of residue to be generated in the plant, monitory plans, potential environmental releases, landfills to be used, and potential markets for the compost. The composting of biosolids is covered under the Clean Water Act (CWA) under the section Standards for the Use or Disposal of Sewage Sludge (40 CFR Part 503).

In addition to state regulations and federal regulations for biosolids, the EPA is empowered to regulate point source discharges into United States waters through the National Pollutant Discharge Elimination System (NPDES). These regulations are also part of the CWA (Title 33, Chapter 26, 1311, USC). This regulation includes confined animal feed operations (CAFOs). CAFOs are facilities with over 1000 animal units (e.g., 1000 head of beef cattle, 700 head of dairy cattle, 2500 pigs over 55 pounds, 125,000 broilers) that are confined on site for over 45 days. Even if an animal feed operation does not meet this definition, it is categorized as a CAFO for purposes of the CWA if it discharges manure or waste water into a natural or man-made ditch, stream, or other waterway. CAFOs are regulated under the CWA because they can potentially release pollutants (e.g., nitrogen, phosphorus, organic matter, pathogens, hormones, antibiotics, ammonia) into the environment. Excess nitrogen and phosphorus can, in turn, contribute to low levels of dissolved oxygen, eutrophication, or toxic algal blooms; conditions harmful to human health. Nitrogen can also contaminate drinking water obtained from ground water. Decomposing organic matter in the water can also reduce oxygen levels and result in fish kills.

Pathogens from these sources can foul drinking water and impair human health or create a food safety issue if the manure is used to fertilize the crops at the wrong time in the growth cycle. Pathogens can also result in some shellfish bed closures.

RELATED ENTITIES
United States Environmental Protection
Agency (EPA)
Acronyms
CAFO: Confined Animal Feed Operations
CWA: Clean Water Act
EPA: United States Environmental Protection Agency
NPDES: National Pollutant Discharge
Elimination System
IM.-_GLO:AWEW/01Oct10:02n1.jpg_PHOTO (COLOR): Visitors at a Composting
Plant Canadian Press 2007_gl_

FURTHER READING
Al-Daher, R., Al-Awadhi, N., Yateem, A., Balba, M. T., & Elnawawy, A. (2001). Compost soil piles for treatment of oil-contaminated soil. *Soil Sediment Contamination*, 10(2), 197-209. Retrieved July 27, 2009, from EBSCO Online Database Academic Search Complete. http://search.ebscohost.com/login.aspx?direct=true&db=a9h&AN=9510975&site=ehost-live

Barker, A. V. (2001). Evaluation of composts for growth of grass sod. *Communications in Soil Science & Plant Analysis*, 32(11/12), 1841-1860. Retrieved July 27, 2009, from EBSCO Online Database Academic Search Complete. http://search.ebscohost.com/login.aspx?direct=true&db=a9h&AN=8534609&site=ehost-live

Beranek, W. (1992). Solid waste management and economic development. *Economic Development Review*, 10(3), 49-51. Retrieved July 27, 2009, from EBSCO Online Database Business Source Complete. http://search.ebscohost.com/login.aspx?direct=true&db=bth&AN=9603222099&site=ehost-live

Brinton, W. F. Jr. (2005, 29 November). Sustainability of modern composting: Intensification versus costs & quality. Retrieved July 27, 2009, from Woods End Laboratories Website. http://www.woodsend.org/pdf-files/sustain.pdf

Brodie, H. L., Carr, L. E., & Condon, P. (2000). A comparison of static pile and turned windrow methods for poultry litter compost production. *Compost Science & Utilization*, 8(3), 178-189. Retrieved July 27, 2009, from EBSCO Online Database Academic Search Complete. http://search.ebscohost.com/login.aspx?direct=true&db=a9h&AN=3566227&site=ehost-live

Confesor, R. B. Jr., Hamlett, J. M., Shannon, R. D., & Graves, R. E. (2009). Potential pollutants from farm, food and yard waste composts at differing ages: Leaching potential of nutrients under column experiments. Part II. *Compost Science & Utilization*, 17(1), 6-17. Retrieved July 27, 2009, from EBSCO Online Database Academic Search Complete. http://search.ebscohost.com/login.aspx?direct=true&db=a9h&AN=37220598&site=ehost-live

Confesor, R. B. Jr., Hamlett, J. M., Shannon, R. D., & Graves, R. E.(2008). Potential pollutants from farm, food and yard waste composts at differing ages: Leaching potential of nutrients under column experiments. Part I - physical and chemical properties. *Compost Science & Utilization,* 16(4), 6-17. Retrieved July 27, 2009,from EBSCO Online Database Academic Search Complete. http://search.ebscohost.com/login.aspx?direct=true&db=a9h&AN=36188318&site=ehost-live

Dawson, G. F. & Probert, E. J. (2007). A sustainable product needing a sustainable procurement commitment: The case of green waste in Wales. *Sustainable Development*, 15(2), 69-82. Retrieved July 27, 2009, from EBSCO Online Database Business Source Complete. http://search.ebscohost.com/login.aspx?direct=true&db=bth&AN=24560658&site=ehost-live

Dimambro, M. E., Lillywhite, R. D., & Rahn, C. R. (2007). The physical, chemical and microbial characteristics of biodegradable municipal waste derived composts. *Compost Science & Utilization,* 15(4), 243-252. Retrieved July 27, 2009, from EBSCO Online Database Academic Search Complete. http://search.ebscohost.com/login.aspx?direct=true&db=a9h&AN=27937474&site=ehost-live

Donoghue, J. & Fisher, A. (2008). Activism via humus: The composters decode decomponomics. *Environmental Communication,* 2(2), 229-236. Retrieved July 27, 2009, from EBSCO Online Database Communication & Mass Media Complete. http://search.ebscohost.com/login.aspx?direct=true&db=ufh&AN=33299389&site=ehost-live

El-Mashad, H. M., van Loon, W. K. P., Zeeman, G., Bot, G. P. A., & Lettinga, G. (2003). Reuse potential of agricultural wastes in semi-arid regions: Egypt as a case study. *Reviews in Environmental Science & Biotechnology,* 2(1), 53-66. Retrieved July 27, 2009, from EBSCO Online Database Environment Complete. http://search.ebscohost.com/login.aspx?direct=true&db=eih&AN=15193546&site=ehost-live

Francou, C., Poitrenaud, M., & Housot, S. (2005). Stabilization of organic matter during composting: Influence of process and feedstocks. *Compost Science & Utilization,* 13(1), 72-83. Retrieved July 27, 2009, from EBSCO Online Database Academic Search Complete. http://search.ebscohost.com/login.aspx?direct=true&db=a9h&AN=16724792&site=ehost-live

Kahn, B. A., Hyde, J. K., Cole, Janet C., Stoffella, P. J., & Graetz, D. A. (2005). Replacement of a peat-lite medium with compost for cauliflower transplant production. *Compost Science & Utilization,* 13(3), 175-179. Retrieved July 27, 2009, from EBSCO Online Database Academic Search Complete. http://search.ebscohost.com/login.aspx?direct=true&db=a9h&AN=18441767&site=ehost-live

Kriipsalu, M. & Kerner, Ü. (2006). Waste farming as opportunity for entrepreneurial activities. Management Theory & Studies for Rural Business & Infrastructure Development, 7, 83-85. Retrieved July 27, 2009, from EBSCO Online Database Business Source Complete. http://search.ebscohost.com/login.aspx?direct=true&db=bth&AN=23720596&site=ehost-live

Lisney, R., Riley, K., & Banks, C. (2004). From waste to resource management: Part 2. *Management Services,* 48(1), 6-12. Retrieved July 27, 2009, from EBSCO Online Database Business Source Complete. http://search.ebscohost.com/login.aspx?direct=true&db=bth&AN=11834845&site=ehost-live

Litterick, A. M., Harrier, L., Wallace, P., Watson, C. A., & Wood, M. (2004). The role of uncomposted materials, composts, manures, and compost extracts in reducing pest and disease incidence and severity in sustainable temperate agricultural and horticultural crop production - a review. *Critical Reviews in Plant Sciences,* 23(6), 453-479. Retrieved July 27, 2009, from EBSCO Online Database Academic Search Complete. http://search.ebscohost.com/login.aspx?direct=true&db=a9h&AN=15642790&site=ehost-live

Maynard, A. A. (2000). Applying leaf compost to reduce fertilizer use in tomato product. *Compost Science & Utilization,* 8(3), 203-209. Retrieved July 27, 2009, from EBSCO Online Database Academic Search Complete. http://search.ebscohost.com/login.aspx?direct=true&db=a9h&AN=3566244&site=ehost-live

McClintock, N. C., & Diop, A. M. (2005). Soil fertility management and compost use in Senegal's Peanut Basin. *International Journal of Agricultural Sustainability,* 3(2), 79-91. Retrieved July 27, 2009, from EBSCO Online Database Sustainability Reference Center. http://search.ebscohost.com/login.aspx?direct=true&db=sur&AN=21656932&site=ehost-live

Meunchang, S., Panichsakpatana, S., & Weaver, R. W. (2005). Tomato growth in soil amended with sugar mill by-products compost. *Plant & Soil,* 280(1/2), 171-176. Retrieved July 27, 2009, from EBSCO Online Database Academic Search Complete. http://search.ebscohost.com/login.aspx?direct=true&db=a9h&AN=19870995&site=ehost-live

Ohio University. (2009). Office of sustainability: The composting project at Ohio University. Retrieved 27 July 2009 from Ohio University Website. http://www.ohio.edu/sustainability/Compost.htm

Rahmani, M., Hodges, A. W., & Kiker, C. F. (2004). Compost users' attitudes toward compost application in Florida. *Compost Science & Utilization,* 12(1), 55-60. Retrieved July 27, 2009, from EBSCO Online Database Environment Complete. http://search.ebscohost.com/login.aspx?direct=true&db=eih&AN=12687560&site=ehost-live

Striebig, B., Jantzen, T., Rosden, K., Dacquisto, J., & Reyes, R. (2006). Learning sustainability by design. *Environmental Engineering Science,* 23(3), 439-450. Retrieved July 27, 2009, from EBSCO Online Database Environment Complete. http://search.ebscohost.com/login.aspx?direct=true&db=eih&AN=21491381&site=ehost-live

United States Environmental Protection Agency. (1997a,

October). Innovative uses of compost: *Bioremediation and pollution prevention.* Retrieved July 31, 2009, from EPA Website. http://www.epa.gov/epawaste/conserve/rrr/composting/pubs/bioremed.pdf

United States Environmental Protection Agency. (1997b, October). Innovative uses of compost: Disease control for plants and animals. Retrieved July 31, 2009, from EPA Website. http://www.epa.gov/epawaste/conserve/rrr/composting/pubs/disease.pdf

United States Environmental Protection Agency. (1997c, October). Innovative uses of compost: Erosion control, turf remediation, and landscaping. Retrieved July 31, 2009, from EPA Website. http://www.epa.gov/epawaste/conserve/rrr/composting/pubs/erosion.pdf

United States Environmental Protection Agency. (1999, July). Organic materials management strategies. Retrieved July 31, 2009, from EPA Website. http://www.epa.gov/epawaste/conserve/rrr/composting/pubs/omms.pdf

United States Environmental Protection Agency. (2000, September). Biosolids technology fact sheet: In-vessel composting of biosolids. Retrieved July 31, 2009, from EPA Website. http://www.epa.gov/owm/mtb/invessel.pdf

United States Environmental Protection Agency. (2009, 6 May). How did 70 billion pounds of manure become a valuable resource? Retrieved July 31, 2009, from EPA Website. http://www.epa.gov/region09/waste/features/manure/

Walker, P., Williams, D., & Waliczek, T. M. (2006). An analysis of the horticulture industry as a potential value-added market for compost. *Compost Science & Utilization*, 14(1), 23-31. Retrieved July 27, 2009, from EBSCO Online Database

Academic Search Complete. http://search.ebscohost.com/login.aspx?direct=true&db=a9h&AN=20399733&site=ehost-live

Wright, A. L., Provin, T. L., Hons, F. M., Zuberer, D. A., & White, R. H. (2007). Soil micronutrient availability after compost addition to St. Augustine grass. *Compost Science & Utilization*, 15(2), 127-134. Retrieved July 27, 2009, from EBSCO Online Database Academic Search Complete. http://search.ebscohost.com/login.aspx?direct=true&db=a9h&AN=25339205&site=ehost-live

The Editors

SEE ALSO: Recycling Technology

Conservation

Humanity's footprint is being felt around the world. As the global population continues to increase, the natural resources necessary to sustain life continue to decline. Fresh water, fossil fuels, and arable land are just a few of the natural resources that must be properly managed to sustain a global population that may reach 9.1 billion by the year 2050, as predicted by the United Nations.

BACKGROUND

The planet Earth may be unable to support future increases in population unless, on a worldwide scale, humans begin to conserve and reduce their rates of consumption and increase efforts to recycle resources for new uses. Moreover, the current global economy is no longer sustainable and is destroying the environment and providing little to support the globally impoverished. Internationally, governments and activists have begun to work together to establish policies that protect the environment and the sustainability of life while concomitantly fostering harmonious economic growth.

CONSERVATION

"Conservation" defined generally refers to the use of resources found in the natural environment in such a way that the resources will serve humans effectively and will be available to humans for as long as possible. Therefore, it does not refer to the indefinite "preservation" of resources in their natural state. Quantitatively, effective conservation could be said to involve obtaining the maximum use for the maximum number of people.

The Earth can be viewed as a life-support system composed of four major subsystems through which energy flows and matter cycles. The subsystems are the atmosphere, biosphere, lithosphere, and hydrosphere, referring to gases, life systems, rock and mineral materials, and water, respectively. As energy flows and matter cycles within and among these subsystems, they interact as component parts to compose the Earth's ecosystem (an ecosystem may be defined as a community of plants, animals, and other organisms interacting in an environment). Humans alter the natural cycling of energy and flow of matter in the Earth's ecosystem. We extract things from natural systems, convert them into what we perceive as more useful products, and then return them to the natural environment in different forms and physical states. In order to achieve more desirable energy conversions, we also use energy from the environment. Natural resources are all of the things that humans take from the environment to help satisfy their needs and wants.

RESOURCES AND RESERVES

All the matter and energy on Earth make up its "stock." Natural resources are subsets of this stock that help humans meet their energy and material needs. Those natural resources that are available in a usable form and at an affordable price under prevailing technology and socioeconomic conditions make up "reserves." For example, uranium was not a part of human energy reserves until the technology to capture and control the flow of nuclear energy was developed. Agrofuels produced from plant resources and biofuels developed from recently lifeless plant and animal materials are other examples of the marriage between natural resources and technology to meet energy demands for such uses as powering vehicles and heating buildings.

Natural resources may be classified as renewable, nonrenewable, and perpetual. Renewable resourcesRenewable resources are those that can be reproduced at a rate equal to or greater than the rate of consumption. Renewable resources are replenished through natural, physical, and biogeochemical cycles. Examples of renewable resources are forest and soil. They are conserved when they are used and reused at a rate, and in such a way, that does not destroy their sustainability. This does not mean that they cannot be depleted; it means that the rate of consumption does not exceed the rate at which they are replenished over an extended period.

Nonrenewable resources, on the other hand, are those for which the rate of consumption exceeds the rate of renewal. They are exhaustible, cannot be replenished, and exist in fixed amounts. Nonrenewable resources, such as minerals and fossil fuels, are conserved by more thorough exploitation of their deposits and more efficient use. Some can be recycled or reused. Recycling involves collecting and reprocessing a resource, while reuse involves using a resource again in the same form. The reprocessing of used aluminum cans into new cans is an example of recycling. Washing beverage bottles before using them again is an example of reuse. Other nonrenewable resources, such as coal and oil, are gone forever once they are used.

Perpetual resources, such as water, wind, tides, and solar energy, continue to flow throughout the Earth's ecosystem whether humans use them or not. Therefore,

they are sometimes called flow resources. Even when their quality is altered they generally continue to flow within the Earth's ecosystem, making them inexhaustible. However, man is affecting the flow of some of these resources, such as water, and the recent harnessing of wind resources to produce energy is leading some scientists to suggest that altering the flow of wind with multiple, large turbines may lead to climate change.

CONSERVATION VS. PRESERVATION

Preservation vs. conservation of natural resources means using things found in the natural environment wisely. In a more quantitative sense, it means sustainability of the natural resources by obtaining the maximum use for the maximum number of people without compromising future needs. It does not imply that resources should be entirely preserved for use later; rather, it means that they should be employed in a way that serves humans as well and as long as possible. Although preservation is closely associated with some aspects of conservation, the two approaches are different, as "preservation" means the complete protection of natural resources from human disturbance. It is true that to conserve some resources is to preserve them: We conserve natural resources such as ecosystems, for example, by restricting their use and protecting them from being altered, because their value is diminished if they are not retained in their original state. However, we conserve most resources when we use them in a certain way, not when we leave them idle.

HISTORICAL PERSPECTIVE

Not until technology developed significantly, and the world's human population reached a certain size, did human exploitation of the environment begin to have significant effects. Until that time, conservation of resources was simply not an issue. For most of humankind's existence, people lived a simple hunter-gatherer existence, obtaining just enough food to survive. Most people lived in small groups—fifty or fewer people—that had little effect on resources or the environment. They made simple tools and weapons. Many groups were nomadic, migrating with the seasons and following game animals. The shift from a hunting-and-gathering society to a sedentary one began about ten thousand years ago. People began breeding animals and cultivating wild plants, thereby having a greater impact on the environment. Slash-and-burn cultivation involved cutting down trees and other vegetation, leaving the cut vegetation on the ground to dry, and then burning it to enrich the soil. Farmers were "subsistence farmers," producing only enough to feed their families.

With the invention of the metal plow about seven thousand years ago, agriculture could be practiced on a larger scale. Animals were used to pull the plows, increasing crop productivity and making the cultivation of new soils possible. Forests were cut and grasslands were plowed—soil erosion and degradation of wildlife habitats inevitably began to follow on a small scale. Occasional food surpluses were produced for sale or storage. Surpluses allowed the development of urban cultures by releasing people from the farm. By the nineteenth century, urbanization and the Industrial Revolution were having profound impacts on the environment and the rate of resource consumption.

HISTORY OF THE CONSERVATION MOVEMENT
In 1864, George Perkins Marsh published *Man and Nature: Or, Physical Geography as Modified by Human Actions*. Marsh's book, which claimed that humanity could no longer afford to continue wastefully exploiting natural resources, is thought by some to mark the beginning of the conservation movement. However, American Indians must also be given credit as one of the first peoples to practice sustainable natural resource use. In 1878, John Wesley Powell completed *A Report on the Lands of the Arid Region of the United States*. Powell's study of the geomorphology and arid landscape transformations in the Colorado River basin was grounded in scientific methodology and called for the creation of a federal agency to survey and map all U.S. lands. In 1879, the United States Geological Survey was created for this purpose. At the beginning of the twentieth century there was growing concern that resource mismanagement could have tragic future consequences. These concerns were based on scientific findings associated with the exploitation and depletion of timber. In 1907, the Inland Waterways Commission, headed by U.S. Forest Service chief Gifford Pinchot, reported that the use and control of water would have an impact on other resources, including timber, soil, wildlife, and minerals. Pinchot's views on resource management greatly influenced forest and water management policies in the United States.

During the Great Depression of the 1930's, the Franklin Delano Roosevelt administration instituted a number of programs in the United States that addressed natural resource problems and helped create employment. In the wake of the severe drought and wind erosion in the Dust Bowl (1930's), the Public Works Administration initiated the Prairie States Forestry Project. Its goal was to establish a shelter belt of trees and shrubs from the Texas panhandle to the Canadian border in North Dakota. This project was designed to reduce wind erosion on rangeland and cropland. Other efforts included the creation of the Tennessee Valley Authority (TVA) and the Civilian Conservation Corps (CCC). The TVA was an innovative water resource management program that involved comprehensive regional planning. Though confined to the Tennessee River and its tributaries, it provided a model for total resource management. The aim of the CCC was to provide employment while repairing some of the damage that had resulted from past exploitation of natural resources and neglect of the environment. Workers constructed bridges, roads, and fire lanes for the development of recreational facilities; conducted tree-planting programs; instituted soil- and water-erosion control projects; made lake and stream improvements; and participated in flood control projects.

Many of these early conservation practices in the United States spread to other countries and, over time, several international conservation organizations were formed, including the United Nations Environment Programme, the International Union for the Conservation of Nature, and the World Wildlife Fund. After World War II, nations focused on resource-related problems, many times creating agencies to assess the impact that the war had on forest and natural resources. Moreover, the use of atomic bombs in the war—and the widespread nuclear testing that occurred in the 1950's—exposed ecosystems to significant levels of radiation. This situation marked the beginning of the modern conservation movement.

THE MODERN CONSERVATION MOVEMENT
Although the United States is credited as the front-runner of the early conservation movement through its linking of ecology with conservation and resource management practices on public lands, during the modern conservation movement, especially in the 1980's, the United States focused on economic growth and deregulation, sacrificing conservation. Nevertheless, the efforts of the Worldwatch Institute and older organizations such as the Sierra Club, the Audubon Society, and Friends of the Earth kept the general citizenry aware of environmental and resource-related issues and their consequences.

In 1962, Rachel Carson, in her book *Silent Spring*, cautioned the public against the indiscriminate use of chemical pesticides. She argued that persistent substances

343

released into the environment move throughout the food chain, concentrating over time, while pests may develop a resistance to the poisons. By the 1960's, pollution from industrial and vehicular sources was beginning to be recognized as a global issue, as industrialized nations increased their spoliation and depletion of natural resources. In the United States, President John F. Kennedy introduced a number of natural resource initiatives aimed at preserving wilderness areas, developing marine resources, reserving shorelines for public use, expanding outdoor recreation, formulating plans for developing water resources and developing actions against water pollution, and encouraging the development of substitutes for resources in short supply. Also, he organized the Youth Conservation Corps to provide a workforce to implement the program. By the 1970's, during the administration of President Richard M. Nixon, the United States had begun to adopt environmental laws such as the Clean Air Act and created the Environmental Protection Agency as its enforcement agency. The first Earth Day to celebrate sustainable use of natural resources was in 1970.

The international community came together to discuss the environment for the first time in 1972. The United Nations held the Conference on the Human Environment in Stockholm, Sweden. This conference, which came to be known as the Stockholm Convention, resulted in the creation of the United Nations Environment Programme. The 1987 publication of the *Brundtland Report* (also known as the *Our Common Future*) by the United Nations World Commission on Environment and Development was one of the first documents to take on the issue of sustainable global development in modern times in a manner similar to that espoused by Pinchot in earlier times. The goal of the *Brundtland Report* was to foster global economic development that is conservation-oriented and economically balanced.

In 1980, another international organization became active in conservation. The International Union for Conservation of Nature (IUCN) published World Conservation Strategy (IUCN). The purpose of this publication, and one of the ongoing goals of the IUCN, was to assist developing nations in conservation planning to protect and maintain natural resources: air, water, soil, forests, and animals.

Since 1992, the international community and world leaders have continued to come together regularly to discuss global environmental problems. At the 1992 United

Nations Conference on Environment and Development held in Rio de Janeiro, Brazil, much of the discussion concerned the *Brundtland Report*. This conference, which came to be known as the "Rio Earth Summit," focused on dire predictions concerning global warming, climate change, the ozone hole; concerns about the depletion of natural resources, loss of habitats, and biodiversity; and continued concerns with resource pollution and depletion, especially forests and marine resources. Some experts at the Rio Summit suggested that society had to choose between economic development and conserving the environment. Although governments have been unwilling to make an either/or choice, one outcome of the Rio Earth Summit was the ratification by many nations of various international agreements to resolve some of the issues discussed at the Summit. For example, the Summit led to the ratification of the Montreal Protocol (1987), which concerns depletion of ozone by man-made chemicals, and the 1992 Kyoto Protocol, to limit industrial emissions that may be affecting global climate change.

Sustainable development became the main topic of discussion at the U.N. 2002 Earth Summit, held in Johannesburg, South Africa. Many world leaders came together to promulgate international regulations to address such environmental problems as improving air and water quality; improving food access, agricultural productivity, and sanitation in developing countries; and developing strategies and economic incentives to cope with international environmental issues related to war, poverty, and disease.

Although the United States has not been a signatory to some of the latter-day environmental protocols, environmental conservation organizations, including the Sierra Club, and individuals, such as former U.S. vice president Al Gore, alert the public to environmental issues. Gore won the 2007 Nobel Peace Prize together with the U.N. Intergovernmental Panel on Climate Change for their efforts in getting out the conservation message on global climate change. International organizations continued the conservation movement in preparation for the 2012 Earth Summit.

POPULATION AND RESOURCE CONSUMPTION
Population growth is a major factor when considering the time it will take to deplete the Earth's nonrenewable resources. A resource is considered economically depleted after 80 percent of its known reserves have been exploited, because at that point the resource becomes too

expensive for wide use. As the world's population grows, the rate of resource exploitation grows. More production is necessary to satisfy the needs and wants of larger populations: More materials are needed, more energy is consumed, and more pollution is created.

Ecologists have come to realize that the Earth is a huge ecosystem with a definite carrying capacity. That is, there is a limit to the number of people that can be supported by the Earth. The rate of resource depletion is a function both of the rate of population growth and of the rate of consumption of resources per person. More resources are consumed per individual in wealthy countries than in poor countries. As poor countries strive to develop, greater pressures are placed on the Earth to provide resources and to assimilate wastes. Overpopulation occurs when there are too many people for the available resources or when population growth exceeds economic growth; such conditions ultimately begin to cause damage to the Earth's life-support system.

WATER RESOURCES: THE NEXT GREAT CONFLICT
The availability and purity of water may be the next great natural resource issue facing the world, and control of water resources could lead to serious conflict. Water not only is necessary to sustain life and health but also is needed for food production and various industrial uses. Water resources continue to be polluted; rivers have dried up and have been dammed, thus reducing downriver flows to wetlands and floodplains; underground water supplies from aquifers have been used faster than they are replenished with rainfall; and development is destroying wetlands and other water resources and converting them, in some cases, to deserts. Because the global society has always relied on water as a renewable resource, it has continued using management policies that are no longer viable. In order to maintain human and wildlife populations, habitats, and health, and in order to ensure that there are sufficient water resources to sustain food production, water resource management policies must change.

OTHER NATURAL RESOURCE ISSUES
Other global natural-resource issues concern extractions from the Earth: minerals, precious metals, and gems such as diamonds; oil and gas drilling; and coal mining. Some of the methods used for these extractions and the consequences of accidents and spills have raised the global consciousness about their impact on the environment. A search for renewable resources to replace many

of these nonrenewable resources is under way within the global community.

Also controversial is the negative environmental impact of outdated rangeland management techniques, uncontrolled timber harvesting, forest destruction, and mismanaged disposal and dumping. Many developed nations suffer from wasteful consumerism and overuse of natural resources, such as those that provide energy. Government structures to foster conservation are lacking in most developing countries, and in many industrialized nations government leaders and the public are unwilling to make genuine efforts to conserve vital and dwindling natural resources, especially if they negatively impact economic growth. Scientists predict that these abuses of the environment and overuse of natural resources can no longer continue at their present rate if we want to preserve the future of humanity.

ECONOMICS AND CONSERVATION
Government and resource management plays an important part in the balancing of resource conservation and resource exploitation. Continued growth in the use of a nonrenewable resource can occur only for a number of years before the resource is depleted. As a resource becomes scarce, the price increases, making it less affordable and reducing the rate of consumption. This is a self-regulating process that makes conservation more practical as resources become more scarce in a market-driven system.

Effective conservation programs often require governmental influence, regulation, or incentives. Since most resources are associated with property, governmental agencies that regulate land, businesses, and private citizens all make decisions that affect resource consumption. The general aim of many decision makers is to maximize the return on investments; conservation must therefore be profitable within a reasonable time for people to practice it voluntarily. In a free enterprise system, resource exploitation produces income from the land and provides much of the incentive for land ownership. Thus, resource exploitation is likely to win out over conservation if there are no incentives to conserve.

Conservation practices must be congruent with economics. Conservation programs are not effectively executed when economic necessity or opportunity intervenes. For the most part, conservation is good for the economy over the long term, because it improves the efficiency of production systems. However, because modern economic growth has not been balanced and has not conserved natural resources, more drastic measures may be necessary to control future growth.

One of the more controversial proposals to combat economic growth issues facing the environment are taxes on carbon-related energy sources. Another highly debated policy recommendation is over emission trading, or cap-and-trade. Controlled ownership of resources through vehicles such as trusts to avoid depletion of natural resources—mostly nonrenewable resources—is another proposal being debated. Those involved in national and global political and social debate must become serious in reaching a consensus for resolving the many environmental issues facing the world and recommend sustainable policies that bring together economists and environmentalists in working for the same achievable goals regarding future growth. However, no matter what policies are eventually adopted, one of the main goals of balancing economic growth with conservation must be continued public awareness. The public and organizations are more likely to become supportive partners for sustainable economic growth if they are provided with not only information on economic growth and its effect on the environment, but also feasible, market-driven solutions.

ASSESSING THE FUTURE

Experts attempting to assess the future of natural resources are divided in their opinions. Positions range from optimistic to direly pessimistic to somewhere between the two extremes. Those who believe that technology can and will solve human problems have reason to be optimistic, and, to a great extent, history supports this view. Whenever humans experience shortages, they turn to technology for solutions—either developing more efficient ways of finding, extracting, and using resources or finding substitutes for them.

On the other hand, technology may not be able to continue solving all humankind's problems—at least not in a timely enough manner to avoid a crisis. The primary basis for the pessimistic argument is that increases in resource consumption rates, coupled with an increase in population, may not allow enough time to find technological solutions to resource shortages. Furthermore, the heavy modern dependence on nonrenewable resources is certain to cause resource shortages.

A more moderate view of the resource future suggests that, although there is good reason for concern, humankind has sufficient time to avoid a major crisis if we begin moving toward a sustainable society now. A sustainable society is one that allows humanity to meet its needs today without compromising its environment and future needs. Sustainability almost certainly requires that people in developed countries begin to live a lifestyle that includes more conservation and recycling, a greater dependence on renewable and perpetual resources than on nonrenewable resources, population control, and more self-discipline. This view embraces the ecological approach to resource management and employs the multiple-use concept. For example, forest conservation not only provides timber but also preserves a habitat for plants and animals; it can serve to help manage water resources, prevent flooding and soil erosion, and provide recreational areas. When we reach sustainability, most of humankind's material and energy needs will be provided by renewable and perpetual resources that should last indefinitely if properly managed.

The ecological approach is holistic. Based on the philosophy that all things in the natural environment are interlaced through a complex system of feedback loops, it implies that the whole is functionally greater than the sum of its parts. This approach to resource management requires an understanding and anticipation of the consequences of human actions throughout the ecosystem. ConservationSustainable development

FURTHER READING

Castillon, David A. *Conservation of Natural Resources: A Resource Management Approach.* 2d ed. Madison, Wis.: Brown Benchmark, 1996.

Chiras, Daniel D., and John P. Reganold. *Natural Resource Conservation: Management for a Sustainable Future.* 10th ed. Upper Saddle River, N.J.: Pearson Prentice Hall, 2009.

Degregori, Thomas R. *The Environment, Our Natural Resources, and Modern Technology.* New York: John Wiley & Sons, 2008.

Freyfogle, Eric T. *Why Conservation Is Failing and How It Can Regain Ground.* New Haven, Conn.: Yale University Press, 2006.

Greenland, David. *Guidelines for Modern Resource Management: Soil, Land, Water, Air.* Columbus, Ohio: C. E. Merrill, 1983.

Greiner, Alfred, and Will Semmler. *The Global Environment, Natural Resources, and Economic Growth.* New York: Oxford University Press, 2008.

Harper, Charles L. *Environment and Society: Human Perspectives on Environmental Issues.* 4th ed. Upper Saddle River, N.J.: Pearson/Prentice Hall, 2008.

Jakab, Cheryl. *Natural Resources (Global Issues)*. North Mankato, Minn.: Smart Apple Media, 2008.

Knight, Richard L., and Courtney White, eds. *Conservation for a New Generation: Redefining Natural Resources Management*. Washington, D.C.: Island Press, 2009.

Krupp, Fred, and Miriam Horn. *Earth: The Sequel—The Race to Reinvent Energy and Stop Global Warming*. New York: W. W. Norton, 2008.

Loeffe, Christian V., ed. *Conservation and Recycling of Resources: New Research*. New York: Nova Science, 2006.

Miller, G. Tyler, Jr. *Resource Conservation and Management*. Belmont, Calif.: Wadsworth, 1990.

Parson, Ruben L. *Conserving American Resources*. 3d ed. Englewood Cliffs, N.J.: Prentice-Hall, 1972.

Raven, Peter H., Linda R. Berg, and David M. Hassenzahl. *Environment*. 6th ed. Hoboken, N.J.: Wiley, 2008.

Scott, Nicky. *Reduce, Reuse, Recycle: An Easy Household Guide*. White River Junction, Vt.: Chelsea Green, 2007.

Conservation International. http://www.conservation.org/Pages/default.aspx

International Union for Conservation of Nature. http://www.iucn.org/

The Nature Conservancy. http://www.nature.org/

United Nations Environment Programme. http://www.unep.org/

World Resources Institute. http://www.wri.org/

World Wildlife Fund. http://www.panda.org/

Worldwatch Institute. http://www.worldwatch.org/

Jasper L. Harris, updated by Carol A. Rolf

SEE ALSO: Organic Food Industry; Recycling Technology; Renewable Energy Resources

Fracking and tar sand fuels

Hydraulic fracturing (fracking) is the process of drilling and injecting fluid into the ground at high pressure in order to fracture shale rocks to release natural gas. This is a controversial issue because, as the level of carbon dioxide in the atmosphere continues to rise, portending hotter temperatures and a more unstable climate, fracking adds greenhouse gases to the atmosphere, and leaves behind strip-mined lands that have been compared to moon-scapes (in Alberta) and an increasing number of earthquakes in areas.

INTRODUCTION

While exploitation of tar sands has brought prosperity to Alberta, it requires a form of strip mining that scars the earth in ways that will not be quickly nor easily repaired. Opponents also assert that oil sands are a relatively new form of fossil fuel — the last thing the Earth needs when carbon-dioxide levels in the atmosphere have risen to more than 400 parts per million, more than 40 per cent above peak pre-industrial levels, with damage to climate, as well as rising seas and oceanic acidity. On a local level, many people worry about oil spills in fragile areas such as the Nebraska Sand Hills that could contaminate the Ogallala aquifer in an area where water is scarce. This aquifer supplies 78 per cent of public water and 83 per cent of irrigation water in Nebraska, almost a third of the irrigation water used in the United States.

Fracking has brought prosperity to North Dakota and Oklahoma, but also has been linked to earthquakes and water pollution. Until recent years, earthquakes were very rare in Oklahoma, which is not a seismically active area for natural reasons. Earthquakes, some as strong as 5.6 on the Richter scale, became more common, increasing from an average of two a year (3.0 or greater) until 2008, to 20 in 2009, 42 in 2010, and 585 in 2014, triple the number in California. If all earthquakes are included, Oklahoma experienced more than 5,000 that year (Galchen, 2015).

BENEFITS OF FRACKING AND TAR SANDS

The oil industry asserts that consumers will receive a secure source of vital energy from fracking and tar sands that does not depend on volatile Middle Eastern markets. Fracking, the tar sands industry, and its transportation pipelines provide employment. About 20 per cent of Alberta's gross domestic product stems from tar sands mining and refining, and fracking has brought widespread prosperity to North Dakota, Oklahoma, and other U.S. regions. Tar sands also provide tax revenue through an Alberta provincial carbon tax. The technology of refining tar sands into oil also has become more efficient during the last twenty years, as carbon emissions from its mining operations have declined about 25 per cent since 1990. In support of the Keystone XL and other pipelines, TransCanada asserts (with statistical support) that transport of oil by pipeline is much safer than by train.

TAR SANDS PRODUCTION

According to NASA, the Alberta tar sands fields, which were first mined in 1967, are "the world's largest oil sands deposit, with a capacity to produce 174.5 billion barrels of oil—2.5 million barrels of oil per day for 186 years" (Athabasca Oil Sands, 2011). The United States as a whole consumes 15 to 20 million barrels of oil per day. Environmental activist Bill McKibben has called tar sands mining and the Keystone XL the "fuse to the biggest carbon bomb on the planet" (Tollefson, 2013). "Saying that the tar sands are not necessarily worse than coal is like saying that drinking arsenic is not necessarily worse than drinking cyanide," said geophysicist Raymond Pierrehumbert of the University of Chicago. He said that fully developing the tar sands could by itself, even if combustion of coal stopped, to warm the Earth an additional 3.6 degrees Fahrenheit by century's end — to a degree that climate scientists warn could be catastrophic (Koch, 2014).

Tar sands are a mixture of clay and sand with bitumen, a thick, low-grade form of petroleum similar to asphalt. According to Thomas Homer-Dixon, who teaches global governance at the Balsillie School of International Affairs, "Tar sands production is one of the world's most environmentally damaging activities. It wrecks vast areas of boreal forest through surface mining and subsurface production. It sucks up huge quantities of water from local rivers, turns it into toxic waste and dumps the contaminated water into tailing ponds that now cover nearly 70 square miles" (Homer-Dixon, 2013).

"If Canada proceeds [with oil-sands development], and we do nothing, it will be game over for the climate," James Hansen, retired head of NASA's Goddard Institute for Space Studies and author of Storms of My Grandchildren, wrote in the New York Times:

"Canada's tar sands, deposits of sand saturated with bitumen, contain twice the amount of carbon dioxide emitted by global oil use in our entire history. If we were to fully exploit this new oil source, and continue to burn our conventional oil, gas and coal supplies, concentrations of carbon dioxide in the atmosphere eventually would reach levels higher than in the Pliocene era, more than 2.5 million years ago, when sea level was at least 50 feet higher than it is now. That level of heat-trapping gases would assure that the disintegration of the ice sheets would accelerate out of control. Sea levels would rise and destroy coastal cities. Global temperatures would become intolerable. Twenty to 50 percent of the planet's species would be driven to extinction. Civilization would be at risk.... If this sounds apocalyptic, it is. (Hansen, 2012).

The concentration of carbon dioxide in the atmosphere has risen from 280 parts per million to slightly more than 400 p.p.m. over the last 150 years, as of 2014. The tar sands contain enough carbon — 240 gigatons — to add 120 p.p.m. Tar shale, similar to tar sands found mainly in the United States, contains at least an additional 300 gigatons of carbon. If we turn to these dirtiest of fuels, instead of finding ways to phase out our addiction to fossil fuels, there is no hope of keeping carbon concentrations below 500 p.p.m. — a level that would, as earth's history shows, leave our children a climate system that is out of their control (Hansen, 2012)."

FRACKING AND EARTHQUAKES

The oil industry in Oklahoma maintains that the increasing number of quakes is a natural problem. United States Geological Survey Geologist William Ellsworth, however, said: "We can say with virtual certainty that the increased seismicity in Oklahoma has to do with recent changes in the way that oil and gas are being produced" (Galchen, 2015, 35). Nearly without exception, the stronger earthquakes by fracking disposal wells, in which brackish water in large amounts (totaling billions of barrels) are pumped into the ground after having been brought up during mining of oil shales underground. Other states (Ohio, Arkansas, Texas, Colorado, and Texas, among others) in areas not noted for earthquakes also have been recording increasing numbers in fracked areas where waste water has been poured back into the earth, although none in the numbers that by 2015 were shaking Oklahoma with an average of two quakes per day.

Late in April, 2015, the United States Geological Survey released a map identifying 17 regions with significant levels of earthquake activity that it attributed to oil and gas operations, mainly waste-water disposal from fracking. By far the greatest concentration of earth-moving incidents was located by the USGS in Oklahoma. This map was released two days after Oklahoma's own state-run Geological Survey issued a map of its own, and acknowledged for the first time that the state's rapid rise in earthquakes within a few years could be traced to oil waste-water disposal initiated by the fracking boom.

FURTHER READING

"Athabasca oil sands. (2011, November 30). *NASA Earth Observatory*. Retrieved from:http://earthobservatory.nasa.gov/IOTD/view.php?id=76559&src=eoa-iotd This satellite survey includes views of oil sands mining.

Galchen, R. (2015, April 13). "Weather underground." *New Yorker*, 34-40. This report describes Oklahoma earthquakes that have been attributed to disposal of water used in fracking.

Hansen, J. (2012, May 9). "Game Over for the Climate." *New York Times*. Retrieved from:http://www.nytimes.com/2012/05/10/opinion/game-over-for-the-climate.html Hansen, a renowned climate scientist, asserts that full exploitation of tar (oil) sands will drive global warming past tolerable limits.

Homer-Dixon, T. 2013, March 31). "The tar sands disaster." *New York Times*. Retrieved from: http://www.nytimes.com/2013/04/01/opinion/the-tar-sands-disaster.html This opinion piece argues that tar sands mining is ruining Native American lands in Alberta.

Koch, W. (2014, March 10). Would Keystone pipeline unload "carbon bomb" or job boom? *USA Today*. Retrieved from: http://www.usatoday.com/story/news/nation/2014/03/01/keystonexls-myths-debunked/5651099/ This report develops the debate over the economic and environmental effects of oil transported from Alberta through the United States.

Kolbert, E. (2007, November 12). Unconventional crude: Canada's synthetic-fuels boom. *New Yorker*, 46-51. Kolbert, a veteran environmental writer, visited Alberta and reported on the boom in unconventional crude.

Tollefson, J. (2013, August 8). Climate science: A line in the sands. *Nature* 500:136-137. http://www.nature.com/news/climate-science-a-line-in-the-sands-1.135150 This scientific survey dissects the effects of unconventional oil mining on climate.

Bruce E. Johansen

See Also: Alternative Fuels (Wind, Solar, Ethanol); Biofuels; Conservation; Nonrenewable Energy Resources; Renewable Energy Resources.

Genetically modified foods

Genetically modified foods are produced through the application of recombinant DNA technology to crop breeding, whereby genes from the same or different species are transferred and expressed in crops that do not naturally harbor those genes. While GM crops offer great potential for food production in agriculture, their release has spurred various concerns among the general public.

THE TECHNOLOGY

Genetically modified (GM) foods are food products derived from genetically modified organisms (GMOs). GMOs may have genes deleted, added, or replaced for a particular trait; they constitute one of the most important means by which crop plants will be improved in the future. The advantage of using genetic engineering is quite obvious: It allows individual genes to be inserted into organisms in a way that is both precise and simple. Using molecular tools available, DNA molecules from entirely different species can now be spliced together to form a recombinant DNA molecule.

The recombinant DNA molecule can then be introduced into a cell or tissue through genetic transformation. When a particular gene that codes for a trait is successfully introduced to an organism and expressed, that organism is defined as a transgenic or GM organism. Transgenic organismsgenetically modified foods

Most of the GM crops in production thus far have modified crop protection characteristics, mainly improving protection against insects and competition (herbicide resistance). Some have improved nutritional quality and longer shelf life. Yet others under development will lift yield caps previously not possible to overcome by conventional means. Because of the direct access to and recombination of genetic material from any source, the normal reproductive barrier among different species can now be circumvented. All these modifications offer great potential for creating transgenic animals and plants useful to humankind, but GMOs also pose the possibility of misuse and unintended outcomes.

CONCEIVABLE BENEFITS OF GM FOODS

The potential benefits of using genetic engineering to develop new cultivars are evident. Crop yields can be increased by introducing genes that increase the crop's resistance to various pathogens or herbicides and enhance its tolerance to various stresses. The increased food supply is vital to support a growing population with shrinking land. One well-known example is the introduction of the Bt gene from the bacterium Bacillus thuringiensis to several crops, including corn, cotton, and soybeans. When the Bt gene is transferred to plants, the plant cells produce a protein toxic to some insects and hence become resistant to these insects. The grains of Bt maize were also found to contain low mycotoxin, thus exhibiting better food safety than non-GM corns. Another example is the successful insertion of a gene resistant to the herbicide glyphosate, reducing production costs and increasing grain purity.

Food quality can be improved in other ways. Soybeans and canola with reduced saturated fats (healthier oil) have been developed. Alterations in the starch content of potatoes and the nutritional quality of protein in maize kernels are being developed. More precise gene transfer is also being used to produce desirable products that the plant does not normally make. The potential products include pharmaceutical proteins (for example, vaccines), vitamins, and plastic compounds. "Golden rice" has been engineered to produce significantly higher vitamin A precursors. This GM rice plays an important role in alleviating vision loss and blindness caused by vitamin A deficiency among those who consume rice as their main staple food. Attempts are being made to increase nitrogen availability, a limiting factor in crop production, by transferring genes responsible for nitrogen fixation into crops such as wheat and maize. In addition, the reduction in the use of fertilizers, insecticides, and herbicides for GM crops not only saves billions of dollars in costs but also alleviates the damage to wild organisms and ecosystems.

CONCERNS ABOUT GM FOODS

Like any other technological innovation, genetic engineering in crop breeding and production does not come without risk or controversy. Some of the common questions raised by consumers include concerns over what plant and animal organisms they are now putting into their bodies, whether these are safe, whether they have been tested, why they are not labeled as GM foods, and whether GM foods might not contain toxins or allergens not present in their natural counterparts. Although most of these questions are understandable, the public uproar concerning the GM crops and other foods, particularly in Great Britain and Europe, are, from a scientific standpoint, an overreaction. Most of the general public does not understand much about the genetic engineering

technology, and scientists need to increase their efforts to educate the public.

Second, most people are not aware of the strict regulations imposed on GM research and active safeguards by most governments. In the United States, research and chemical analyses by many scientists working with the Food and Drug Administration(FDA), the U.S. Department of Agriculture (USDA), or independently have concluded that biotechnology is a safe means of producing foods. Thousands of tests over fifteen years in the United States, along with the consumption of GM foods in the United States for four years, have revealed no evidence of harmful effects related to GM foods. Most food safetyFood safety problems arise from handling (for example, microbial contamination), for GM and non-GM foods alike.

A third reason for the societal concern is rooted in negative media opinion, opposition by activists, and mistrust of the industry. Most current complaints about GM foods can be categorized into three major areas: the possible detrimental health effects, the potential environmental threats such as "superweeds," and the social, economic, and ethical implications of genetic engineering. Some activists have taken extreme measures, such as destroying field plots and even firebombing a research laboratory. Although the majority of the public do not agree with the extreme measures taken by some activists, some continue to push for mandatory labeling of all foods whose components have derived from GMOs. Activist groups and media also continue to create myths and release misinformation regarding GM foods: GMOs have no benefit to the consumer, they may harm the environment, they are unsafe to eat, the only beneficiary of GM foods is big corporations, GM crops do not benefit small farmers, or they will will drive organic farmers out of business.

BROADER ISSUES IN BIOTECHNOLOGY

Although some concerns are genuine—particularly ecological concerns regarding gene flow from GM plants to wild relatives—one should not ignore the fact that safety is a relative concept. Agriculture and animal husbandry have inherent dangers, as does the consumption of their products, regardless of GM or non-GM foods. In response to the demands of activist groups, the European Union (EU) and its member states adopted strict regulations over the import and release of GMOs. GM crops and foods are being subjected to more safety checks and tighter regulation than their non-GM counterparts. Through extensive studies and analyses, both the USDA and the EU have found no perceptible difference between conventional and GM foods. Of course, one cannot ensure consumers of absolute, zero risk with regard to any drug or food product, regardless of how they are produced. The demand for zero risk is more of an emotional reaction than realistically possible. Mandatory labeling on all GM foods is both impractical and technically difficult and would drive food prices to much higher levels than consumers are willing to pay. Farmers and the food industry would have to sort every GMO and store and process them separately. Realizing the complexity, federal agencies like the FDA and USDA have recommended a voluntary labeling system by which the organic and non-GM food products can be marked for consumers who are willing to pay the premium.

WHERE DO WE GO FROM HERE?

Development of new crops is vital for the future of the world. Since conventional breeding cannot keep up with the population explosion, biotechnology may be the best tool available to produce a greater diversity and high quality of safe food on less land, while conserving soil, water, and genetic diversity. To ensure the safety and success of GM crops, scientists and regulators will need to have open and honest communications with the public, building trust through better education and more effective regulatory oversights. In the meantime, the media will also need to convey more credible, balanced information to the public.

As Nobel laureate Norman Borlaug, father of the Green Revolution, stated, "I now say that the world has the technology that is either available or well advanced in the research pipeline to feed a population of 10 billion people. The more pertinent question is: Will farmers and ranchers be permitted to use this new technology?"

FURTHER READING

Borlaug, Norman E. "Ending World Hunger: The Promise of Biotechnology and the Threat of Antiscience Zealotry." *Plant Physiology* 124, no. 2 (October, 2000): 487-490. The father of the Green Revolution and Nobel Peace Prize winner speaks of his unwavering support for GMOs.

Cummins, Ronnie, and Ben Lilliston. *Genetically Engineered Food: A Self-Defense Guide for Consumers.* 2d rev. ed. New York: Marlowe, 2004. Examines the scientific, political, economic, and health issues related to genetically engineered food. Argues that the new food technology has not been adequately tested for safety and that genetically engineered food is being sold without proper labeling.

Fedoroff, Nina V., and Nancy Marie Brown. *Mendel in the Kitchen: A Scientist's View of Genetically Modified Foods.* Washington, D.C.: Joseph Henry Press, 2004. Argues that genetically modified foods are safe, nutritionally enhanced products that can fill a major vitamin deficiency in the Third World. Describes the technology of food engineering, maintaining that the risks associated with this technology are trivial.

Fresco, Louise O. "Genetically Modified Organisms in Food and Agriculture: Where Are We? Where Are We Going?" Keynote Address, Conference on Crop and Forest Biotechnology for the Future, September, 2001. Falkenberg, Sweden: Royal Swedish Academy of Agriculture and Forestry, 2001. Fascinating and informative perspectives on GM foods by a European Union scientist.

Heller, Knut J., ed. *Genetically Engineered Food: Methods and Detection.* 2d updated and enl. ed. Weinheim, Germany: Wiley-VCH, 2006. Covers methods and applications of genetically engineering food, including transgenic modification of production traits in farm animals, fermented food production, and the production of food additives using filamentous fungi. Examines legal issues regarding genetic engineering. Describes methods for detecting genetic engineering in composed and processed foods.

Potrykus, Ingo. "Golden Rice and Beyond." *Plant Physiology* 125, no. 3 (March, 2001): 1157-1161. The originator of the wonder rice presents scientific, ethical, intellectual, and social challenges of developing and using the GMOs. Illuminating and insightful.

Ronald, Pamela C., and Raoul W. Adamchak. *Tomorrow's Table: Organic Farming, Genetics, and the Future of Food.* New York: Oxford University Press, 2008. Examines the debate about genetically engineered food and how it might affect the future food supply, weighing arguments for and against technologically created food.

WEB SITES OF INTEREST

Agbios.http://www.agbios.com/main.php. Contains a database of safety information on all genetically modified plant products that have received regulatory approval, information on the implementation of biosafety systems, and a searchable library of biosafety-related citations in key topic areas.

AgBioWorld.org. http://www.agbioworld.org. Advocates the use of biotechnology and GM foods.

Agriculture Network Information Center. http://www.agnic.org. Offers information on agricultural topics, including transgenic crops.

Physicians and Scientists for Responsible Application of Science and Technology. http://www.psrast.org. Developed for the general reader, this site discusses the risks of genetically modified foods. Topics include a general introduction to the topic and "Alarming Facts About Genetically Engineered Foods."

Transgenic Crops. http://cls.casa.colostate.edu/TransgenicCrops/index.html. This richly illustrated site provides information on genetically modified foods, including new developments, the history of plant breeding, the making of transgenic plants, government regulations, and risks and concerns. This site is also available in Spanish.

World Health Organization. http://www.who.int/foodsafety/publications/biotech/20questions/en. A list of twenty questions and answers that provides an objective overview of the issues surrounding genetically modified foods.

Ming Y. Zheng

SEE ALSO: Becoming a Green Consumer; Buying Local; Organic Food Industry

Greywater

Greywater (also called Graywater, or sullage) is formerly used water from homes, office buildings, and factories (as opposed to sewage from toilets, called "blackwater"). Greywater includes run-off from sinks, showers and baths, as well as washing of clothes and dishes, as well as various industrial processes. With the advent of recent widespread drought, especially a multi-year, intense erosion of water supplies in California and elsewhere in the United States Southwest, greywater is receiving attention for its re-use potential. Greywater recycling systems are being developed and patented for use by individual houses in areas where drought has intensified. As of 2015, roughly 8 million greywater systems in the United States were in use. A complete home greywater system can collect up to 40 gallons of water per person per day, or about half of what many people use, according to a report in the Los Angeles Times *(Stevens and Grad, 2015).*

INTRODUCTION

Use of greywater has been adapted in many countries, from aiding in restoration of wetlands in Norway to re-use of water in Frankfurt, Germany office buildings, and schools in India. The fastest-growing market, however, has been drought-stricken California, where severe water rationing has forced nearly everyone to take a crash course in water conservation.

With new designs, household greywater is gathered separate from sewage (toilet) water so that it can be used on site without fear of contamination that requires treatment of sewage water at a remote location. If greywater is stored, however, it must be considered perishable and used within a short time because it contains organic solids that may putrefy. Recycled greywater should never be used for drinking. Greywater also may be treated with various filters (membrane bioereactors, sand, and lava, for example).

Greywater is widely enough used to be subject to the International Plumbing Code, which, for example, allows water from bathtubs and showers to be re-used for flushing toilets in much of Europe, as well as Australia, and in sections of the United States that subscribe to it. Such use may reduce household water use by about 30 per cent. Use of a cleaning tank to segregate floating and sinking biological contaminants is advised. A device may be timed to flush automatically so that greywater will not be stored past a time when it may putrefy and become hazardous, usually 24 hours. Grey water is meant to be used. Without daily evacuation, anaerobic bacteria may grow. Users of greywater also should avoid re-use of water containing bleach, artificial dyes, and chlorine, which is used as a base in many household cleaners and solvents. Such things raise the salt level in soil and kill plants, especially at the germination stage. Greywater used on soils may be mixed with gypsum (calcium sulfate) to reduce acidity.

With these safeguards greywater also may be used where potable water used for drinking and cooking is not required, such as watering lawns and flushing toilets. Re-use of greywater reduces demand for freshwater as well as sewage-processing services, providing a more environmentally sustainable system, in addition to a reduction in use of fresh water from lakes, streams, and aquifers.

Devices also have been developed (called "drainwater heat recovery") to recover heat from water used in dishwashers, showers, or some industrial processes, taking what would have been wasted heat and putting it to use.

Incoming cold water flows through a heat exchanger, saving roughly half the cost of heating it.

GREYWATER AT GROUND LEVEL

Ability to use greywater may be restricted in jurisdictions that classify all waste water as sewage. In such areas, greywater treatment is usually required through a central sewage system or household septic tank. Adoption of the Uniform Plumbing Code, which allows greywater to be separated from sewage, has generally taken place in areas with persistent water shortages that provide an incentive for conservation, such as Wyoming, California, Utah, and New Mexico. California has made accommodation of greywater a priority not only because of intense drought, but also because of state policy that favors ecologically sustainable planning that will reduce emissions of greenhouse gases. California has added a section on "Non-Potable Water Reuse Systems" to its state plumbing code.

The more complicated systems for use of greywater may require separation of blackwater and greywater waste lines in a structure, something that can be designed into new construction, but may require expensive, reconstructed plumbing in an existing house or business, often involving addition of a sub-surface greywater system. Greywater installation also may involve modification of existing septic systems.

The *Los Angeles Daily News* provided a sketch of a homeowner who uses greywater to alleviate that area's historic drought:

"In the backyard of Penny Pengra's home in Glendale, California, there are no signs of the historic drought that has ravaged Southern California for the past three years.

'My plants are crazy awesome,' says the 40-something who works in television, crediting her lush, green backyard oasis to the affordable, low-tech grey water system she had installed last year (Barrera, 2014)."

The systems vary from low-tech, inexpensive gravity-flow systems with no pumps or filters to the self-cleaning ReWater, which is called the "Rolls Royce of grey water systems" (Barrera, 2014). Pengra's system is the most basic. It guides used shower water to her plants with an assist from gravity. Her system required no permit, inspection or fees, and little construction. A free diagram is available at http://greywatercorps.com. "Filters can be pretty gross so we tend to stick to really low-tech systems that have no filters and just bigger pipes so there's no clogging issues," said Leigh Jerrard, a licensed architect who founded Greywater Corps in 2009, and installs

residential grey water systems in Southern California (Barrera, 2014).

An analysis in *Off the Grid News* agreed with Jerrard – keep it simple if possible: "Although there have been zero reports of illnesses caused by grey water recycling, it does not mean that we should not exercise care when implementing grey water systems, especially when those systems are home projects with little or no filtration involved. Avoid using pumps and complicated filtering systems as much as possible. These require a lot of maintenance and cleaning, not to mention the unnecessary drain on electricity. A system that allows grey water to naturally flow downwards is much more efficient" (Ultimate Guide, n.d.).

FURTHER READING

Albrechtsen, H., Binning, P., and Rygaard, M. (2010). Increasing urban water self sufficiency: new era, new challenges. *Journal of Environmental Management*, 92(1), 185. Retrieved from http://0-go.galegroup.com.libcat.lafayette.edu/ps/i.do?&id=GALE|A239692841&v= 2.1&u=east55695&it=r&p=AONE&sw=w. This article focuses alternatives to fresh water resources on a policy level.

Barrera, Sandra.(2014, October 30). "For good or bad, grey water systems becoming more popular due to drought." *Los Angeles Daily News.* http://www.dailynews.com/lifestyle/20141030/for-good-or-bad-grey-water-systems-becoming-more-popular-due-to-drought. This piece contains brief descriptions of greywater use in Los Angeles.

Godfrey S., Labhasetwar P., and Wate S. (2009). Greywater reuse in residential schools in Madhya Pradesh, India -- A case study of cost-benefit analysis. *Resources, Conservation & Recycling* 287, retrieved May 22, 2015 from: http://0- go.galegroup.com.libcat.lafayette.edu/ps/i.do?&id=GALE% 7CA194627792&v=2.1&u=east55695&it=r&p=AONE&sw=w. Greywater has been put to use in a school setting in India, as described in this paper.

Stevens, M. and Grad, S. (2015, April 15). "L.A. pushes to use shower, bathwater to combat drought." Los Angeles Times. http://www.latimes.com/local/lanow/la-me-ln-la-pushes-to-use-shower-bath-water-to-combat-drought-20150415-story.html. This newspaper account describes simple, practical greywater systems that have been installed in drought-stricken Southern California.

"Ultimate guide to re-using grey water." (n.d.) Off-the-grid news. Accessed May 21, 2015. http://www.offthegridnews.com/how-to-2/ultimate-guide-to-re-using-grey-water/. This practical guide focuses on low-tech gravity systems.

Bruce E. Johansen

SEE ALSO: Conservation; Recycling; Nonrenewable Energy Resources; Renewable Energy Resources

Hybrid vehicles

Hybrid vehicle technologies use shared systems of electrical and gas power to create ecologically sustainable industrial and passenger vehicles. With both types of vehicles, the main goals are to reduce hazardous emissions and conserve fuel consumption.

DEFINITION AND BASIC PRINCIPLES

As the word "hybrid" suggests, hybrid vehicle technology seeks to develop an automobile (or, more broadly defined, any power-driven mechanical system) using power from at least two different sources. Before and during the first decade of the twenty-first century, hybrid technology emphasized the combination of an internal combustion engine working with an electric motor component.

BACKGROUND AND HISTORY

Before technological development of what is now called a hybrid vehicle, the automobile industry, by necessity, had to have two existing forms of motor energy to hybridize--namely internal combustion in combination with some form of electric power. Early versions of cars driven with electric motors emerged in the 1890's and seemed destined to compete very seriously with both gasoline (internal combustion engines) and steam engines at the turn of the twentieth century.

Although development of commercially attractive hybrid vehicles would not occur until the middle of the twentieth century, the Austrian engineer Ferdinand Porsche made a first-series hybrid automobile in 1900. Within a short time, however, the commercial attractiveness of mass-produced internal combustion engines became the force that dominated the automobile industry for more than a half century. Experimentation with hybrid technology as it could be applied to other forms of

transport, especially motorcycles, however, continued throughout this early period.

By the 1970's the main emerging goal of hybrid car engineering was to reduce exhaust emissions; conservation of fuel was a secondary consideration. This situation changed when, in the wake of the 1973 Arab-Israeli War, many petroleum-producing countries supporting the Arab cause cut exports drastically, causing a nationwide gas shortage and worldwide fears that oil would be used as a political weapon.

Until 1975 government support for research and development of hybrid cars was tied to the Environmental Protection Agency (EPA). In that year (and after at least two unsatisfactory results of EPA-supported hybrid car projects), this role was shifted to the Energy Research and Development Administration, which later became the Department of Energy (DOE).

During the decade that followed the introduction of Honda's Insight hybrid car in 1999, the most widely recognized commercially marketed hybrid automobile was Toyota's Prius. Despite some setbacks in sales in 2010 following major recalls connected with (among other less dangerous problems) the malfunctioning anti-lock braking system and accelerator devices, the third-generation Prius still held a strong position in total hybrid car sales globally going into 2011.

HOW IT WORKS

"Integrated motor assist," a common layperson's engineering phrase borrowed from Honda's late-1990's technology, suggests a simple explanation of how a hybrid vehicle works. The well-known relationship between the electrical starter motor and the gas-driven engine in an internal combustion engine (ICE) car provides a (technically incomplete) analogy: The electric starter motor takes the load needed to turn the crankcase (and the wheels if gears are engaged) until the ICE itself kicks in. This overly general analogy could be carried further by including the alternator in the system, since it relieves the battery of the job of supplying constant electricity to the running engine (recharging the battery at the same time).

In a hybrid system, however, power from the electric motor (or the gas engine) enters and leaves the drivetrain as the demand for power to move the vehicle increases or decreases. To obtain optimum results in terms of carbon dioxide emissions and overall fuel efficiency, the power train of most hybrid vehicles is designed to depend on a relatively small internal

FASCINATING FACTS ABOUT HYBRID VEHICLE TECHNOLOGIES

The basic technology that is being used, albeit in perfected form, in post-2000 hybrid vehicles was first used to manufacture a working hybrid car more than one hundred years ago.

Consideration of total weight of a hybrid vehicle is so important that engineers devote major attention to possible innovations for any and all hybrid electric vehicle (HEV) components. The most obvious component that undergoes changes from one generation of HEV to the next involves ever-more-efficient modes of supplying electrical energy.

Technological use of hybrid power systems need not, probably will not, be limited to land transportation. It is possible that aviation--a transport sector that went from conventional to jet engines in the middle of the 20th century--could become considerably more economical and ecological by a combination of power sources.

Many major cities, especially in Europe (most notably Paris) have fleets of municipal bicycles that can be checked in and out for inner-city use by individuals physically capable and desirous of peddling. It is to be hoped that a next stage--hourly rentals of small HEVs, especially those with major electrical power sources--will follow when production of "basic" (markedly less expensive) hybrid vehicles becomes feasible.

As more and more sophisticated hybrid-power procedures are developed, the possibility of using different forms of fuel, and eventually bypassing dependence on petroleum, and even biofuels, is a long-range goal of hybrid technology.

Using regenerative braking, engineers are able to recover electric energy from the magnetic field created when braking results and store it in the HEV's battery for future use.

---

combustion engine with various forms of rechargeable electrical energy. Although petroleum-driven ICE's are commonly used, hybrid car engineering is not limited to petroleum. Ethanol, biodiesel, and natural gas have also been used.

In a parallel hybrid, the electric motor and ICE are installed so that they can power the vehicle either individually or together. These power sources are integrated by automatically controlled clutches. For electric driving, the clutch between the ICE and the gearbox is disengaged, while the clutch connecting the electric motor to the gearbox is engaged. A typical situation requiring simultaneous operation of the ICE and the electric motor would be for rapid acceleration (as in passing) or in climbing hills. Reliance on the electric motor would happen only when the car is braking, coasting, or advancing on level surfaces.

It is extremely important to note that one of the most vital challenges for researchers involved in hybrid-vehicle technology has to do with variable options for supplying electricity to the system. It is far too simple to say that the electrical motor is run by a rechargeable battery, since a wide range of batteries (and alternatives to batteries) exists. A primary and obvious concern, of course, will always be reducing battery weight. To this aim, several carmakers, including Ford, have developed highly effective first-, second-, and even third-generation lithium-ion batteries. Many engineers predict that, in the future, hydrogen-driven fuel cells will play a bigger role in the electrical components of hybrids.

Selection of the basic source of electrical power ties in with corollary issues such as calculation of the driving range (time elapsed and distances covered before the electrical system must be recharged) and optimal technologies for recharging. The simplest scenario for recharging, which is an early direct borrowing from pure-electric car technology, involves plugging into a household outlet (either 110 volt or 220 volt) overnight. But, hybrid-car engineers have developed several more sophisticated methods. One is a "sub-hybrid" procedure, which uses very lightweight fuel cells, mentioned above, in combination with conventional batteries (the latter being recharged by the fuel cells while the vehicle is underway). Research engineers continue to look at any number of ways to tweak energy and power sources from different phases of hybrid vehicle operation. One example, which has been used in Honda's Insight, is a process that temporarily converts the motor into a generator when the car does not require application of the accelerator. Other channels are being investigated for tapping kinetic-energy recovery during different phases of simple mechanical operation of hybrid vehicles.

APPLICATIONS AND PRODUCTS

Some countries, especially Japan, have begun to use the principle of the hybrid engine for heavy-duty transport or construction-equipment needs, as well as hybrid systems for diesel road graders and new forms of diesel-powered industrial cranes. Hybrid medium-power commercial vehicles, especially urban trolleys and buses, have been manufactured, mainly in Europe and Japan. Important for broad ecological planning, several countries, including China and Japan, have incorporated hybrid (diesel combined with electric) technology into their programs for rail transport. The biggest potential consumer market for hybrid technology, however, is probably in the private automobile sector.

By the second decade of the twenty-first century, a wide variety of commercially produced hybrid automobiles were on European, Asian, and American markets. Among U.S. manufacturers, Ford has developed the increasingly popular Escape, and General Motors produces about five models ranging from Chevrolet's economical Volt to Cadillac's more expensive Escalade. Japanese manufacturers Nissan, Honda, and Toyota have introduced at least one, three, and two standard hybrid models, respectively, to which one should add Lexus's RX semi-luxury and technologically more advanced series of cars. Korea's Hyundai Elantra and Germany's Volkswagen Golf also competed for some share of the market.

One of the chief attractions to Toyota's hybrid technology has usually been its primary goal of using electric motors in as many operational phases as possible. The closest sales competitor in the United States to the Prius (mainly for mileage efficiency) was Chevrolet's Volt.

At the outset of 2011, Lexus launched an ambitious campaign to attract attention to what it called its full hybrid technology(as compared with mild hybrid) in its high-end RX models. A main feature of the full hybrid system, according to Lexus, is a combination of both series and parallel hybrid power in one vehicle. Such a combination aims at transferring a variable but continuously optimum ratio of gas-engine and electric-motor power to the car. Another advance claimed by Lexus's full hybrid over parallel hybrids is its reliance on the electric motor only at lower speeds.

Early in 2011, Mercedes-Benz also announced its intention to capture more sales of high-end hybrids by dedicating, over a three-year period, more research to improve the technology used in its S400 model. Audi, a somewhat latecomer, unveiled plans for its first hybrid, the Q5, to appear in European markets late in 2011.

As fuel alternatives continue to be added to the ICE components of HEVs, advanced fuel-cell technology could transform the technological field that supplies electrical energy to the combined system.

IMPACT ON INDUSTRY

Given the factors of added cost associated with designing and producing hybrid vehicles, private companies, both manufacturers and research institutions, are more likely to enter the field if they can receive some form of governmental financial assistance. This can be in the form of direct subsidies, tax reductions, or grants. Similarly, institutions of higher learning, both public and private, frequently seek outside sources of funding for specially targeted research activities. Major national laboratories that are not tied to academic institutions, such as the Argonne National Laboratory near Chicago, also submit research proposals for grants. Private foundations that favor ecological research, particularly reduction of carbon dioxide emissions and alternative methods for producing electrical energy, can also be approached for seed money.

In the United States in 2010, hybrid vehicles made up only 3 percent of the total car sales. If this is a valid indicator, only a much bigger sales potential is likely to induce manufacturers to fund research that could bring to the market more fuel-efficient hybrid-technology cars at increasingly attractive prices. Major vested interests on the potentially negative side are: the gigantic ICE automobile industry itself, which is resistant to changes that require major new investment costs, and the fossil-fuel (petroleum) industry, which holds a near monopoly on fuels supplying power to automobiles, including diesel, and, in some cases, ethanol, around the world.

Future expansion in the number of hybrid cars might also cause important changes in the nature of equipment needed for various aspects of hybrid refueling and recharging—equipment that will eventually have to be made available for commercial distribution. At an even more local level, hiring specialized and, perhaps, higher-paid mechanics capable of dealing with the more advanced technical components of hybrid vehicles may also become part of automotive shops' planning for as-yet unpredictable new directions in their business.

CAREERS AND COURSE WORK

Academic preparation for careers tied to HEV technology is, of course, closely tied to the fields of electrical and mechanical engineering and, perhaps to a lesser degree, chemistry. All of these fields demand course work at the undergraduate level to develop familiarity not only with engineering principles but with basic sciences and mathematics used, especially those used by physicists. Beyond a bachelor's degree, graduate-level preparation would include continuation of all of the above subjects at more advanced levels, plus an eventual choice for specialization, based on the assumption that some subfields of engineering are more relevant to HEV technology than others.

The most obvious employment possibilities for engineers interested in HEV technology is with actual manufacturers of automobiles or heavy equipment. Depending on the applicant's academic background, employment with manufacturing firms can range from hands-on engineering applications to more conceptually based research and design functions.

Employment openings in research may be found with a wide variety of private- sector firms, some involving studies of environmental impact, others embedded in actual hybrid-engineering technology. These are too numerous to list here, but one outstanding example of a major private firm that is engaged on an international level in environmentally sustainable technology linked to hybrid vehicle research is ABB. ABB grew from late-nineteenth-century origins in electrical lighting and generator manufacturing in Sweden (ASEA), merging in 1987 with the Swiss firm Brown Boveri. ABB carries on operations in many locations throughout the world.

Internationally known U.S. firm Argonne National Laboratory not only produces research data but also serves as a training ground for engineers who either move on to work with smaller ecology-sensitive engineering enterprises or enter government agencies and university research programs.

Finally, employment with government agencies, especially the EPA, the DOE, and Department of Transportation, represents a viable alternative for applicants with requisite advanced engineering and managerial training.

SOCIAL CONTEXT AND FUTURE PROSPECTS

Although obvious ecological advantages can result as more and more buyers of new vehicles opt for hybrid cars, a variety of potentially negative socioeconomic factors could come into play, certainly over the short to medium term. The higher sales price of hybrids that were available toward the end of 2010 already raised the question of consumer ability (or willingness) to pay more at the outset for fuel-economy savings that would have to

be spread out over a fairly long time frame--possibly even longer than the owner kept the vehicle. It is nearly impossible to predict the number of potential buyers whose statistically lower purchasing ability prevents them from paying higher prices for hybrids. Continued unwillingness or inability to purchase hybrids would mean that a proportionally large number of used older-model ICE's (or brand-new models of older-technology vehicles) would remain on the roads. This socioeconomic potentiality remains linked, of course, to any investment strategies under consideration by industrial producers of cars.

How is one to know which companies worldwide are developing new, economically attractive applications for forthcoming hybrid cars?

The European digital news service EIN News, established in the mid-1990's, provides (among dozens of other categories of information) a specific subsection on hybrid vehicle technology and marketing events, including exhibitions, to its subscribers.

Subscribers from all over the world can obtain up-to-date information on hybrid technology from the Detroit publication *Automotive News* and *Automotive News Europe* and *Automotive News China*. There are, of course, many different marketing congresses (popularly labeled automotive shows) all over the globe, where the latest hybrid technology is introduced and different manufacturers' models can be compared.

In the United States, the Society of Automotive Engineers (SAE) is an important source of up-to-date information for ongoing hybrid vehicle research for both engineering specialists and well-informed general readers.

FURTHER READING
Bethscheider-Kieser, Ulrich. *Green Designed: Future Cars.* Ludwigsburg, Germany: Avedition, 2008. Presents European estimates of technologies that should be compared with the hybrid gas-electric approach to fuel economy.

Clemens, Kevin. *The Crooked Mile: Through Peak Oil, Hybrid Cars and Global Climate Change to Reach a Brighter Future.* Lake Elmo, Minn.: Demontreville Press, 2009. As the title suggests, issues of hybrid car technology need to be placed in a very broad ecological context, where even bigger issues (downward decline in world oil reserves, climate change) may necessitate emphasis on new possible technological solutions.

Lim, Kieran. *Hybrid Cars, Fuel-cell Buses and Sustainable Energy Use.* North Melbourne, Australia: Royal

Australian Chemical Institute, 2004. Provides an idea of technologies and programs imagined in other countries.

Society of Automotive Engineers. *1994 Hybrid Electric Vehicle Challenge.* Warrendale, Penn.: Society of Automotive Engineers, 1995. Reports published by thirty American and Canadian college and university engineering laboratories on their respective HEV research programs.

WEB SITES

Electric Auto Association: http://www.electricauto.org
Electric Drive Transportation Association: http://www.electricdrive.org
Society of Automotive Engineers: http://www.sae.org
U.S. Department of Energy
Clean Cities: http://www1.eere.energy.gov/cleancities

Byron D. Cannon

SEE ALSO: Alternative Fuels (Wind, Solar, Ethanol); Biofuels

Nonrenewable energy resources

Sufficient, reliable sources of energy are a necessity for industrialized nations. Energy is used for heating, cooking, transportation, and manufacturing. Energy can generally be classified as nonrenewable and renewable. More than 85 percent of the energy used in the world is from nonrenewable supplies. A nonrenewable energy resource is a natural resource that cannot be replaced on a scale that can sustain its consumption rate. These resources often exist in a fixed amount and are consumed much more quickly than nature can create them.

PROS AND CONS OF NONRENEWABLE SOURCES

There are both pros and cons to the use of nonrenewable sources of energy. Among the attractive aspects of nonrenewable sources is that they are cheap and easy to use. People can easily fill up their car and other motor vehicle tanks. Moreover, a small amount of nuclear energy can produce a large amount of power. Nonrenewable sources are considered cheap from the standpoint of the cost of converting their energy into forms we can use.

However, nonrenewable sources will someday be depleted, because they are being used at a rate faster than the eons of geologic time required to form them. Therefore, we must use our endangered resources

carefully to create more renewable sources of energy. Moreover, the speed at which nonrewables are being used can have serious environmental changes. Nonrenewable sources undergo combustion to release their energy for use, but at the same time they release toxic gases into the air, a major cause of global warming. Finally, since these sources are going to expire soon, their cost to consumers is soaring.

Sufficient, reliable sources of energy are a necessity for industrialized nations. Energy is used for heating, cooking, transportation, and manufacturing. Energy can generally be classified as nonrenewable and renewable. More than 85 percent of the energy used in the world is from nonrenewable supplies. A nonrenewable energy resource is a natural resource that cannot be replaced on a scale that can sustain its consumption rate. These resources often exist in a fixed amount and are consumed much more quickly than nature can create them.

The major categories of nonrenewable energy sources are the fossil fuels(oil, natural gas, and coal, including petroleum products such as gasoline, diesel fuel, and propane), and nuclear power (nuclear energy). Fossil fuels are continually produced by the decay of plant and animal matter, but the rate of their production is extremely slow, much slower than the rate at which we use them—thus they are nonrenewable. Nuclear energy is also considered nonrenewable in that it uses a relatively rare metal, uranium-235. Nonrenewable energy sources come out of the ground as liquids, gases, and solids. Crude oil and petroleumoil (petroleum) is the only commercial nonrenewable fuel that is naturally in liquid form. Natural gas and propane are normally gases, but coal and uranium ore are solid.

OIL AND PETROLEUM PRODUCTS

Crude oil or liquid petroleum is a fossil fuel that is refined into many different energy products: gasoline, diesel fuel, jet fuel, and heating oil, for example. Oil forms underground in rocks, such as shale, which is rich in organic materials. After the oil forms, it migrates upward into porous reservoir rock, such as sandstone or limestone, where it can become trapped by an overlying impermeable cap rock. Wells are drilled into these oil reservoirs to remove the gas and oil. More than 70 percent of oil fields are found near tectonic plate boundaries, because the conditions there are conducive to oil formation.

More than 50 percent of the world's oil is found in the Middle East; sizable additional reserves occur in North

America. Most known oil reserves are already being exploited, and oil is being used at a rate that exceeds the rate of discovery of new sources. If the consumption rate continues to increase and no significant new sources are found, oil supplies could be exhausted by about 2040.

Despite its limited supply, oil is a relatively inexpensive fuel source. It is preferred over coal as a fuel source because an equivalent amount of oil produces more kilowatts of energy than coal. It also burns cleaner, producing about 50 percent less sulfur dioxide. However, the burning of oil contributes significantly to environment problems and atmospheric pollution in the form of carbon dioxide, carbon monoxide, sulfur dioxide, and nitrogen oxide emissions. These greenhouse gases pollute the air and contribute to global warming.

OIL SHALE AND TAR SANDS

One source of oil, oil shale and tar sands, is currently among the least utilized of fossil fuel sources. Oil shale is sedimentary rock with very fine pores that contain kerogen, a carbon-based, waxy substance. If shale is heated to 490 degrees Celsius, the kerogen vaporizes and can then be condensed as shale oil, a thick, viscous liquid. This shale oil is then further refined into usable oil products. Production of shale oil requires large amounts of energy, however, for mining and processing the shale. Indeed, about half a barrel of oil is required to extract every barrel of shale oil. The largest tar-sand deposit in the world is in Canada and contains enough material (about 500 billion barrels) to supply the world with oil for about 15 years. However, because of environmental concerns and high production costs, these tar sands are not being fully utilized.

NATURAL GAS

Natural gas production is often a by-product of oil recovery, as the two commonly share underground reservoirs. Natural gas is a mixture of gases, the most common being methane (CH_4). It also contains some ethane (C_2H_5), propane (C_3H_8), and butane (C_4H_{10}).

Natural gas is usually not contaminated with sulfur and is therefore the cleanest-burning fossil fuel. After recovery, propane and butane are removed from the natural gas and made into liquefied petroleum gas (LPG). LPG is shipped in special pressurized tanks as a fuel source for areas not directly served by natural gas pipelines (such as rural communities). The remaining natural gas is further refined to remove impurities and water vapor and is then transported in pressurized pipelines.

Natural gas is highly flammable and odorless. The characteristic smell associated with natural gas is actually that of minute quantities of a smelly sulfur compound (ethyl mercaptan) that is added during refining to allow consumers to smell the gas should it leak from pipes and thus pose a hazard.

The use of natural gas is growing rapidly. Besides being a clean-burning fuel source, natural gas is easy and inexpensive to transport, once pipelines are in place. In developed countries, natural gas is used primarily for heating, cooking, and powering vehicles. It is also used in a process for making ammonia fertilizer. The current estimate of natural gas reserves is about 100 million metric tons. At current usage levels, this supply will last an estimated 100 years. Most of the world's natural gas reserves are found in Eastern Europe and the Middle East.

COAL

Coal is the most abundant fossil fuel in the world, with estimated reserves of 1 trillion metric tons. Most of the world's coal reserves exist in Eastern Europe and Asia, but the United States also has considerable reserves. Coal formed slowly over millions of years from the buried remains of ancient swamp plants. During the formation of coal, carbonaceous matter was first compressed into a spongy material called peat, which is about 90 percent water. As the peat became more deeply buried, the increased pressure and temperature turned it into coal.

Different types of coal resulted from differences in the pressure and temperature that prevailed during formation. The softest coal (about 50 percent carbon), which also has the lowest energy output, is called lignite. Lignite has the highest water content (about 50 percent) and relatively low amounts of smog-causing sulfur. With increasing temperature and pressure, lignite is transformed into bituminous coal (about 85 percent carbon and 3 percent water). Anthracite (almost 100 percent carbon) is the hardest coal and also produces the greatest energy when burned.

Currently, the world is consuming coal at a rate of about 5 billion metric tons per year. The main use of coal is for power generation, because it is a relatively inexpensive way to produce power. Coal is used to produce more than 50 percent of the electricity in the United States. In addition to electricity production, coal is sometimes used for heating and cooking in less developed countries and in rural areas of developed countries. If consumption continues at the current rates, reserves will last for more than 200 years.

Coal mining creates several environmental problems. Coal is most cheaply mined from near-surface deposits using strip-mining techniques. Strip mining causes considerable environmental damage in the form of erosion and habitat destruction. Subsurface mining of coal is less damaging to the surface environment, but it is much more hazardous for miners because of tunnel collapses and gas explosions. The burning of coal results in significant atmospheric pollution. The sulfur contained in coal forms sulfur dioxide when burned. Harmful nitrogen oxides, heavy metals, and carbon dioxide are also released into the air during coal burning. The harmful emissions can be reduced by installing scrubbers and electrostatic precipitators in the smokestacks of power plants. The toxic ash remaining after coal burning is also an environmental concern and is usually disposed into landfills.

RADIOACTIVE FUEL

The use of nuclear technology requires a radioactive fuel. Uranium ore is present in the ground at relatively low concentrations and is mined in 19 countries. Uranium is used to create plutonium; uranium-238 is fissionable and can be transmuted into fissile plutonium-239 in a nuclear reactor. Nuclear fuel is used in nuclear power stations to create electricity. Nuclear power provides about 6 percent of the world's energy and 13–14 percent of the world's electricity. Nuclear technology is a volatile and contaminating source of fuel production, with the expense of the nuclear industry predominantly reliant on subsidies.

In most electric power plants, water is heated and converted into steam, which drives a turbine generator to produce electricity. Fossil-fueled power plants produce heat by burning coal, oil, or natural gas. In a nuclear power plant, the fission of uranium atoms in the reactor provides the heat to produce steam for generating electricity.

Originally, nuclear energy was expected to be a clean and cheap source of energy. Nuclear fission does not produce atmospheric pollution or greenhouse gases, and its proponents expected that nuclear energy would be cheaper and last longer than fossil fuels. Unfortunately, because of construction cost overruns, poor management, and numerous regulations, nuclear power has become much more expensive than predicted. The nuclear accidents at Three Mile Island in Pennsylvania (1979) and Chernobyl in the Ukraine (1986) raised concerns about the safety of nuclear power. Furthermore, the problem of safely disposing spent nuclear fuel remains unresolved.

SUSTAINABLE DEVELOPMENT

It is our responsibility to use scarce nonrenewable energy resources judiciously and sustainably, so that we do not contribute to their fast depletion. Although today's society will remain dependent on nonrenewable energy resources for the next few decades, the development of alternative energy sources and the technology to harness them at the nascent stage should be our aim. Also, we need to have proper technology in place and devise newer methods to eliminate the negative environmental impact of fossil fuels. Overexploitation of nonrenewables will lead to excessive pollution and rising threats of global warming. The judicious use of nonrenewables can save us from an energy crisis in the immediate future until we develop alternative sources.

FURTHER READING

Deffeyes, Kenneth S. *Hubbert's Peak: The Impending World Oil Shortage.* Princeton, NJ: Princeton University Press, 2008.

Heinberg, R., and D. Lerch, eds. *The Post Carbon Reader: Managing the 21st Century's Sustainability Crises.* Healdsburg, CA: Watershed Media, 2010.

Kaur, Ravnit. "Five Non-Renewable Sources." January 18, 2011. http://www.brighthub.com/environment/renewable-energy/articles/100982.aspx#ixzz1IIW0EsYG.

Maugeri, Leonardo. *Beyond the Age of Oil: The Myths, Realities, and Future of Fossil Fuels and Their Alternatives.* Westport, CT: Praeger, 2010.

University of California. "Non-Renewable Energy Sources." http://cnx.org/content/m16730/latest/.

U.S. Department of Energy. "Energy Sources: Nonrenewable." http://www.eia.doe.gov/kids/energy.cfm?page=nonrenewable_home-basics.

Reza Fazeli

SEE ALSO: Conservation; Renewable Energy Resources

Organic food industry

The organic food industry produces food grown and processed without pesticides, food additives, and genetically modified organisms

INTRODUCTION

The organic food movement began in response to the twentieth-century introduction of chemicals and pesticides to the food industry to increase yield. The organic food industry grew steadily in the United States after the passage of the Organic Foods Production Act of 1990, which helped set strict standards for organic food production. In the 2000s, many Americans, inspired by new books and films on food production and consumption, began seeking alternatives to the conventional food supply chain, including organic foods.

The Organic Foods Production Act of 1990 implemented national organic standards and established the National Organic Standards Board. The board makes recommendations to the National Organic Program (NOP) of the United States Department of Agriculture (USDA) to help regulate the organic food industry. The NOP, established in 2000, is in charge of developing and regulating organic food standards, which ensure that companies use the correct practices when growing and producing organic products. The NOP verifies that the players within the organic food industry—including farmers, ranchers, distributors, and processors—comply with these standards and become certified by accredited agents.

The organic food industry is heavily regulated by the USDA, which frequently inspects and audits organic companies to ensure that regulations are followed and organic products are labeled correctly. All organic products must carry the USDA organic seal, which verifies that the product is at least 95 percent organic or has been made with certified organic ingredients. The seal means the crops have been harvested without exposure to radiation, sewage sludge, synthetic fertilizers, pesticides, or genetically modified organisms. The seal also ensures that animals are raised according to standards that protect their health and well-being. Farmers raising livestock cannot use antibiotics or growth hormones and must feed the animals a 100 percent organic diet. The animals must also be provided with an outdoor pasture. Animals that have been cloned do not qualify as organic products

LABELING

As awareness of food production methods grew in the 2000s, food labeling became an important issue. Consumers often had difficulty understanding the differences between the profusion of labels and health claims, especially those denoting organic and nonorganic food products. In addition to carrying the USDA organic seal, products from livestock—including meat, eggs, and milk—may also have other labels regulated by the USDA. Products that contain any of these various labels may or may not be organic. If a product is labeled "natural," for example, but does not contain a USDA organic seal, it is not an organic product. Products that are 70 percent organic can carry the label "made with organic ingredients" but cannot bear the USDA organic seal.

Animal products could bear a number of different labels in addition to or instead of organic. A product labeled "free range" means that the livestock was permitted unlimited access to indoor/outdoor areas and fresh food and water. "Cage-free" means the livestock was not kept in caged areas, but was permitted unlimited access to indoor areas. Products labeled "natural" do not contain any artificial ingredients and are minimally processed. This labeling applies to meat and egg products only. "Grass-fed" livestock are fed primarily grass. Unlike organic grass-fed livestock, these animals may be fed grass that has been treated with pesticides and may be given antibiotics and/or hormones. A "no-added hormones" label means that the livestock has been raised without the use of hormones or steroids. Other labels, such as "pasture-raised" and "humane," may or may not be regulated by non-USDA independent certifying organizations.

INDUSTRY GROWTH

The organic food industry grew steadily through the 2000s in the United States to become one of the fastest-growing segments in the food market. According to the Organic Trade Association, organic foods accounted for almost $14 billion in sales in 2005. By the following year, this number had risen to $17.7 billion. Sales continued to increase, even when the US economy entered a recession during the late 2000s. In 2009, organic foods accounted for $26.6 billion in US sales and $54.9 billion in global sales. The United States led the global market in organic food sales, with Germany and France not far behind.

The wider availability of organic foods at large grocery chains was cited as one of the main reasons for the continued increase. At first, organic foods could be found only at small specialty grocery stores and farmers markets. People also began choosing more organic products because of an increased awareness of health issues, the environmental impact of food manufacturing, and food and animal safety concerns.

IMPACT

During the 2000s, people increasingly chose organic products because they believed these products were better for both their health and the environment. Organic foods do not contain potentially toxic chemicals such as pesticides, which can leave a residue on produce and affect its taste and appearance. Organic foods also do not contain food additives, such as artificial sweeteners, colorings, flavorings, and preservatives. Organic farmers are prohibited from using chemical pesticides, which can wash from farmlands into waterways where they may contaminate the water supply and soil, kill wildlife, and destroy vegetation. Instead, organic farms use such practices as hand weeding and crop rotation, which are designed to benefit the environment and reduce pollution.

FURTHER READING

Dunn-Georgiou, Elisha. *Everything You Need to Know about Organic Foods*. New York: Rosen, 2002. Print. Traces the development of the organic food movement in the United States and outlines the parameters set for food to be considered organic by the USDA.

Fromartz, Samuel. Organic, Inc.: *Natural Foods and How They Grew*. Orlando: Harcourt, 2006. Print. Tracks the changes in Americans' awareness of the food they consume and looks at the sources of organic food.

Langley, Andrew. *Is Organic Food Better?* Chicago: Heinemann, 2009. Print. Looks at the range of opinion on and facts about organic foods. Good starting place for discussing the topic of organic foods.

"Organic Foods: Are They Safer? More Nutritious?" *Mayo Clinic*. Mayo Foundation for Medical Education and Research, 7 Sept. 2012. Web. 26 Nov. 2012. Provides medical research on organic foods, including information on nutrition and health.

Organic Trade Association. "Quick Overview: Organic Agriculture and Production." *Organic Trade Association*. Organic Trade Assn., 16 Feb. 2011. Web. 21 Nov. 2012. Provides information about the organic trade industry and how organic food is produced.

Angela Harmon

SEE ALSO: Buying Local, Genetically Modified Foods

Recycling technology

The environmental movement, which has been growing steadily since the 1940's, has brought increasing attention to the need to change the public and industrial practices that have enormous environmental costs. Managing the vast amounts of waste produced in a consumer society is a prodigious challenge that is exacerbated by the closing and non-replacement of landfill-waste dump sites. One important aspect of the green attitude is to reduce the level of consumption of virgin planetary resources by reusing and recycling products. While citizens are being called upon to reduce, reuse, and recycle, it is generally recognized that efficient recycling requires the application of new technologies. The major targets for residential recycling programs, which now exist in most cities of the developed world, have traditionally been glass and aluminum containers, paper products, certain types of plastics, and plant and yard waste. However, as technologies are further developed and industries find profitable ways of recycling and reusing waste, recycling programs are being extended to include rubber, a variety of metals, asphalt shingles, and electronics.

DEFINITION AND BASIC PRINCIPLES

Recycling is the process of returning previously manufactured products to a raw material state to be utilized afresh for the manufacture of new products. The purpose of recycling technologies is to discover new ways to extend this practice into new material fields. In keeping with the mantra of the global environmental movement—reduce, reuse, recycle—recycling is a crucial aspect of the global environmental justice movement because recycling reduces pollution by reducing the amount of landfill waste and the amount of waste destroyed in incinerators, both of which add to greenhouse gases. Recycling conserves natural resources, which would otherwise be relied upon for the manufacture of new products. Recycling also reduces pollution by reducing manufacturing energy consumption, since less energy is required to recycle a product than to make a new one from virgin materials.

BACKGROUND AND HISTORY

The creation of industries focused on reusing previously manufactured products grew out of an increasing awareness of the effects of industrialization and urbanization on the planet's atmosphere, waters, and land. The launching of the global environmental justice movement is credited to Rachel Carson, an American marine biologist and conservationist whose book *Silent Spring* (1962) stimulated public awareness of the effects of unrestricted pesticide use in the United States.

People have always reused their possessions, finding new ways to put old things to fresh uses. However, reuse of products had been waning in affluent societies, since the notion of "planned obsolescence" rendered voracious consumption a virtue. The idea was first introduced by New York real estate broker Bernard London and promoted in his 1932 paper, "Ending the Depression Through Planned Obsolescence." London argued that science and business were successfully producing products in factories and fields; inadequate consumption

practices were to blame for the economic woes of the country. Consumers were not buying enough, but London had the answer: Products must be designed to serve only a specific, limited life span. Increased consumption offered the preventative against future economic depressions. Against the traditional Protestant ethic of extreme frugality, London posited that an insatiable appetite for goods was the mark of the good citizen, acting in support of the nation's economic health.

During World War II, Americans had experimented with conservation and recycling as a function of national security. However, in the economic boom following the war, Western middle-class life unapologetically adopted an ethos of consumption, where product value was directly tied to newness and abundance. As environmental

---

FASCINATING FACTS ABOUT RECYCLING TECHNOLOGY

- More than one-half million trees could be saved if every household in the United States replaced just one roll of paper towels with recycled ones.
- Twenty million tons of electronic waste are disposed of in landfills each year. One ton of scrap from discarded computers contains more gold than can be produced from seventeen tons of gold ore.
- Nine cubic yards of landfill can be saved by recycling one ton of cardboard.
- The global recycling industry is worth more than $160 billion and employs more than 1.5 million people.
- It takes five percent of the energy to recycle aluminum compared with mining and refining new aluminum.
- Each year, the United States alone generates more than 160 million metric tons of solid waste.
- In the United States alone, recycling is estimated to save more than 18 million tons of CO_2 each year, equivalent to reducing the number of cars on the roads by approximately 5 million.
- Environmental groups often head the search for new recycling methods and products. In 2006, Earth First engineered a new proprietary tire processing system, which salvages steel, carbon, high-energy gas and oil, as well as

effectively recycles tires. The benefit of the new method is that the tires are burned at a fraction of the temperature needed for pyrolysis, which satisfies very strict emissions regulations while effectively preserving the tire components.

- New recycling technologies, developed by scientists at University College Dublin in 2006, use a bacteria that eats polystyrene foam, commonly known as Styrofoam, and turns it into a usable plastic. The bacteria offer an efficient scheme for recycling the more than 14 million metric tons of Styrofoam produced annually, which has traditionally ended up in landfills.
- In 2009, Motorola unveiled the world's first-carbon neutral cell phone, made from recycled water bottles. The company promised to offset the carbon emissions created during the phone's manufacture by investing in reforestation and renewable resources.
- New York-based Ecovative Design has developed a substitute for pink fiberglass insulation named Greensulate, which is made from rice hulls (agricultural garbage), mushroom fibers (very inexpensive), and recycled paper (readily available). Greensulate repels water, prevents fire, and is resistant to temperature changes. As of 2011, the product still needs to be tested to determine whether it is mold resistant.

problems grew, in the United States and across the planet, the environmental justice movement gained increasing credence among middle-class Americans, and the wastefulness of modern consumer societies became increasingly obvious, intolerable, and shameful to more and more citizens. Across the industrialized West, people began to call upon their governments for regulation of polluting industries, and they began to integrate more sound practices into their private lives. The cultural and social impact of the new public awareness culminated in the establishment of Earth Day in 1970.

Recycling is an important aspect of the modern environmentalism movement, but, in the light of the vast environmental damage done by industry all over the planet, recycling can be undervalued by some environmental activists as having little actual environmental impact. However, one crucial caveat of the environmental justice movement has been to encourage consumers to do their part and institute small lifestyle changes as their personal contribution to the health of the planet. A minor shift in general human consumption behavior, in the context of a globalizing consumerism, suggests that significant benefits can be reaped by reducing, reusing, and recycling old products. The change in public attitudes has forced environmental concerns to the forefront of political debate and contributed to a new ethic that values restraint in consuming. Recycling is a crucial aspect of the new ecological awareness. Recycling has become the fashion, and industry has responded to the new attitudes, finding new applications for the new ethic, creating new business opportunities for profit and development.

HOW IT WORKS
When people and communities recycle, used materials are set aside in recycling bins, collected, and converted into new products. Simple societies have always been avid recyclers, since their access to new products is limited compared with consumer societies. They tend to produce very little waste and place a high premium on the human creativity that reuses old products for new tasks and designs new products from old discards. Most cities in the developed world support the reduce, reuse, and recycle ethic by collecting used products as part of their curbside trash-collection services. The materials may be sorted as they are placed on the recycling trucks or once collected, they may be sorted in substations, where the used products and materials are then sold to dedicated recycling companies to be made into newly valuable commodities for sale in the global marketplace.

Some recycling programs ask residents to separate their recyclables from their trash, which may be collected on different days. To encourage recycling, many Canadian communities have the policy of charging residents for the trash put out for collection but not for their recycling. Residents may be asked to sort and separately bind their recycling into various types of materials—paper products, plastics, glass, Styrofoam, corrugated cardboard, and boxes.

APPLICATIONS AND PRODUCTS
Most recycling programs target for collection previously used household items that are made from paper, cardboard, metal, glass, plastic, and compostable yard wastes. Recycling recovered metals and glass involves a relatively simple procedure: The items are melted down and sold to processing plants that refill the newly formed containers or to manufacturing plants that create new products from the raw materials. Yard waste can be composted with very little investment in equipment, and many families have created their own composting systems. Paper is the most important recycled material, because recycling is simple and saves harvesting new trees. Paper is recycled by mixing with water, and if necessary, de-inking the pulp before reusing it. Plastics recycling, on the other hand, entails an expensive process, whereby differing resins are separated. Since plastics are made from the Earth's dwindling stores of petroleum, they are a favorite target of recycling programs, despite the more complicated processes involved. Plastics can be recycled into a wide range of secondary products, from textiles, such as fiberfill and polyester-like fibers, to plastic toys, recycling bins, and plastic furniture. Recycling of e-waste began in the late twentieth century. Prior to that, television sets, computer monitors, computers and laptops, printers, and microwave ovens had to be disposed of in landfill sites, where they presented a number of health and safety risks, because of the dangerous materials they contain (barium, beryllium, flame retardants, cadmium, hexavalent chromium, lead, mercury, plastics). Moreover, the precious metals used in electronic boards are rare, and thus highly coveted, in their natural state. New industries have cropped up to salvage useful and valuable materials from these sources.

IMPACT ON INDUSTRY
Recycling affects a broad spectrum of industries that used to rely solely on newly harvested raw materials. Since the green ethos has elevated recycling to the sta-

tus of a virtue, recycling technologies have burgeoned as well. As university and corporate research churns out new ideas about how to recycle not only the products consumers discard, but metal from airplanes and ships, electronic products, asphalt from existing roadways and roofing materials, rubber from automobile tires, and methane gas from the decaying refuse in landfills. While recycling is a term generally reserved for metals, glass, papers, and like materials, water can be recycled as well. Water recycling reuses treated wastewater for agricultural and landscape irrigation, industrial processes, toilet flushing, and replenishing groundwater basins. Water is sometimes recycled and reused on-site in industrial facilities, for example, for cooling processes.

The business community works hand in hand with research teams to put the new ideas into practice and to develop new products from recycled materials. In turn, purchasing products stamped with the label, "made from recycled materials," allows consumers to attach themselves to the ethically significant global movement, which promises to save the planet. Recycling stimulates industry at every level, from the curbside-pickup industry to the dedicated recycling companies that break down the various products to their raw-material states to the manufacturing industries that implement the new technologies for fashioning new products from the recycled materials. The search for the most innovative new technology is always a constant challenge in the recycling industry. Companies, research scientists, and environmental groups are racing to come up with better recycling processes and machines, as well as to create new schemes for recycling previously nonrecyclable materials.

Government and University Research. Green technologies represent heavily funded arenas for research. Most research funding comes from two major sources: corporations, motivated mainly by profit, and government, seeking innovative answers to its waste, energy, and pollution problems. Grants for green technologies are primarily awarded to universities or specialized government agencies. A third, more limited, funding source is nonprofit organizations.

Industry and Business. Full-service recycling companies exist in most towns and cities across the developed world. Some of these remain municipally owned but private industries appear to be taking the lead in assuming the responsibility for the residential collection of recyclable materials. RecycleInAmerica is one of the leading recyclers of plastics in the United States, with outlets in all fifty states. Republic Services is another recycling industry leader, providing services for commercial,

industrial, municipal, and residential customers through more than 375 collection companies in forty states and Puerto Rico. Republic also owns or operates more than 223 transfer stations and seventy-eight recycling facilities, serving millions of residential customers in more than 2,800 municipalities. Many industry leaders are joining forces to reach their green goals: The Consumer Electronics Association is teaming up with manufacturers and retailers, such as Panasonic, Best Buy, Sony, and Toshiba, for an industry-wide initiative in e-waste recycling, with a goal of recycling one billion pounds by 2016. This represents triple the e-waste recycled in 2010. The effort focuses on educating consumers about electronics recycling, increasing e-waste recycling collection centers, transparency in reporting progress, and supporting third-party recycler certification.

Major Corporations. Recyclingcompanies.com lists forty-seven global recycling companies and 173 new recycling organizations around the world. Busch Systems of Barrie, Ontario, Canada, is the world's largest supplier of recycling, waste, and compost containers, and has been the industry leader for more than twenty-five years. Based in Connecticut, the Canusa Hershman Recycling Company manages monthly totals of more than 100,000 tons of fiber and 3 million pounds of plastics and other materials. It has a dozen offices and processing facilities in North America and offers a wide range of services to generators and consumers of secondary recyclable materials. Greenstar Recycling is a American paper recycling company that serves a global market. Salvage America is an example of a multi-material recycling company that services industries and municipalities to recycle a great spectrum of materials, including cardboard and paper products, wood pallets, scrap lumber and tree brush, plastics, construction materials, such as concrete, brick, block, and dirt, as well as all metals, ferrous and nonferrous.

CAREERS AND COURSE WORK

On the theoretical side, undergraduate and graduate degrees are offered in the fields of sustainability and environmental studies, which grants students the opportunity to grasp the fundamental scientific concepts that underpin sustainability, understand the policy framework and the political environments in which environmental policy is enacted, create new economic motivations for developing sustainable practices, and analyze and evaluate the consequences of adopting the new technologies. Environmental ethics is a popular course offered in many philosophy departments, business schools, earth science programs, and science and technology studies departments. On the practical side, recycling technologies is an aspect of engineering studies, with varied applications in mechanical, electrical, civil, and systems engineering. Courses in design and materials science look to the creation of new recycling methods and new materials to be targeted for recycling, while civil engineering addresses problems of landfill elimination, road surface recycling, and asphalt shingle recycling.

SOCIAL CONTEXT AND FUTURE PROSPECTS

Throughout the middle decades of the twentieth century, public attitudes in industrialized nations attached virtue to consumption, believing heavy consuming would stimulate the economy and guard societies against economic depressions. Western middle-class life began to locate its identity in products. Through the phenomenon of branding, companies capitalized on this identifying tendency, and advertising convinced consumers that newer, bigger, and more plentiful was better. However, as environmental problems grew more and more evident, in the United States and across the planet, the environmental justice movement gained increasing authority among middle-class Americans, and the wastefulness of modern consumer societies came to be seen as deplorable, irresponsible, and shameful. Across the industrialized West, people began to call upon their governments for regulation of polluting industries, and they began to integrate more sound practices into their private lives. The cultural and social impact of the new public awareness led to the creation of recycling programs in many communities.

Recycling is an important aspect of the modern environmental justice movement. The planet is one component of the triple bottom line (planet, people, and profit), which is a cornerstone of global ethics and the Corporate Social Responsibility movement. In the light of the vast environmental damage still being done by industry all over the planet, recycling is sometimes undervalued by environmental activists, who feel that the biggest offenders are actually governments that need to regulate polluting practices and industries that need to implement environmentally sound manufacturing methods. There is good reason to agree with this activist charge. However, since overconsumption and consumer wastefulness are enormous aspects of the environmental problem, the claim that recycling fails to target the biggest culprits is hardly helpful in changing the public's attitude about its

extravagant lifestyle, which is fast being exported to the developing world. Recycling, as a lifestyle ethos, can and has begun to spill out into the business world, stimulating new recycling industries at every level of public life. It is precisely this change in public attitudes that has forced environmental concerns to the forefront of political debate and contributed to public policy changes in favor of industrial pollutant regulation and recycling in the public realm. Recycling programs in the eleven U.S. states in which deposit legislation forces bottle-return practices have been enormously successful. Recycling is a crucial aspect of the ecological justice movement. Scientists and other experts agree that the future of recycling technologies consists in placing more of various recycling technology sites around the country and throughout the world. As of 2011, it is generally agreed that the process of developing new recycling technologies will move very quickly because so many scientists and business leaders are on board.

However, the biggest boost to recycling technologies comes when governments get onboard, and politicians raise recycling as an issue of importance, which then draws to the subject both media coverage and research funding. The United States, traditionally a slow participant in global ecological concerns, is leading new efforts to explore the possible recycling of commercial nuclear waste, as a potential fuel product. Dangerous materials, such as plutonium, require enhanced security in transporting to, and managing in, recycling plants, but these matters are currently under investigation as recycling technologies spread into broader arenas of application.

FURTHER READING

Crampton, Norman. *Green House: Eco-Friendly Disposal and Recycling at Home*. Lanham, Md.: M. Evans, 2008. Crampton, a career worker in the field of waste prevention, is the widely acclaimed expert on practical information for adopting green habits of disposal.

Friedman, Lauri S., ed. *Garbage and Recycling*. Farmington Hills, Mich.: Greenhaven Press, 2009. Offers comprehensive overview of recycling that is useful in teaching novices about the field and introduces debate and sorts out misinformation about the subject.

Kintisch, Eli. "Congress Tells DOE to Take Fresh Look at Recycling Spent Reactor Fuel." *Science* 310, no. 5753 (December 2, 2005): 1406. This article reports on renewed U.S. plans to recycle commercial nuclear waste into fuel, an increasingly attractive option as a petroleum alternative, but one fraught with many dangers.

Lund, Herbert F. *McGraw-Hill Recycling Handbook.* 2d ed. New York: McGraw-Hill, 2001. Lund offers answers to hundreds of questions about recycling, focusing on how to develop an effective recycling program, given current recycling technologies, strategic goals, public awareness levels, and legislation.

Mancini, Candice, ed. *Garbage and Recycling: Global Viewpoints.* Farmington Hills, Mich.: Greenhaven Press, 2010. Provides international perspective on recycling technologies through a broad collection of primary-source information, including government documents and essays from international magazines and journals. A good resource for comparative studies of recycling attitudes and programs; annotated table of contents, world map, and country and subject indices.

Porter, Richard C. *The Economics of Waste.* Washington, D.C.: RFP Press, 2002. Porter applies economic and ethical analysis to the dangerous aspects of waste disposal and recycling, especially landfills, incineration, illegal disposal, international trade in waste, and disposal and recycling of hazardous materials, revealing the true costs and risks of recycling policies and the complex problems associated with meeting strategic recycling goals, while still protecting human health and the environment.

Scott, Nicky. *Reduce, Reuse, Recycle: An Easy Household Guide.* White River Junction, Vt.: Chelsea Green Publishing, 2007. This book offers a helpful A-to-Z listing of household items, explanations on how to recycle discarded products, suggestions on how to make discards profitable, and information on how to draw upon local resources to get more involved in recycling projects and opportunities in local communities.

WEB SITES

Charitable Recycling Program
http://www.charitablerecycling.com/CR/home.asp
Construction Materials Recycling Association
http://www.cdrecycling.org
Grass Roots Recycling Network
State Recycling Organizations
http://www.grrn.org/resources/sros.html
National Recycling Coalition
http://www.nrcrecycles.org

Wendy C. Hamblet

SEE ALSO: Battery Recycling; Composting; Conservation

Renewable energy resources

Renewable energy is energy derived from regenerative resources. These resources can be fully replenished in a short time period. Renewable energy is generated from elements found in nature and include the use of biomass in fuels such as ethanol, biodiesel, charcoal, and biogas; the use of water or hydropower by means of waterwheels, water mills, run-of-the-river hydroelectricity facilities, hydroelectric dams, tidal power, and wave power; the use of solar energy in solar heating, photovoltaic (PV) systems, and concentrating solar power; the use of wind to drive turbines via windmills; and the use of geothermal energy, the heat energy that emanates from deep inside the Earth. These renewable energy resources, if well explored and developed, can be inexhaustible.

RENEWABLE VERSUS ENVIRONMENTALLY FRIENDLY

Renewable energy generation and use are not by definition environmentally or ecologically friendly. The terms renewable and environmentally friendly are related to different issues. Renewable energy refers to energy generated from regenerative resources. However, the generation of renewable energy can affect the environment and various life forms. Hydropower, for example, is an important type of renewable energy, originating in the motion of water in rivers and the oceans. This water is periodically supplied by rain, and then, via evaporation, is returned to the Earth's atmosphere in a process called the hydrologic cycle. The water from rain therefore is virtually inexhaustible, and it makes hydropower renewable. However, hydroelectric power plants require huge water reservoirs for their operation. The building of dams and the associated flooding of large land areas can cause several environmental impacts. The damming of rivers results in the submersion of extensive areas upstream of the dams, destroying biologically rich lowlands. Aquatic riverine ecosystems change drastically, both upstream and downstream of the dam site. Damming can also have a negative influence on the migration of fish, although this can be mitigated in some cases by installing appropriate fish ladders. Ultimately, however, the alteration of natural ecosystems to make use of renewable hydropower will have an environmental impact that needs to be weighed against the benefits of harnessing renewable energy.

Renewable energy is energy derived from regenerative resources. These resources can be fully replenished in a short time period. Renewable energy is generated from elements found in nature and include the use of biomass in fuels such as ethanol, biodiesel, charcoal, and biogas; the use of water or hydropower by means of waterwheels, water mills, run-of-the-river hydroelectricity facilities, hydroelectric dams, tidal power, and wave power; the use of solar energy in solar heating, photovoltaic (PV) systems, and concentrating solar power; the use of wind to drive turbines via windmills; and the use of geothermal energy, the heat energy that emanates from deep inside the Earth. These renewable energy resources, if well explored and developed, can be inexhaustible.

By contrast, nonrenewable energy resources, such as fossil fuels and nuclear power, are limited, and their use leads to the depletion of those reserves. For much of human history, the kind of energy used to power societies came from renewable resources; however, with the rise of the Industrial Revolution and its use of coal and later oil, nonrenewable fossil fuels became predominant. The foundation of our energy systems on these fossil fuels has made us dependent on a resource that will soon be depleted.

HISTORICAL ASPECTS

Until the 19th century, civilization survived using essentially renewable energy resources, based on firewood and biomass burning for cooking, heating, and building materials. Nowadays, least developed countries are still using essentially these kinds of energy resources.

The use of fossil fuels became dominant in the 20th century and it is still increasing at the beginning of the 21st century. During the Industrial Revolution, the demand for energy increased drastically, and the high use of coal, petroleum, and natural gas led to the large-scale generation of electricity, heat, and fuel. Today, fossil fuels account for more than three-fourths of the energy used in the world. Fossil fuels have higher energy density when compared to the raw biomass. They are easy to extract because huge amounts of these materials are found in a single place, which make them relatively low-cost raw materials. The use of fossil fuels has had a large impact on civilization's industrial development. However, the reduction of fossil fuel usage is an important issue today, mainly for two reasons: The first is related to the depletion of reserves, cost instability, and irregular distribution

of these resources around the world, conditions that have led to many conflicts and wars; the second reason is related to the climate change that is resulting from the emission of greenhouse gases from the burning of these fuels for energy.

WORLD ENERGY SCENARIO

The Renewable Energy Data Book issued in 2009 by the U.S. Department of Energy (DOE), notes that, worldwide, 19 percent of energy consumed comes from renewable sources and 81 percent from nonrenewable resources, of which 78.2 percent are based on fossil fuels and the remaining 2.8 percent on nuclear energy. The renewable sources are divided among traditional biomass energyas renewable energybiomass (13 percent), hydropoweras renewable energyhydropower (3.2 percent), and new renewable sources (2.8 percent), such as small hydropower plants, wind, solar energy, and geothermal energy. In 2009, during the worldwide economic recession, there was a boom in renewable energy. In mid-2010, more than 100 countries focused their energy production on renewable sources, an increase of almost 100 percent compared with 2005.

There has thus been a major shift in the global energy scenario with regard to renewable fuels, with more than half of the efforts to cultivate renewable sources concentrated in developing countries. In 2009, wind power and solar photovoltaic (PV) power had record growth in both Europe and the United States: renewable energy accounted for more than half of new installations in that year. For the second straight year, more money was invested in new renewable energy sources than in new sources of fossil fuels. Globally, Brazil leads the production of sugar-derived ethanol and has also been adding new sources of biomass to its energy matrix. Other countries, such as Argentina, Uruguay, Costa Rica, Egypt, Indonesia, Kenya, Tanzania, Thailand, and Tunisia, are rapidly increasing their market share of renewables. Developing countries already account for half of all countries with some sort of policy to promote renewable energy.

In 1990, wind power was used in only a few countries, but now it plays a role in the energy sources of more than 80 countries. In 2009, China produced 30 percent of the world's wind turbines and 77 percent of the world solar collectors for hot water. Argentina, Brazil, Colombia, Ecuador, and Peru have become Latin America's major biofuel producers, and other renewable technologies are being expanded as well. At least 20 countries in the Middle East, North Africa, and sub-Saharan Africa have active markets for renewable energy. In addition to Europe and the United States, other developed countries, including Australia, Canada, and Japan, are diversifying their renewable technologies. All these changes in the world energy scenario have helped to increase confidence in renewable energy. By the year 2009, the United States had 12 percent of total installed capacity and more than 10 percent of total generation focused on renewable sources.

BIOMASS

The first application of biomass as a source of energy occurred in the early days of humankind, when people learned to use fire to produce heat and cook food. The first evidence that humans cooked food over controlled fires, based on the evolution of human molars, dates to 1.9 million years ago.

Biomass is organic raw material derived, directly or indirectly, from plants as a result of photosynthesis and includes crop residues for cogeneration, forest residues, animal wastes, municipal solid waste, and energy crops such as sugarcane, switchgrass, jatropha, and corn. Photosynthesis is the chemical process plants use to convert energy from sunlight, carbon dioxide, and water into oxygen and organic compounds, especially sugars (stored energy). The use of biomass to generate energy, as a substitute for fossil fuels, mitigates the greenhouse effect, because even though the carbon present in the biomass will be emitted when used as fuel, it comes from plants that previously removed the carbon (as carbon dioxide) from the atmosphere; hence, the "carbon sink" role of the plant has balanced the later combustion of the fuel and emissions from the plant.

Biomass can provide raw material for multiple fuel uses, for the production of heat, electricity, and both liquid and gaseous fuels for transport. We can extract the energy from these various sources of biomass through biochemical processes, chemical reactions, and mechanical technologies to convert biomass into liquid or gaseous fuel. However, a considerable disadvantage of biomass is related to its low energy density when compared with that of fossil fuels. The processing of biomass can require significant energy inputs, which should be minimized to maximize the conversion of biomass and energy recovery.

There are three basic uses of biomass as fuel. These include biofuels, biogas, and thermochemical energy.

Biodiesel and bioethanol are the best-known biofuels available for use in automobiles and other motor vehicles. Biodiesel is produced by transesterification, which is a reversible chemical reaction of vegetable oils or animal fats with alcohols, producing esters (biodiesel) and glycerin. Currently in the world, the most commonly used raw materials to produce biodiesel are canola and sunflower oils. Biodiesel can be mixed with traditional diesel fuel and used in compression-ignition engines without engine adaptations. Sugarcane, maize, wheat, sugar beets, and sweet sorghum can be used as raw materials for the production of bioethanol. These products are rich in sugars or starches, which are converted to alcohol by means of fermentation. Bioethanol production using sugarcane fermentation techniques has been commercially undertaken in Brazil since the 1980s.

Biogas can be produced from any kind of biomass by means of anaerobic microbes (bacteria that live in the absence of oxygen). Pigs, cattle, and chickens reared in confined areas produce a considerable concentration of organic waste matter with high moisture content, which can be use for biogas production. Biogas contains mainly methane and carbon dioxide, along with small amounts of other gases, such as hydrogen sulfide, ammonia, hydrogen, and carbon monoxide, giving it a very bad smell. The wet biomass is fed into an enclosed digestion tank together with a source containing anaerobic microbes; in the tank, anaerobic reactions occur. The remaining solid and liquid residues can be used as fertilizers. The period of time that biomass should remain in the digestion tank can range from a single day to several months. In 1630, it was discovered that decomposing organic matter is capable of producing a flammable gas, and in 1808 it was discovered that the gas contained methane. Biogas can be used as a low-cost fuel for heating and cooking; it can also be converted to electricity and heat or purified and compressed, much like natural gas, to create fuel to power motor vehicles.

Finally gasification and pyrolysis are thermochemical energythermochemical processes in which organic matter is degraded by thermal reactions in the presence of limited amounts of air or oxygen. The major products are biochar (charcoal), bio-oil, or a gaseous product, which can also be burned as fuel. The amount of each of the three products formed is dependent on the type and nature of the biomass input, the type of facility used, and the particular process adopted. Pyrolysis aims to obtain solid and liquid products, whereas gasification produces a gaseous product, composed mostly of hydrogen, carbon monoxide, methane, carbon dioxide, and water vapor.

HYDROPOWER

Hydropower refers to the energy generated through the use of flowing water. From millennia, hydropower has been used for irrigation; notable engineering of water channels has been found in the ancient remains of Egyptian and Mayan civilizations, and the engineering feats of the Roman civilization are well documented. There are many ways to harness the potential and kinetic energy of water to perform work; some examples include the use of waterwheels, water mills, run-of-the-river hydropower plants, hydroelectric dams, tidal power, and wave power.

Hydroelectric power is the electricity generated when water flows through a turbine to a lower level. These turbines, which are flow controlling blades mounted on rotating shafts, are usually located within the dams. The potential energy is stored by dams as a volume of water located behind the dam. As long as water is being released through the dam, it rotates the turbines, which are coupled to generators that then supply electricity to transmission lines. Hydropower plants play a major role in the world's capacity to generate electricity. For example, the Three Gorges Dam in China—the greatest hydropower plant in the world—has more than twice the capacity of the Kashiwazaki-Kariwa Nuclear Power Plant in Japan, which is the nuclear plant with greatest capacity in the world.

Tidal power is the energy that can be extracted from the rise and fall of ocean tides. Extraction of tidal power is simple in theory. The tidal dam, termed a barrage, is built across an estuary and creates an enclosed basin for storage of water at high tide. Turbines in the barrage are used to convert the potential energy, resulting from the difference in water levels, into electrical energy.

Less common types of hydroelectricity are wave power, run-of-the-river hydropower, and marine (or ocean) current power.

SOLAR ENERGY

Most solar energy used on Earth has its origin from the electromagnetic radiation from the sun, including biomass, hydropower, and wind power. However, the term solar power in the context of energy generation is used to refer to the direct conversion of solar radiation to a useful form of energy. Forms of solar power include photovoltaic electricity, solar power tower plants, and solar thermal heating, among other forms.

Although only a very small fraction of the radiation from the sun reaches the Earth, sunlight represents a tremendous source of renewable, greenhouse-gas-free energy. Passage through the atmosphere splits the radiation reaching the surface into direct and diffuse components, reducing the total energy through selective absorption by dry air, water molecules, dust, and cloud layers, while heavy cloud coverage eliminates all the direct radiation. Sunlight is intermittent; it varies diurnally from day to night over a 24-hour period as the Earth rotates. Thus, storage of the energy is a very important factor if it is to be used efficiently and economically.

A typical procedure is to use a solar collector to absorb the solar energy and convert it to thermal energy, which is transferred by heat pipes carrying pumped fluids for low-temperature (less than 100 degrees Celsius) heating or storage. Therefore, the collector should be made of materials with high thermal conductivity and low thermal capacity, such as metals (copper, steel, and aluminum) and some thermal-conducting plastics. The most common collectors are flat, blackened plates, since they convert both direct and diffuse (cloud-mitigated) radiation into heat.

Direct solar radiation can also be focused by a range of concentrating solar power technologies and collected to provide medium- to high-temperature heating. These technologies for concentrating solar power are of three types: parabolic troughs, power towers, and heat engines. The heat generated by the radiation is then used to operate a conventional power cycle, generally by steam-generating techniques similar to those used in conventional power plants. Solar thermal power plants designed to use direct sunlight must be sited in regions with high direct solar radiation.

Another way to use solar power is by means of photovoltaic (PV) conversion. The PV effect is the production of electric potential and current when a system is exposed to light. A solar cell is the PV device, and the light source is the sun. A solar PV cell consists in a semiconductor electrical junction device, which absorbs and converts the radiant energy of sunlight directly into electrical energy. Solar cells may be connected in series and/or parallel to obtain the required values of current and voltage for electric power generation needs. Most solar cells are made from single crystal silicon and have been expensive for generating electricity, but they have found applications. Research has emphasized lowering solar cell cost by improving performance and by reducing the costs of materials and manufacturing. Besides their low efficiency (relative to the percentage of the incident sunlight that is converted into electrical output power) and high costs, solar cells' power generation is limited by the presence or absence of solar radiation. For some applications, the electricity can be stored (in batteries, for example) to supply electricity on cloudy days and during the night.

WIND POWER

Windmills have been used to pump water and perform other kinds of mechanical work for centuries, but they were not used to produce electric power until the late 1800s. A wind power station consists of rotating blades attached to a generator, which is connected to transmission lines.

Wind power does not emit polluting emissions and does not produce unwanted substances that require careful disposal. There appear to be minor environmental impacts associated with the installation of wind turbines, aside from the possible disturbance of wildlife habitat and farming, which for some include the visual impact of a large, multiturbine wind farm on the natural beauty of an area. Wind turbines are not considered to be noisy machines; however, some noise is generated in their operation, and this has led to negative reactions of the public in some areas. Another issue is the coincident location of wind turbines in areas along the migration routes of birds; there have been reports of birds dying after colliding with the rotating blades of wind turbines. However, perhaps the greatest obstacles to wind farms have been that the areas where there is wind are often heavily populated and that the kind of equipment wind farms require is still too expensive.

GEOTHERMAL POWER

Geothermal energy is heat renewable energy from the depths of the Earth. It originates from the Earth's molten interior and from the radioactive decay of isotopes in underground rocks. The heat is brought near the surface by crustal plate movements, by deep circulation of groundwater, and by intrusion of molten magma, originating from a great depth, into the Earth's crust. In some places, the heat rises to the surface in natural streams of steam or hot water, which have been used since prehistoric times for bathing and cooking. Wells can be drilled to trap this heat to supply pools, greenhouses, and power plants. The reservoirs developed to harness geothermal energy to generate electricity are termed hydrothermal

convection systems and are characterized by circulation of water to depth. The driving force is the convection, via the density difference between cold, downward-moving recharge water and heated, upward-moving thermal water. Hot water from a reservoir is flashed partly to steam at the surface, and this steam is used to drive a conventional turbine-generator set.

Geothermal energy tends to be relatively diffuse, which makes it difficult to trap. If it were not for the fact that the Earth itself concentrates geothermal heat in certain regions—typically regions associated with the boundaries of tectonic plates—geothermal energy would be essentially useless.

Geothermal resources are renewable within the limits of equilibrium between off take of reservoir water and natural or artificial recharge. Within this equilibrium, the energy source is renewable for a long period of time. Although geothermal energy may not be technically "renewable," the global geothermal potential represents a practically inexhaustible energy resource. The issue is not the finite size of the resource but the availability of technologies able to trap this kind of energy.

FURTHER READING

Boyle, Godfrey. *Renewable Energy.* New York: Oxford University Press in Association with the Open University, 2004.

Klass, Donald L. *Biomass for Renewable Energy, Fuels, and Chemicals.* San Diego, CA: Academic Press, 1998.

Renewable Energy Policy Network for the 21st Century (REN21). *Renewables 2010 Global Status Report.* Paris: REN21 Secretariat, 2010. http://www.ren21.net/ REN21Activities/Publications/GlobalStatusReport/ tabid/5434/Default.aspx.

Sørensen, Bent. *Renewable Energy: Physics, Engineering, Environmental Impacts, Economics, and Planning.* Burlington, MA: Academic Press, 2011.

Spellman, Frank R., and Revonna M. Bieber. *The Science of Renewable Energy.* Boca Raton, FL: CRC Press, 2011.

U.S. Department of Energy. "2009 Renewable Energy Data Book, August 2010." http://www1.eere.energy. gov/maps_data/pdfs/eere_databook.pdf.

Leonardo Fonseca Valadares

SEE ALSO: Conservation; Nonrenewable Energy Resources

Going Online

Catfishing

"Catfishing" is the creation of false Internet identities to "snare" affection, money, or other things. Some catfish target celebrities whom they never meet. or may be sexual predators posing as hot dates. Catfish may be motivated by revenge, loneliness, or boredom, as well as sexual perversion. The term originated in 2010, from a documentary film, Catfish.

INTRODUCTION

Catfishing has become so popular that web sites exist which aggregate hundreds of fake photos from which a "cat" may choose. Some of them are models (or wannabe models) who want their images spread around the Internet, under anyone's name. As the number of social media sites proliferates, the number of fake traffickers rises as well. With all the electronic tricks now available for enhancing photographs, what one sees may or may not – in fact, in at least some cases, likely isn't – what one gets.

A person is being "catfished" when a seemingly attractive person appears online at random, and initiates conversation. Such people generally refuse to use Skype, on which an image is very difficult to fake. The catfish also generally shies away from telephone conversation or face-to-face communication, at least at first.

The number of people who now use the Internet seeking romantic relationships may exceed 40 million (Doctor Phil, 2015). The Catfish among them tend to target models on-line, becuaase they are attractive, and photographs of them are easily available. A "cat" may even borrow one model's photos and career details to go after another one. Doctor Phil added: "We see car accidents, deaths in the family and cancer a lot in catfish scams. This is very common because the best way to avoid meeting up is by having a traumatic experience. It will make the other person say, 'Oh, my God, don't worry about meeting with me now. I will just wait until you are better.' This is a way of tugging at your heartstrings and making you feel guilty." (Doctor Phil, 2015).

CATFISH, THE FILM

Catfish, directed by Henry Joost and Ariel Schulman, describes a young man named Yaniv (Nev) Schulman as he develops a Facebook conversation with an 8-year old child prodigy (as an artist), Angela (sometimes Abby) Pierce, who sends Nev one of her paintings. The relationships broaden to include her mother, the mother's husband, and Abby's older half-sister Megan, who becomes an object of Nev's on-line affection.

Megan sends Nev MP3s of songs that she says are hers, but he discovers that they all have been copied off YouTube. He later learns that large parts of Abby's art career also have been faked. Nev decides to visit Megan at her home in Michigan. Reality then intrudes: Abby rarely paints at all. Megan has an alcohol problem and has checked into re-hab, or so Nev thinks. Instead, Angela has been posing as Megan over a cellphone. The household includes two severely disabled chidren who require constant care. Angela discloses that she has cancer. Later, these stories collapse as well: Angela has no cancer, and Megan isn't in rehab. She may not even exist. After 1,500 text messages over nine months, Nev is left wondering just what is real and what is fake – and that's the point that the film is making about social media. What is being passed off as reality can change in an instant.

Social media (especially Facebook) encourage people to "curate" their images and use their profiles to gather a circle of friends. The Catfish takes advantage of this and many other platforms to concoct an entirely fictional persona that can be used for entrapment. Given the open and anonymous nature of social media, people can post photos and invent biographical narratives that have little to nothing to do with in-person reality.

The term "Catfish" was first used near the end of the film by its protagonist, Nev Schulman, as a reference to an Internet faker who had been a fisherman: "They used to tank cod from Alaska all the way to China. They'd keep them in vats in the ship. By the time the codfish reached China, the flesh was mush and tasteless. So this guy came up with the idea that if you put these cods in these big vats, put some catfish in with them and the catfish will keep the cod agile. And there are those people who are catfish in life. And they keep you on your toes. They keep you guessing, they keep you thinking, they keep you fresh. And I thank god for the catfish because we would be droll, boring and dull if we didn't have somebody nipping at our fin."

The Internet not only makes personal fakery easy. It also obliterates geographical differences. The young woman who was portrayed in the in pictures that Abby (or Angela) sent to Nev actually was Aimee Gonzales, who is known as a professional photographer and model who lived with her husband and two children in Vancouver, Washington, nowhere near Michigan. Her graphics had been poached off the Internet. Angela, at the height of her activity, had 15 fake Facebook pages, each under a different identity. Gonzales became part of the film, was compensated for her time, and took part in publicizing the documentary.

CRITICAL REACTION TO THE FILM

Given the tenuous nature of reality portrayed in the film, some viewers were skeptical of *Catfish*. Some thought that the film itself was an exercise in what came to be known as Catfishing. In the social-media era, the line between fact and fiction has never been less clear.

The film was generally well-received by critics and viewers as a gripping mystery that explored the important issue of fiction versus reality in social media. *TIME* magazine published a full-page article, written by Mary Pols in its September 2010 issue, saying "as you watch Catfish, squirming in anticipation of the trouble that must lie ahead—why else would this be a movie?—you're likely to think this is the real face of social networking" (Pols, 2010). John DeFore of the *Hollywood Reporter* said that Catfish was "jaw-dropping" and "crowd-pleasing' (DeFore, 2010). Roger Ebert, writing in the Chicago *Sun-Times*, said that *Catfish*, supplied "a severe cross-examination" of this issue and that (contrary to some skeptics), "everyone in the film is exactly as the film portrays them" (Ebert, 2010).

FURTHER READING

Bierly, Mandy (2010, September 3). "'Catfish' clips: A movie you'll be talking about." *Entertainment Weekly*. http://www.ew.com/article/2010/09/03/catfish-documentary-trailer. This is a positive review of Catfish, the movie.

Buchanan, Kyle. (2010, January 29) "Does Sundance sensation Catfish have a truth problem?" *Movieline*. http://movieline.com/2010/01/29/does-sundance-sensation-catfish-have-a-truth-problem/ This critical review asks whether Catfish (the movie) was a vehicle for media fakery.

Carlin, Peter Ames. (2010, October 6). "Aimee Gonzales stars in 'Catfish' -- without being in them movie". *Portland Oregonian*. http://www.oregonlive.com/entertainment/index.ssf/2010/10/aimee_gonzales_stars_in_catfis.html This feature story focuses on the woman whose life was raided without her knowledge in the movie *Catfish*.

Catfish (2010). Quotes. *Covergirl*. IMDb. Accesed May 20, 2015. http://www.imdb.com/title/tt1584016/

quotes This source traces the origin of the phrase "Catfishing."

DeFore, John. (2010, October 14). "Catfish -- film review." *Hollywood Reporter*, http://www.hollywoodreporter.com/review/catfish-film-review-29219. This review praises the engaging nature of the film.

Doctor Phil. "Online dating red flags: Warning signs of a catfish." Accessed May 9, 2015. http://www.drphil.com/articles/article/720. Dr. Phil, the well-known celebrity physician, advises viewers on how to avoid being "Catfished."

Ebert, Roger. (2010, September 22)."Catfish" Chicago *Sun-Times*.http://www.rogerebert.com/reviews/catfish-2010. Ebert, an eminent movie critic, places the film into a social-media context, finding it realistic.

Kaufman, Amy. (2010, October 5). "The woman behind 'Catfish's' mystery". *Los Angeles Times*. http://articles.latimes.com/2010/oct/05/entertainment/la-et-catfish-lady-20101005. This detailed report looks at the documentary *Catfish* in the context of problems with reality on social media.

McHugh, Molly. (2013, August 23). "It's catfishing season! How to tell lovers from liars online, and more." http://www.digitaltrends.com/web/its-catfishing-season-how-to-tell-lovers-from-liars-online-and-more/#ixzz3Zjfrdy77. This Internet site contains advice for the Facebook-smitten.

Pols, Mary. (2010, September 27)."Fish tale: The twisty new documentary Catfish examines how well wereally know the people we meet online." *TIME*. http://content.time.com/time/magazine/article/0,9171,2019606,00.html. Pols looks at the film as a comment on the slippery nature of reality on social media.

Bruce E. Johansen

SEE ALSO: Online Relationships

Computer hacking

Hacking is intrusions, unauthorized access, or attempts to circumvent or bypass the security mechanisms of a computer, computer network, computer program, or information system. Unauthorized access includes approaching, trespassing within, communicating with, storing data in, retrieving data from, or otherwise intercepting and changing computer resources without authorized consent.

SIGNIFICANCE

The financial damage, destruction, and disruption caused by computer hackers worldwide have been tremendous. The incidence and severity of computer hacking have severely worsened since the 1980's, when hackers' primary aims were to steal bandwidth or gain fame in the hacker community. Since 2001, computer hacking has expanded into a global form of white-collar crime motivated by profit, with hackers engaging in data theft, identity theft, computer hijacking, sabotage, extortion, and money laundering for personal financial gain or to fund illegal activities.

The term "hacking" has various meanings, but it is commonly used to refer to forms of intrusion into a computer, computer database, or computer network without authority or in excess of authority. Hackers are criminals who exploit vulnerabilities in computers, information systems, e-mail systems, and digital devices. Hackers routinely break into computer networks through the Internet by "spoofing" the identities of computers that the networks expect to be present.

Hackers may be thieves, corporate spies, or disgruntled individuals; they may work for organized crime organizations or for nations or political groups. Hackers motivated by personal grievances who attack individuals they know or their own companies are the easiest to track down. In contrast, the investigation of hacking and Web-based illegal activities used to finance terrorism is complex, requiring the cooperation of national intelligence agencies. Common to all computer hacking investigations is the use of computer and network forensic tools and techniques to follow digital trails back to the computers used for hacking, to determine the identities of the hackers, or to learn how and why hackers' attacks were successful.

Computer hacking is one type of computer crime that might violate several federal laws in the United States as well as laws in many individual U.S. states. The federal laws under which hacking might be prosecuted include the Computer Fraud and Abuse Act of 1984, the Electronic Communications Privacy Act of 1986, and, depending on whether copies of materials have been made, the Copyright Act.

ELECTRONIC EVIDENCE LEFT BY HACKERS

Although hackers vary in their intentions, all tend to use similar techniques, all of which require expertise in computers and computer networks; those who investigate hacking must have this expertise as well. The first step in hacking is usually to gain access to a networked computer and install an unauthorized hacker program, such as a Trojan horse or backdoor. All computer networks create logs that record the exact times of all attempts to log in, the IP (Internet protocol) addresses of the source computers, the commands that were used, and the programs that were installed. Those logs are valuable sources of information in the investigation of hack attacks unless the hackers covered their tracks by deleting entries from log files. Investigators can examine a computer's registry for stored information on installed software.

Not all hacking involves great technical skill. A hacker can sometimes gain access to a corporate system by calling an employee and pretending to be a coworker who needs help logging in. Because hackers can gain access through authorized accounts, investigators must consider the possibility that a person whose account was used to hack was not the hacker.

TRACING HACKERS' LOCATIONS

Software programs such as Netstat are available that enable investigators to trace hackers'

IP addresses to geographic locations. Hackers often use computers owned by other parties, however, such as those in public libraries or in public Internet cafés. This complicates investigations because such hackers must be prosecuted using evidence they leave on other people's computers. The longer hackers are allowed to compromise particular computers or networks, the more evidence can be collected against them to build solid cases. It is important that law-enforcement investigators are aware of this fact, but in some cases it may be necessary to shut down networks immediately to protect them.

In addition to needing an IP address, investigators need to identify the Internet service provider (ISP) from which an attack originated. Software is available that can reveal this information.

Hackers may try to hide their locations and identities by using software that routes Internet communications through untraceable IP addresses. Determining the IP address of the computer used to launch an attack is an important first step in discovering a hacker's identity. Most often, the IP address will be traceable back to a particular ISP. ISPs usually own "blocks" of IP addresses, in which only the last few digits differ, through which their customers connect to the Internet. These IP addresses are either statically or dynamically assigned, depending on the configuration of the ISP. An IP address of a static cable modem user constitutes a constant, traceable "fingerprint" of both the ISP provider and the specific user's computer terminal.

FURTHER READING

Casey, Eoghan. Digital Evidence and Computer Crime: Forensic Science, Computers, and the Internet. 2d ed.NewYork: Elsevier, 2003. Explains how computers and networks function, how they can be involved in crimes, and how they can be used as sources of evidence.

Kipper, Gregory. Wireless Crime and Forensic Investigation. New York: Auerbach, 2007. Presents an overview of the various types of wireless crimes and the computer forensic investigation techniques used with wireless devices and wireless networks.

Thomas, Douglas, and Brian D. Loader, eds. Cybercrime: Law Enforcement, Security, and Surveillance in the Information Age. New York: Routledge, 2000. Collection of articles covers topics such as criminality on the electronic frontier, hackers, cyberpunks, and international attitudes toward hackers. Points out mistakes that law-enforcement personnel and prosecutors sometimes make during the investigation of computer crimes.

Thomas, Timothy L. "Al Qaeda and the Internet: The Danger of 'Cyberplanning.'" Parameters: U.S. Army War College Quarterly 33 (Spring, 2003): 112-119. Discusses how the Internet is used to support and fund terrorism.

U.S. Department of Justice. Criminal Division. Federal Guidelines for Searching and Seizing

Computers and Obtaining Electronic Evidence in Criminal Investigations. Washington, D.C.: Government Printing Office, 2002. Explains the guidelines developed by the Justice Department's Computer Crime and

Intellectual Property Section in conjunction with an informal group of federal agencies known as the Computer Search and Seizure Working Group.

Volonino, Linda, Reynaldo Anzaldua, and Jana Godwin. Computer Forensics: Principles and Practice. Upper Saddle River, N.J.: Prentice Hall, 2007. Explains the use of investigative tools and procedures to maximize the effectiveness of evidence gathering. Chapter 10 discusses how investigators track down hackers and conduct large-scale investigations.

Linda Volonino

SEE ALSO: Protecting Your Computer

Online relationships

Online relationships have been a source of discontent between parents and adolescents since the Internet first entered our lives, and with good reason! We have all heard the horrid and tragic accounts of teens being lured to meet a "friend" they met online, only to discover this "friend" was a dangerous stranger whose intent was to victimize and harm. But is this an accurate depiction of the current climate of adolescent online relationships? Research into the online lives of today's teens paints a different, more positive picture. However, online relationships are not without their caveats.

INTRODUCTION

Technology has become an integral part of most everyone's lives, especially today's youth. The creation of MySpace in 2003 was the beginning of a social media phenomenon that very few could have predicted. By 2006, MySpace had become the most popular social network in the world. Many similar sites followed, such as Facebook, but also different types of technology became popular with adolescents including instant messaging, e-mail, text messaging, blogs, video and photo sharing, interactive video games, and virtual reality environments. These are all technological tools that adolescents use to engage in various types of online relationships.

Researchers have studied, and continue to study, these various types of technologies, as well as what types of relationships teens tend to form online.

These studies can inform us as to the safety of online relationships and provide parents and teens with a guide for understanding the importance of these relationships and ways to engage in them in healthy and safe ways.

THE PROGRESSION OF SOCIAL TECHNOLOGY AND ONLINE RELATIONSHIPS

The early years of social technology were very basic. The desktop computer was the main tool used and chat rooms were the popular choice where people would go to interact socially. Chat rooms were usually populated with people unknown to the user. Strangers. This is where the negative stigma of online relationships originated.

In addition, it was believed the majority of adolescents who chose to fulfill their social needs via online activities rather than real world interactions, were often those who suffered from social awkwardness or were socially marginalized for one reason or another.

Over time, much has evolved. We are no longer tethered to our desktop computers. We can now access various types of social technology via laptops, cell phones, tablets, and video gaming systems. Many of these new devices allow teens to be mobile and more secretive in their online activities.

The variety of social technologies has evolved as well. In addition to chat rooms and sites such as MySpace and Facebook, we have Intstagram, YouTube, Snapchat, Skype, FaceTime, virtual worlds like Second Life, online gaming, instant messaging, texting, email, and more.

As the technology has changed, so has the way adolescents use it. No longer are they mostly meeting and engaging in relationships with strangers online. It is now more popular to use social media to connect with established, offline friends as a means to enhance those relationships.

REASONS ADOLESCENTS ENGAGE IN ONLINE RELATIONSHIPS

Research tells us that all types of adolescents participate in social media, extroverts and introverts alike. With various personality types come various motivations for participation. Teens who are more outgoing use social media to enhance their existing relationships. They use various forms of online technology to make offline plans with friends, to communicate with friends when not together, to stay in touch with friends they don't see often, and to share the day-to-day details of their lives as well as to self-disclose more personal details about themselves.

Teens who are more socially shy find it easier to form new relationships online as they may feel more comfortable emailing, texting, or using instant messaging systems to communicate rather than engaging in face-to-face encounters. Like their extroverted peers, they also use online technology to self-disclose information about themselves they most likely would not share in face-to-face communication.

All teens may feel more comfortable exploring personal issues online with strangers as opposed to doing so with offline friends or family members. To meet this need, there are chat rooms and support groups where relationships are formed around a common theme. Teens may find supportive communities where they can discuss topics such as eating disorders, self-harming behaviors, chronic illnesses, sexuality concerns, and most any topic a teen may feel embarrassed to discuss face-to-face.

In addition to forming friendships or finding support online, many teens and adolescents use online technologies to find or enhance romantic relationships. Those already in offline romantic relationships use all types of online technologies to communicate, share pictures, and deepen their relationship. This is not without problems. As many have learned the hard way, information sent online is often permanent and cannot be controlled by the sender. This can result in intimate texts, pictures, and other communications being seen or shared with those not intended, including, at times, parents. Adolescents need to remember once they post information online it is out there forever, therefore, they must be careful what they post. A good rule of thumb is to ask yourself, "Would I be okay with my parents or someone else's parents seeing this?" before you hit send.

The increase in teen dating sights and apps such as Tinder and Omegle have led to a resurgence of teens looking for and finding new romantic relationships online, usually with strangers. Some of these sights encourage sexual dialogue inappropriate for adolescents. Some also encourage people to meet in person.

This can be dangerous since there are few safeguards in place to prevent interactions with those looking to victimize teens.

Developmental psychologist, Erik Erikson, is well known for his work on stages of development. According to Erikson, identity development is the main task of adolescence. The Internet, with it anonymity, various group and chat room options, and its facilitation of self-disclosure and self-exploration can assist adolescents with this developmental task. However, more research is needed to determine which tasks are facilitated in a healthy way and which are not.

THE GOOD, THE BAD AND THE UGLY OF ADOLESCENT ONLINE RELATIONSHIPS

As with most things in life, there are pros and cons to adolescent online relationships. Studies have found improvements in social media technologies over the years concerning safety, privacy settings, and the types of online relationships formed. However, dangers still exist and teens and parents need to be aware so they can take steps to minimize them. How can you stay safe?

- Understand and use the site's privacy settings. Most social media applications have them, but they vary from site to site and often change. Learn how the privacy settings work and be sure to limit who can view your information.

- Always let someone in your offline world know if you are talking to someone online that you don't know well.

- Beware of solicitation from hate groups. In addition to racist and sexist slurs sometimes found in poorly monitored chat rooms and discussion groups, some hate groups use the Internet to increase its membership by seeking out vulnerable adolescents who are searching for a sense of belonging. Report solicitation of this nature to a parent or other trusted adult, and to authorities.

- Be careful not to let online relationships reduce the quality and quantity of your offline relationships. Both are important. This includes relationships with family members. Make time to communicate with people face-to-face.

- As with offline relationships, be wary of strangers you meet online. Never meet a stranger in person without discussing it with your parents or another trusted adult. There are safe ways to meet your online friends in person. Take precautions.

- Sleep is important too. Many adolescents spend bedtime hours interacting with their online friends, foregoing needed sleep. A survey conducted by Teenage Research Unlimited found the hours between midnight and 5 a.m. are popular times for online communication, especially for those involved in romantic relationships. This results in sleep deprived teens who then have difficulty functioning the next day. Make sleep a priority.

- Beware of "social media depression". Remember that those who post on social media are often posting the highlights of their life. They don't usually post their disappointments, but remember that everyone has them. It's not fair to compare your life in its entirety to someone's highlights on social media. You will often come away feeling sad and unfulfilled. Likewise, adolescents often judge their self-worth based on how many "friends", "followers", "likes", or "shares" they get online. If you find yourself, or your child, becoming negatively affected by social media, it's time to take a break and do more face-to-face interacting.

- Most importantly, once you post something online you give up your control over it. Others have the ability to copy, save, share, and alter your text, photos, and videos. Parents, friends, teachers, school administrators, potential employers or colleges may be able to learn things about you that you'd prefer to have private. If you want something private, don't post it on social media.

THE FUTURE OF ONLINE RELATIONSHIPS

It is almost impossible to predict what the future will bring in terms of social media and online adolescent relationships. New types of technology and social media apps are continually being created. What is popular today may be quickly replaced by something new tomorrow. We need to be informed about new technologies, but also proceed with caution. And always remember to make face-to-face communication a priority.

FURTHER READING

Conway, P. (2015, March 4). "15 Apps and Websites Kids Are Heading To After Facebook. *Commonsense Media.* Retrieved from: https://www.commonsensemedia. org/blog/15-apps-and-websites-kids-are-heading-to-after-facebook?utm_source=030615%20Parent%20 Default#. This article discusses fifteen apps popular with today's teens. It separates the apps into four categories: texting apps, micro-blogging apps and sites, self-destructing/secret apps, and chatting, meeting, and dating apps and sites. In addition to providing an overview of the app or site, it also has a "what parents need to know" section for each.

McCarthy, C. (2013, September 30). "Online Dating For Teens? Why Parents Need To Talk About Online Relationships". *Huffington Post.* Retrieved from: http:// www.huffingtonpost.com/claire-mccarthy-md/online-dating-for-teens_b_3682486.html. This article discusses the different types of relationships teens may encounter online, romantic and otherwise. It also provides parents with sensible advice for navigating online relationships and their teens.

Spoon, M. (n.d.). "What's Social Media Depression— and Might I Have It? *HowStuffWorks.* Retrieved from: http://health.howstuffworks.com/mental-health/depression/questions/social-media-depression2.htm. This article defines social media depression, describes symptoms to look for, and what to do if you think you have it.

Taylor, J. (2013, February 27). Are online relationships healthy for young people? *Psychology Today.* Retrieved from: https://www.psychologytoday.com/blog/the-power-prime/201302/are-online-relationships-healthy-young-people. This article discusses the pros and cons of online relationships, giving particular attention to meeting new people online and forming relationships with them. The author addresses what is healthy and harmful, the affect on a teen's long-term development, and what parents can do to help ensure their children have positive experiences with online relationships.

Barbara Flor

SEE ALSO: Attention-Seeking Behavior; Peer Pressure; Social Media and Etiquette

Protecting your computer

Computers are everyday devices; however, they need to be protected in different ways than many other common devices. Computers require protection from physical hazards to which they are more susceptible than other items, such as dust, humidity, and electrical surges. Additionally, computers need to be protected from damage or intrusion by unauthorized users, programs, computer viruses, and other malicious activity to which they are susceptible without the owner's knowledge.

INTRODUCTION

Originally, computers were very expensive, complicated, and difficult to use devices designed to perform calculations and data manipulations much faster than possible manually by humans. Scientists, engineers, and businessmen at laboratories, universities, corporations, military, and government facilities operated computers. But, by the late twentieth century, computers had become more commonly available and were being operated by people with little concern for computer security. This change in computer use provided opportunities to those intending to do harm. Early issues with computer security involved unauthorized computer access and pranks in the form of computer programs that caused computers to perform harmless tasks. However, the harmless pranks evolved into malicious harmful tasks with computer files damaged or erased, or the computer rendered inoperable. Unauthorized access evolved from computer users attempting to gain access to computers for curiosity's sake to criminals attempting to gain access to computers to do damage or to steal information. Early computers were rarely connected to other computers, so intrusions and malevolent programs were passed from one another through shared files. As computers become more interconnected, though, intrusions became more common and more difficult to detect and prevent. Furthermore, cyber-criminals (the term used to describe persons committing crimes by computer) became more interested in controlling computers and stealing computer data than in committing pranks, destructive or non-destructive. Cyber-criminals began to write malevolent computer programs that could be inserted into computers and computer networks giving them access to the computers and the data stored on them and passed back and forth on the network between computers.

PHYSICAL PROTECTION

Computers are complex electronic devices. Their sophistication makes them useful, but it also makes computers vulnerable to several hazards that are often overlooked. Computers have to plug into power outlets. Even laptops and tablets, designed for portability, need to plug in to charge their batteries. But, spikes in voltage in the building's wiring can damage the sensitive electronics in computers. Small changes in voltage can occur due to interference from other devices plugged into wall outlets nearby, such as power tools or vacuum cleaners. Modern computers typically can handle small voltage fluctuations. However, large voltage spikes, such as those caused by a lightning strike or a transformer failure can sometimes irreparably damage a computer. Unplugging a computer during a thunderstorm is a simple solution, but another solution is to plug the computer into a surge protector that is then plugged into the electrical outlet. Surge protectors are designed to protect against voltage spikes.

Other physical hazards affecting computers include environmental factors such as heat, dust, humidity, and vibration. Humidity and heat can affect the electronics of computers. Heat, in particular, can cause computers to fail. Thus, it is important to maintain proper ventilation for the computer and not to expose it to excessive heat. Fans and vents on a computer should never be blocked. Laptops should be placed on hard smooth flat surfaces for best ventilation. Improper airflow over time might significantly shorten the life of a computer. Humidity can cause corrosion and interfere with computer operation after extended exposure. Dust, vibration, and impact, though are hazards that affect hard drives in computers. Modern hard drives are less susceptible to dust than older drives, but excessive dust should be avoided. Vibration and impact shock, though, can still damage hard drives, except for solid state hard drives. Solid-state drives are also not susceptible to dust damage. For these reasons, solid state drives, rather than the more common disk drives, are sometimes used in computers most susceptible to shaking, dropping, and dust, such as computers in industrial and construction settings.

When computer failures happen, files on the computers are often unrecoverable. Therefore, it is important to always remember to backup files. If files are backed up, either to portable media or to online storage before a computer failure, then the files can be still be accessed after the computer is repaired or replaced. Backups should occur on a frequent basis, because anything stored on the computer since the last backup is in danger of being lost if the computer fails. Very important documents and files should always be saved in more than one place as a backup to the backup.

SOFTWARE AND INTRUSION PROTECTION

Protecting computers from physical hazards is similar to protecting other electronic devices from similar hazards. Computers, however, are also susceptible to malevolent software. Rogue programmers, or hackers, began writing unauthorized software shortly after large numbers of people began to use computers. The early forms of such software inserted copies of itself into other programs, similar to the way that biological viruses replicate in living cells. Thus the term "computer virus" was coined for these programs. Though many modern rogue programs operate less like viruses than the original ones, the term computer virus is used to describe all manner of rogue programs. Some computer viruses delete files or interfere with computer operation while others attempt to steal passwords or data stored on computers. The best defense for personal computers against viruses is to make sure that current up-to-date anti-virus software is running on the computer. Anti-virus software works to recognize virus programs and to block their operation. However, anti-virus software does not stop all viruses. Anti-virus software only stops known viruses, so new viruses sometimes escape detection and can infect a computer, sometimes even disabling the anti-virus software's ability to later remove the virus.

A second defense against viruses is to avoid them in the first place. Classic viruses can attach themselves to files, so limiting downloading, copying, or looking at files except from a trusted source is a form of virus protection. It is especially important to only download files and programs from trusted sources. Email attachments can also carry viruses. Opening the email can infect the computer,

and some email viruses can then email themselves to other people. Anti-virus software can protect against known email viruses, but the best defense is to simply not open attachments unless they are expected. Some viruses can also be embedded in web pages, and simply viewing the web page can infect a computer. Sometimes virus-like programs, called malware, can be installed on a computer that will attempt to steal information or alter computer operation or access. Much malware is blocked by good anti-virus software, but sometimes separate anti-malware software is required to block or remove malware. Some malware is installed through web browsers, so such malware can be avoided by avoiding looking at only trusted and reputable web sites.

Computers are also susceptible to electronic intrusion and eavesdropping through networks connections. It is therefore important to have a firewall on the computer. A firewall is a program that controls incoming and outgoing databases on predefined rules, limiting what can be installed by an untrusted source, or what data an untrusted external computer can download from the computer with the firewall. Many modern operating systems include basic firewall protection, but more robust firewalls can be installed from third-party sources providing additional intrusion protection.

Network connections are the primary weakness for computer security problems involving intrusions and data theft. Firewalls and anti-virus software provide important layers of protection for computers. However, private information is routinely passed back and forth on networks, such as passwords, credit card numbers, and other sensitive information. Even if anti-virus and firewall software protect the computer from intrusion, cyber-criminals can still eavesdrop on the computer communications and capture the information being exchanged, putting the computer user at risk. To minimize this risk, ensure that when using a web browser to transmit information that the connection in encrypted (signified by a "https" prefix to a web page). But, web browser encryption is only part of computer networking security. If a computer uses a wireless router to connect to the internet, then it is important to use an encryption between the computer and the router in order to block other computers from being able to intercept the communication. This typically requires the use of a passkey to connect to the router. Such encryption is common with home and business routers, and it is important to use it. However, public open connections are often not encrypted in the same manner, permitting passwords and private information passed over the networks to be viewed by persons who have the proper equipment to eavesdrop on the communication. Thus, private information should never be shared over public, non-encrypted Wi-Fi networks.

Sophisticated cyber-criminals discover and exploit security flaws in operating systems, web browsers, firewalls, and anti-virus software. Companies that produce these products offer software patches and updates to ensure that their products are safe and secure whenever security holes are discovered. Therefore, it is important to frequently update software, particularly the protective software such as anti-virus and firewall programs. But, all software that interacts with files, such as office software, operating systems, web browsers, plug-ins, music players, and video players can also be exploited by sophisticated cyber-criminals. Thus, all software should be regularly updated, especially when the updates are designed to fix security flaws. Updates can be scheduled to occur at times when the computer is otherwise not being used so as to minimize the impact on computer performance while it is updating, and many programs can be set to check for updates automatically.

CONCLUSION

Computers are important tools in modern life; therefore, they should be cared for and protected. Physical protection of computers, of course, involves taking care of them and avoiding dropping or hitting them, but it also involves protecting them from excessive heat, cold, humidity, or dust. Proper ventilation is an important tool to prolonging the life of a computer. Computers also require protection from electrical hazards through the use of surge protectors. Besides physical protection, computers also require software protection, in the form of anti-virus software and firewalls. But, anti-virus software and firewalls can only do so much. It is also important to make sure that connections are secure and encrypted, and it is important to remember to never share any information over open connections that should remain private. It is also important to make sure that the computer is up-to-date with all installed software.

FURTHER READING

Geier, E. (2014) "7 easy tips to extend your PC's life span" *PC World*, 32, 6, 23 – 27. This is a very short article in a common periodical with basic tips to protect a home computer from hazards, both physical and software.

Geier, E. (2012) "The ultimate PC security toolbox" *PC World*, 30, 12, 87-93. This is an easy to follow article about basic computer security, focusing on virus protection and intrusion prevention for home computers.

Goodman, M. (2015) *Future crimes : Everything is connected, everyone is vulnerable and what we can do about it.* New York: Doubleday. More than just computer protection, this book covers vulnerabilities for all manner of computerized electronic devices.

Gregory, P. (2004) *Computer viruses for dummies.* Hoboken, NJ: Wiley. A bit dated, but this book gives a very easy to understand overview of viruses and how they affect computers.

Raymond D. Benge, Jr.

SEE ALSO: Computer Hacking

Social media addiction

Social media addiction represents a constellation of uncontrollable, impulsive, and damaging behaviors caused by persistent social media usage that continues despite repeated negative consequences.

BACKGROUND

The rise in popularity of social media websites, such as Facebook and Twitter, has spawned an age of social media consumption that is difficult to quantify. Rather than point to specific numbers or trends in everyday use, perhaps a better way of considering the effect of social media on society is to consider that two professional journals now chronicle the ongoing relationship with social media. The new journals are the *Journal of Social Media* and the *Journal of Cyberpsychology and Behavior,* both of which are relevant to studies of the effects of social media on human behavior.

Facebook, for example, has changed the way that people communicate and maintain social relationships, both in productive and nonproductive ways. Twitter has become a global vehicle through which people collect, report, and share the news of the moment. Communicating with other people has become easier and more immediate, while the boundaries, rules, and language that govern this communication have become more convoluted. As a result, research aimed at how and why people find themselves using social media (and technology in general) is on the rise.

Furthermore, features of one's personality that predict heavy (or limited) social media use are under investigation. So too are the merits of what widely interconnected, online relationships mean for face-to-face communication, intimacy, and privacy.

THE HUMAN RELATIONSHIP WITH TECHNOLOGY

Social media researcher Sherry Turkle has been exploring the interaction of human relationships and technology for decades. Her work has developed a collective understanding of how human beings interface with a technology and society. Her seminal works applying self and interpersonal theories to social media relationships were predictive and formative. Turkle has shown that technological advances have made it virtually impossible to isolate oneself from complex interpersonal relationships. Additionally, technology has done as much to challenge self-representation as it has challenged interpersonal relationships. In so doing, the ways in which one's real life aligns with one's virtual life are telling and have become useful fodder for ongoing research.

PSYCHOLOGICAL ADDICTION? LONELINESS, ANXIETY, SHYNESS

Because of the long-held assumption that social media helps to foster meaningful, online relationships, and because of the ease through which one can build a relationship with someone previously unknown to them, three psychological concerns in particular are now being studied: loneliness, anxiety, and shyness. No consensus exists on how these factors intersect with one's proclivity for social media (or for social media addiction), though there are a few interesting points to highlight.

First, research has shown a clear line of preference between people who self-identify as "lonely" and people who self-identify as "anxious"; specifically, lonely people prefer face-to-face communication (they find that social media lacks intimacy), whereas anxious people prefer electronic modes of communication. As such, loneliness has come to be better understood as something self-representational (with concerns hovering around issues of the self rather than of a specific fear of others or of socializing with others). Anxious people prefer social media because of the anonymity involved, making it easier to rationalize possible disapproval while having more

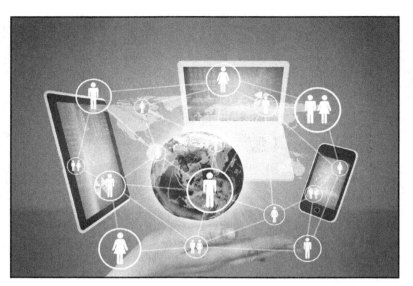

Photo: iStock

control over how the other person experiences them. Lonely people seek levels of intimacy that, while possible through social media, are not easily attainable.

Second, shyness is not something that inhibits social media usage despite the likelihood that shy people will experience the same minimal amount of social contact online as they would otherwise. Despite reported difficulty maintaining online relationships, shy people report heightened satisfaction in their virtual worlds. This is likely because they are spending a greater amount of time seeking, surveying, and considering positive social encounters while online. Additionally, social media provide a rather safe and secure outlet for heightened social interaction.

Third, the issue of locus of control has come under scrutiny as it relates to potential social media addiction. Specifically, research has examined closely the types of reinforcements experienced by heavy social media users. People are less likely to become addicted to social media if they feel that they have control over their own lives (both online and off), whereas people are more likely to be addicted to social media if they feel as if others have greater control over them (both online and off).

Turkle's analysis of the Internet (and social media) as seductive is especially relevant here, particularly when one considers the fluid nature of a person's experience of social media. That is, a person can update, alter, change, or redefine his or her online identity in the click of a button.

FURTHER READING

Beard, Keith W. "Internet Addiction: A Review of Current Assessment Techniques and Potential Assessment Questions." *Cyberpsychology and Behavior* 8.1 (2007): 7–14. Print. A useful article for those looking to initiate research in this particular area. Examines the relevant methodological issues important to research into social media (as well as some of the common challenges).

Chak, Katherine M., and Lous Leung. "Shyness and Locus of Control as Predictors of Internet Addiction and Internet Use." *Cyberpsychology and Behavior* 7.5 (2004): 559–70. Print. Examines at internal versus external reinforcement factors and how they affect one's proclivity for social media usage. Relates well to Turkle's work on self and interpersonal theory, challenges several notions about shyness and social media, and captures ongoing dilemmas in research methodology.

Chia-Yi, Mba, and Feng-Yang Kuo. "A Study of Internet Addiction through the Lens of the Interpersonal Theory." *Cyberpsychology and Behavior* 10.6 (2007): 799–804. Print. Of particular interest in this article is the exploration of the negative correlation found between addiction and interpersonal relationships. Also explores reasons underlying addictive behaviors.

Lam, Lawrence T., et al. "Factors Associated with Internet Addiction among Adolescents." *Cyberpsychology and Behavior* 12.5 (2009): 551–55. Print. Attempts to identify relevant risk factors for addiction in a younger population. Of particular concern are adolescents who are male, dissatisfied with their family, and have recently experienced a stressful event.

Muise, Amy M., Emily Christofides, and Serge Desmarais. "More Information Than You Ever Wanted: Does Facebook Bring out the Green-Eyed Monster of Jealousy?" *Cyberpsychology and Behavior* 12.4 (2009): 441–44. Print. Counterbalances research suggesting long-term positive benefits of social media usage. Concerned with how social media can potentially introduce one to more jealousy-provoking information than would ordinarily be available.

Orr, Emily S., et al. "The Influence of Shyness on the Use of Facebook in an Undergraduate Sample." *Cyberpsychology and Behavior* 12.3 (2009): 337–40. Print. A good example of the type of research being conducted to better understand how increasing social media usage intersects with shyness.

Rosen, Larry D. iDisorder: *Understanding Our Dependency on Technology and Overcoming Our Addiction*. New York: Palgrave, 2012. Based on decades of research and expertise in the psychology of technology. Offers clear explanations for why many people are addicted to technology, including social media.

Stevens, Sarah, and Tracy Morris. "College Dating and Social Anxiety: Using the Internet as a Means of Connecting to Others." *Cyberpsychology and Behavior* 10.5 (2007): 680–88. Print. This article examines whether or not high levels of social anxiety (specifically, dating anxiety) are related to heightened social media usage.

Turkle, Sherry. "Whither Psychoanalysis in Computer Culture." *Psychoanalytic Psychology* 21.1 (2004): 16–30. Print. This article explores three competing (though related) theoretical orientations that help explain the human relationship with technology.

WEBSITES OF INTEREST

Center for Internet Addiction
http://www.netaddiction.com
Internet Addiction Guide
http://psychcentral.com/netaddiction

Joseph C. Viola

SEE ALSO: Online Relationships

Social media and etiquette

Social Media includes the use of online frameworks to communicate, educate, socialize, and connect with others along a continuum. Teens and young adults utilize these resources but lack the education to do so appropriately. Etiquette and safety are essential tools to utilize when exploring and experiencing social media. Without a code of conduct or rules to follow, anyone can divulge misinformation or inappropriate content leading to long-term consequences. Resources exist to lend support to teens, young adults, parents, and families on how to navigate social media sites.

INTRODUCTION

High school and college students spend the majority of their time exploring social media sites—posting, liking, and viewing other online members' pages and comments. This has significantly increased over the last few years with teens and young adults utilizing these sites for networking, connecting with others, messaging, and sending pictures. These are just a few of the common occurrences on social media platforms. Negative occurrences include bullying, disgracing their jobs, sending nude pictures, or humiliating other individuals all of which can destroy a reputation. It is important young adults are responsible and learn the appropriate etiquette and safety when it comes to social media.

Social media is a major aspect of human connection, and it is essential for college and high school students to develop skills to portray themselves appropriately online. Many resources have created tips and tools to help direct proper use of social media sites. Improper use of social media can impact future endeavors as many employers scan social media sites for inappropriate images and comments that can provide background on each individual being interviewed. Young adults do not need any negative portrayal of their character, especially online, as they begin to progress through life and develop their career. Knowing the resources that provide education on etiquette and safety for networking sites can protect one's dignity now, and in the future.

SOCIAL MEDIA ETIQUETTE

Etiquette or in this case 'netiquette' is rules of social behavior that drive interaction across online networks. Multiple resources have provided guides to help navigate what should or should not be done online. The three main focuses are picture content, posted comments, and accessibility. If youth are able to tackle these subjects successfully then they will represent themselves appropriately and will less likely fall into common pitfalls of bullying, dishonesty, and poor social behavior.

PICTURE CONTENT

A profile picture should be a direct representation of the page owner, either with a picture of the owner or an image the owner feels represents one's self well. Pictures should be age-appropriate and lack discriminatory or degrading content. One blog mentioned that each owner should take a step back after posting a picture and ask themselves what their mother would think of this. It may curb the need to post degrading pictures that misrepresent who they are. Also, it may help to remember that it is necessary to represent the others in the picture appropriately as well. Pictures should be about truth, honesty, and a dignified expression of their content. Remember

that you will never be the only one seeing these pictures, so post them wisely.

POSTED COMMENTS

A common mistake made by teens and young adults is over-communication. Over-communication is the concept of posting too much content most of which is irrelevant. This will likely mean different things to different people. However, imagine scrolling through an online feed and commenting on every post or frequently clicking the 'like' button. The question is whether or not it was necessary to do so. Was the post relevant to your well-being or thoughts at that specific time? Was it necessary to let others know how you felt on that subject? These are the questions that should be asked before posting or responding online.

THINK is often used as an acronym to help answer the above questions. It stands for: truth, helpfulness, inspiration, necessary, and kind. These qualities should be considered when posting online. If the content falls under one of these it is more likely to be valuable online content. Perception is important when posting comments, because individuals want to be perceived as they truly are. How others read and react to their comments dictates how they are perceived. Being mindful of this can help guide their internal decision to post. Following the THINK principle in posting promotes positivity and builds a general framework to follow when posting to social media.

It is essential not to forget to give credit where credit is due. If posting a quote or even a statement from another friend remember to acknowledge the original author. This demonstrates your integrity and also shows respect to the original author. Being respectful is extremely important on online networks.

ACCESSIBILITY

Accessibility refers to other's access to your online content on different networking sites. Privacy settings exist on each of the online venues, but often are not changed by users. However, one should not rely solely on default privacy settings to protect their social media content. Content posted on social media is often public information and is viewed by more than those on your friend's list. Common ways to avoid invasion of privacy is to friend those who are truly friends, and separate your professional and personal profiles.

Anyone on your friends list can read the content posted on your timeline and many times if a friend is tagged in the post, it can also be read by their friends. Some sites allow individuals to specify who can read posts while others do not. It is important to know what each site allows. Examine privacy settings to explore how friends and non-friends can view your content. For example, potential employers are becoming technically savvy and view the social media accounts of their potential employees. Although they are not on your friend's list, if your content is public they will be able to view it. Therefore, it is important for your online profile to be an authentic and positive image of yourself.

Lastly, having separate professional and personal profiles can make many issues obsolete. You may choose to have your coworkers connect with you on professional networks like LinkedIn, while your family and friends connect with you on Facebook. Although potential employers can still search for you on either social networks, having separate profiles allows you to keep your professional connections professional instead of having them as friends on sites that are less inhibiting.

SOCIAL MEDIA SAFETY

Aside from participating in appropriate 'netiquette', it is also necessary to learn techniques for online safety. These tools are critical because of the vital information we share and the amount of time we spend on social networking sites. Online safety falls into two categories, general safety and avoiding unsafe environments.

General safety includes managing passwords, using security software, and limiting personal information online. These three are particularly important because of the potential for hacking, unwanted exposures to the public, and for knowing how to manage your online presence. Each social media site requires information to sign-up, but it is important to provide only what is necessary. The more personal information you provide such as your phone number or address, the more vulnerable you possibly become to hacking or unwanted exposure.

Adjusting your privacy and security settings on the site is another avenue of protection. Take the time to review these settings and change them to provide the highest level of protection. Also, do not forget about your password, as this is the ultimate key to online information. Each password should be different for each social media site. This can be difficult to do, but is significant for protecting data. Longer and more complex passwords are more difficult for hackers to decode. Hackers prey on those who have simple passwords or use their favorite color or dog's name as passwords. Complexity includes

adding lowercase, uppercase, and symbols to a password with at least six to eight characters. Remember not to share passwords with others. However, teens may consider or be required to share their password with their parents for safety reasons.

Additionally, security software for a home network or computer adds another layer of defense. These are easily purchased at electronic stores or even online. Creating a safe online presence can be challenging but necessary.

Social media can often be an avenue for bullying, harassing, or even just an unsafe environment. People can only control their own actions; therefore it is vital to create a positive online environment. Avoid making negative comments and avoid over- sharing as discussed above. Have a confidant that can make suggestions on directions to go if bullying or harassing begins, and even if friend requests appear from unknown people. The confidant can be a best friend, family member, or parent, and can offer suggestions on how to approach each situation. Others may not always be kind on social media, but that does not mean engaging in that behavior is appropriate. Positive social behaviors can lead to a decrease in negative outcomes.

CONCLUSIONS

Navigating social media in terms of etiquette and safety takes time, skill, and knowledge. Talking about it with others can help solidify choices and increase knowledge. Managing privacy and security settings can set an individual's page apart from others. It provides more control and decreases the opportunity for others outside of the friends list to have access to the page. Avoiding over-communication and negativity will go a long way in social media. Be truthful, maintain integrity, and consider separating professional and personal ventures. These tools are important in establishing 'netiquette' and staying safe on social media.

FURTHER READING

Gottsman, D. (2015, March 11). Social media etiquette for college students and young professionals. *Huffington Post*. Retrieved from: http:// http://www. huffingtonpost.com/diane-gottsman/social-media-etiquette-fo_1_b_6838796.html. This article provides tips on social media etiquette for young adults, especially those beginning to navigate the business world and find jobs. It discusses concepts to consider when posting or joining a social media site and reminds this audience that employers can see what you post.

National Cyber Security Alliance. (n.d.). Social Networks. Retrieved on May 26, 2015 from StaySafeOnline.org website: http://www.staysafe-online.org/stay-safe-online/protect-your-personal-information/social-networks. This website is a great resource for social media information, both on etiquette and safety. It provides blogs reviewing online information for specific social media sites as well as general information for teens, young adults, and parents regarding he social media wave. It purposefully focuses on staying safe online and provides resources on how to do just this with security software and how to navigate the sites one currently engages on.

Pulido, M. (2013, March 22). Social media gone awry: Tips for teens to stay safe. *Huffington Post*. Retrieved from: https://www.huffingtonpost.com/mary-l-pulido-phd/social-media-gone-awry-ti_b_2923603.html. This article provides basic tips for teens to follow on what to and not to post by exploring appropriate and inappropriate content. The author provides tips on how to change what might already be posted and to encourage thinking before posting. The article also talks about safety measures to take if meeting someone offline that you met online.

Lenhart, A., Madden, M., Smith, A., Purcell, K., Zickuhr, K, & Rainie, L. (2011, November 9). Teens, kindness, and cruelty on social networking sites: How American teens navigate the new world of digital citizenship. *Pew Research Center: Internet, Science, & Tech*. Retrieved from: http://ww.pewinterest.org/2011/11/09/teens-kindness-and-cruelty-on-social-network-sites/. This article references a study done by the Pew Research Center of teen social media use. It provides statistics behind the number of teens using social media and some of the situations they have encountered on social media such as harassment or bullying. It also compares these statistics to the adult population and identifies some common responses to negative situations..

Oriaku A. Kas-Osoka & Emmanuel L. Chandler

SEE ALSO: Catfishing; Changing Passwords; Computer Hacking; Interpersonal Communication; Online Relationships

Spam and scams

The 200 billion e-mail messages sent and received each day worldwide present all sorts of frontiers in thievery.

Once upon a time, it was said that some rob you with a gun, and others do it with a fountain pen. Today, more money is stolen with computer keyboards than with guns and fountain pens combined. Some scams even commit identity theft by claiming to eliminate it, by offering phony "anti-fraud" software – free, a click away. Forewarned is forearmed, and a few precautions can avoid massive rip-offs.

INTRODUCTION
E-mail users may be greeted by a supposed International Monetary Fund agent and "United Nations Diplomat" who says that he was husbanding a $4 million inheritance in the e-mail recipient's name at Hartsfield International Airport. The same morning, the same recipient might hit the numbers in the British lottery, or so an email suggests. Just call this number, or click on this link, and have your checking account routing number handy.

Scammers also have been committing tax fraud using the telephone as well as the keyboard. Fake IRS "agents" sternly lecture anyone they can reach that they owe a huge sum in back taxes and will soon be hauled off to prison by local police if the "debt" is not promptly pay up on a pre-paid debit card.

According to the Associated Press, by mid-March, 2015, the IRS-scamsters, some of whom were calling or spamming from overseas (obvious when a caller referred to the "Internal Revenue Department"), had targeted at least 366,000 people, of whom at least 3,000 had taken the bait, and coughed up about $15.5 million, usually on pre-paid debit cards or wire transfers, as the scamsters demanded. Some of these scams had been traced to call centers in India. By 2015, this form of fakery topped the IRS' "Dirty Dozen" list of tax scams. By 2015, according to the Federal Trade Commission, tax scams comprised fully one third of the identity theft complaints in its database – that is, 100,000 of 330,000.

E-mail users have been forced to hack their way through hundreds of offers for various "services" they do not want, like having a personal carnival midway and whorehouse annex camped on their desks, with a mile-long line of barkers shouting for attention. Some of the offers are silly: buy an acre of the back side of the Moon? ($29.95, major credit card accepted).

One subject line read: "Tired of Fake Promises for Money?" The text then pledged that anyone who quit his or her day job and made a few phone calls from home could make "$6,000 to $20,000 in a month. Another asked, "What if you could make $20,000 in one click? Another one implored, "Earn $24,000 in 24 hours!" And another: "One hundred grand in 100 days!!!…We'll pay you to do next to nothing!"

A UNIVERSE OF SCAMS

The Nigerian money scam is also known as a "419" after its number in the Nigerian government's criminal code. The scammer says he is a government official, an affluent business owner, or a spouse of a deceased person with an estate who will transfer a large sum of money (perhaps several million dollars) into your bank account if you pay a fee or taxes. Any "fees" will be stolen, but that's just the beginning. Having acquired bank account numbers, these will be drained as well.

The Nigerian money scam now comes in many varieties, from anywhere in the world. One Nigerian moneyman titled his spam "Divine Will" invoking Jesus Christ. Others involve offers of money from international bodies, such as the United Nations, the International Monetary Fund, or various banks. It may invite participation in an investment partnership, or collection of an inheritance, lottery winnings, and so forth. Anyone who takes the bait by replying will be told to forward a sum of money, perhaps a few thousand dollars, to guarantee payment of hundreds of thousands, even millions. The guarantee, once delivered, will then disappear. Many "419" schemes steal reputable aliases. One claimed to have been posted by Ban Ki-Moon, secretary general of the United Nations on June 5, 2015, by way of "Zenith Bank Compensation Unit." It offered $350,000 as well as free anti-scam software.

One such scam claimed, under the name of Barclays Bank in London, to offer $15 million from an "inheritance fund" with the Nigerian National Petroleum Corporation in conjunction with the Ministry of Finance of the Federal Republic of Nigeria. The huge amount on offer, as well as tortured grammar and spelling errors are something of a giveaway. This one went to lengths to stress that the $15 million would be transmitted at no charge – just send account numbers and international clearance codes. Related to the Nigerian money scam are emails claiming that the recipient has won a foreign country's lottery but must pay "taxes" or "customs duties" to collect the prize. Any money will be stolen, and any bank-account numbers will be used to drain the target's accounts.

"Phishing" attacks claim affiliation with familiar businesses or other organizations, bank, or e-mail payment services (such as PayPal), instructing anyone who receives it to "update" an account or have it shut down. This is actually a form of identity theft designed to get access to credit card numbers, bank accounts, and other assets.

The world of spam scams has its own terminology, which describes how it works. An address harvester, for example, a robot or "spider" will "crawl" websites for addresses at which to aim messages, making lists for sale to spammers. It may seek symbols (such as @), which appear in many types of e-mail addresses. "Adware" includes software that many free programs install on your computer without permission that will send your address to advertisers that send "popup" ads or other commercial material.

"Attachments" may contain material required to activate malicious programs ("malware") that act as "Trojan horses" to hijack computers and commit identity theft by hackers who invade computer systems and steal massive amounts of personal data. Hijacking has been defined as "an attack whereby an active, established session is intercepted by an attacker who wants to abuse your session. Hijacking can occur both via the Internet as well as locally, i.e. if a user leaves a computer unprotected making it possible for a spammer to pretend his mails are coming from someone else" (Spam and scam, 2015). Hackers, through use of malware installed on computers by users who have clicked on attachments, have seized a "zombie" computer. Never click on an unknown attachment.

"Spoofing" involves faking identity, "when a spammer or scammer fakes his origin or pretends to be someone else i.e. of a sent mail, where the header is made to appear from someone other than who it really is. This is often the case when someone sends phishing mails, making it look like it came from a legitimate sender to try to trick you" (Spam and scam, 2015). One form of this trick hijacks users' email address books and then sends messages that the sender is in trouble (imprisoned in a foreign country, for example) in an attempt to get money, which is then directed to the scammer.

FURTHER READING

Apter, Andrew (2005). *The Pan-African nation: Oil and the spectacle of culture in Nigeria*. Chicago, IL: University of Chicago Press. This book provides cultural context for Nigerian money scams.

Spam and scam glossary. (2015). Spamfighter. http://www.spamfighter.com/SPAMfighter/FAQ_Glossary.

asp. This list contains a guide to the language of spamming and scamming.

"Ten common spam scams." IT Business Edge. http://www.itbusinessedge.com/slideshows/show.aspx?c=83258&slide=2. This list describes some of the most common spam scams and how to avoid them.

Bruce E. Johansen

SEE ALSO: Changing Passwords; Computer Hacking; Protecting Your Computer

Grief and Loss

Accidents

An occurrence in a sequence of events that produces unintended injury, death, or property damage. "Accident" refers to the event, not the result of the event. "Unintentional injury" refers to the result of an accident and is the preferred term in the health community for accidental injury.

CAUSES AND SYMPTOMS

Unintentional injury continued to be the fifth leading cause of death in the United States as of 2000, exceeded by heart disease, cancer, stroke, and chronic obstructive pulmonary diseases (asthma, pneumonia, and influenza). In 2000, injuries had a financial impact on the average American household of approximately $4,600. Individuals and households sustain this loss by paying higher prices for goods and services and higher taxes or through direct, out-of-pocket loss. The leading cause of unintentional injury and death remains motor vehicle accidents, followed by poisoning, falls, drowning, and burns. Other injuries and deaths result from air transportation accidents, weather, and major disasters.

As of 2000, motor vehicle unintentional injuries, including those from automobile and motorcycle accidents, remained the leading cause of injury and death in the United States in individuals aged one to thirty-eight. Males between fifteen and twenty-one accounted for 60 percent of the deaths from automobile crashes. Not wearing seat belts in automobiles and not wearing helmets while operating other vehicles can lead to serious head trauma and death. Falls are a serious problem for seniors and the leading cause of death in people sixty-five and older.

Broken bones, cuts, bruises, and whiplash are the most common injuries in accidents involving one or more vehicles. More serious injuries from vehicles, sports, and falls include trauma to the head and neck; spinal cord injuries; knee injuries; eye injuries and blindness; comminuted, compression, and compound fractures; hip fractures; severed limbs; and severe burns.

Vehicle accidents are those caused by automobiles and motorcycles and cause more serious injuries, such as head trauma, spinal cord injuries, blindness, and burns. Self-propelled vehicles, bicycles, scooters, skateboards, and in-line skates are also included in this group and produce less serious injuries, such as cuts, bruises, and simple fractures.

Head injuries are always considered serious. They cause more deaths and disabilities than any other neurologic condition before the age of fifty and occur in 70 percent of all unintentional injuries. They are the leading cause of death in men and boys up to thirty-five years of age. Motorcycle head injuries are most serious in those who do not wear helmets. Upon impact, the rider is thrown toward the ground at accelerated speeds, causing severe blunt force trauma, especially to the head.

The brain fits loosely within the skull so that blunt force to the skull or violent shaking of the head back and forth causes the brain to bounce off the skull. This violent brain movement causes bruising, tearing, and bleeding between the brain tissue and the skull.

There are two types of brain injury, diffuse and focal. Diffuse is most common and includes concussion. One-third of those who die from brain injury die from diffuse brain injury. An injury victim can have a concussion without losing consciousness and have no visible signs of trauma on the head, such as a bump or cut. If signs of amnesia, impaired attention, distractibility, and changes in cognitive functioning (knowing information such as one's immediate location) are temporary after concussion, this may imply the patient has had no structural damage. This does not, however, indicate the severity of the injury. A CT (computed tomography) scan or MRI (magnetic resonance imaging) is used to diagnose the extent of diffuse and focal brain injuries. Careful examination by a neurosurgeon is necessary.

Focal brain injury involves a specific area of the brain. This includes brain contusions that occur from a direct blow to the head (and are similar to other external bruises); ischemia, which is damage to the brain tissue due to a reduction in the flow of blood to the brain; infarction, which causes affected brain tissue to die from lack of blood supply; and pressure which is caused by the brain tissue swelling from the trauma.

A direct blow to the head can cause an epidural hematoma, which is bleeding between the skull and the brain membranes. This occurs quickly and causes unconsciousness at the time of injury, perhaps a lucid interval, and then coma. Subdural hematomas cause bleeding that occurs slowly within the brain tissue, are frequently complicated by contusions of the brain tissue, and carry a significant risk of death even with surgery. A favorable outcome with any brain injury depends on rapid and careful transportation to a hospital for diagnosis and treatment.

Bicycle, scooter, skateboard, and in-line skate injuries are sustained in falls. About half of these occur to hands and arms, one-third to head and face, and one-third to legs and feet, including fractures and dislocations. Other injuries include lacerations requiring stitches, cuts and bruises, and strains and sprains. Fatalities may occur when a victim collides with an automobile.

Sports injuries are generally to ligaments, muscles, and joints. More serious sports injuries include concussions, broken bones, and spinal cord injuries. Knee injuries can be sustained in vehicular and sports accidents and falls. Most severe knee injuries occur in competitive sports accidents, particularly football. The most common are ligament or cartilage tears and traumatic arthritis. A "blown out knee" is a tear of the anterior cruciate ligament, one of four principal ligaments in the knee and most important for stability of the knee.

Unintentional injuries from falls are most common in patients aged fifty-five to seventy-five and are the primary cause of fatal injury for people aged sixty-five and older. Approximately 60 percent of fatal falls occur in the home, 30 percent in public places, and 10 percent in institutions. Hip fractures are the most serious injury sustained from falls. The impact on the injured individual's quality of life can be devastating. Most patients cannot return home or live independently after a hip fracture. Aseriously injured patient requires a caregiver on duty twenty-four hours a day, which can be costly. Lack of mobility causes severe depression, especially for someone who had been active. Climbing to reach an object is not the cause of most falls in older adults, but rather vision problems, poor lighting, slippery surfaces, wearing house shoes with soft soles, balance problems resulting from disease or medication, and clutter such as papers or magazines on the floor.

Poison is any substance that produces disease conditions or tissue injury, or otherwise interrupts natural life processes when in contact with or absorbed into the body. Most poisons taken in sufficient quantity are lethal. A poison, depending on the type, may attack the surface of the body or, more seriously, internal organs or the central nervous system.

Poisoning is a leading cause of accidents resulting in unintentional injury and death. These agents include illicit drugs (street drugs and those not prescribed by a physician), medicines (over-the-counter and prescribed drugs), mushrooms, eggs, shellfish, and gases or vapors. Poisons are usually classified by effects as corrosives, irritants, or systemic or nerve poisons (narcotics).

The American Association of Poison Control Centers estimates that 2.5 million poison cases, fatal and nonfatal, were reported during 2000. These incidents have nearly tripled in the last thirty years. This may be due to the increase in the use of illegal street drugs.

Common results of poisoning include burns to the skin or eye tissue, or to mucous membranes of the mouth, throat, esophagus, stomach, and other parts of the body with which a caustic poison might come in contact when swallowed or inhaled; central nervous stimulation or depression; cerebral edema; renal (kidney) and/or hepatic (liver) failure; brain damage; and death.

Corrosives are strong acids or alkalies that, when swallowed, burn the skin or lining of the mouth, throat, and stomach, causing bloody vomiting. Ammonia is an example of a common household corrosive. Irritants (such as iodine, arsenic, and laxatives) act directly on the mucous membrane, causing inflammation and gastrointestinal upset with pain and vomiting. Irritants can be absorbed slowly and become cumulative until they take effect suddenly, causing serious illness or death. Central nervous system poisons (narcotics) affect the heart, liver, lungs, and kidneys, as well as the respiratory and circulatory systems. Examples of household narcotics include alcohol, turpentine, cyanide, and strychnine (found in some pesticides). Botulin toxin, the bacteria that causes botulism (food poisoning), is one of the most dangerous poisons known and is included in this group. Asphyxiants include gas poisons such as carbon monoxide. Gases, when inhaled, get into the bloodstream and prohibit the body from properly absorbing oxygen. Blood poisoning, or septicemia, is included in this category. Microorganisms get into the bloodstream through a wound or infection, also preventing, in advanced stages, proper oxygen absorption. Smoke from house fires is an asphyxiant and causes most fire-related deaths.

Deaths from residential fires are second only to those occurring as the result of automobile accidents. In 2000 alone, five thousand people were killed in house fires. Most accidents causing burns can be avoided by preventing the cause. Burns are the most devastating of all unintentional injuries, causing red and painful areas on skin with blisters, scarring, contractions of skin resulting in a decrease in motion, dehydration, shock, damage to lungs from inhalation of smoke and hot air, and loss of skin that can be traumatic and lifethreatening.

TREATMENT AND THERAPY

Simple fractures, those bones broken with little or no displacement, can be set in the hospital emergency room or clinic by a general or orthopedic surgeon. A cast is applied to hold the bones in place until they grow together again. The patient is usually asked to come back in six weeks for new X rays and probable cast removal. Comminuted fractures (bone broken into fragments), compression fractures (damage to soft tissue at site), and compound fractures (bone protruding through skin) require surgery. These fractures may cause deformity of the limbs if extensive and if surgical intervention cannot return the bone fragments to proper alignment. In some compression or comminuted fractures, a steel plate is attached with screws through healthy bone above and below the fractured area, and a cast is applied. Traction may be required and the patient kept hospitalized and immobile for several weeks. Physical therapy may be required to regain strength and mobility in the legs or motion in the joints of the upper extremities.

Skull fractures are easier to diagnose and treat. A simple linear skull fracture, depending on the location, often requires no intervention except hospitalization for observation. A skull fracture that goes deeper than the thickness of the skull requires surgical evaluation.

Any foreign objects or objects impaled in a victim's head will be removed only in the operating room by a neurosurgeon, with the patient being kept for at least a twenty-four hour observation. Patients who have had severe head wounds often require extensive physical and psychological therapy. Personality changes can occur, causing the patient to exhibit agitated behaviors, anger, and the inability to cope with everyday activities. Relearning normal bodily functions, such as speech, walking, and writing, becomes a series of frustrating, monumental tasks. Behaviors can be so uncontrolled that confinement is necessary so that there is no danger to the patient or others. Medications combined with psychotherapy and physical therapy can typify the long road back to normalcy. Some patients never fully recover.

Repair to an injured knee is done under general anesthesia. Instruments are inserted into the knee joint through several small punctures. While viewing the ligaments through the arthroscope, the surgeon can repair or remove damaged tissue. If torn, the anterior cruciate ligament can be rebuilt. Most arthroscopic surgery is performed on an outpatient basis. Meniscal cartilages are the "shock absorbers" between the femur (thighbone) and the tibia (large leg bone) at the knee joint. A tear in the meniscal cartilage is the most common knee injury requiring surgical intervention. Arthroscopic surgery is done on an outpatient basis, and the patient is allowed to walk on the affected leg as soon as it feels comfortable. Physical therapy may be recommended for both anterior cruciate ligament and meniscal cartilage tears. Chances of returning to competitive sports are quite good, even for those who play professionally.

Poisoning should be treated immediately but with the direction of a health care professional. Most poison cases can be handled in the home after consulting a poison control center. In most cases of poisoning, ingestion of large quantities of water or milk (dilution) is called for. Sometimes an emetic is administered. Some common household emetics include a tablespoon of salt dissolved in warm water or two tablespoons of mustard dissolved in a pint of warm water. Vomiting must never be induced in a person who has swallowed a corrosive poison. An antidote is given for ingestion of corrosives, which neutralizes the chemical, absorbs it, or prevents it from being absorbed. Transport to a local hospital is always necessary.

The first forty-eight hours are important in burn treatment. When admitted to the hospital for severe burns, patients require stabilization of breathing and replacement of fluids to prevent dehydration and shock. Wounds are debrided in surgery to promote blood flow to healthy tissue underneath the wound. Grafts may be required. Surgical dressings soaked in antibiotics are applied to prevent infection. Many surgeries may be required until the grafts cover all the burned areas. Medical staff work to develop pain management strategies specific to each person's suffering. Physical and occupational therapy, though painful, must not be avoided. Burn injury places the patient at risk for severe loss of motion. Exercise, nutrition, and emotional support are important factors in helping the burn patient to heal.

PERSPECTIVE AND PROSPECTS

There are three major ways to prevent accidents: education, making the home and workplace safer, and banning dangerous activities and equipment. Air bags have helped tremendously to eliminate many types of injuries in automobiles, and many lives have been saved. Whiplash, head and neck trauma, and eye injuries have been less serious since air bags have been installed in automobiles. With bicycle riders especially, wearing a helmet is the single most effective safety device available to reduce fatal injury to the brain and disfiguring injury to the face from crashes. The best investment against bicycle, scooter, skateboard, and in-line skate injuries is protective gear.

New technologies and advanced training in sports medicine for health care professionals have greatly advanced complete recovery for unintentional injuries received in competitive sports. Artificial turf, though easier to care for, causes many knee and back injuries from slipping. Biotechnology has made great advances in providing safer equipment for sports participants, more effective imaging technology (such as magnetic resonance imaging, or MRI, and computed tomography, or CT, scanning equipment) for diagnosing all injuries, and physical therapy techniques and equipment to help those who have disabling injuries such as those involving the spinal cord. New materials and designs for limb prostheses are aiding those who have lost limbs to lead normal lives, even in competitive sports. There have been several examples of runners being competitive despite a leg or foot prosthesis. Pharmaceutical research is making advances in medications that can control pain without being addictive, for those with behavior problems and depression resulting from severe head trauma.

For seniors, a simple screening test can accurately identify those who are most likely to fall. Constant review and adjustment of medications by a physician are musts for preventing side effects such as dizziness, drowsiness, or disorientation. Installing grab bars in the shower and around the toilet, installing rails on both sides of the stairs, increasing lighting throughout the home and encouraging its use, and removing tripping hazards have been very effective in preventing falls. Most important for seniors is the encouragement of regular exercise to improve strength and balance.

Measures to prevent poisoning include labeling of household products, elimination of lead from gasoline, use of carbon monoxide detectors, and improved monitoring of exposure to toxic elements within industry and throughout the environment. The telephone number of a poison control center should be posted at home and in the workplace. More than 50 percent of accidental poisonings in 2000 happened in the home and involved such products as aspirin, barbiturates, insecticides, and cosmetics. Awareness, safety, and education are the keys to preventing accidents involving poisons. Improvements in burn care have resulted in fewer deaths and better infection control. Technological advances in the provision of skin substitutes, improved monitoring techniques, surgical instrumentation, and better understanding of

the underlying metabolic changes have all contributed to successful therapy.

FURTHER READING

Beers, Mark H., et al., eds. *The Merck Manual of Diagnosis and Therapy.* 18th ed. Whitehouse Station, N.J.: Merck Research Laboratories, 2006. The sections on burns, poisoning, and bites and stings are very complete and informative resources for the lay reader, if a bit technical. Includes pictures, charts, and graphs.

English, Peter. *Old Paint: A Medical History of Childhood Lead-Paint Poisoning in the United States to 1980.* New Brunswick, N.J.: Rutgers University Press, 2001. Chapters include "Lead Poisoning Before 1920," "The Scientific Study of the American Workplace," "Peeling and Flaking Paint: A 1950s Transformation," and "New Therapies: Industry and Public Health Responses."

Gronwall, Dorothy, Philip Wrightson, and Peter Waddell. *Head Injury: The Facts-A Guide for Families and Care-Givers.* 2d ed. New York: Oxford University Press, 1998. Examines common wounds and injuries of the brain and the process of rehabilitation.

Matthews, Dawn D., ed. *Household Safety Sourcebook: Basic Consumer Health Information About Household Safety.* Detroit, Mich.: Omnigraphics, 2002. A comprehensive and accessible handbook detailing the prevention and treatment of common household accidents, including those caused by fire, chemicals, water, electricity, and home equipment and appliances.

Monafo, W.W. "Initial Management of Burns." *New England Journal of Medicine* 335 (1996): 1581-1586. A technical article but accessible to the lay reader with some medical knowledge.

National Center for Emergency Medicine Informatics. http://ncemi.org. Site provides Web links, frequently asked questions, bibliographies, and articles.

National Safety Council. *Injury Facts* 2005-2006. Itasca, Ill.: Author, 2006. Complete injury statistics without much text, offering good facts and topic organization.

Nestle, Marion. *Safe Food: The Politics of Food Safety.* Updated ed. Berkeley: University of California Press, 2010. Examines foodborne microbial illnesses that plague American consumers as part of its range of topics, arguing that the food industry acts in its own economic self-interest rather than out of concern for the public welfare.

Roberts, Anthony H. N. "Burn Prevention: Where Now?" *Burns* 26, no. 6 (August, 2000). Accessible to general readers and includes applicable information.

Virginiae Blackmon

SEE ALSO: Death and Dying; Drowning; Road Rage; Texting and Driving

Coping with terminal illness: Part I

Terminal illness is perceived as a catastrophic threat to the continued existence of the self, one's relationships, and all that is valued in this life. Successful coping depends on available medical, personal, social, and spiritual resources. The hospice movement has introduced a humane and holistic approach to the support of the dying, treats the family as the unit of care, and is an alternative to the traditional, medical model.

INTRODUCTION

A terminal illness cannot be cured and, therefore, is recognized by the person dying as a catastrophic threat to the self, to the individual's relationships, and to the body. In terms of the model of coping proposed by Richard Lazarus and Susan Folkman, death is the perceived threat or stressor causing stress and is evaluated by primary appraisal; the response or coping strategy depends on the person's secondary appraisal of available physical, psychological, social, and spiritual resources. The relationship between the perception of threat and the coping response is dynamic in that it changes over time. For example, the threat of death varies with physical or psychological deterioration and calls for changing strategies during the period of dying.

Anxiety and fear are typical of any crisis; however, when faced with the overwhelming crisis that death poses, a dying person is flooded with death anxiety or mortal fear of dying. Two classic views of death anxiety are Freudian and existential. Sigmund Freud believed that it was impossible to imagine one's own death and that "death anxiety" is really fear of something else, whereas the existentialists believe that awareness of mortality is a basic condition of human existence and is the source of death anxiety. In 1996, Adrian Tomer and Grafton Eliason offered a contemporary "regrets" model, where death anxiety is a function of how much one regrets not having accomplished what one had hoped to accomplish in light of the time left. A major criticism of their work is that achievement takes precedence over social relationships and other sources of meaning. In 2000, Robert J. Kastenbaum proposed an edge theory, where

the response to extreme danger is distinct from the ordinary awareness of mortality. He suggested that death anxiety is the consequence of a heightened awareness of potential disaster at the edge of what is otherwise known to be relatively safe.

Thanatology, the study of death and dying, focuses on the needs of the terminally ill and their survivors. Some thanatologists distinguish between fear of the process of dying and fear of the unknown at death. For example, the Collett-Lester Scale, established in 1994, operationalizes these ideas by offering four subscales: death of self, death of others, dying of self, and dying of others. A major problem with studies of death anxiety is that researchers typically employ self-report questionnaires that measure conscious attitudes. In general, the construct validity of questionnaires is reduced when anxiety is confounded with unconscious denial or when death is confounded with dying.

HOSPICE AND PALLIATIVE CARE

From the beginning of the twentieth century until the 1970s, Americans with terminal illnesses usually died in hospitals. Medical treatment focused on pathology; control of pain with narcotics was limited, as most physicians were worried about consequent drug addiction. Efforts to save lives were machine-intensive and often painful. The psychological, social, and spiritual needs of the person were not as important as the heroic effort to preserve life at any cost. When Dame Cicely Saunders, a British nurse and physician, opened St. Christopher's Hospice in London in 1967, she introduced holistic reforms that treated both the dying person and his or her family and included regular administrations of morphine for the amelioration of pain. It was discovered that control of pain is better when dosing at regular intervals and that the total dosage may be less than if drugs are offered only in response to severe, acute pain. Saunders was a profound inspiration to the international hospice movement, as well as to the new field of palliative medicine. The goal of palliative care is to relieve pain and symptoms and is different from traditional, curative care.

Initially, hospices were based in hospitals; however, toward the end of the twentieth century, home-based care became common. A full-service program provides an interdisciplinary team of a physician, social worker, registered nurse, and pastor or counselor; round-the-clock care is available. Furthermore, after death, support services are offered to grieving families. In the United States, the National Hospice Reimbursement Act of

1983 offered financial support for full-service hospice care. A local hospice is an important coping resource for someone who chooses to forgo traditional medical treatment. It offers a means for preserving some control of the environment, as well as for maintaining personal dignity. Most important, a peaceful, pain-free death is possible.

STAGES OF DYING

About the time that the international hospice movement was gaining momentum, an important book titled *On Death and Dying* (1969) was published in America by the psychiatrist Elisabeth Kübler-Ross. She presented transcripts of interviews with dying patients who were struggling with common end-of-life concerns. What gripped American readers was her call for the treatment of dying people as human beings and her compelling, intellectual analysis of dying as a sequence of five stages: denial and isolation, anger, bargaining, depression, and acceptance. However, according to Robert J. Kastenbaum, there is no real empirical verification of her stage theory. Specifically, dying need not involve all stages and may not proceed in the sequence described by Kübler-Ross. Therapists point out that depression and anxiety are ever present but change in intensity—sometimes manageable, sometimes overwhelming. Although theoreticians argue about the scientific status of Kübler-Ross's stage theory, clinicians use her ideas to tailor therapeutic regimens depending on the current needs of their patients. One way to evaluate current status is in terms of how the patient is coping with various threats and challenges posed by dying.

The "stages" of dying may be thought of as emotion-focused coping behaviors for responding to death, a stressor that cannot be changed. In contrast, problem-focused coping behaviors are appropriate when an aspect of the stressor can be changed. When a dying mother is too weak to care for a child, she copes with the problem of her weakness by arranging for child care. When a husband is worried about the financial security of his wife, he draws up a will.

Denial is usually the first response to the shocking news of terminal illness. Denial of one's impending death is a way of coping with the threat of losing one's self and key relationships. The loss of one's self is characterized by the loss of what one values as personally defining. For example, death implies the ultimate loss of strength or of the capacity for meaningful work and ushers in a radical, unwanted change of self-concept. However, denial allows an acceptance of the facts at a slower, more

manageable rate and is a way to cope emotionally with death anxiety.

Anger is a common venting response once denial is no longer consuming. (Other venting strategies include crying, yelling, sarcasm, and recklessness.) The private or public expression of anger is evidence that the person has moved beyond complete denial toward the recognition of death as a real threat.

Bargaining with fate or some higher power is a futile but common coping strategy, whereby the person tries desperately to restore body integrity and self-concept. The efforts are sometimes heroic, as when a person has accepted that he or she is dying but tries to maintain some version of prior meaningful activities. The scope is limited and the places may change, but relationships and activities critical to self-concept continue for as long as possible.

Depression is marked by sorrow, grief for current and future losses, and diminished pleasure. It is different from the anxiety that arises when a person fears that what is necessary for an intact self is jeopardized; in contrast, depression occurs when the dying person is certain that he or she has lost what is necessary. Depression is the most common psychological problem in palliative-care settings. However, when ordinary depression becomes major, the treatable condition is often unrecognized and patients suffer needless emotional pain. Minor depression, an expected coping behavior, may be adaptive, whereas major depression is maladaptive and requires medical intervention.

Acceptance of a terminal condition is viewed by many clinicians as a desired end-state because the possibility of a peaceful death comes with acceptance. The person has not given up emotionally but has reached a point of choosing not to struggle for survival. Therapists of various kinds interpret acceptance in the light of a particular worldview or theoretical paradigm. For example, the transpersonal counselor sees acceptance as evidence of an intrapsychic transformation of the self to a higher level of consciousness.

OTHER COPING STRATEGIES

Dying presents many threats and challenges, including psychological and spiritual distress, pain, exhaustion, loss of independence, loss of dignity, and abandonment. In addition to depression and anxiety, guilt is a response to believing that one must have been a bad person to deserve such a fate or that one risked one's health in a way that brought on the illness. Sometimes people feel guilty because of anger and sarcasm vented on hapless family members, friends, helpers, or a higher power. Thoughts of suicide may occur when depression is severe enough or if the pain is intolerable. Not all people suffer all these assaults, but each requires a strategy for coping.

It is not uncommon for friends and relatives to pull away from the dying person because of their own anxiety and discomfort. Witnessing the physical and emotional distress of a valued person poses a threat to successful, day-to-day management of mortal fears; one way to cope is by ignoring the dying. Unfortunately, physical or emotional distancing causes dreadful isolation and a sense of abandonment just when social support is most critically needed. The terminally ill in such a predicament may cope by turning to a pastoral counselor, therapist, self-help group, or local hospice.

Each type of therapist has a different focus. A psychoanalyst might encourage frank discussions of fears and anxieties. A cognitive behavioral therapist might focus on changing maladaptive behavior by modifying negative thought patterns. A humanistic-existentialist might encourage a life review to help consolidate the patient's perceptions of the meaning of life and as a way to say "good-bye." A transpersonal counselor might focus on facilitating a meaningful transformation of self in preparation for death. A primary goal of therapy of any kind with dying patients is to promote physical and psychological comfort. Often, the therapist is an advocate acting as a liaison between the patient and the hospice, hospital, family, or friends. The therapist may provide helpful psychoeducational interventions, such as alleviating distress about an upcoming medical procedure by informing the patient about the rationale for the procedure, the steps involved, the predictable side effects, and the prognosis or forecast for the outcome. When the therapist also educates the family, the quality of their support is enhanced, thereby improving the well-being of the patient.

SELF-HELP GROUPS

Self-help groups provide significant mutual support to the terminally ill and to those in mourning. They are available in professional and nonprofessional settings. They are usually composed of peers who are in a similar plight and who, therefore, are familiar with the depression, anxiety, and guilt associated with dying. Access to a new, primary group counteracts common feelings of alienation and victimization by offering the opportunity for meaningful social support and information. Mutual disclosure reduces feelings of isolation and abandon-

ment by building a community of peers. Sharing successful strategies for coping with secondary losses triggered by terminal illness restores hope. (For example, group members may know how to cope with the disfigurement of mastectomy or with confinement to a wheelchair.) Group participants also encourage one another to be active partners in their own medical care. Unreliable patterns of communication and reluctance to talk about dying are common outside the group; however, group members talk to one another openly, thereby reducing the dismay associated with patronizing exchanges with doctors and nurses or the silence of family and friends.

RELIGIOUS AND SPIRITUAL COPING

Psychologists emphasize the ways in which adversity may be conquered or controlled, but not every stressor is controllable. Certainly, dying brings into sharp relief the fact that humans are ultimately powerless in the face of death. At the end of life, people often turn to religion or spirituality for answers as to the purpose of their lives, the reasons for suffering, the destination of their souls, the nature of the afterlife—whether a life everlasting exists. Coping theorists may reduce the function of religion to "terror management," but others believe that the experience of the sacred cannot be understood empirically and that religion is more than an elaborate coping mechanism.

The psychologist of religion Kenneth I. Pargament studied the relationship between religion and coping. He defined religion functionally in terms of a search for significance in the light of the sacred. He described a typical Christian belief system involving the event (in this case, death), the person, and the sacred. Core beliefs are that God is benevolent, the world is just or fair, and the person is good. Dying jeopardizes the balance of this belief system; to cope, people turn to religious reframing as a way of conserving the significance or value of their core beliefs. For example, people facing a seemingly pointless death reframe its significance—death becomes an opportunity for spiritual growth or enlightenment; this preserves the beliefs that the person is good and that God is benevolent. Others reframe the nature of the person as being sinful; otherwise, why does suffering exist? The result is that belief in a just world is preserved. Some reframe their beliefs regarding the sacred and consider God as punishing. However, several researchers have found that only a small proportion of people attribute their suffering to a vengeful, punishing God. Another way to reframe the nature of God is to reconsider his omnipotence. People may conclude that a loving God is constrained by forces in nature. This reframed belief preserves the idea that God is good.

Dying is not always the occasion for spiritual crisis; people of deep Christian faith find solace in their relationship with God or with their understanding of the transcendent. The psychiatrist Harold G. Koenig reports in *The Healing Power of Faith* (1999) that faith, prayer, meditation, and congregational support mitigate fear, hopelessness, and the experience of pain. For people committed to a Christian religious or spiritual belief system, God or spirit is a source of peace and hope while dying.

FURTHER READING

Balk, David E. *Dealing with Dying, Death, and Grief During Adolescence.* New York: Routledge, 2014. Print.

Cook, Alicia Skinner, and Kevin Ann Oltjenbruns. *Dying and Grieving: Life Span and Family Perspectives.* 2nd ed. Fort Worth: Harcourt Brace, 1998. Print.

Kastenbaum, Robert J. *Death, Society, and Human Experience.* 11th ed. Boston: Pearson, 2014. Print.

Kessler, David. *The Needs of the Dying: A Guide for Bringing Hope, Comfort, and Love to Life's Final Chapter.* New York: Harper, 2007. Print.

Kübler-Ross, Elisabeth. *On Death and Dying.* 1969. Reprint. New York: Routledge, 2009. Print.

Lair, George S. *Counseling the Terminally Ill: Sharing the Journey.* Washington, DC: Taylor & Francis, 1996. Print.

Miller, Glen E. *Living Thoughtfully, Dying Well: A Doctor Explains How to Make Death a Natural Part of Life.* Harisonburg: Herald, 2014. Print.

Pargament, Kenneth I. *The Psychology of Religion and Coping: Theory, Research, and Practice.* New York: Guilford, 2001. Print.

Tanja Bekhuis

SEE ALSO: Anger; Death and Dying; Grieving and Guilt; Loss of a Friend; Loss of a Parent or Guardian; Loss of a Sibling; Helping Friends Cope; Meditation

Coping with terminal illness: Part II

On the first day of his senior year in high school a young man hung back after class to talk to his English teacher. As he approached the desk she said: "Is there anything I can help you with today?" The young man said: "No, but there is something I have to tell you." She replied: "OK, What is it?" Looking her right in the eye he said: "I have a terminal illness." She paused, taking in the magnitude of his statement, and after a moment said: "I am sorry to hear that. Is there anything I can do?" "No," he said, "except to act like we never had this conversation." She smiled and nodded. "Sure, I can do that. But if things change and I can do anything else, you'll let me know, OK?" He left the class room and went to his next class and when it was over, he stayed back to talk to his Chemistry teacher.

INTRODUCTION

There is probably nothing adolescents dislike more than being singled out, or for things to seem out of the ordinary. The desire to have friends in your peer group and fit in with others is probably most strongly experienced by people at this stage of life than at any other time during the life span. Knowing you have a terminal illness is challenging, regardless of a person's age, but in adolescence, there are some features of this experience that make it especially difficult. However, if the young adult is allowed to participate in his or her health care decisions and has the support of friends, family and other persons in their lives, the last portion of a life, made shorter than expected by incurable illness, can be a time of personal growth and community engagement.

TERMINAL ILLNESS IN RELATIONSHIPS

Terminal illness is defined as a chronic medical condition in which the prognosis for recovery is unlikely and the patient is expected to live for no longer than 6 months to a year. Especially for teenagers, this can be a very difficult idea to make sense of due to the general sensibility that adolescents have that they are invincible. The resulting cognitive dissonance, (which is a theory that says when humans experience tension because of two opposing thoughts happening at the same time they will try to take action to reduce the tension by whatever means possible) can have significant psychological impacts. In addition to having to deal with the illness itself, the possibility of a great deal of physical pain, and the sense that one has no control over their own body, the time remaining might also be complicated by changing interpersonal relationships and the potential financial hardships such an illness can cause for families.

How well the teen will manage all of these difficult and rapidly changing circumstances is often determined by how much social support the individual has and how well he or she is able to accept the support which is offered. Psychologists such as John Bowlby and Mary Ainsworth have written about the concept of "attachment" and have provided some insights into how a child's earliest bonding with their primary caregiver has an impact on relationships formed at later stages of life. They say most people fall into one of three categories of attachment styles, with those who form secure early attachments most able to negotiate social interactions throughout the life course. Those who experience either ambivalent or avoidant attachments in infancy tend to have a more difficult time with other relationships, but some individually are resilient and can overcome their early problems with attachment and form quality interactions later on. Both those who come to relationships easily and those who are resilient will find that they are better able to face the great existential dilemma of terminal illness with somewhat less trouble than those who struggle with attachment issues. These individuals might even experience the period of preparing for their death as a time of personal growth. The psychologist Judith Herman has written: "Just as basic trust is the developmental achievement of earliest life, integrity is the developmental task of maturity." She sees the interconnected nature of integrity and trust as the foundation for a caretaking relationship that "completes the cycle of generations and regenerates the sense of human community that trauma destroys."

Some teens may find that dealing with terminal illness becomes a time in which they undertake and accomplish tasks they had only dreamed of doing, previously. It also might be a period of spiritual or intellectual engagement, particularly if they are confined to bed and yet are clear minded and able to be engaged in these pursuits. Community members, especially religious leaders such as a priest, rabbi, imam or guru may be called upon to assist teens with questions of a spiritual nature. In-home schooling or tutoring may become necessary and young people should be encouraged to keep up academically for as long as is practical.

Another time that adolescents might be have to deal with terminal illness is when the ill person is someone they care about. This could be an ill parent, grandparent, sibling, friend or other important person in their life. If the person is elderly and would be nearing a logical end of life but becomes ill in a way that takes some months to a year between onset and death, watching that person's condition deteriorate can be stressful and anxiety causing. The situation is much more difficult when the ill person is the parent or other primary caregiver that the teen relies upon for a loving and nurturing relationship. Issues of terminal illness when the teen is in a relationship with another young person who is ill can be a source of confusion. Questions like "Why does this person have to go so young?" And even "Why them and not me?" are almost inevitable in these cases. Survivor guilt can add additional stressors for the entire family during what is already a difficult period. This can be further complicated by the normal adolescent need to define their own identity and begin to pull away from parental authority, especially if the teen is required, by the needs of the family, to take on additional responsibilities at home due to the absence of parents while visiting hospital or hospice.

LACK OF SUPPORT

One of the things that may happen when either a teen is ill or they are facing the illness of a loved one is that they might find some of the people they considered to be their friends are not spending as much time with them as before. Many people have a hard time being present during times of loss and grief because it raises questions for them about their own mortality, which may be something they are not ready to face. As a result, the affected teen may find themselves alone and lonely. It is at these times that the people closest to the adolescent need to be especially available. Emotional support and just taking the time to do things that the teen enjoys can be very valuable under these circumstances. Consider referring the young person, if they are under 18 years old, to the Make a Wish Foundation which grants wishes to youths over 2 1/2-years-old with a life-threatening medical condition. These experiences have been proven to enhance state of mind, improve health status, and even strengthen communities.

It is not uncommon for emotions like anger, guilt, sorrow, helplessness, loneliness and denial to be felt when someone is terminally ill. It is important that teens be allowed to express their feelings and have them respected. It may be necessary for the family to attend family therapy to find solutions for managing these emotions if they become overwhelming or disruptive. When death comes in unanticipated ways and may take some time following diagnosis, there may or may not be the chance to come to terms with the impending death. Terminal illness comes with many logistical, financial, and emotional strains. Graphic images of decline and death may linger and be intrusive, traumatic memories. If symptoms of Post-Traumatic Stress manifest, these need proper intervention by a trauma-informed therapist.

COPING

Anticipating death, whether it is one's own or that of a loved one, has psychological consequences because the world may no longer seem safe and stable and people feel powerless to alter the outcome. Young people tend to cope better with exposure to terminal illness when they know they are loved, supported, and feel the freedom to ask questions, especially if it is about their own care. There may come a time when decisions about staying at home, going to hospice or palliative care and/or being hospitalized become important determinations to be made and including teens in these decisions will help them to feel empowered. This is true even if, ultimately, the care they need is not available at their desired facility. Just being allowed to voice their preferences can have a significant impact upon psychological wellness. It is also important to consider the wishes of adolescents regarding how they want to be remembered and memorialized. They may also have come to some conclusions about the level of care they want; how much relief of pain they desire, and other medical matters. Using a document such as "Voicing My Choices: A Planning Guide for Adolescents and Young Adults" may be helpful in guiding such a conversation and allowing the teen to record their last wishes. Families that are able to engage in such conversations will likely fare better following the death of the teen because they will know they provided the respect and dignity that all people deserve as they come close to the end of their lives.

At some point teens who are terminally ill may come to terms with their situation. If they reach this stage of acceptance they will especially need the loving support of their families and friends, and those others may not have yet come to the same acceptance. For many people, acceptance is a state that takes some time following death, with an appropriate time of mourning. These differences in experience by the one who is dying and those around him or her can be stressful in and of themselves. The most important thing to remember is that it is the dying person who matters most at these times and being able to set aside one's own condition to be present with

the one who has only a limited time left to live is the priority, however painful this may be. Saying goodbye will inevitably be difficult for all concerned but it can also be very healing. Depending on the limitations that the illness may cause, planning sufficient time for teens to have a final visit with as many people as they wish to speak with one last time is an organizational task that extended family and friends can help with, so that immediate family do not have to carry the full burden. Including young children as a greeter for visitors can help siblings and other youngsters in the teen's life feel valued and cherished under very trying circumstances. Judith Herman has said that "healthy children will not fear life if their elders have integrity enough not to fear death." In the case of teens that are living with a terminal illness, they are experiencing profound physical illness. Nevertheless, their psyches can be helped when the adults in their lives face the challenges of the impending death fearlessly and with integrity. The reality is that young people do die, they are not invincible, and mortality must be faced. Young people will manage these tasks so much more smoothly with the aid of their loved ones than they will in actual or emotional isolation.

One type of intervention that can be used to assist everybody involved and need not be done with professional assistance, although that option does exist, is to use some of the much written about techniques that fall under the category of "mindfulness." There are many books and recordings available to guide individuals choosing to explore the deep breathing and relaxation exercises which can be used cognitively, or which can easily incorporate a spiritual element. The advantage of these practices, which can be done alone or in groups, is that they do not have to cost anything at a time when finances may already be strained. Mindfulness has been proven to improve brain function, is calming, and if done in a group can enhance the filial or community bonds between individuals.

Teens who are facing death should be encouraged to be as active physically and mentally as is reasonable, given their condition. Being allowed to slip into boredom or depression wastes what little time they have. Continuing successes and project completions foster meaning and are affirming of the life they are still living. Caution should be taken to watch for signs that teens with terminal illness are having suicidal thoughts or are engaging in self-destructive behaviors. As long as they are alive, life is a precious gift and they should be aided in living each and every day to its and their fullest potential.

FURTHER READING

"Dying Young: Managing A Terminal Illness As a Teen". http://teendiaries.net/article/dying-young-managing-terminal-illness-teen. An excellent, brief blog entry from the Teen Diaries which honestly discusses fear, the stages of grief, teens engaging in negative and very harmful acts in order to cope, spirituality and more with some great photos of beautiful, although ill, adolescents. The Teen Diaries is working to transform the lives of teen girls nationwide and there is much more on this blog site that young women, especially, might find of interest, including videos, merchandise and DRadio "Where Hip Pop and Teen Culture Collide!" The blog has a strong ethnocultural emphasis.

Online Mindfulness-Based Stress Reduction, http://palousemindfulness.com/selfguidedMBSR.html. Eight-week long online Mindfulness-Based Stress Reduction (MSBR) course is modeled on the program founded by Jon Kabat-Zinn at the University of Massachusetts Medical School; includes guided practices, with videos and additional articles. No one says you have to do every module or that you must complete it in 8 weeks, but the whole package is there, for free.

"30 Questions To Ask Yourself Before You Die", http://www.rebellesociety.com/2013/07/17/30-questions-to-ask-before-you-die/. Thirty intriguing questions posed by 30 year old Andrea Balt on the Rebelle Society: Creatively Maladjusted blog. A few may not be apropos to teens, but the majority are more than suitable queries for teens, especially those facing the death of a loved one or their own impending death. Andrea's goal is to "reflect the wholeness of the human experience by combining Art & Health + Mind & Body + Darkness & Brilliance into a more alive, unabridged and unlimited edition of ourselves."

"Voicing My Choices: A Planning Guide For Adolescents and Young Adults". http://www.agingwithdignity.org/voicing-my-choices-thanks.php. An online preview version (cannot be printed) is available on the Web site of Aging with Dignity, the organization that also produced the adult version entitled "Five Wishes." There is an online form to request a free paper copy. This planning guide is designed for use with young adults under the age of 18 and is therefore not a legally binding Living Will. It includes sections on comfort and support, medical care and treatment decisions, who should be told, spiritual thoughts, remembrance, what to do with belongings, a section for writing letters called "My Voice" and a glossary.

Wright, K. (2004). "Personal Reflection: The Patient as Teacher". *Journal of Palliative Medicine.* 7(5), pp. 718-719. Retrieved from http://online.liebertpub.com/doi/abs/10.1089/jpm.2004.7.718?journalCode=jpm. A very brief but insightful personal reflection on the lessons about love, support and dying that a young man was able to share with his doctor during the 5 years he was under her care, from age 14 to 19, for HIV /AIDS.

Rebekah Tanner and Karen Wolford

SEE ALSO: Anger; Death and Dying; Grieving and Guilt; Loss of a Friend; Loss of a Parent or Guardian; Loss of a Sibling; Helping Friends Cope; Meditation

Death and dying

Medicine determines that death has occurred by assessing bodily functions in either of two areas. Persons with irreversible cessation of respiration and circulation are dead; persons with irreversible cessation of ascertainable brain functions are also dead. There are standard procedures used to diagnose death, including simple observation, brain-stem reflex studies, and the use of confirmatory testing such as electrocardiography (ECG or EKG), electroencephalography (EEG), and arterial blood gas analysis (ABG). The particular circumstances—anticipated or unanticipated, observed or unobserved, the patient's age, drug or metabolic intoxication, or suspicion of hypothermia—will favor some procedures over others, but in all cases both cessation of functions and their irreversibility are required before death can be declared.

Between 60 and 75 percent of all people die from chronic terminal conditions. Therefore, except in sudden death (as in a fatal accident) or when there is no evidence of consciousness (as in a head injury which destroys cerebral functions while leaving brain-stem reflexive functions intact), dying is both a physical and a psychological process. In most cases, dying takes time, and the time allows patients to react to the reality of their own passing. Often, they react by becoming vigilant about bodily symptoms and any changes in them. They also anticipate changes that have yet to occur. For example, long before the terminal stages of illness become manifest, dying patients commonly fear physical pain, shortness of breath, invasive procedures, loneliness, becoming a burden to loved ones, losing decision-making authority, and facing the unknown of death itself.

As physical deterioration proceeds, all people cope by resorting to what has worked for them before: the unique means and mechanisms which have helped maintain a sense of self and personal stability. People seem to go through the process of dying much as they have gone through the process of living—with the more salient features of their personalities, whether good or bad, becoming sharper and more prominent. People seem to face death much as they have faced life.

Medicine has come to acknowledge that physicians should understand what it means to die. Indeed, while all persons should understand what their own deaths will mean, physicians must additionally understand how their dying patients find this meaning.

In 1969, psychiatrist Elisabeth Kübler-Ross published the landmark *On Death and Dying*, based on her work with two hundred terminally ill patients. Though the work of Kübler-Ross has been criticized for the nature of the stages described and whether or not every person experiences every stage, her model has retained enormous utility to those who work in the area of death and dying. Technologically driven, Western medicine had come to define its role as primarily dealing with extending life and thwarting death by defeating specific diseases. Too few physicians saw a role for themselves once the prognosis turned grave. In the decades that followed the publication of *On Death and Dying*, the profession has reaccepted that death and dying are part of life and that, while treating the dying may not mean extending the length of life, it can and should mean improving its quality.

Kübler-Ross provided a framework to explain how people cope with and adapt to the profound and terrible news that their illness is terminal. Although other physicians, psychologists, and thanatologists have shortened, expanded, and adapted her five stages of the dying process, neither the actual number of stages nor what they are specifically called is as important as the information and insight that any stage theory of dying yields. As with any human process, dying is complex, multifaceted, multidimensional, and polymorphic.

Well-intentioned, but misguided, professionals and family members may try to help move dying patients through each of the stages only to encounter active resentment or passive withdrawal. Patients, even dying patients, cannot be psychologically moved to where they are not ready to be. Rather than making the terminally

ill die the "right" way, it is more respectful and helpful to understand any stage as a description of normal reactions to serious loss, and that these reactions normally vary among different individuals and also within the same individual over time. The reactions appear, disappear, and reappear in any order and in any combination. What the living must do is respect the unfolding of an adaptational schema which is the dying person's own. No one should presume to know how someone else should prepare for death.

COMPLICATIONS AND DISORDERS

Kübler-Ross defined five stages of grief. Denial is the first stage defined by Kübler-Ross, but it is also linked to shock and isolation. Whether the news is told outright or gradual self-realization occurs, most people react to the knowledge of their impending death with existential shock: Their whole selves recoil at the idea, and they say, in some fashion, "This cannot be happening to me." Broadly considered, denial is a complex cognitive-emotional capacity that enables temporary postponement of active, acute, but in some way detrimental, recognition of reality. In the dying process, this putting off of the truth prevents a person from being overwhelmed while promoting psychological survival. Denial plays an important stabilizing role, holding back more than could be otherwise managed while allowing the individual to marshal psychological resources and reserves. It enables patients to consider the possibility, even the inevitability, of death and then to put the consideration away so that they can pursue life in the ways that are still available. In this way, denial is truly a mechanism of defense.

Many other researchers, along with Kübler-Ross, report anger as the second stage of dying. The stage is also linked to rage, fury, envy, resentment, and loathing. When "This cannot be happening to me" becomes, "This is happening to me. There was no mistake," patients are beginning to replace denial with attempts to understand what is happening to and inside them. When they do, they often ask, "Why me?" Though it is an unanswerable question, the logic of the question is clear. People, to remain human, must try to make intelligible their experiences and reality. The asking of this question is an important feature of the way in which all dying persons adapt to and cope with the reality of death.

People react with anger when they lose something of value; they react with greater anger when something of value is taken away from them by someone or something. Rage and fury, in fact, are often more accurate descriptions of people's reactions to the loss of their own life than is anger. Anger is a difficult stage for professionals and loved ones, more so when the anger and rage are displaced and projected randomly into any corner of the patient's world. An unfortunate result is that caregivers often experience the anger as personal, and the caregivers" own feelings of guilt, shame, grief, and rejection can contribute to lessening contact with the dying person, which increases his or her sense of isolation.

Bargaining is Kübler-Ross's third stage, but it is also the one about which she wrote the least and the one that other thanatologists are most likely to leave unrepresented in their own models and stages of how people cope with dying. Nevertheless, it is a common phenomenon wherein dying people fall back on their faith, belief systems, or sense of the transcendent and the spiritual and try to make a deal—with god, life, fate, a higher power, or the universe. They ask for more time to help family members reconcile or to achieve something of importance. They may ask if they can simply attend their child's wedding or graduation or if they can see their first grandchild born. Then they will be ready to die; they will go willingly. Often, they mean that they will die without fighting death, if death can only be delayed or will delay itself.

At some point, when terminally ill individuals are faced with decisions about more procedures, tests, surgeries, or medications or when their thinness, weakness, or deterioration becomes impossible to ignore, the anger, rage, numbness, stoicism, and even humor will likely give way to depression, Kübler-Ross's fourth stage and the one reaction that all thanatologists include in their models of how people cope with dying.

The depression can take many forms, for indeed there are always many losses, and each loss individually or several losses collectively might need to be experienced and worked through. For example, dying parents might ask themselves who will take care of the children, get them through school, walk them down the aisle, or guide them through life. Children, even adult children who are parents themselves, may ask whether they can cope without their own parents. They wonder who will support and anchor them in times of distress, who will (or could) love, nurture, and nourish them the way that their parents did. Depression accompanies the realization that each role, each function, will never be performed again. Both the dying and those who love them mourn.

Much of the depression takes the form of anticipatory grieving, which often occurs both in the dying and

in those who will be affected by their death. It is a part of the dying process experienced by the living, both terminal and nonterminal. Patients, family, and friends can psychologically anticipate what it will be like when the death does occur and what life will, and will not, be like afterward. The grieving begins while there is still life left to live.

Bereavement specialists generally agree that anticipatory grieving, when it occurs, seems to help people cope with what is a terrible and frightening loss. It is an adaptive psychological mechanism wherein emotional, mental, and existential stability are painfully maintained. When depression develops, not only in reaction to death but also in preparation for it, it seems to be a necessary part of how those who are left behind cope to survive the loss themselves. Those who advocate or advise cheering up or looking on the bright side are either unrealistic or unable to tolerate the sadness in themselves or others. The dying are in the process of losing everything and everyone they love. Cheering up does not help them; the advice to "be strong" only helps the "helpers" deny the truth of the dying experience.

Both preparatory and reactive depressions are frequently accompanied by unrealistic self-recrimination, shame, and guilt in the dying person. Those who are dying may judge themselves harshly and criticize themselves for the wrongs that they committed and for the good that they did not accomplish. They may judge themselves to be unattractive, unappealing, and repulsive because of how the illness and its treatment have affected them. These feelings and states of minds, which have nothing to do with the reality of the situation, are often amenable to the interventions of understanding and caring people. Financial and other obligations can be restructured and reassigned. Being forgiven and forgiving can help finish what was left undone.

Kübler-Ross's fifth stage, acceptance, is an intellectual and emotional coming to terms with death's reality, permanence, and inevitability. Ironically, it is manifested by diminished emotionality and interests and increased fatigue and inner (many would say spiritual) self-focus. It is a time without depression or anger. Envy of the healthy, the fear of losing all, and bargaining for another day or week are also absent. This final stage is often misunderstood. Some see it either as resignation and giving up or as achieving a happy serenity. Some think that acceptance is the goal of dying well and that all people are supposed to go through this stage. None of these viewpoints is accurate. Acceptance, when it does occur, comes from within the dying person. It is marked more by an emotional void and psychological detachment from people and things once held important and necessary and by an interest in some transcendental value (for the atheist) or god (for the theist). It has little to do with what others believe is important or "should" be done. It is when dying people become more intimate with themselves and appreciate their separateness from others more than at any other time.

EXISTENTIAL CONSIDERATIONS

Every person will eventually die, and the fact of death in each life is one that varies by culture in terms of its meaning. For some cultures, dying is seen as the ultimate difficulty for dying people and their loved ones. For other cultures, it is seen as not difficult at all, but more so like passing on to another realm of existence. In Western cultures, however, dying has very much become a medical process, and it is often a process filled with challenging questions. Patients ask questions that cannot be answered; families in despair and anger seek to find cause and sometimes to lay blame. It takes courage to be with individuals as they face their deaths, struggling to find meaning in the time that they have left. Given this, in Western medicine, a profession that prides itself on how well it intervenes to avoid outcomes like death, it takes courage to witness the process and struggle involved in death. Working with death also reminds professionals of their own inevitable death. Facing that fact inwardly, spiritually, and existentially also requires courage.

Cure and treatment become care and management in the dying. They should live relatively pain-free, be supported in accomplishing their goals, be respected, be involved in decision making as appropriate, be encouraged to function as fully as their illness allows, and be provided with others to whom control can comfortably and confidently be passed. The lack of a cure and the certainty of the end can intimidate health care providers, family members, and close friends. They may dread genuine encounters with those whose days are knowingly numbered. Yet the dying have the same rights to be helped as any of the living, and how a society assists them bears directly on the meaning that its members are willing to attach to their own lives.

Today, largely in response to what dying patients have told researchers, medicine recognizes its role to assist these patients in working toward an appropriate death. Caretakers must determine the optimum treatments, interventions, and conditions which will enable such a death to occur. For each terminally ill person, these should be unique and specific. Caretakers should respond to the patient's needs and priorities, at the patient's own pace and as much as possible following the patient's lead. For some dying patients, the goal is to remain as pain-free as is feasible and to feel as well as possible. For others, finishing whatever unfinished business remains becomes the priority. Making amends, forgiving and being forgiven, resolving old conflicts, and reconciling with one's self and others may be the most therapeutic and healing of interventions. Those who are to be bereaved fear the death of those they love. The dying fear the separation from all they know and love, but they fear as well the loss of autonomy, letting family and friends down, the pain and invasion of further treatment, disfigurement, dementia, loneliness, the unknown, becoming a burden, and the loss of dignity.

The English writer C. S. Lewis said that bereavement is the universal and integral part of the experience of loss. It requires effort, authenticity, mental and emotional work, a willingness to be afraid, and an openness to what is happening and what is going to happen. It requires an attitude that accepts, tolerates suffering, takes respite from the reality, reinvests in whatever life remains, and moves on. The only way to cope with dying or witnessing the dying of loved ones is by grieving through the pain, fear, loneliness, and loss of meaning. This process, which researcher Stephen Levine has likened to opening the heart in hell, is a viscous morass for most, and all people need to learn their own way through it and to have that learning respected. Healing begins with the first halting, unsteady, and frightening steps of genuine grief, which sometimes occur years before the "time of death" can be recorded.

FURTHER READING

Becker, Ernest. *The Denial of Death.* New York: Free Press, 1997. Written by an anthropologist and philosopher, this is an erudite and insightful analysis and synthesis of the role that the fear of death plays in motivating human activity, society, and individual actions. A profound work.

Cook, Alicia Skinner, and Daniel S. Dworkin. *Helping the Bereaved: Therapeutic Interventions for Children, Adolescents, and Adults.* New York: Basic Books, 1992. Although not a self-help book, this work is useful to professionals and nonprofessionals alike as a review of the state of the art in grief therapy. Practical and readable. Of special interest for those becoming involved in grief counseling.

Corr, Charles A., Clyde M. Nabe, and Donna M. Corr. *Death and Dying, Life and Living.* 6th ed. Belmont, Calif.: Wadsworth/Cengage Learning, 2009. This book provides perspective on common issues associated with death and dying for family members and others affected by life-threatening circumstances.

Forman, Walter B., et al., eds. *Hospice and Palliative Care: Concepts and Practice.* 2d ed. Sudbury, Mass.: Jones and Bartlett, 2003. A text that examines the theoretical perspectives and practical information about hospice care. Other topics include community medical care, geriatric care, nursing care, pain management, research, counseling, and hospice management.

Kübler-Ross, Elisabeth, Ed. *Death: The Final Stage of Growth.* Reprint. New York: Simon & Schuster, 1997. A psychiatrist by training, Kübler-Ross brings together other researchers' views of how death provides the key to how human beings make meaning in their own personal worlds. Addresses practical concerns over how people express grief and accept the death of those close to them, and how they might prepare for their own inevitable ends.

Kushner, Harold. *When Bad Things Happen to Good People.* 20th anniversary ed. New York: Schocken Books, 2001. The first of Rabbi Kushner's works on finding meaning in one's life, it was originally his personal response to make intelligible the death of his own child. It has become a highly regarded reference for those who struggle with the meaning of pain, suffering, and death in their lives.

McFarlane, Rodger, and Philip Bashe. *The Complete Bedside Companion: No-Nonsense Advice on Caring for the Seriously Ill.* New York: Simon & Schuster, 1998. A comprehensive and practical guide to caregiving for patients with serious illnesses. The first section deals with the general needs of caring for the sick, while the second section covers specific illnesses in depth. Includes bibliographies and lists of support organizations.

Paul Moglia

SEE ALSO: Grieving; Guilt; Loss of a Friend; Loss of a Parent; Loss of a Sibling

Grieving

Grieving is the usual, expected reaction to loss. After a loss, a normal process occurs in grieving, involving feelings such as anger and sadness, followed by reassessment and reorganization of oneself and one's perspective. Some bereaved individuals experience prolonged or extreme grief reactions, commonly referred to as "complicated grief." In these cases, grief may be associated with depression, physical illness, and heightened risk of mortality. Some losses, such as miscarriage or loss of a lover, are not widely recognized, leading to an experience known as "disenfranchised grief."

INTRODUCTION

Much of life depends on successful adaptation to change. When that change is experienced as a loss, the emotional and cognitive reactions are properly referred to as "grief." When the specific loss is acknowledged by a person's culture, the loss is often met with rituals, behaviors that follow a certain pattern, sanctioned and choreographed within the culture. The term "bereavement" is applied to the loss of a significant person (such as a spouse, parent, child, or close relative or friend). In this case the grief and the sanctioned rituals are referred to as "mourning," although some writers use the terms "mourning" and "grieving" as synonyms.

Reaction to a loss often depends on whether the loss is experienced as central as opposed to peripheral to the self, with more central losses exerting greater impact on the people's ability to function. People who have experienced an important loss may experience obsessive thoughts about who or what was lost, a sense of unreality, a conviction that they were personally responsible for the loss, a sense that there is no help or hope, a belief that they are bad people, and a sense that they are not able to concentrate and remember. Searching for and even perceiving the lost person (often in a dream) are not uncommon.

People's emotional response may at first be engrossing. Shock, anger, sadness, guilt, anxiety, or even numbness are all possible reactions. Crying, fatigue, agitation, or even withdrawal are not unusual. Some people find it difficult to accept or absorb the reality of the loss in a reaction known as "denial." Depending on cultural, family, and individual traditions, some people suppress, repress, and deny part of their awareness, grief reaction, or both.

The centrality of loss within the self is also related to its circumstances. If people are prepared for the loss, they have made themselves less vulnerable to the loss of that person, place, or object in a process known as "anticipatory grief." This is experienced, for example, by those caring for terminally ill patients, as well as by the patients themselves. Although some argue that grief that is anticipated may be less challenging than that following an unexpected loss, the experience of grieving for someone and caring for that person at the same time can be extremely challenging.

HISTORY OF GRIEF STUDIES

The study of grief as a scholarly concern was started by an essay, "Mourning and Melancholia," written in 1917 by the Austrian founder of psychoanalysis, Sigmund Freud. In it, Freud proposed that hysteria (a disorder of emotional instability and dissociation) and melancholia are symptoms of pathological grief. He indicated that painful dejection, loss of the ability to love, inhibition of activity, and decrease in self-esteem that continue beyond the normal time are what distinguish melancholia from mourning (the pathological from the normal). In melancholia, it is the ego (or self) that becomes poor and impoverished. In the pathological case, the damage to self is becoming permanent instead of being a temporary and reversible deprivation.

The study of grief as a normal process of loss evolved over two-and-a-half decades. It was not until 1944 that psychiatrist Erich Lindemann published a study based mostly on interviews with relatives of victims of the Cocoanut Grove nightclub fire in Boston in 1942. He characterized five different aspects of the grief reaction. Each of the five was believed by Lindemann to be normal. Each would give way as the individual readjusted to the environment without the deceased, formed new relationships, and released the ties of connection with the deceased. Morbid or pathological grief reactions were seen as distortions of the normal patterns. A common distortion had to do with delay in reacting to the death.

In these cases, the person would either deny the death or continue to maintain composure and show little or no reaction to the death's occurrence. Other forms of distorted reactions were overactivity, acquisition of symptoms associated with the deceased, social isolation, repression of emotions, and activities that were detrimental to the person's social status and economic well-being. Examples of such detrimental activities might be getting drunk, being promiscuous, giving away all one's money, and quitting one's job.

In the early 1950s, British psychoanalyst and physician John Bowlby began to study loss in childhood, usually with children who were separated from their mothers. His early generalization summarized the child's response in a threefold way: protest, despair, and detachment. From his later work, which included adult mourning, he came to the conclusion that mourning follows a similar pattern whether it takes place in childhood, adolescence, or adulthood. In his later work, he specified wide time frames for the first and second phases and expanded his threefold description of the process to identify four phases of mourning. All four phases overlap, and people may go back for a while to a previous phase. These phases were numbing, which may last from a few hours to a week and may be interrupted by episodes of intense distress or anger; yearning and searching for the lost figure, which may last for months and even for years; disorganization and despair; and reorganization to a greater or lesser degree.

What was new and interesting about the fourth phase is Bowlby's introduction of a positive ending to the grieving process. This is the idea of reorganization, a positive restructuring of the person and the individual's perceptual field. This is a striking advance beyond Lindemann's notion that for the healthy person, the negative aspects of grieving would be dissipated in time.

Meanwhile, in the mid-1960s, quite independently of Bowlby, Swiss-born psychiatrist Elisabeth Kübler-Ross was interviewing terminally ill patients in Chicago. She observed closely, listened sensitively, and reported on their experiences in an important book, *On Death and Dying* (1969). Her work focused on the experiences of the terminally ill.

Kübler-Ross was there as patients first refused to believe the prognosis, as they got angry at themselves and at others around them, as they attempted to argue their way out (to make a deal with God or whoever might have the power to change the reality), as they faced their own sadness and depression, and finally as they came to a sense of acceptance about their fate. (Her idea of acceptance is similar to Bowlby's concept of reorganization.) From her interviews, she abstracted a five-stage process in which terminally ill patients came to deal with the loss of their own lives: denial and isolation, anger, bargaining (prayer is an example), depression, and acceptance.

THE PROCESS

The grief process is complex and highly individualized. It is seldom as predictable and orderly as the stages presented by Bowlby and Kübler-Ross might imply. Studies conducted by psychologist Janice Genevro in 2003 and Yale University researchers in 2007, as well as a survey of Canadian hospices in 2008, contradict the stage theory of grief altogether and suggest that grief is actually a complex mix of recurring emotions and symptoms that eventually alleviate. The duration of intense grief is quite variable, which can be a source of frustration to bereaved individuals who just want to know when their intense grief will end. Some people take a while to fully realize their loss. In a process known as "denial" or "disbelief," the grieving itself may be delayed. In a normal grief process, bereaved people eventually reach acceptance and accomplish reassessment and reorganization of their lives.

Grieving is the psychological, biological, and behavioral way of dealing with the stress created when a significant part of the self or prop for the self is taken away. Austrian endocrinologist Hans Selye made a vigorous career defining stress and considering the positive and negative effects that it may have on a person. He defined stress as "the nonspecific response of the body to any demand made upon it." Clearly any significant change calls for adjustment and thus involves stress. Selye indicated that what counts is the severity of the demand, and this depends on the perception of the person involved.

COMPLICATED GRIEF OR DEPRESSION?

Researchers and practitioners are beginning to understand the antecedents and consequences of complicated grief. To some extent, the likelihood of complicated grief depends on the nature of the loss. Losses that are unexpected and those involving sudden or violent death or suicide are especially problematic, as are those associated with childhood abuse or neglect. Individuals who are socially isolated, who were abused or neglected as children, who had a difficult emotional relationship with the deceased, or who lack resilience are particularly vulnerable to complicated grief. Prior history of mental illness, religion, gender, age, and social support are other factors. Between 10 and 20 percent of individuals experiencing a loss exhibit complicated grief reactions. Apart from its negative emotional attributes, this type of grief reaction is associated with higher rates of illness and suicide. In 2013, the American Cancer Society estimated that major clinical depression develops in up to 20 percent of bereaved persons, diagnosable after two months of extreme symptoms such as delusions, hallucinations, feelings of worthlessness, or dramatic weight loss.

Clinical trials suggest that cognitive behavioral therapy or complicated grief treatment may be helpful for those experiencing complicated grief. There is also limited evidence for using antidepressant medications for treating complicated grief, though the outcomes were not as good as those for people with clinical major depression unrelated to grief.

The Diagnostic Statistical Manual of Mental Disorders (DSM) long stated that clinicians should rule out grief due to a recent loss (within the first few weeks after the death) before making a diagnosis of depression or an adjustment disorder. The fifth edition (DSM-5), published in 2013, eliminates this "bereavement exclusion," generating a great deal of controversy. The American Psychiatric Association states that the reasons for the change are that bereavement often lasts one to two years, not less than two months, and that major depression can be triggered by bereavement, particularly in those who have personal or family histories of depression. Proponents argue that bereavement is merely another stressor like unemployment or divorce and therefore should be considered similarly in diagnosing a patient. Many critics warn that normal grief reactions will be pathologized and patients given unnecessary treatment, particularly antidepressants.

CULTURAL AND SOCIAL INFLUENCES

Because loss is such a regular part of life, a person's reaction to it is likely to be regulated by family and cultural influences. Religious and cultural practices have developed to govern the expected and acceptable ways of responding to loss. Many of these practices provide both permission for and boundaries to the expression of grief. They provide both an opportunity to express feelings and a limit to their expression. Often a religion or culture will stipulate the rituals that must be observed, how soon they must be concluded, how long they must be extended, what kind of clothing is appropriate, and what kinds of expressions are permissible and fitting. They also provide a cognitive framework in which the loss may be understood and, perhaps, better accepted—for example, framing the loss as God's will.

The funeral home industry has been subject to criticism for profiting from the ubiquity of death. In part as a result, several organizations have sprung up to deliver affordable alternatives to traditional funeral arrangements, such as cremation, home-based funeral services, and green (environmentally sensitive) burials.

Toward the end of the twentieth century, professional interest in grief and grief counseling began to grow. The Association for Death Education and Counseling was founded in 1976 to provide a forum for educators and clinicians addressing this concern. Major journals such as Omega and Death Studies provide sources for research on grief and loss.

FURTHER READING

American Cancer Society. *Coping with the Loss of a Loved One*. Atlanta: American Cancer Society, 4 Feb. 2013. PDF file.

Bowlby, John. *Loss: Sadness and Depression*. London: Tavistock Inst., 1980. Print.

Doka, Kenneth J. "Grief and the DSM: A Brief Q&A." *HuffPost Healthy Living*. TheHuffingtonPost.com, 29 May 2013. Web. 21 May 2014.

Freud, Sigmund. "Mourning and Melancholia." *Collected Papers*. Vol. 4. London: Hogarth, 1956. Print.

"Grief, Bereavement, and Coping with Loss." *National Cancer Institute*. US Dept. of Health and Human Services, National Institutes of Health, 6 Mar. 2013. Web. 21 May 2014.

Harvey, John H., ed. *Perspectives on Loss: A Sourcebook*. Philadelphia: Taylor, 1998. Print.

Konisberg, Ruth Davis. "New Ways to Think about Grief." *Time*. Time, 29 Jan. 2011. Web. 21 May 2014.

Lindemann, Erich. "Symptomatology and Management of Acute Grief." *American Journal of Psychiatry* 101 (1944): 141–48. Print.

Marrone, Robert. *Death, Mourning, and Caring*. Pacific Grove: Brooks/Cole, 1997. Print.

Mitford, Jessica. *The American Way of Death Revisited*. Rev. ed. New York: Knopf, 1998. Print.

Parkes, Colin Murray, and Holly G. Prigerson. *Bereavement: Studies of Grief in Adult Life*. 4th ed. New York: Routledge, 2010. Print.

Worden, M. *Grief Counseling and Grief Therapy: A Handbook for Mental Health Professionals*. 3rd ed. New York: Springer, 2008. Print.

Everett J. Delahanty, Jr.; updated by Allyson Washburn

Guilt

The psychoanalytic and psychological concept of guilt has received extensive attention. Guilt, the feeling of tension when violating a moral code, is one of the significant ideas in psychoanalytic theory. Its psychological understanding has changed over time and continues to evolve.

INTRODUCTION

The concept of guilt has played an important role in the development of human behavior and culture since the early days of civilization. More recently, there has been a focus on the psychological understanding of guilt. One of the first people to write extensively about the psychological meaning of guilt was the Austrian founder of psychoanalysis, Sigmund Freud. His writings from the 1890s to the 1930s provide the basic foundation of the contemporary understanding of guilt. Guilt is the feeling of tension when one feels that one has violated a moral code by thought, action, or nonaction. It is considered to be a type of anxiety. The unpleasant feeling of guilt usually prompts the guilty person to take some type of action to relieve the tension.

Freud believed that guilt starts in early childhood as a result of the child's fear of being punished or of losing the love of the parent through misbehavior. Freud stressed that the most significant event in establishing guilt is the Oedipus complex. At the age of four or five, Freud hypothesized, the male child wants to kill his father and have sex with his mother. In the counterpart to this, sometimes called the Electra complex, the female child wants to kill her mother and have sex with her father. The child becomes anxious with these thoughts and attempts to put them out of his or her consciousness. As a result of the Oedipus complex, the child develops a conscience, which represents inner control and morality. There is the ability to recognize right from wrong and to act on the right and refrain from doing wrong. Freud would later use the concept of the superego to explain conscience. The superego represents the parental thoughts and wishes that have been internalized in the child. Now the internal superego can monitor the morality of the child, and guilt can be generated when the superego is displeased.

An important distinction is to be made between normal guilt and neurotic guilt. Normal guilt is experienced when one has acted in such a way as to violate one's moral code. A person then usually takes some action to relieve the guilt. Neurotic guilt relates to thoughts or wishes that are unacceptable and cause anxiety. These thoughts are pushed out of consciousness, so that the person feels guilt-ridden but is not aware of the source of the guilt. There is no relief from the guilt. In neurotic guilt, the thought is equated with the deed.

ORIGIN

The origin of guilt can be traced back to childhood. In human development there is a long period in which the baby is dependent on the parent. The young baby cannot survive without someone providing for its care. As the baby begins to individuate and separate from the parent, ambivalent feelings are generated. Ambivalent feelings are opposing feelings, typically love and hate, felt for the same person. The child begins to worry that these hateful feelings will cause the parents to punish him or her or remove their love. With this fear of parental retaliation, the child becomes guilty when thinking or acting in a way that might displease the parents.

The Oedipus complex dramatically changes this situation. The dynamics of this complex are based on the play by the Greek playwright Sophocles, in which Oedipus murders his father and takes his mother as his wife, unaware that they are his parents. When Oedipus finds out the truth, he blinds himself and goes into exile. Freud believed the Oedipal situation to be a common theme in literature. He also discussed the play *Hamlet* (1603) by the English playwright William Shakespeare. At the beginning of the play, Hamlet's uncle has killed Hamlet's father and married Hamlet's mother. There is the question as to why Hamlet hesitates in killing his uncle, and Freud attributed this indecision to Hamlet's Oedipus complex. Freud argued that Hamlet had thoughts of killing his father and having sex with his mother, and Hamlet's uncle only put into action what Hamlet had thought. Hamlet's guilty desires prevent him from taking any action. Freud believed that the Oedipus complex can exist throughout one's life. People can feel guilty about separating from their parents or achieving more than their parents, as this can unconsciously represent killing them off.

Freud's examination of neurotic guilt led him to the concept of unconscious guilt. Neurotics experience guilt but are not sure what they are guilty about. Freud first noticed this attitude in obsessive patients. These patients tended to be perfectionistic and overly conscientious, and yet they were wracked by guilt. Freud believed them to be feeling guilty about thoughts and wishes they had pushed out of consciousness, that is, Oedipal wishes. Freud observed the paradox that the more virtuous a person, the more the person experiences self-reproach and guilt as temptations increase.

Freud's final writings on guilt highlighted its importance for civilization. He wrote that guilt enabled people to get along with others and form groups, institutions, and nations. Without the ability to curb impulses, particularly aggression, society would suffer. Freud did feel that humans pay a price for this advance in civilization, in that there is a loss of personal happiness due to the heightening of the sense of guilt.

HISTORY

Writing in the 1930s, child psychoanalyst Melanie Klein argued that the Oedipus complex started much earlier in the child's development than Freud had suggested. She believed that it started toward the end of the first year of life and centered primarily on the mother. The baby hates the mother for withdrawing the breast during feeding. The baby then feels guilty and worries that the mother will no longer breast-feed. Klein felt that the baby would want to relieve its guilt by making amends to the mother, causing it to show concern and care for the mother. Klein felt that this was the most crucial step in human development, the capacity to show concern for someone else. Guilt is thus seen as a critical ingredient in the ability to love.

The psychoanalyst Franz Alexander further advanced understanding of guilt. He wrote that feeling guilty can interfere with healthy assertiveness. The guilty person may need excessive reassurance from other people. When the guilty person is assertive, he or she fears retaliation from others. Alexander also wrote about the concept of guilt projection. This term refers to situations in which people who tend to be overly critical induce guilt in other people.

The psychoanalyst Erik H. Erikson also wrote on the theme of guilt interfering with assertiveness. He formulated a theory of eight stages of human development, focusing primarily on early development. The fourth stage of development, around the age of four to five, is called guilt/initiative. The child must successfully repress Oedipal wishes to avoid feeling excessive guilt. The child can then proceed with normal initiative.

Another perspective on guilt is the concept of existential guilt, discussed by American psychiatrist James Knight. Existential guilt is the failure to live up to one's expectations and potentialities. It can lead to questioning one's existence and to states of despair until personal meaning can be established.

Erich Fromm expanded the concept of guilt in order to better understand group psychology. He wrote that there are essentially two types of conscience: authoritarian and humanistic. Authoritarian conscience is the voice of internalized external authority. It is based on fear and danger. It is afraid of displeasing authority and actively seeks to please authority. Authoritarian conscience can lead to immoral acts committed as the individual conscience is given over to this higher authority. Humanistic conscience is one's own voice expressing one's own true self. It is the essence of one's moral experience in life. It includes integrity and self-awareness.

CURRENT STATUS

Since 1960, there has been a significant change in the views of psychoanalytic theory on guilt. The psychoanalyst Hans Loewald wrote extensively about guilt. He considered that guilt does not necessarily lead to punishment; sometimes punishment is sought to evade guilt. Bearing the burden of guilt makes it possible to master guilt by achieving a reconciliation of conflicting feelings. Guilt is thus seen not as a troublesome feeling but as one of the driving forces in the organization of the self. Guilt plays a critical part in developing self-responsibility and integrity.

The American psychoanalyst Stephen Mitchell, writing in 2000, expanded on Loewald's ideas. Mitchell concerned himself with the concept of genuine guilt. He believes it is important to tolerate, accept, and use this feeling. People need to take responsibility for the suffering they have caused others and themselves. People particularly hurt those they love, but by taking personal responsibility for their behavior, they can repair and deepen their love.

GUILT AND SHAME

Throughout the 1990s, there were a number of writings about the concept of shame and its relation to guilt. Shame is experienced as a feeling of inadequacy in the self. There can be physical, psychological, or emotional shame.

The American psychoanalyst Helen Lewis wrote extensively about this topic. She believed that shame includes dishonor, ridicule, humiliation, and embarrassment, while guilt includes duty, obligation, responsibility, and culpability. A person can feel both guilt and shame.

FURTHER READING

Akhtar, Salman, ed. *Guilt: Origins, Manifestations, and Management*. Lanham: Aronson, 2013. Print.

Carveth, Donald L. *The Still Small Voice: Psychoanalytic Reflections on Guilt and Conscience*. London: Karnac, 2013. Print.

Freeman, Lucy, and Herbert S. Strean. *Understanding and Letting Go of Guilt*. Northvale: Aronson, 1995. Print.

Joseph, Fernando. "The Borrowed Sense of Guilt." *International Journal of Psychoanalysis* 81.3 (2000): 499–512. Print.

Lewis, Michael. *The Rise of Consciousness and the Development of Emotional Life*. New York: Guilford, 2014. Print.

Piers, Gerhart, and Milton B. Singer. *Shame and Guilt: A Psychoanalytic and a Cultural Study*. New York: Norton, 1971. Print.

Reilly, Patrick. *The Literature of Guilt: From Gulliver to Golding*. Iowa City: U of Iowa P, 1988. Print.

Rodogno, Raffaele. "Gender and Shame: A Philosophical Perspective." *Gender and Emotion*. Ed. Ioana Latu, Marianne Schmid Mast, and Susanne Kaiser. Bern: Lang, 2013. 155–70. Print.

Tangney, June Price, and Ronda L. Dearing. *Shame and Guilt*. New York: Guilford, 2004. Print.

Tournier, Paul. *Guilt and Grace: A Psychological Study*. San Francisco: Harper, 1983. Print.

Daniel Heimowitz

Helping friends cope

Loss impacts everyone at some point in life. When it strikes during the teen years it can be especially challenging to deal with. Teens may think they should be able to handle their grief and loss reactions now that they are nearing the age of independence but that is sometimes when they need the most support. Teens are most likely to turn to peers or friends for close support. In addition they are likely to reach out to members of their immediate or extended families who can be a primary source of support in a time of grief and loss. Spirituality can also be a major part of the healing process.

INTRODUCTION

The adolescent years are a time of growing independence. This is the period of life when, according to Erik

Erikson, the accompanying psychosocial stage of development focuses on identity versus role confusion. This is where a teen begins to develop their own sense of competencies related to goals and purpose in life. There is a risk of identity foreclosure according to the psychosocial developmental theory of Erikson when events interfere with this process. Identity foreclosure can lead to a lack of exploration of possible roles. However challenges such as experiencing a major loss during this period can also help us achieve a stable identity if they are resolved in an adaptive way. Erikson studied development over a lifespan and identified key crises during each stage that if we work through correctly would help us with the progression to the next stage of development and its psychosocial challenges. Adolescents are trying to become their own person and to work to identify their own strengths weaknesses and interests as well as goals for the future. (See the book by David Balk in the section on further reading for more information on the impact of loss on identity development.) During this time of life that Erikson called a moratorium, it's also possible to have more emotional intensity about changes in our lives. Anxiety and depression can be common and can accompany loss and grief reactions. Coping with these feelings of grief and loss can be challenging. There are generally two types of coping: adaptive and maladaptive. Adaptive coping involves being able to access social and spiritual support and engage in problem solving to come up with solutions to move towards acceptance regarding the feelings of loss. Maladaptive coping involves turning to substance use or other unhealthy behaviors that only complicate one's life and makes healing from loss even harder.

To experience loss one must first have experienced attachment. Attachment bonds are what make a relationship important to us. John Bowlby wrote about attachment and loss and the despair that can come with experiencing the loss of an important attachment figure. We not only become attached psychologically and emotionally from the very beginning of life to our primary caregiver (usually our mothers) or to any significant caregiver, but also we become attached physiologically. Our bodies produce oxytocin which is a bonding hormone. It can feel like we are going through withdrawal when we lose an important person to whom we were attached. These powerful feelings of grief and loss can be overwhelming if we don't have coping skills in place.

TYPES OF GRIEF AND LOSS SITUATIONS

Loss can be triggered by the anticipation of a future ending of something significantly important to us. For example someone might anticipate that when they graduate from high school they will miss all their friends when they all go off to various colleges or jobs. Life will never be the same. The feeling is bittersweet because it is both a time of excitement and of loss. Loss in this example, includes the loss of the routine of going to that particular school with that particular schedule and the loss of those contacts and supports as they were configured in that setting. For example maybe someone was on a high school sports team, an academic team, and a member of a band. If all of those activities for that time and place terminate when graduation occurs there will be multiple losses that are experienced. Loss will also include the new responsibilities that come with having reached a milestone such as moving on to undergraduate work at college or a new job. One way of coping with these kinds of changes is to approach them gradually. Some students will go for one or more weekends to a college for a visit to start to acclimate to the change. This may help make the transition less difficult and more gradual. Another way of coping is to make very concerted efforts to stay in touch with those persons who mean the most to us. Even if it's not possible to physically visit those who are important to us we can keep in touch frequently through texting, Skype, old-fashioned phone calls and some planned visits especially around the holidays.

Loss of place can be experienced in immigrant teens or teens who are refugees and have to leave not only their home but also their country of origin to flee to a safer or more stable environment. This loss of place has many aspects – feeling longing not only for those who were left behind, but also for the places where one had many memories of perhaps better times but also some not so happy times. In the words of a displaced teen from Africa, "When I first went to Tanzania everything was different. We had lived in the city; it was a "normal life" like it is here. There I had to go daily to get water in a bucket that I carried on my head back to the tin shelter. Now, when I think about what I miss most when I think about Africa as a place, rather than the lost relationships it is Tanzania I think of. I even miss going to carry water sometimes. Because I was so young when all that happened in the Congo and I don't really know the details or why it happened. So, I think of the landscape as I knew it in the camp, and of course, I miss the food and the pace of life. Here it is the city. It took a long time to get used to it here, even though my life in the Congo was much as it is here. But if you asked me what I miss most, it is that here I have no friends my own age unless they also speak Swahili."

Loss can also be triggered by the breakup of a relationship that was romantic in nature. The more significant the relationship was and the longer it had lasted the more painful the ending is likely to be. It is helpful to realize that most people experience at least one major romantic breakup in their lifetime if not more. We eventually learn to carry forward what was special about that relationship and eventually come to a resolution and refer to it as a learning experience for future relationships.

Loss can be triggered by having to move away from friends when one's family must relocate for a job or perhaps military reassignment. It can take a good six months to reestablish connections and attachments in a new location. Until those are in place, it can be a lonely time.

Loss of a friend is an example of a loss that teens may experience. Teens may lose friends to car or other accidents such as drug or alcohol related fatalities and in the unfortunate instances of school shootings that occur periodically in our society. In some cases teens will experience multiple losses of this nature and they can be hard to reconcile particularly when you lose someone so early in their life. There can be anger and frustration associated with these types of losses. School counselors often make concerted efforts to form healing communities to help students memorialize and grieve these losses.

The loss most often associated with grief is the sudden absence of a loved one due to death or divorce (which is sometimes experienced as a death of a relationship). Parental loss in a young person's life is perhaps one of the most impactful and significant types of loss and can be overwhelming for a young person to deal with. Life will never be the same once someone loses one or more of their parents. It is especially important to get support and even consider getting grief counseling with loss of a parent. Anxiety and depression are common reactions to parental loss. There can be a concern over another issue that needs to be worked through; the concern over forgetting that parent over the course of time. Communities may have support groups for teens who can meet with other teens in the same situation. Family member loss and sibling loss also may require extra support from others, relatives and counselors to assist survivors in utilizing healthy coping strategies during the grief process.

Loss of a loved one to suicide or a peer to suicide is a form of loss that is a particularly stressful. This type of loss can be associated with disenfranchised grief where others are not quite sure how to reach out to assist. Fortunately some communities have suicide survivor support groups. These can be extremely helpful when you realize you are not alone and are able to observe how others have dealt with this type of heartbreaking loss. Additional counseling may be advised after such a traumatic loss.

The loss of a pet can be just as significant as a loss of a significant person in one's life. As humans we often become attached to our pets as if they were a person. Finding others who understand this type of loss would be key in getting the kind of support one would need when one loses a pet. Some schools may have support groups that could be beneficial in healing from this type of loss.

STAGES OF GRIEF

Everyone goes through the grieving process a little bit differently. There are some stages of grief that have been recognized for some time. These include denial, anger, bargaining, depression and acceptance. Elizabeth Kubler-Ross wrote about the stages of grief initially to describe someone going through their own terminal illness and facing death. Later, these stages have been applied to the grief process overall. In our society a lot of the initial grieving takes place in the company of others such as in the rituals surrounding wakes or funerals and activities in the days immediately thereafter. Teens are unique in that in today's world they may have other tools or resources to express their grief. Anniversaries can reactivate that sequence of grieving. It is important to have a way to recognize those anniversary reactions. Social media may be one of these outlets. Some young and not so young people, when they have lost a person who meant a great deal to them, have created a memorial to the lost loved one such as a Facebook page where they post their feelings, thoughts and memories. This provides another outlet for social support where others can post memories feelings and thoughts as well. It is a way to honor the memory of those who are no longer with us. These types of virtual communities perpetuate across time and help others to recognize anniversaries related to the loss.

STRATEGIES

Education about the grief process is important and is the first step in being able to understand grief and loss. Understanding is the first part of healing. Support is the second part of healing from loss. Although there may be stages to the grieving process, there can be wide variation in coping with loss and no one person grieves the same as another person. There is no right way or wrong way to grieve. Recovering from loss takes time (sometimes years). The pain never stops, it only decreases in intensity. Initially some will need to take a few personal days from school or work to honor the loss. Notifying school advisement centers of a loss can help as they can let teachers or others know of your absence. Other strategies include resuming one's routine and trying to stay busy which will allow a person to gradually move forward emotionally when they are ready. Most people will still feel the sadness of the loss when they recall memories and that will be normal going forward.

Research on coping has shown that the type of coping that is the healthiest is coping that involves direct problem-solving strategies as opposed to coping that is primarily emotion-focused. Keeping busy, taking time out for self-care, seeking social support from friends and loved ones are all healthy strategies for healing from grief. New research on meditation with mindfulness strategies (deep breathing, elements of yoga and focused attention) have been found to be helpful for some of individuals recovering from grief. Having a strong sense of spirituality and a spiritual community for healing can also facilitate the grieving process.

FURTHER READING

Balk, D. E. (2014). *Dealing With Death, Dying and Grieving During Adolescence.* New York: Routledge. The author of this informative book elaborates on Erikson's theory as it relates to identity formation during the teen years and the positive and negative effects when loss occurs during this period. It also provides chapters on coping skills for handling loss in the teen years.

Christ, G.H., Siegel, K. & Christ, A.E. (2002). Adolescent grief, "It never really hit me until it actually happened...". *Journal of the American Medical Association*, 288:10. This article goes into depth about stages of grief and signs of grief in teens and children of all ages. It pays particular attention to parental loss and how to help youth cope during this difficult time.

griefspeaks.com retrieved 5/15/15. Grief Speaks is a website with a lot of resources including worksheets on how to set up a social support system after loss. This website has practical tools for healing from grief.

Shuttleworth, J. (n. d.) *Grief Retreat For Teens: Hospice Wellington Welcomes Youth Struggling With Loss.*

Guelph Mercury. A story about a retreat for grieving teens in Canada. See also: http: www.hospicewellington.org Retrieved 5/16/15.

Sjoqvist, S. (2007). *Still Here With Me: Teenagers and Children On Losing A Parent.* Philadelphia, PA: Jessica Kingsley Publishers. A thoughtful anthology of the experiences of thirty-one children and teenagers who have lost a parent. Retrieved 5/15/15 from https://books.google.com › books

Turner, M. (2006). *Talking With Children and Young People About Death and Dying.* (2d ed.) London: Jessica Kingsley. This is a resource book on grief, bereavement and loss tailored for children and young people

http://www.whatsyourgrief.com/helping-a-teenager-deal-with-grief-2/ retrieved 4/20/15. This resource is a website that parallels the grief of teens with that of adults. It takes an informed approach in terms of unique developmental and emotional considerations in teens. It speaks of the rituals and etiquette following the loss of a person. It gives particular information on how to best support teens who have experienced loss.

Karen Wolford and Rebekah Tanner

SEE ALSO: Accidents; Death and Dying; Loss of a Friend; Loss of a Parent or Guardian; Loss of a Sibling; Separation and Divorce: Children's Issues; Teenage Suicide

Loss of a friend

Grief is a strong emotion that impacts everyone who is fortunate to have someone who brings friendship and joy to their lives. Therefore, that makes grief something everyone experiences at one time or another. Perhaps one might identify the emotion as a consequence for having enjoyed the understanding, comfort, companionship, support, or love that embraces a meaningful relationship. As adolescents become more and more independent from family, they depend increasingly on their peers for emotional support. They have increased empathy and a special closeness – I can tell my friend anything and she will understand. We even know what each other is thinking! It would not be an overstatement or exaggeration to suggest that the death of a friend can be traumatic.

Very young children experience loss when they misplace or lose their favorite blanket or teddy bear. They cry, search, and feel their life is simply not the same without the object of their affection that once helped make everything in the world seem a little brighter. The old raggedy bear or blanket was always standing ready to hug when lonely, afraid, confused, happy, or sad. It went everywhere with me … and now, it's gone! The young child probably gave the object a nickname that mimicked a feeling of endearment.

Similarly, the intense emotions what accompany losing a friend are normal. Everyone responds differently to loss; however it's clear that we all experience grief when we wake-up to find our world is turned upside down after the moment when we learn we lost a friend. The loss of a friend in adolescence may evoke the most intense feelings we have ever experienced as someone who is in the early stages of life's journey. Those emotions can cause great distress, despair, confusion, and everything we defined as truth "turns on a dime." We are faced with our own mortality. Our sense that death is for old people is shaken and the feelings that accompany that realization may require counseling intervention.

INTRODUCTION

Adults may suggest that we need to prepare for the death of someone we love. We were told that our friend had a terminal illness, but hospital visits, disclosed or leaked information, and the passage of time before their passing, didn't cushion the pain. It still hurts even though you saw all the side effects when witnessing their struggle to beat the disease.

Sometimes, we begin to grieve the loss of a friend before their death. For example, we may experience *anticipatory grief* when we learn our friend's chemotherapy treatments are not successful and the cancer is spreading. We begin the grieving process as we foresee their death and how the loss will impact our lives. In other words, we begin to miss them before they are gone.

The death of a young person often comes without notice, it's sudden, traumatic, and without warning. A car accident takes the life of a friend moments after meeting at the local gym, a sports event, or on the way home from a fun vacation with family. Sadly, a friend may take their own life, leaving friends feeling abandoned, angry, guilty, and helpless. Grieving the loss of a friend who commits suicide is probably the most difficult. Survivors are left with so many unanswered questions, feelings of guilt, and further anger and rage. *How could you do this to me!*

Research documents that we go through stages when we grief the loss of a friend. Grief comes in waves, steps or stages can vary, as well as intensity. Everyone does not experience grief in the way same. The manner and order in which we move through the grief process is also unique. The stages may serve as guidelines to help us have a better understanding of what we are feeling and enhance our ability to eventually find comfort and peace. A positive outcome would be to heal, continue our journey, forever changed, but renewed in hope. We deserve to be happy. Grief becomes bearable, the pain lessons, the waves of emotions are less intense, and we allow ourselves to feel joy again. The following figure illustrates a tide format that serves to introduce the Stages of Grief and remind readers that the strong emotions that accompany grief come in waves:

GRIEVING THE LOSS OF A FRIEND: THE CELL PHONE
Shock and Denial:

One bright sunny day, you return home from school to find that your cell phone is missing from your backpack. You search all the carefully zipped pockets over and over again because it's not possible that it could be gone … *you're shocked!* You always secure it in the same place and why would today be any different than any other day? You depend on it being exactly where you put it and this must be a coincidence, there must be a simple explanation. You believe that the result will be positive if you simply continue your search. Of course, the cell phone will reappear, and all will be well again. It is too much to digest at the moment. You persist in reminding yourself that for some reason you are looking in the wrong place and the reality of it actually being lost must be a mistake. Now, your sense of urgency and dread begins to increase … *this can't be happening!* I'll look again, really deep this time … it will appear … *it doesn't.*

Anger:

You begin to panic. *Why is this happening to me?* The cell phone is overflowing with all your most valuable personal data, identification, phone numbers, photos, personal website access codes, appointments, calendar events, birthdates, text messages, reminders, and everything else that helps make life easier and *defines who you are.* It helped you feel connected to the world and everyone in it. Your cell phone offered instant access to everything that represented what was important to you, and now it's missing. You begin to question how you are going to get through the next minute, hour, day, week, or month without something that meant so much. You become angry and fearful because now you feel lost, and your life is spiraling out of control without your phone. *How could I be so stupid! If only I had been more careful … it wouldn't have happened!* Intense feelings often emerge without warning, unexpectedly, and tears accompany the surge, all normal responses. Tears are part of the healing process, perhaps a way of cleansing away some pain so as to eventually make way for more joy and hope.

Bargaining and Depression:

Routine day-to-day activities are impacted. It's hard to concentrate. You wish you could feel normal again and change what happened. It doesn't seem fair that the whole world is going about its business while your life is in such turmoil and in shambles. *No one else could possibly feel the way I do!* It's like living in a bad dream and you can't wake up. You feel sad, especially because many of the lost photos and silly selfies were taken standing next to your best friend who died in an unfortunate car accident. Also, saved voicemails and text messages were vivid reminders. Some things are irreplaceable and you would do anything to get those amazing memories and bits of your life back. Seemingly little things trigger intense emotions like an empty locker in the school

hallway, a vacant classroom chair, songs, places, smells, and sounds. *I can't stop thinking about it!* Many events were documented in your cell phone, but you have the power to retrieve them in your memories. Some things remain safe no matter the harshness of reality.

Acceptance and Hope:

Little by little, grief remains, but the emotional pain and wave of emotions soften and become bearable. You replace your new cell phone with new memories, numbers, appointments, text messages, voicemails, access codes, favorites, icons, songs, apps, and search engines. Your life is beginning to come back together again, but it's not necessarily the same. It's not the same cell phone and it will take time to enter all the data that will help give you a sense that things are returning to normal. In the mean time, you begin your journey to move forward having learned from the experience.

Most importantly, you learned that you can survive a difficult time of incredible grief and loss. This does not mean you forget all the good things that were once entered in your cell phone that made it so important in your life. It takes time to come to a place of hope. Now, you can tell your story and retrieve fond memories of

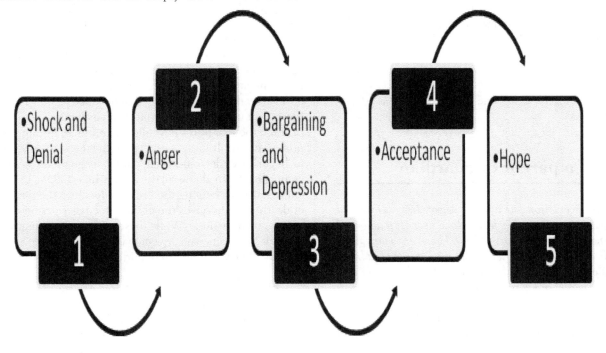

Figure 1.

your friend without shedding tears … you are on your way to recovery.

It is not a sign of weakness to seek assistance during your journey to healing. Grief counselors are prepared to support you and discuss your feelings as you move through the process. Two things they do best … listen and understand.

FURTHER READING

Fitzgerald, H. (2003). *The grieving child: A parent's guide*. New York: Simon & Schuster. This book is clear in the ways that are helpful for children.

www.grief.com. The goal of the website is to provide tools and resources to help guide readers through difficult situations and loss.

Kübler-Ross, E., & Kessler, D. (2014). On grief and grieving: Finding the meaning of grief through the five stages of loss. New York: Scribner. Ten years after the death of Elisabeth Kübler-Ross, this commemorative edition of her final book combines practical wisdom, case studies, and the authors' own experiences and spiritual insight to explain how the process of grieving helps us live with loss. This book includes a new introduction and resources section.

www.therapistaid.com. The website offers free worksheets, guides, videos, and articles for mental health counselors.

Jane Piland-Baker and Thomas E. Baker

SEE ALSO: Anger; Death and Dying; Grieving and Guilt; Teenage Suicide

Loss of a parent or guardian

Grief is an emotion felt when a person has experienced the death of someone they love or hold dear. It is a normal and natural response to the loss. There are many ways people can experience grief, including feelings of sadness, low energy, and fear for the future. When the person who died is a parent or guardian, many people, especially children and teenagers, will feel this loss to a greater extent than they might if the death were that of a friend or extended family, such as an aunt or uncle. Social or cultural influences often have an impact on how a person outwardly grieves. In the United States, where there are few rituals to mark death, the grieving child or adolescent may have fewer opportunities to express the depth of emotion that comes with the loss of a parent or guardian. It is important to allow children and teenagers to both express their grief and to understand that there is no right or wrong way to grieve.

INTRODUCTION

In 1969, Elisabeth Kubler-Ross outlined her observations of stages of grief in her landmark book, *On Death and Dying*. The stages include denial, anger, bargaining, depression and acceptance. Most individuals who experience grief can expect to feel any or all of these stages. The stages are not necessarily steps through which the person progresses, but are rather an understanding of different emotions and thoughts the grieving person can have at any time during the grief process. People, including children or teenagers, can move back and forth among the stages, or can feel a combination of these thoughts, beliefs or feelings.

RESPONSES OF CHILDREN AND TEENAGERS TO DEATH

For most of us, death is the ultimate mystery, and this is especially the case for children and adolescents. Many young people are exposed to death regularly through the media. They may have seen movies or TV shows where an actor dies in one episode or movie, but is alive and well in another. Video games sometimes include eliminating (killing) a target, but when the teenager returns to the game at another time, the character who was killed off in an earlier game may need to be killed again. Thus, there is an unreal quality about death as being final. Explaining the death to the young person in an age appropriate, yet truthful way is crucial for the teenager or child to begin to understand their parent or guardian is not coming back. By doing so, the adult who is talking to the child assists in helping the child understand the nature of death, but also gives the child or teenager permission to talk about the loss. While these conversations may be difficult for adults who are going through their own grief process, they will open up opportunities for the child to grieve as well.

Children and teenagers do not grieve in the same way as adults, and should not be expected to (Wolfelt, 2001). Children sometimes express their dismay and then appear to be quite happy when they return to play. The grief will come up at different times, especially on noteworthy days such as the child's birthday or other holidays celebrated by the family where the loss of the parent is especially apparent. It is not unusual for young children to regress to a stage prior to the death as a way to return to a safer more secure time (Worden, 2009). Children will sometimes develop behavior problems where none existed before as they try to come to grips with the ultimate abandonment that is death. They may not have the words to express their feelings, and may even need help identifying feelings of sadness, anger, hurt or fear (Grollman, 1990).

Teenagers sometimes become sullen or isolated as a way to cope with their feelings of unreality or denial about the death. Adolescence is a time of many changes, when the teenager is trying to develop an identity and to become more independent of the parents. Often a time of great conflict, the teenager may have been having fights with the parent or guardian who has died. While this is a normal part of the developmental process, the teenager may not understand it as such, and might feel extraordinary guilt for the parent's death. Most teenagers have not experienced a loss of a parent or guardian, and for the teen who is going through the grieving process, there can be difficulty finding support. The teenager, feeling he or she must stand out because of the grief, can't understand why others don't "get it" (Wolfelt, 2004). If there are not supportive adults in the teenager's life, lack of empathy from peers can complicate the grieving. Teens may express their distress by acting out, doing poorly in school, becoming depressed or hopeless, resulting in suicidal thoughts (Freudeberger & Gallagher, 1995).

With the loss of a parent or guardian, children and teens might be anxious or fearful about the future. This is especially true if the loved one who died was the primary financial support for the family (Wolfelt, A.D. 2001). Reassurance that the family will come through this intact, even if there have to be some changes to the lifestyle, can mitigate these fears. Reassurance of this type by adults gives the child or teen permission to relax and feel his or her feelings.

IT MATTERS WHAT TYPE OF DEATH IT WAS

If a parent or guardian has been sick for any length of time, children and teenagers may have begun the mourning process prior to the death. Society seems to allow people to mourn these deaths with less judgment, although there can be statements that marginalize the grief, such as "You knew this was going to happen." In the case of accidents, there can be speculation on causes, adding shame or the need to defend the loved one after the death. Suicides are also still stigmatized by some people, which stifles the grief process. Teens and children often don't know how to talk about a death due to suicide, nor do they know how to handle morbid curiosity that can accompany this type of death. Murder or violent death can also open up the doors for judgment, stigmatization, or morbid curiosity. Young people who have lost a parent or guardian to a sudden or violent death or to suicide will need places they can safely talk about the death. In the case of a death due to suicide, the young person may experience greater anger or despair. They can struggle with feelings of unworthiness because the parent or guardian chose to abandon them. While adults often feel they should shield the child from the information associated with sudden or violent deaths, young people need to be informed in age-appropriate language about what has happened. If they don't hear the story from the trusted adults in their lives, they will ultimately hear it elsewhere, and could end up feeling they can't trust the people in their life they need the most. Both children and teenagers need to make meaning of the events in their lives, and when they are unable to talk to family members about death, the meaning they make might be that it is not okay to talk about the loved one. This can make the grieving process longer, or can complicate losses they experience later in life.

Regardless of the type of death, it is important for children and adolescents to know they did not "cause" the death. Depending on the age and maturity level of the child or teenager, there can be some fears that either arguing with the parent or wishing they would die caused the person to die. The death or a parent or guardian rocks the child or teenager's world, and shatters safety and security. Adding guilt to the mix will only make things worse. The surviving parent or other adults in the family have the responsibility for initiating conversations that will allow the young person to express feelings of guilt or responsibility for the death. Adults in the family will want to monitor the depth of the teenager's feelings, and may need to contact a mental health professional to help the teen work through his or her fears and emotions.

WHAT CHILDREN AND TEENAGERS CAN DO TO GRIEVE

There is often some controversy about whether or not young people should attend funerals. The reality is that funerals or celebrations of life are one of the few ways death is acknowledged in our society. Thus, the decision whether or not the child or teenager should attend a funeral should be discussed with them. Regardless of whether they go to the funeral or not, there are other ways young people can honor the loss of the parent or guardian, while they acknowledge the reality of the loss. Making a memory book with pictures, drawings and writings can be a way of dealing with the loss, as can making a memory box with mementos associated with the parent who has died. Planting plants is a living reminder of the person who has died. Teenagers and children often had special activities they did with the parent or guardian who has died. Doing some of these things in honor of the loved one can be a way to not only honor the deceased, but a way to recognize life goes on. Small ceremonies at significant times after the death can help acknowledge the feelings a teen or child has at these times.

CONCLUSION

When a young person loses a parent or guardian, they are losing one of the strongest bonds in life (Wolfelt, 2001). This can have a lifelong effect on the child or teenager (Freudenberger & Gallagher, 1995). Young people who have lost a parent or guardian sometimes have trouble later in life with relationships. Because they can feel abandoned by the parent or guardian who died, they have difficulty developing the trust that is essential to close relationships. How the surviving parent or other adults in the family respond to the child can have a positive impact on how the child or teenager grieves. A child or teen who is given permission to grieve, and to do so in his or her own individual way is more likely to accept the death and express feelings openly and honestly. While the child or teen may not "get over" the death of a parent or guardian, they will adjust to the loss on their own timetable.

FURTHER READING

Fitzgerald, H. (1992). *The Grieving Child: A Parent's Guide*. New York, NY: Fireside Books. This book offers advice to parents and other adults on helping the child cope with death.

Freudenberger, H.J., Gallagher, K.M. (1995). "Emotional Consequences of Loss For Our Adolescents". *Psychotherapy* (32), 150-153. Scholarly article that talks about the emotional, behavioral and psychological effects of the death of a parent during adolescence.

Grollman, E.A. (1990). *Talking To a Child About Death: A Dialogue Between Parent and Child*. Boston, MA: Beacon Press. This book, with read-along sections for children is a guide for parents and caregivers on how to talk to children about death.

Haine, R.A., Ayers, T.S., Sandler, I.N. & Wolchik, S.A. (2008). "Evidence-based Practices For Parentally Bereaved Children and Their Families". *Professional Psychology: Research and Practice*, 39, 113-121. Scholarly article that discusses the parent-child relationship and makes recommendations for helping children whose parent has died grieve appropriately.

Kubler-Ross, E. (1969). *On Death and Dying*. New York: Scribner. Landmark book that identifies the stages of grief and describes them.

The Grief Recovery Institute (2015). Why society will use any word but grief. Recovered from https://www.griefrecoverymethod.com/blog/2013/07/why-society-will-use-any-word-grief-grief-recovery-can-help-dealing-ptsd. This article talks about the impact of society on how people understand they can grieve.

Walsh, F. & McGoldrick, M. (Eds.). (2004). *Living Beyond Loss: Death In The Family*. (2d ed.). New York: WW. Norton & Company. Book with chapters by authorities on grief and loss that discusses the impact of death in the family, including children, suggesting ways to address the loss.

Wolfelt, A.D. (2001). *Healing A Child's Grieving Heart: 100 Practical Ideas For Families and Friends*. Fort Collins, CO: Companion Press. This short book offers suggestions for ways parents and adult friends of the family can help the child cope with grief.

Wolfelt, A.D. (2004) *A Child's View of Grief: A Guide for Parents, Teachers and Counselors*. Fort Collins, CO: Companion Press. A book with helpful hints on how significant adults in a child's life can respond to a child's grief.

Worden, J.W. (2009). *Grief Counseling and grief Therapy: A Handbook For the Mental Health Practitioner*. (4th ed.). New York: Springer. This book intended for the mental health professional, offers practical information and insight into how to help individuals cope with grief and loss.

Janice Tedford

SEE ALSO: Accidents; Death and Dying; First Steps to Counseling; Grieving and Guilt; Resiliency

Loss of a sibling

"Grief is an irrational process. It has discordant and disorienting effects which defy the rational process of a "normal" way of being in the world. Yet within its devastating context, and given the heroic work of integrating the event into the mental, emotional, physical and spiritual being, its effects are entirely rational" (Pryce, 2012).

The goal of this "heroic work" for survivor siblings is the consolidation of identity which arises from reconciliation, resilience and / or post-traumatic growth. The ways in which this goal might be arrived at will vary depending on the circumstances surrounding the loss, the intensity and duration of grief expression, ethnocultural considerations, and the needs of the individual.

INTRODUCTION

Most people, if asked, would say the most tragic loss of any in the human experience is the loss felt by a parent when a child of theirs has died. However, the loss a young person experiences when a sibling dies or is lost to them by some other means is profound beyond words. Yet, the degree of loss and the depth of grief experienced by siblings is often not acknowledged or recognized. The death of a young person seems to be off-time, reminding others of their own fragile mortality. To then discuss such a loss with another young person seems like throwing salt on the wound. However, research on many types of irrevocable losses shows that families with good avenues of interconnected communication raise surviving siblings into adulthoods that can bear loss fairly well. Some teens who feel they are not well supported by their family or their community following the loss of a sibling; or those who have stoic, silent or otherwise unavailable parents may find themselves using maladaptive or dysfunctional coping mechanisms. These teens may have trouble forming solid adult relationships later in life. Some, having become parents later in life, reported that they were hypervigilant, or overprotective of their own children. They remained burdened by issues of safety and security. Good communication appears to be a key element in empowering young people to achieve successful identity consolidation following the loss of a sibling. Another important element is forgiveness.

Machajewski and Kronk (2013), reported that an estimated 73,000 children (persons under the age of 18) die each year in the United States and that an estimated 83% of them leave behind one or more sibling survivor.

They wrote, "Very often the physically and emotionally exhausted parents are mourning the loss of a child and may be unable to meet the needs of the surviving sibling." For the surviving sibling this situation can result in tremendous loneliness. Not only do they feel alienated from their parents, but their friends are likely unable to understand what they are going through. In addition, because the young survivor is grieving, a process that "encompasses the internal thoughts and feeling that are given to the loss of a loved one" in order to "reconcile a future life without the lost sibling" they may find that things which were once important have become trivial (Machajewski & Kronk, 2013). This distancing from peers, especially for adolescents, can result in intense feelings of alienation, of not being understood, or of being different from those around them. At a developmental stage in life when young adults usually "play out who they want to be and decide who they do not want to be" within a "geography of emotions," many of which are being experienced for the first time, the "sudden trauma at this stage interrupts development toward a cohesive and stable self" (Goodman, 2013). Because trauma causes specific biological reactions in the brain and body there can be disruptions in memory, concentration, and somatic difficulties. It is not uncommon for these siblings to see their grades slip, although with some survivors, grades actually improve. This is often because feeling uncomfortable with the social circle they previously enjoyed they redirect their attentions to their studies in order to stay busy and therefore, not have to think about the sibling they are mourning. While the apparent outcome seems positive, the coping mechanism may not be, in actuality.

For some young people, and especially for females, the loss of a sibling has been found to be more profound than the loss of a parent (Worden, Davies & McCowen, 1999). The reason for this may be that with siblings the relationship tends to be more "egalitarian and is supposed to last longer than the parent-child relationship" (Robinson & Mahon, 1997 cited in Grief & Bowers, 2007). There are many ways that young people might react following the actual or seemly irrevocable loss of a sibling to death by accident, illness, suicide, or murder; to the loss of a sibling who is missing, abducted, runaway or thrownaway; or who has been separated from other siblings by adoption, foster care, or an extended imprisonment; or due to political conditions such as war, genocide or refugee status; or, as in the famous case in 1961, when Michael Rockefeller was lost at sea. These reactions might include anger, shame, guilt, disbelief, misbehaving, regression to an earlier state of developmental functioning, sexual promiscuity, self-inflicted harm, substance use, abuse or addiction, aggression or violence toward others, withdrawal, clinginess, emotional sensitivity, crying, numbness or dissociation. Many researchers who have studied grief in children and youth report that demonstrations of grief are often delayed, as compared to the adults experiencing the same loss, and as a result of this, mourning, which is "the process of adjusting to a loss" often takes longer (Worden, 2002 cited in Grief & Bower, 2007).

BRIEF CASE STUDY: MARY ROCKEFELLER MORGAN

Mary Rockefeller Morgan is a New York City based psychotherapist, author, and producer of documentaries. She is also the twin sister of Michael Rockefeller. She has written extensively about her life, family relationships, and healing following the loss of her brother when they were both 23 years old. Because the Rockefeller family was well connected politically and had significant wealth at their disposal, the search for Michael was extensive and thorough, but was ultimately, unsuccessful. Mary accompanied her father, Nelson, 4-time governor New York (from 1959 – 1973), who would later be appointed to the Vice Presidency by Gerald Ford following Nixon's resignation, to New Guinea for the 10-day long search. She writes of the unrelenting presence of media reporters and her feeling of being invaded after the family received word of Michael's disappearance. She puts this tragedy in the context of her family's dynamics at the time. Her father, just 2 months earlier, had announced that he was divorcing her mother and would be remarrying. Mary's trauma regarding this loss of relationship between her parents was further compounded by the way her mother greeted her following the trip to New Guinea when she said, "You must get a hold of yourself, Mary. The one thing we cannot do now is cry" (Morgan, 2012). For more than two decades Mary would be told to get on with her life by people who did not seem to understand the depth and profundity of grief that the unresolved loss of her twin had caused her. Then, in her late 40's Mary made a decision to spend time alone on an extended wilderness walk in the Rocky Mountains. She used this walk in a way that is similar to the Vision Quest tradition of some Native American Peoples, seeking clarity and life purpose. By the time she returned from this spiritual exercise, she had decided to resume her education and study to become a psychotherapist. In that

work she has made a specialty of counseling twinless siblings. Following the catastrophe at the World Trade Center (which was one of the building projects her father initiated as governor of NY) she sought out the 46 individuals who had lost a twin on September 11, 2001. Under a grant-funded project she led a group with the 11 who were living in New York. There were expressions of anger, regret and guilt, and of sharing happy memories. "The feeling of extreme loneliness coming from their loss and the misunderstandings of family and friends were appreciated and understood." What Mary shared in common with this group of twins was, as in the case of her brother, "these twins would have no physical closure, the bodies of their twins were never found" (Morgan, 2012).

BRIEF CASE STUDY: ELAINE PRYCE

Elaine Pryce is a British educator and mental health professional who has worked in intercultural education, family counseling and therapeutic interventions in grief and loss trauma. As the author of *Grief, forgiveness, & redemption as a way of transformation* (2012) she writes from her own experience of having been both a subsequent birth after her parents had endured the loss of an infant daughter, and of having been the 16 year old present at the moment her 4 year old brother died of drowning. She describes her family in the immediate aftermath of this tragedy in this way, "My mother blamed me and would not have me near her; my older brother raged that it was all my fault. My father buckled like a gravely wounded deer, quietly broken with grief" (Pryce, 2012). Later, she describes her older sister's coping mechanism, who, like their mother, "caged their sorrow with fury's bile" (Pryce, 2012). Pryce reports that while her "immediate family never recovered" she was fortunate that her extended family, and in particular her maternal grandmother, provided shelter and solace. She also found support in the country chapel where her family worshipped, "These simple, working people of faith and integrity, not educated, nor articulate in bereavement, nevertheless were gently present in its byways" (Pryce, 2012). But it was her own experience of facing the "unnerving challenge" of going across a deep ravine by way of a bridge made of vines and bamboo, early in her career in Papua New Guinea, that became symbolic of her decision to "continue with the journey, wherever it took me" (Pryce, 2012). Acknowledging that the journey was not finished there, that other difficulties and uncertainties would likely arise, she addresses those who grieve in this way, "— but the energy of vision is focused upward and ahead rather than downward and behind. We have gazed with despair into the low reaches of the valley and have discovered that this is not the whole landscape. There is also sky" (Pryce, 2012). For Pryce, this new vision became possible through forgiveness, not only of others, but of herself. She quotes Dag Hammarskjold, "At some moment I did answer "Yes" to Someone or Something, and from that hour I was certain that my existence was meaningful" (Pryce, 2012) and it is this meaning which provides an answer to the sorrowing self for whom the "extent of the grief is a tribute paid to the person who is still loved, who has left the griever utterly bereft of the mutuality of that love. The meaningless felt is an existential dilemma, since it is love that gives life meaning" (Pryce, 2012).

CONCLUSION

The sad truth is that many young people who grieve the loss of a sibling often have to manage their pain on their own. One unfortunate aspect of the search for meaning which is brought about by that pain is that language often lacks ways for them to accurately describe their experience. If Isak Dinesen is correct when she says, "All sorrows can be born if you put them in a story" and the Gaelic expression, "My story and yours are the same, but it is in my soul that the story is" can be applied to this circumstance, then there is one word often used in discussions of death that is profoundly unhelpful: ACCEPTANCE.

Sibling survivors have a hole in the middle of their lives that is shaped like the brother or sister they have lost. The wind that whips through it can be as vast as the territory of a hurricane and as acute and powerful as a tornado, all at once. This hole is a wound for which total healing is probably impossible. The best such siblings can realistically hope for is an experience of grace, whereby the hole scars over, and the wind calms to a gentle breeze. Nevertheless, the hole is a permanent feature of their lives. Asking or demanding them to accept that, or implying that they can or should just get back to normal, is unhelpful and potentially cruel. Once a young person has irreversibly lost a sibling, their life is never, ever *normal* again.

One way families, communities and others involved in the lives of sibling survivors can help is by creating age and culturally appropriate rituals of remembrance. Adults should be sensitive to the fact that these rituals may need repetition and evolution as the young person continues to age and develop. For some siblings, a transitional object which may be something they either shared with their sibling or that is given to them from their sibling's belongings might become a focal point in directing affect and consolidating an identity filled with forgiveness, remembrances, bittersweet joy, graces, and as Victor Frankl has said, "tragic optimism". Or, put in terms of life choices, as Elizabeth Neeld has written in *Seven choices: Taking the steps to new life after losing someone you love* (1990), to make the "integrative choice to continue to make choices – that is the nature of life --and to feel freedom from the domination of grief" (*Neeld cited in Harvey, 2002*).

FURTHER READING

American Foundation for Suicide Prevention. The focus of this organization is education, research and prevention. The quality and quality of the resources they produce are rich and excellent. When dealing with younger siblings their booklet entitled *Child survivors of suicide: A guidebook for those who care for them* focuses on children under age 10 and is organized as "Day One," "Week One," "Month One," and "Year One." Also highly recommended is After a suicide: A toolkit for schools. The entire Website is well worth exploring. http://afsp.org

Morgan, M.R. (2014). *When grief call forth the healing: A memoir of losing a twin.* New York: Open Road Media. Also see her earlier book (2012) entitled Beginning with the end: A memoir of twin loss and healing. NY: Vantage Point. The material quoted herein comes from a "Two minute memoir" in the July / August, 2012 (pp. 30 – 33) edition of *Psychology Today* which is adapted from Beginning with the end and is entitled "A loss like no other." Morgan's site has additional biographical information, a section on grieving and links to additional resources. She asks the challenging question, "How do you survive and heal the loss the person closest to you? A spouse, a sibling, a twin?" and answers her own question in this way, "Healing does not mean forgetting the person who has died. It means forming a new relationship to that person and being able to lead a new and meaningful life." http://www.whengriefcallsforththehealing.com

Office of Juvenile Justice and Delinquency Prevention. A major study was carried out in 1999 and published in 2002 which was written by Hammer, Finkelhor, and Sedlak under the auspices of the U.S. Department of Justice, Office of Justice Programs, Office of Juvenile Justice and Delinquency Prevention entitled: National incidence studies of missing, abducted, runaway and throwaway children. Although somewhat dated now, it remains the seminal work in the field. This and other documents like it can be found here, some are available in e-book format. http://www.ojjdp.gov/publications/index.html

Pryce, E. (2012). *Grief, forgiveness & redemption as a way of transformation.* Wallingford, PA: Pendle Hill Pamphlets, #416. An online PDF of this pamphlet does not seem to be available; however it can be purchased for $7.00. The entire series of Pendle Hill Pamphlets dates back to 1934 and covers a wide range of topics with several, in addition to this one, focusing on trauma, death, grieving and loss. Some of the pamphlets are now available for Kindle or Nook. http://www.pendlehill.org/product/grief-forgiveness-redemption-way-transformation/

Regen, S. (2012). *Forgiveness.* Handout on forgiveness used by the Alternatives to Violence Project – New York, in which forgiveness is defined as "something I choose to do within myself so I can go forward (or backward) into relationship with love" (as per Betsy Griscom). This brief compilation of information includes ideas on how to achieve forgiveness, a mindfulness meditation upon forgiveness, secular, Old and New Testament quotations about forgiveness, the entire text of Reinhold Niebuhr's "Serenity Prayer," and more, including a substantial bibliography of additional resources. http://avpny.org/files/Forgiveness%20handouts%20Sue%20Regen%2002.13.pdf

Rebekah Tanner

SEE ALSO: Anger; Death and Dying; Grieving and Guilt; Teenage Suicide

Romantic breakups

Teenage love and inevitable breakups are a universal experience. Developmental aspects of teen relationships, reasons for breakups, two models of recovery - stages of grief and loss and an addiction model, lessons learned, tips for recovery and how to identify when grieving has turned to depression are all covered here.

INTRODUCTION
There is nothing like the magical and heady feeling of a first love, and nothing more devastating than the first romantic breakup. One major developmental milestone for teens is experiencing romantic relationships. These are new and different kinds of relationships for teens. Dating, holding hands, and kissing are exploration grounds for physically and emotionally intimate experiences. Finding someone special to hang out with and share dreams, fears and feelings with can be wonderful, intense and compelling. Romantic relationships are places where teens experiment with sexuality and sexual experiences, and explore different aspects of themselves and their identities. Given the rapid changes in moods and attitudes, high level of sensitivities and feelings of vulnerability, teen relationships can be very dramatic. When these relationships end, as they inevitably do, breakups can be devastating for one or both partners.

DEVELOPMENTAL STAGES OF ADOLESCENCE AND EXPERIENCING BREAKUPS
Mid-adolescence (ages 13 - 15) Having a boyfriend or girlfriend is a developmental achievement that functions as a symbol of being more grown up and socially complete. Being part of a couple often enhances your status among your peer group. A great deal of the social life in middle school revolves around who has a crush on whom, whether the object of the crush is equally interested, who will tell Jack that Jill wants to go out with him, which couples are an item, who is breaking up with whom, etc. A great deal of the gossip at lunch and recess, notes passed between friends, and Facebook postings surround these issues. At this stage, the girls tend to take the pairing more seriously, while boys can be slower to mature, and often see it as more casual. Breaking up at this stage, often referred to as "being dumped", can be more challenging from the vantage point of the loss of identity and social standing than the loss of love and intimacy.

Late adolescence (ages 15-18) In this stage, romantic relationships are more a function of attachment, sexual attraction, meaningful companionship, and emotional intimacy, and as such create more powerful romantic attachments than young people have known before. Many couples in this stage become so focused on each other, that they ignore other friendships and interests, creating a different kind of loss for their other peers.

When a late adolescent couple has been deeply in love, depression or aggressive reactions can follow a breakup. For many adolescents, this is the first loss of its kind. Looking at how the rejected party has managed the pain of past losses, can help predict how the young man or woman will cope. If the teen feels that all that is valuable in their life has been lost with this relationship, depression and/or rage can result. For some the pain will be turned inwards, and for others, the pain of rejection might be turned outward and result in retaliation, which can range from spreading rumors, to using social media to humiliate or attack the reputation of the lost partner, to verbal harassment and even to physical attack.

Independence stage (18-23) During this phase, the tasks of adulthood are more on the adolescent's radar screen; looking to settle down and focus on the future, including meaningful work and finding love. Relationships during this stage can be longstanding and deep, and the breakups can be devastating requiring many months to heal.

REASONS FOR TEEN BREAKUPS

When romantic partners in a couple find themselves having difficulty meeting disparate needs of the individuals in the pair, the stage is set for a breakup. This can occur when one person in the couple needs more together time, while the other wants more separate time, or when one or both become jealous and mistrustful, or life intervenes, with one person heading away to college, and the other remaining local or not yet finished with high school. Conflict can emerge, and the couple may not be able to sustain the relationship. One of the pair may feel overly controlled and wish for more freedom, and one or both may become disenchanted with the relationship. Their commitment may not withstand their competing needs and wishes. Other scenarios in which teen relationships breakup include: one person becoming romantically involved with someone else, feeling they've come together too young and wish to experience other relationships, differences in their comfort level with sexual activity, parental involvement, and mismatches in personality styles leading to intense couple dynamics. In other cases, the breakup may blindside one of the pair, and may feel entirely mysterious and incomprehensible.

TWO MODELS OF CONCEPTUALIZING RECOVERY FROM A TEEN BREAKUP

Model of Grief and Loss

The ending of a relationship has been compared to the death of a loved one. Dr. Elisabeth Kubler-Ross has written a classic work entitled *"On Death and Dying"* (1969) about the stages of recovering from the death of a loved one. Grieving the breakup of an important

love relationship has been conceptualized as a loss akin to a death, and these stages (with some slight modification) can be applied to what a young man or woman goes through following a breakup.

The stages of grief that follow any loss, including romantic breakups don't progress in any predictable time frame and can cycle back and forth. These can take place over the course of minutes, days, weeks, months or years, and one can regress and move forward. In the beginning it can feel very shaky, and without firm ground to stand on one can feel strange and disconnected from themselves and/or others. The task is to learn how to move forward without that partner in your life, and find the ways to fill in the space that has been left in the absence of the relationship. Taking the risk of loving means opening yourself up to the pain of grieving, which is a universal experience and part of being alive. Knowing that you are not alone can help you ride it out. These grieving experiences build the foundation for handling other inevitable losses that will come throughout one's life, and also lead the way to new beginnings.

Stages of grief and loss in recovering from a breakup

1. **Denial:** In this stage there is a numbness and kind of shock. It is difficult to wrap your head around the idea that the relationship is breaking up. The teen feels that this can't be happening, that this relationship you have invested so much into is ending, and that this person won't be in your life in the same way. By not facing the ending, one postpones the need to grieve, and may hold onto unrealistic hope that the relationship is reparable.

2. **Bargaining:** In the Bargaining stage, you begin to think of the 'what ifs', and the 'if onlys'. You promise to fix everything that you have done wrong, attempt to repair the relationship at all costs, and may beg to try again. It is painful to face the thought of life without your partner. The future is completely unknown, and that is frightening. Often one of the partners places the entire blame upon themselves and does not realistically evaluate the reasons that the relationship ended, and both partners' contribution. Bargaining can give you the illusion of control, but often leaves one in the position of having the reality of the breakup crash down on them over and over again.

3. **Relapse:** Some teens cannot bear the pain of the breakup and succeed in convincing their ex to try again. Sometimes this happens more than once, and some relationships have serial breakups and makeups before ending. The person who has taken all the responsibility for the breakup is sometimes alone in trying to make it work and sustain the relationship. Without some help to resolve the problems and/or communication issues that led to the breakup, it is highly unlikely that the relationship will succeed. Even though the pain of ending is temporarily relieved, the issues have not been resolved, and are likely to resurface.

4. **Anger:** While the initial feelings following a breakup may be dominated by anxiety and fear of the unknown, at some point feelings of anger will set in. The anger allows you to begin to stand up for your own needs and understand that perhaps you were treated poorly or unfairly and deserve better treatment. The anger may be directed at your ex, at yourself or at the situation, or possibly at the world. The anger empowers you, and can mobilize you to begin to look towards your future. Being able to access the anger is a sign that you are moving through the stages of grief, and can help you begin to make some changes in your life and be proactive in creating a life that doesn't revolve around this relationship.

5. **Initial Acceptance**: Both partners in a relationship have to come to a place of accepting the breakup and establishing some boundaries for their future interactions with each other. These define the new 'rules' of the relationship. One person may be struggling to maintain these boundaries having recognized that the relationship is over and isn't meant to continue. The person who may have wanted to avoid the breakup may come to realize that it is inevitable and ultimately for the best.

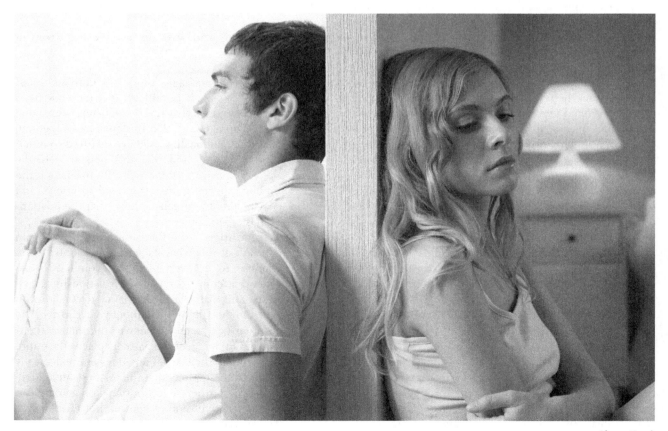

Photo: iStock

6. **Redirected Hope and Moving towards Acceptance:** A big milestone in the process of grieving a lost relationship comes when you begin to believe that you can envision the future without your ex and be ok. This allows you to move forward and maintain some hope and optimism for your future.

Model of Addiction

Psychological and Neurological Similarities between Romantic Relationships, Heartbreak, and Addiction

Recent research has suggested that love, heartbreak, and addiction are similar psychologically. Burkett and Young, (2012) state that from "initial encounters to withdrawal," the experience of love leads to experiences of "exquisite euphoria, loss of control, loss of time, and a powerful motivation to seek out the partner" and that the experience of getting over a former partner is likened to withdrawal from an addiction. Many aspects of recovering from a romantic loss are consistent with the criteria of substance abuse, including "a persistent desire or unsuccessful efforts to cut down or control substance use" and spend "a great deal of time ...us[ing] the substance, or recover[ing] from its effects."

There is also evidence that suggests that attachment, love, and addiction share commonalities in brain regions and neurochemical activity (Burkett and Young, 2012). The neurochemicals dopamine, opioids, oxytocin, corticotrophin-releasing hormones, and arginine vasopressin are seen to be highly involved in both drug addiction and romantic relationship bonding. The presence of withdrawal symptoms in both substance disorders and breakups, and the finding that the same hormones are activated during both withdrawal processes supports the concept that going through a breakup and suffering from an addiction share underlying physiological commonalities.

Understanding breakups through the addiction model can lead to clinical interventions similar to those used in recovery from an addiction, including psycho-education, self-monitoring triggering experiences, abstinence, and using the support of a sponsor.

PUTTING IT IN PERSPECTIVE

Each relationship is an opportunity to learn about parts of yourself and who you are in intimate relationships. While the endings of romantic relationships can feel devastating at the time, many are necessary losses (just like falling down helped you learn to walk) and will help you grow as a young adult. Each time you are in a deep relationship with another person, you take a risk of being known and being hurt. Falling in love is a good risk to take, because we open ourselves up to another person, and deepen our own rich experience of learning how to love ourselves and others. If we don't take this risk in life, we lose the opportunity to experience these magic feelings and learn things about ourselves and others that we can only learn by allowing ourselves to be vulnerable and intimate. In the words of Albert Lord Tennyson "Tis better to have loved and lost, than never to have loved at all".

With each new partner, foundation skills for new relationships are developed. We have the chance to explore aspects of who we are. We can also learn about the qualities we value and want to look for in our next romantic partner, as well those that we want to avoid. Part of growth as adults includes learning about what kind of romantic partner we are. We also learn about things that are important to someone we love and it broadens our world. We learn about the hopes and dreams of someone else, and begin to share our own. We learn empathy and compassion; to accept the quirks and habits of someone else, and feel that our own are accepted. Antoine de St.-Exupery explores the nature of love in his well-known work, "The Little Prince". "If you love a flower that lives on a star, it is sweet to look at the sky at night. All the stars are a-bloom with flowers..." This quote captures the notion that when we love another, we expand our universe to include elements that are valued by and thus remind us of our partners.

LESSONS LEARNED

"What doesn't kill you makes you stronger"

As we grow, we learn that change is an inevitable part of life. Most teenage relationships will not last forever. Breakups are one of those life experiences that help build resilience and strengthen the muscles that allow one to deal with change. Throughout life we all will face changes and transitions. Some will be planned and anticipated like a graduation, or starting a new job, and others will be sudden and unexpected. The more experience one has with coping with change, the more one will be able to face changes and use them to foster growth.

In addition, we learn about what aspects of our own behavior we may need to modify to sustain an intimate relationship with another person. We may need to hone our own ability to listen or attune to another person and understand their needs as different from our own.

The ability to deal with change is called resilience. Resilience can help refocus one's energies in a healthy and productive way. You may learn that you have more emotional strength than you thought you had. It is something you can build and develop. Learning how to cope with change and weather losses is a skill that you will call on many times throughout your life, and being able to count on your resilience will allow you to move out of your comfort zone and open up your world even further.

Tips for getting through a relationship breakup

- Be kind and compassionate to yourself
- Give yourself lots of tender loving care
- Look at what you learned from that relationship—what would you want in a future relationship, what aspects don't you want
- Reconnect with your friends and get support from them as well as family members
- Seek professional counseling if you find that you are not recovering after a period of time and it is interfering with your functioning in school or work and with friends.
- Engage in activities that keep you active and allow you to heal
- Accept your single status
- Know that time heals, and what feels raw and unbearable will not always be so painful
- Don't be afraid of your feelings

SIGNS THAT YOU ARE DEPRESSED AND WHAT TO DO

At the time of the relationship breakup, it can feel as if the world is coming to an end. You may have feelings of desperation and even feelings of wanting to end it all because you can't bear the pain. If months go by and you still feel the intense feelings of hurt and despair, have thoughts of hurting yourself, find yourself isolating, crying and having difficulty sleeping, feel sad all the time, you may be experiencing depression that will require professional help. Speaking to a trusted adult, your medical doctor, a parent or relative, coach, guidance counselor or clergyman will help steer you towards the appropriate professional support.

Remember Alexander Graham Bell's old phrase, "As one door closes, another door opens…"

FURTHER READING

Burkett, J. P., & Young, L. J. (2012). "The Behavioral, Anatomical and Pharmacological Parallels Between Social Attachment, Love and Addiction". *Psychopharmacology*, 224(1), 1-26. This article reviews the literature and studies that have been done comparing love, attachment and drug addiction.

Durayappah, A. (2011, February 23). "5 Scientific Reasons Why Breakups Are Devastating". *Huffington Post*. Retrieved from: http://www.huffingtonpost.com/adoree-durayappah-mapp-mba/breakups_b_825613.html This article reviews five reasons why people have so much difficulty moving on from a breakup. Discussion focuses on how the physiological responses following rejection and recovering from a breakup can be similar to trying to overcome a drug addiction.

Furman, W., and Shaffer, L. (2003). *The Role of Romantic Relationships in Adolescent Development*. In Florsheim, P. (Ed.) Adolescent romantic relations and sexual behavior: Theory, research and practical implications (pp 3-22). Mahwah, NJ: Lawrence Erlbaum Associates. This chapter discusses the role of earlier relationships with family and peers in the development of teenage relationship, and also focuses on how romantic and sexual relationships can encourage or inhibit achieving the normal developmental tasks of adolescence.

Heussner, K.M. (2010, July 8). "Addicted To Love? It's Not You, It's Your Brain. *ABC News*. Retrieved from: http://abcnews.go.com/Technology/addicted-love-brain/story?id=11110866 This article focuses on the similarities between romantic break-ups and suffering from an addiction. The author discusses the benefits of applying treatment techniques for addiction to individuals suffering from heartbreak.

Kubler-Ross, E. (1969) *On Death and Dying*. New York: Macmillan. This classic work details the stages of grieving deaths and losses, which can be applied to the work required to recover from a broken relationship.

Lachmann, S. (2013, June 4). "How To Mourn A Breakup To Move Past Grief and Withdrawal. *Psychology Today*. Retrieved from: http://www.psychologytoday.com/blog/me-we/201306/how-mourn-breakup-move-past-grief-and-withdrawal This article focuses on the physical and emotional withdrawal symptoms that many people going through a breakup experience. The author provides examples of ways individuals can overcome the acute withdrawal symptoms.

Lachmann, S. (2014, June 10) "The 7 Stages of Grieving a Breakup. Understanding Your Emotional Response to Breakup Can Help You Feel Less Alone". *Psychology Today*. Web log post. Me Before We. This article amends Kubler-Ross's stages of grieving a death to incorporate aspects of grieving a romantic breakup.

Lauren Behrman

SEE ALSO: Addictive Personality and Behaviors; Attachment Issues; Depression; Ending an Unhealthy Relationship; Peer Pressure; Resiliency; Separation Anxiety; Self-Esteem

Teenage suicide

The teen years are bursting with all the changes and adaptations that come as you transition from childhood to becoming a young adult. It's an exciting time! Many fresh experiences and the budding of youth can challenge unexplored emotions and underdeveloped coping skills. It can be the earliest time you experience significant loss of your first love or some other life event that creates emotional turmoil and confusion. Your journey thus far has given you little preparation or understanding that you can survive loss, betrayal, personal defeat, or unkind comments and taunting from bullies that hurt you to the core. You are strong enough – but, maybe you don't know it yet. That's understandable – but, it's not okay to hurt yourself.

The reasons behind adolescent suicide or attempted suicide are likely multi-faceted. The rate of suicide and attempts increases greatly during the teen years. Some teenagers may feel, hopeless, helpless, and unlucky. It's not about today's weather report– we all have bad days. It's about their emotional climate.

INTRODUCTION

Your friendships are significant and peer approval appears crucial to everyday life. There's a lot going on at home – and some of it may not be good. In fact, it may seem unbearable. Everything seems to be collapsing around you and you might feel like SpongeBob SquarePants:

"Help me, I'm so ashamed! I'm spiraling! I'm spiraling! (Patrick slaps SpongeBob) Thanks, Patrick. (Patrick is about to slap him again, but SpongeBob stops him) It's ok, Patrick. Spiraling, over!"

We all feel like we're spiraling at one time or another. Sometimes teens feel depressed or angry. This is especially true when dealing with the pressures of school,

friends, relationships, and family. Without warning or preparation a crisis may emerge. The event may be especially upsetting and your emotions begin to spiral out of control. An impulse emerges that moves you toward making a life altering decision, and at that moment, it might seem like the only solution to stopping the pain. You don't want to die and wish someone would stop you from hurting yourself – will someone please listen to me!

Now, we really have a problem – and something that could trigger an unfortunate event.

Depression can affect many areas of a teenager's life and outlook about their future. Those with intense feelings of depression, emotional pain, or irritability may begin to think about suicide. Even small problems may seem like too much to handle. Their resiliency, decision-making, and problem-solving skills are not surfacing quickly enough – therefore immediate intervention is necessary and may be lifesaving. Suicidal emotions come in waves and someone needs to send for a lifeguard – now! The undertow is too strong even for an experienced swimmer and it's pulling them down. Maybe you are the only person who hears the perfect storm coming because you're listening and can sound the alert.

DO IT!

If you or someone you know has been thinking about suicide or hurting themselves, seek help immediately. Suicide may seem like the only choice – it's not. Those who talk about suicide are most likely to attempt or commit suicide. Hopefully, someone will listen to them when they drop hints. The hints could be restrained or obvious. Listen to their words – they may often be warning those around them.

Some outward displays of warning behaviors can be observed. For example, multiple superficial cuts on the wrists for no apparent reason – perhaps practice? No matter the case, take action. Having information that someone is contemplating suicide is not something that you promise to keep a secret. The appropriate step is to support them in getting the help they need. In addition, do not be afraid to ask if your friend is talking about hurting themselves or thinking about suicide – say the words.

That's really hard! Yes, but not as hard a losing a friend or family member. Most suicides are preventable. We don't hear about those statistics – but, that's the good news!

Suicide rates differ among male and females. Teenage females think about and attempt suicide about twice as often as males. They tend to attempt suicide by over-dosing on drugs or cutting themselves. However, males die by suicide about four times more often than females – they tend to use more lethal methods, such as firearms, hanging, or jumping from heights.

According to the Centers for Disease Control and Prevention (CDC) suicide is the third-leading cause of death for (fifteen-to-twenty-four year-olds), after accidents and homicide. At least twenty-five attempts are made for every completed teen suicide.

A good friend often knows if someone is going through tough times. Perhaps they recently experienced a failed relationship, started using drugs, alcohol, or the police get calls to come to their home for domestic violence. These events can trigger suicidal ideation in someone who is already feeling depressed and showing warning signs. You know that another member of your friend's family committed suicide last year and he was taken, at least once, to the hospital for an overdose. Those who attempt suicide are likely to attempt it again – that's serious! He is being treated for depression, taking anti-depressants, and stashing pills in his bedroom drawer, no one notices.

One particular friend, a senior, is totally infatuated and thinks he's in love with the football team's most popular cheerleader. He discloses that life would not be worth living without her. You wish that he would not tell you those things, but really try to listen because he's your friend and you want to help. He usually talks more openly when you don't make judgments about what he says and he does most of the talking.

I can live with that. He would do the same for me – we trust each other.

However, right now, there's a lot of pressure for everyone – finals, grades, and graduation. It's all unfolding at the same time and your friend just learned that his girlfriend wants to take a break from their relationship and date other guys for the summer. She says maybe they can stay friends – you know this is not good news!

Your friend's response is immediate and concerning. Now, he doesn't want to do any of the things you used to do together, says he can't sleep, and just sits in his room – isolated from everyone. You are also concerned about his reckless driving. He gives you his most prized possession and comments that he won't need it any longer.

In addition, he is no longer interested in going for a run with you on the high school track. You always

seemed to get along, but now he appears agitated whenever you try to make suggestions – even the simplest conversation ends up in an argument. It's exhausting, and you never know what kind of mood he will be in!

You are concerned and encourage him to talk like he always has done in the past – but, something is different this time. What's worse is you remember the day his dad showed you his gun collection and where he hides the cabinet key. Your friend smokes pot and you notice burn marks on his forearm.

Finally, he breaks down and discloses that he feels life is not worth living without his girlfriend and the idea of her being with someone else is just too much. You take a risk and ask him if he is thinking about hurting himself or committing suicide. He answers – Yes.

Peer support is essential to assisting teenagers in trouble, and at the crossroads of emotional traffic. Adolescents who consider seeking help are more likely to reach for someone they know and trust. Friends can serve as the conduit for coordination and referral to counseling and treatment. You can tell someone like your school counselor. Peer support can provide the critical link to saving a life. This is not the time to make a promise to keep a secret. The twin feelings of hopelessness and helplessness reinforce each other.

Denial, loyalty, and the fear that you are betraying confidences all represent obstacles to preventing suicide. These barriers are deterrents to saving the life of a friend, peer, or family member. Take action and do not remain passive. All threats are to be taken seriously. Do not dismiss statements or warning signs as simple adolescent melodrama to be ignored. Their emotions will not allow them to make good decisions and they need direction. Do not leave them alone. If you feel you're in immediate danger of hurting yourself, you can also go to the emergency department at your local hospital. It's not a sign of weakness to ask for help. Having a bad day, or even a few bad days, does not mean you have a bad life. You don't have to feel that way. Help is available.

Would you be willing to ask, listen, and tell to save a life?

FURTHER READING

No matter what problems you are dealing with, http://www.suicidepreventionlifeline.org/ wants to help you find a reason to keep living. By calling 1-800-273-TALK (8255) you'll be connected to a counselor at a crisis center in your area, anytime 24/7. http://

www.suicide.org/suicide-hotlines.html offers state hotline numbers.

http://store.samhsa.gov/product/SMA12-4669: *Preventing Suicide: A Toolkit for High Schools Assists* high schools and school districts in designing and implementing strategies to prevent suicide and promote behavioral health. The kit includes tools to implement a multi-faceted suicide prevention program that responds to the needs and cultures of students.

Cobain, B., & Verdick, E. (2012). *When nothing matters anymore: A survival guide for depressed teens.* Minneapolis, MN: Free Spirit Pub. Things you can do right now and in the future to help yourself feel better - and ways to stay healthy, strong, and positive

Hurlbut, J., & Wood, P. (2011). *Teenage suicide: A cultural tragedy of adolescence* (2nd ed.). Fairbanks, AK; Pristine's Professional Press. The authors examine the potential of a community counseling approach for adequately preparing adolescents for their future places in society.

Schab, L. (2008). *Beyond the blues: A workbook to help teens overcome depression.* Oakland, CA: Instant Help Books. This book provides a comprehensive approach to treating depressed teens. The 40 illustrated activities include helping teens be more assertive, finding ways to make friends, handling conflicts, and dealing with sad and difficult feelings.

Jane Piland-Baker and Thomas E. Baker

SEE ALSO: Antidepressants; Cutting and Self-Mutilation; Dealing with Bullying; Dealing with Peer Pressure; Intervention; Depression; Domestic Violence; Parent-Teen Relationships and Conflict; Resiliency